Handbook of Topical Drug Treatment in Dermatology

Rebecca M. Law
Howard I. Maibach
Editors

Handbook of Topical Drug Treatment in Dermatology

Springer

Editors
Rebecca M. Law
School of Pharmacy and Faculty of Medicine (Discipline of Family Medicine)
Memorial University of Newfoundland
St. John's, NL, Canada

Howard I. Maibach
Department of Dermatology
University of California San Francisco (UCSF)
San Francisco, CA, USA

ISBN 978-3-031-93615-9 ISBN 978-3-031-93616-6 (eBook)
https://doi.org/10.1007/978-3-031-93616-6

This Springer imprint is published by the registered company Springer Nature Switzerland AG
The registered company address is: Gewerbestrasse 11, 6330 Cham, Switzerland

In Remembrance

Aaron B. Lerner MD PhD

(September 21, 1920–February 3, 2007)

Dr. Lerner was the first Chair of the Department of Dermatology at Yale University. He was a renowned dermatologist, researcher, and professor. He is known for his discovery of melatonin in 1958, where he led a team of researchers to isolate and to name the hormone melatonin. He also isolated MSH (melanocyte-stimulating hormone). He was also an expert in inherited diseases, in particular vitiligo, where he developed a skin transplantation therapy. Upon retirement in 1991, he was named a Professor Emeritus of Dermatology.

Wayne P.F. Gulliver MD FRCP(C)

(March 4, 1958–September 5, 2025)

Dr. Gulliver was one of the lead researchers on the team who discovered the HLA-Cw6 gene for psoriasis, and put Newfoundland and Labrador genetic research on the world map. He was a renowned dermatologist, researcher, professor, and a leader in psoriasis. He received many awards and accolades throughout his prestigious career including the Albert Neisser award, considered the "Nobel Prize" of Dermatology. Always leading by example, he embraced many leadership roles including being the first Chair of Medicine at Memorial University who was from Newfoundland and Labrador.

Preface

The concept for this book was conceived in Howard Maibach's home office during one of Rebecca Law's numerous visits. Howard has an enormous home office/library with hundreds of his treasured textbooks and publications. He has already published a systemic drug treatment in dermatology handbook with Sarah Wakelin (currently in its third edition), so clearly a topical drug treatment in dermatology handbook would make a suitable companion textbook.

Thus began the recruitment of authors with expertise in specific dermatologic conditions, and authors with expertise in one specific dermatologic category of drugs, or even in one specific drug treatment. With the intent of also providing a learning experience for students and a teaching experience for their mentors, some of our authors have involved their students, residents, and/or fellows in preparation of their chapters.

The handbook is in two sections. The first section includes foundational chapters discussing general principles such as factors affecting percutaneous absorption, extemporaneous compounding, pharmacogenomics, factors affecting topical therapy in pediatrics and geriatrics, and systemic considerations when topical drug treatments are used. The second section includes chapters of drug monographs grouped either by disease state (e.g., acne, atopic dermatitis) or drug classification (e.g., antibiotics, corticosteroids) or stand alone (e.g., sirolimus). There is cross-referencing between chapters.

The chapters have been reviewed and edited by the editors and by Springer. FDA drug monographs and LexiComp/LexiDrug drug monographs are consistent reference sources for each drug monograph chapter, in addition to specific additional references and readings for each drug treatment.

The editors' hope is to provide a handbook that will be useful to clinicians and educators. We welcome corrections or comments regarding this book.

St. John's, NL, Canada — Rebecca M. Law
San Francisco, CA, USA — Howard I. Maibach

Acknowledgments

We thank Springer and in particular Michelle Tam, Jeffrey Taub, Marie Felina Francois, Kavitha Manikannan, Rekha Muthusamy, Shanjini Rajasekaran and Patricia Gutierrez for their involvement with the publication of the first edition of this handbook.

Contents

Contributors

Parsa Abdi Faculty of Medicine, Memorial University of Newfoundland, St. John's, NL, Canada

Susuana Adjei Center for Clinical Studies, Webster, TX, USA

Jack L. Arbiser Department of Dermatology, Emory University School of Medicine, Winship Cancer Institute, Atlanta Veterans Administration Health Center, Atlanta, GA, USA

Paola A. Baker Department of Dermatology, Emory University School of Medicine, Atlanta, GA, USA

Erin Bartholomew Department of Dermatology, Eastern Virginia Medical School, Norfolk, VA, USA

Enzo Berardesca Dr. Phillip Frost Department of Dermatology and Cutaneous Surgery, Miller School of Medicine, University of Miami, Miami, FL, USA

Eric Beresford Formerly with Nobelpharma America, LLC, Bethesda, MD, USA

Sreedevi Boggarapu Formerly with Nobelpharma America, LLC, Bethesda, MD, USA

Gilbert J. Burckart Office of Clinical Pharmacology, Office of Translational Sciences, Center for Drug Evaluation and Research, US Food and Drug Administration, Silver Spring, MD, USA

Anuk Burli Department of Dermatology, Stanford University School of Medicine, Redwood City, CA, USA

Drake Carter Chicago Medical School, Rosalind Franklin University of Medicine & Science, North Chicago, IL, USA

Chavy Chiang Department of Dermatology, University of Rochester Medical Center, Rochester, NY, USA

Mimi Chung University of Alabama at Birmingham, Birmingham, AL, USA

Brian W. Connor Schweiger Dermatology Group, New York, NY, USA

Stephen Coombs School of Pharmacy, Memorial University, St. John's, NL, Canada

Faculty of Medicine, Discipline of Family Medicine, Memorial University, St. John's, NL, Canada

Sarah J. Currie Faculty of Medicine, Memorial University of Newfoundland, St. John's, NL, Canada

Le Hanh Dung Do Roger Williams Medical Center, Providence, RI, USA

Arian Farahani Medical Science Liaison at Nobelpharma America, LLC, Bethesda, MD, USA

Aileen Feschuk Faculty of Medicine, Memorial University of Newfoundland, St. John's, NL, Canada

Elimika Pfuma Fletcher Office of Clinical Pharmacology, Office of Translational Sciences, Center for Drug Evaluation and Research, US Food and Drug Administration, Silver Spring, MD, USA

Larisa J. Geskin Department of Dermatology at Columbia University Irving Medical Center, New York, NY, USA

Meghan T. Greene Faculty of Medicine, Memorial University of Newfoundland, St. John's, NL, Canada

Marwa Hakimi Department of Dermatology, University of California San Francisco (UCSF), San Francisco, CA, USA

Christina Huang Sidney Kimmel Medical College, Thomas Jefferson University, Philadelphia, PA, USA

Nadia Kashetsky Department of Dermatology and Skin Science, Faculty of Medicine, University of British Columbia, Vancouver, BC, Canada

Kiha Kim Faculty of Medicine, Memorial University, St. John's, NL, Canada

Bradley D. Kwinta Department of Dermatology at Columbia University Irving Medical Center, New York, NY, USA

Rebecca M. Law School of Pharmacy and Faculty of Medicine (Discipline of Family Medicine), Memorial University of Newfoundland, St. John's, NL, Canada

Wilson Liao Department of Dermatology, University of California San Francisco (UCSF), San Francisco, CA, USA

Mahan Maazi Faculty of Medicine, University of British Columbia, Vancouver, BC, Canada

Howard I. Maibach Department of Dermatology, University of California San Francisco (UCSF), San Francisco, CA, USA

Lisa E. Maier Department of Dermatology, UW Medicine, Seattle, WA, USA

Sean Mangion UniSA: Clinical and Health Sciences, University of South Australia, Adelaide, SA, Australia

Therapeutics Research Centre, Basil Hetzel Institute of Translational Health Research, The Queen Elizabeth Hospital, Woodville, SA, Australia

Sydney Medical School, The University of Sydney, Camperdown, NSA, Australia

Austinn C. Miller Center for Clinical Studies, Webster, TX, USA

Mai A. Ngo California Department of Toxic Substances Control, Sacramento, CA, USA

Victoria Nguyen School of Pharmacy, University of Waterloo, Kitchener, ON, Canada

Linda B. Ou Sunnybrook Health Sciences Centre, Toronto, ON, Canada

Aaron Park Acelyrin Inc., McLean, Virginia, USA

Michael Pham Sr. Director, Head of Medical Affairs at Nobelpharma America, LLC, Bethesda, MD, USA

Dirk B. Robertson Department of Dermatology, Emory University School of Medicine, Atlanta, GA, USA

Sheeva Shahinfar Texas A&M University College of Medicine, Bryan, TX, USA

Chinmay Shukla Office of Clinical Pharmacology, Office of Translational Sciences, Center for Drug Evaluation and Research, US Food and Drug Administration, Silver Spring, MD, USA

Maggie Shukla Compounding Wellness Sterile Lab, Mount Pearl, NL, Canada

Taylor Skinner Faculty of Medicine, Memorial University of Newfoundland, St. John's, NL, Canada

Laurie A. Temiz Department of Dermatology and Cutaneous Surgery, University of South Florida, Tampa, FL, USA

Center for Clinical Studies, Webster, TX, USA

Stephen K. Tyring Center for Clinical Studies, Webster, TX, USA

Department of Dermatology, University of Texas Health Science Center, Houston, TX, USA

Amanda Tzenov Faculty of Medicine, Memorial University of Newfoundland, St. John's, NL, Canada

Heather Warren Compounding Wellness Sterile Lab, Mount Pearl, NL, Canada

Jason Ya Department of Dermatology, Stanford University School of Medicine, Redwood City, CA, USA

Abbreviations

ACEI	Angiotensin-converting enzyme inhibitor
ADR	Adverse drug reaction
ALP	Alkaline phosphatase
ALT	Alanine aminotransferase
aPTT	Activated partial thromboplastin time
AST	Aspartate aminotransferase
BID	Twice daily
BP	Blood pressure
°C	Celsius (Centigrade)
CA	Cancer
Ca	Calcium
CDC	Centers for Disease Control and Prevention
CFU	Colony-forming unit
CK	Creatine Kinase
Cl_{cr}	Creatinine clearance
cm	Centimeter (centimetre)
CNS	Central nervous system
CO	Cardiac output
COPD	Chronic obstructive pulmonary disease
CXR	Chest X-ray
ECG	Electrocardiogram
EEG	Electroencephalogram
EENT	Eyes, ears, nose, throat
ESR	Erythrocyte sedimentation rate
ETOH	Ethanol
°F	Fahrenheit

FDA	Food and Drug Administration (United States)
G6PD	Glucose-6-phosphate dehydrogenase
GFR	Glomerular filtration rate
GI	Gastrointestinal
Gtt	Drops
H/A	Headache
Hb_{A1C}	Hemoglobin A_{1C}
HCTZ	Hydrochlorothiazide
HEENT	Head, eyes, ears, nose, throat
IBW	Ideal body weight
kJ	Kilojoule
L	Liter (Litre)
MRSA	Methicillin-resistant *Staphylococcus aureus*
MRSE	Methicillin-resistant *Staphylococcus epidermidis*
MTX	Methotrexate
NRTI	Nucleoside reverse transcriptase inhibitor
NS	Normal saline
NSAID	Nonsteroidal anti-inflammatory drug
NSCLC	Nonsmall cell lung cancer
NTG	Nitroglycerin
N/V	Nausea & vomiting
OCT	Optical coherence tomography
OD	Once daily or right eye
OS	Left eye
OTC	Over-the-counter
OU	Each eye
PCN	Penicillin
PDE	Phosphodiesterase
pH	Hydrogen ion concentration
QID	Four times daily
RADT	Rapid antigen detection test
RCT	Randomized controlled trial
RNA	Ribonucleic acid
RSV	Respiratory syncytial virus
RT-PCR	Reverse transcriptase—polymerase chain reaction
SC	Subcutaneous
SC_r	Serum creatinine
SG	Specific gravity

SGOT	Serum glutamate oxaloacetic transaminase
SGPT	Serum glutamic pyruvic transaminase
SIADH	Syndrome of inappropriate antidiuretic hormone secretion
SJS	Stevens-Johnson syndrome
SPF	Sun protection factor
TB	Tuberculosis
TEN	Toxic epidermal necrolysis
TID	Three times daily
TMP/SMX	Trimethoprim-sulfamethoxazole
TSH	Thyroid-stimulating hormone
TTP	Thrombotic thrombocytopenic purpura
T_x	Treatment
UV	Ultraviolet

Part I

General Principles

20 Clinically Pertinent Factors/Observations for Percutaneous Absorption in Humans

1

Rebecca M. Law, Mai A. Ngo, and Howard I. Maibach

Contents

R. M. Law (✉)
School of Pharmacy and Faculty of Medicine (Discipline of Family Medicine), Memorial University of Newfoundland, St. John's, NL, Canada
e-mail: rlaw@mun.ca; rlawUCSF@gmail.com

M. A. Ngo
California Department of Toxic Substances Control, Sacramento, CA, USA

H. I. Maibach
Department of Dermatology, University of California San Francisco (UCSF), San Francisco, CA, USA
e-mail: howard.maibach@ucsf.edu

R. M. Law, H. I. Maibach (eds.), *Handbook of Topical Drug Treatment in Dermatology*,
https://doi.org/10.1007/978-3-031-93616-6_1

Introduction

Clinicians routinely use the topical route to administer medications with minimal consideration of details: If there is an approved topical formulation, then obviously absorption through the skin should work. But is percutaneous absorption that simple? What factors are involved for a medication—or for that matter, for any chemical—to be percutaneously absorbed? What can enhance or reduce topical absorption? We consider these factors when using the topical administration route as they may affect drug efficacy and/or toxicity and hence patient outcome. What follows is evidence-based; the interested reader is encouraged to access the 62 reference citations for the evidence behind this discussion of skin absorption (not mucous membranes). Furthermore, textbooks providing in-depth discussions of percutaneous absorption are available as reference sources. The reader is referred to the extensive literature on percutaneous penetration enhancers in the 5-volume series by Dragicevic N, Maibach HI. Ed. Percutaneous Penetration Enhancers Chemical Methods in Penetration Enhancement. Springer. ISBN 978-3-662-47039-8.

Factors in Percutaneous Absorption

What questions should we ask when using a topical medication? Consider at least 20 factors. In 1983, we suggested a ten-factor guide in percutaneous absorption based on observations from in vitro and in vivo comparisons [1], which was expanded to 15 [2] in 2012, modified in 2013 [3, 4], with clinical relevance and complexities added in 2017 [5]. To aid the clinician or student, 20 factors affecting topical absorption are presented here in practical terms, including clinical implications. Questions asked are as follows:

What Are the Relevant Physicochemical Properties of the Medication/Chemical?

Particle Size/Molecular Weight Smaller molecules are often more easily absorbed; most topical medications are less than or around 500 Daltons in size/molecular weight with few exceptions. Topical calcineurin inhibitors are efficacious despite larger particle sizes (tacrolimus [Protopic] at MW 822 Dalton and pimecrolimus [Elidel] at MW 810 Dalton) [3].

Lipophilicity The outer skin layer (stratum corneum) are corneocytes with cell membranes consisting of lipids, with proteins and water. Lipophilic drugs (and lipophilic chemicals) will be more readily absorbed than hydrophilic substances [6]. However, highly lipophilic substances may be less well absorbed than moderately lipophilic compounds.

pH The pH of the environment will determine the proportion of drug or chemical that is ionized versus unionized. Skin membrane proteins are basic in nature. It is the unionized form of a drug or chemical that passes through membranes. Thus, drugs and chemicals that are primarily in their unionized form in a basic pH environment will be optimally absorbed. Since basic drugs will have a greater proportion in unionized form than acidic drugs in a basic environment, therefore, basic drugs will be absorbed better than acidic drugs. Less ionization leads to increased lipid solubility and passage through membranes [7].

pKa pKa is a measure of a chemical's acid strength and provides details of the dissociation of an acid in aqueous solution. Since there is a specific pKa for each substance that relates to pH, knowing the pKa of a drug becomes a useful predictor of percutaneous drug absorption [7].

Partition Coefficient (P) The partition coefficient is the ratio of concentrations of a substance in a mixture of two immiscible phases at equilibrium. This ratio is therefore a measure of the difference in solubility of the substance in these two phases. There are two partition coefficients of relevance to percutaneous absorption: the oil-to-water partition coefficient (i.e., octanol:water P) and the partition coefficient for cream or ointment to the stratum corneum (i.e., formulation:skin P). Hydrophobic drugs or chemicals will have a high octanol:water P and will be mainly distributed to hydrophobic areas such as the lipid bilayers of cell membranes, whereas hydrophilic drugs or chemicals (with low octanol:water Ps) will be mainly distributed to aqueous areas such as serum. The partition coefficient between a cream/ointment and the stratum corneum will depend on the product formulation. Thus, knowing the partition coefficients of a drug or chemical for various immiscible phases may be a useful predictor of percutaneous drug absorption and/or drug partitioning between biologic systems, which can include solids such as bone (i.e., blood:bone P).

What Effects Do the Vehicle/Formulation of the Product Have on Drug Absorption?

Occlusive Vehicles *Occlusive vehicles* often aid absorption by increasing hydration [8]. *Water-based* vehicles are nonocclusive and are less helpful for topical drug absorption, but they allow water-soluble drugs to dissolve in higher concentrations, which may offset the nonocclusive aspect.

Oil-Based *Oil-based vehicles* are occlusive and act as humectants to enhance drug penetration. Thus, for example, a betamethasone dipropionate 0.1% ointment will generally have greater potency than a betamethasone dipropionate 0.1% cream (note that changing salt forms may affect potency—e.g., betamethasone dipropionate 0.1% cream is more potent than betamethasone valerate 0.1% cream). Although *alcohol-based or acetone-based* vehicles are less occlusive and have a skin-drying effect, they may enhance solubility of some drugs and thereby augment dermal absorption.

The *pH of the vehicle* may alter the unionized:ionized drug ratio, thus affecting drug absorption, since it is the unionized form of the drug, which most efficiently crosses through the skin. Other *excipients* (i.e., inactive ingredients) in the vehicle such as surfactants may have been purposely added to enhance solubility and hence drug absorption.

What Effects Do the Conditions of Drug Exposure (Dose, Duration, Surface Area, and Frequency of Exposure) Have on Drug Absorption?

Intuitively, greater *dose*, longer *treatment duration*, larger *surface area of application*, and greater *frequency of reapplication* (once up to three or four times a day) should all increase the amount of drug absorbed, and they generally do. However, (although the experimental data remains sparse), with corticosteroids, a high single exposure (hydrocortisone 40 ug/cm^2) substantially increases absorption over one-third of the dose (13.3 ug/cm^2) applied either once or three times in 1 day, there was no statistically significant difference seen with increasing frequency of reapplication [9]. With multiple dosing over many days, there is currently insufficient experimental data to provide a general predictive statement.

In addition, the *body surface area-to-body weight ratio (BSA:BW)* is important as this may affect drug toxicity, since drug doses are usually based on body weight (with a few exceptions such as in oncology). In particular, newborns have a BSA:BW ratio at least twice that of adults, so that topical drug doses—even when adjusted for body weight—will still cover a larger % BSA than in adults. Thus, newborns are at greater risk of systemic drug toxicity from topical application of drugs or chemicals. It is partially for this reason that sun protection in newborns less than 6 months of age does not include the use of sunscreens/sunblocks, even the physical (mineral-based) sunblocks like titanium dioxide. (Recommendations by the American Academy of Pediatrics for sun protection in this population include sun avoidance, using a stroller cover, wearing lightweight long pants, long-sleeve shirts and hats with wide brims that shade the neck etc.)

Also, note the following: (a) There may be residual drug remaining on and in the skin even if the dose is wiped off—that is treatment duration may be unknowingly extended; (b) repeated exposure over time may lead to chronic toxicity manifestations, such as corticosteroid-induced skin atrophy; (c) inadvertent chemical/drug exposure may occur via transfer from one person to another, for example, a mother wearing sunscreen and holding her infant with bare arms (further discussed in section "Can medications or chemicals be transferred from one person to another through skin contact, clothing, or contact with an inanimate surface?" below).

Do the Skin Appendages (Hair Follicles, Sebaceous Glands, Apocrine, and Eccrine Sweat Glands) Have a Role in Topical Drug Absorption?

Yes they do. Skin appendages that originate in the dermis are *subanatomical pathways*, whereby drugs and chemicals can be transported through the skin. Diffusion of chemicals through skin appendages is termed "*shunt diffusion.*" Hair follicles can contribute to the total skin surface area for drug absorption. Skin appendages are especially important for the penetration and skin storage of larger molecules (e.g., proteins), as discussed in section "How does substantivity and binding to the different skin components affect topical absorption?" below. Little data exists regarding transport through the eccrine, apocrine, and sebaceous glands.

How Do the Skin Sites of Application Affect Absorption?

There is marked *regional variability* in absorption: absorption rates vary at different anatomical skin sites—in general, faster if hair follicles are present in large numbers and somewhat slower if the stratum corneum is thick. More specifically, the scrotum has the highest rate of topical absorption due to having both a very thin stratum corneum and a rich blood supply. The next highest body areas for absorption are the forehead, scalp, and neck. These regional differences may partially relate to skin thickness and the number of cell layers in the stratum corneum. Body areas with the lowest topical absorption rates include the palms and soles.

What Population Variability Factors Affect Topical Absorption?

Ethnicity Although the skin is approximately equally thick in persons of different pluralistic societies, the stratum corneum in blacks has more cell layers and a higher lipid content than in whites [10]. These differences may lead to absorption differences. In addition, blacks and Hispanics have stronger irritant reactions than whites to sodium lauryl sulfate [11, 12], a surface-active agent often found in non-medicated and medicated shampoos. (Note that experimental data in comparing blacks and Hispanic skin is limited, and there is conflicting data. The interested reader can obtain more information from two textbooks detailing these points: Berardesca E, Leveque J-L, Maibach HI. Ethnic Skin and Hair 1st ed. CRC Press. Dec 2019. ISBN 9780367389994; and earlier edition Nov 2006 ISBN 978-0849330889 Skin irritation may lead to inflammation and enhanced absorption of topical agents.)

Age Age can significantly affect topical absorption. Aged skin is drier with less skin surface lipids [13]. It is also thinner and more friable—skin aging is associated with progressive dermal atrophy including atrophy of the skin's capillary network, resulting in a gradual reduction of blood supply to the skin [13]. All of these changes may potentially affect topical absorption. Overall, it paradoxically appears that the *permeability barrier function* of the skin is increased as we age. In particular, percutaneous absorption of less lipophilic substances (e.g., hydrocortisone, benzoic acid, acetylsalicylic acid, and caffeine) is reduced, while more lipophilic substances (e.g., testosterone and estradiol) are not [13].

However, increased friability may result in broken skin, resulting in the loss of permeability barrier function and increased percutaneous absorption.

At the other end of the age spectrum, that is, infants and children, topical absorption may be increased. In the preterm baby, the permeability barrier function of the skin is not yet intact. Prenatal skin undergoes developmental stages in utero (including permeability barrier development, e.g., proteolipid layer and pilosebaceous units), but some functions are not fully developed even in the neonate [14]. Importantly, the acid mantle is developed in the first 4 weeks after birth, and skin surface pH of both term newborns and premature neonates is less acidic than that of children and adults [15]. Newborn skin has higher permeability than topical agents. Pediatric skin is thinner, potentially allowing for an increase in the rate and amount of drug absorbed. In fact, pediatric and in particular neonatal and infant skins have skin surface conditions different from adult skin surface conditions, which may enhance absorption [16].

Skin hydration naturally differs with age. Although at birth the skin surface is rougher and drier compared with older children, within the first 30 days, the skin smoothens, and skin hydration increases [16, 17]. During the next 3 months, skin hydration continues to increase then exceeds that found in adults [17–19]—perhaps relating to sweat gland maturation in function [20]. The stratum corneum in infants 3–12 months of age is significantly more hydrated compared to adult skin [16, 17]. These factors may increase the potential for drug and chemical toxicities in neonates, infants, and children, and this should be kept in mind whenever the topical route is used. For example, increased topical absorption and toxicity have been reported in infants with the use of rubbing alcohol [21, 22], boric acid powders [23], and hexachlorophene baths, emulsions and soaps [24, 25]—thus, their use should be minimized. The evidence that rubbing enhances percutaneous penetration has recently been reviewed [26]. The preterm infant may be at even greater risk—even medications that are not normally administered topically due to their physicochemical characteristics may be absorbed enough to be efficacious or cause toxicity. For example, a theophylline gel (17 mg spread over an area 2 cm in diameter) applied to the abdomens of premature infants produced therapeutic serum theophylline concentrations [27].

How Do Skin Surface Conditions Affect Topical Drug Absorption?

Hydration Hydration is crucial (as discussed above with age comparisons). Well-hydrated skin often promotes topical absorption, and it is for this reason that occlusion is often intentional in product formulation, for example, ointments are often more potent than creams or lotions, also mentioned earlier, since occlusion creates a humectant effect. Formulation or application changes resulting in potency differences should be remembered when prescribing (e.g., clobetasol or hydrocortisone). For example, a tenfold increase in hydrocortisone absorption was seen when occlusion was applied for 24 h after topical administration [2, 28].

Skin Temperature Skin temperature also affects topical absorption: an increase in skin temperature—such as a febrile state or sometimes even when a heating pad is present—may increase topical absorption. For example, skin temperature at 40 °C increases the transdermal delivery of testosterone and fentanyl [29].

Skin pH The *skin pH* may affect topical absorption: a less acidic skin pH may enhance absorption. The normal stratum corneum is typically acidic and hence favors transport of chemicals and drugs whose pKas allow for greater unionized forms in an acidic environment. Abnormal stratum corneum frequently has higher pH (i.e., a more basic environment), and this would favor the penetration of chemicals and drugs whose pKa allows for greater unionized forms in a basic environment. Thus, the acid mantle of the intact adult skin (pH 4–5) would be an absorption barrier to most basic drugs and some acidic drugs.

Skin pH elevations can occur with occlusion [30] or with a change in the skin microbiome (e.g., caused by prolonged occlusion [30]). Even 1 day of occlusion (with plastic wrap) can cause a 10^4 increase in bacterial count (most significantly with Coagulase negative *Staphylococci*), resulting in a corresponding increase in skin pH [30]. With 4 days of occlusion the skin pH can change from acidic to neutral (4.38–7.05) [30].

Skin Surface Topography The *skin surface topography* can also affect topical absorption, since it affects lateral spread of drug or chemical (see section "How does lateral spread affect percutaneous absorption?").

How Does Skin Health and Skin Integrity Affect Topical Absorption?

Be cognizant that *any skin damage or trauma*—be it mechanical, chemical, biocidal, or clinical disease—may potentially enhance topical absorption [5, 31], and the effects may be more significant for hydrophilic (water-soluble) substances than lipophilic (oil-soluble) substances [31]. These effects are not only demonstrated in in vivo human studies measuring penetration through damaged or diseased skin [31], but also enhanced absorption has also been shown in in vitro studies using human models of damaged or diseased skin [32]. Even mild skin trauma such as adhesive tape stripping (which removes stratum corneum layers) may significantly enhance absorption. For example, penciclovir absorption was increased by 1300-fold and acyclovir absorption by 440-fold through tape stripping (to glistening but not broken skin) [33]. Skin compromised by sodium lauryl sulfate (a surfactant) was more permeable to various polyethylene glycols (of different molecular weights) [34].

Skin Diseases Skin diseases such as psoriasis and atopic dermatitis [35] also compromise skin integrity, and and topical drugs and chemicals may be absorbed faster and in greater amounts. There is some complexity though. For example, in atopic dermatitis (AD) patients (when compared to healthy individuals), increased absorption occurred not only through lesional skin but also through non-lesional skin [35–37]. Although non-lesional AD skin is "normal-appearing," it still responds to petrolatum applied to it—by increasing stratum corneum thickness, reducing

T-cell infiltrates, upregulating antimicrobial peptides, etc. [35]. And both lesional and non-lesional skin of AD patients have higher *Staphylococcus aureus* levels than healthy controls, which correlates with disease severity [38].

However, it is AD patients with clinically active disease who demonstrated increased skin absorption (in both lesional and non-lesional skin)—patients with clinically inactive disease did not [36, 39, 40]. Furthermore, skin absorption increases significantly with the severity of AD [36, 41, 42].

Practically, this means that topical medications are better absorbed during dermatologic disease flare-ups—thus, (a) becoming more effective at that time, a useful phenomenon; (b) being potentially less effective when used as maintenance therapy, especially if intermittent (twice weekly) regimens are used, thus patient monitoring and follow-up during periods of inactive disease would be important; and (c) systemic toxicity from topical medications may be significantly increased during disease flare-ups, especially if higher potency agents within a class of medications are used (e.g., corticosteroids). Furthermore, absorption of and potential systemic toxicity of *any* chemical touching the skin may be similarly increased during a skin disease flare-up, such as in AD.

How Does Substantivity and Binding to the Different Skin Components Affect Topical Absorption?

Substantivity Substantivity can be defined as the adherence of chemicals to the stratum corneum, that is more like adsorption. In practical terms, the substantivity of a sunscreen (as an example) would be that sunscreen's ability to remain effective during prolonged exercise, sweating, or swimming, and this may be a property of the active ingredient, the vehicle, or both. Obviously, the greater the substantivity, the greater the potential efficacy and systemic toxicity of a topical formulation that is meant for local/topical treatment or prevention (e.g., sunscreens, antibacterials, and antifungals).

Binding Binding can occur to various other skin proteins, lipids, or other substances, which have differing binding sites and chemical affinities [3]. Thus, binding is drug- or chemical-specific. Bindings to different skin components (such as eccrine and apocrine sweat glands and hair follicles) are also important to consider as the bound drug or chemical may serve as a skin reservoir. Further, drugs or chemicals stored in skin reservoirs may be absorbed systemically, potentially causing prolonged pharmacologic effect or toxicity. This is an area of current decontamination research, as bound substances may not be easily washed off or otherwise removed [3, 4]. (Washing is further discussed in section "Does washing affect topical absorption?".)

How Does Topical Application Result in Systemic Distribution of the Drug or Chemical?

Systemic Distribution First, drugs or chemicals are adsorbed to the superficial skin surface (substantivity being an issue here). Second, drugs or chemicals may penetrate and bind to various skin proteins, lipids, skin appendages, and other substances (binding affinity being an issue here). Third, drugs or chemicals penetrate deeper into the lower dermis where there is a vascular blood supply and partition into the bloodstream for systemic circulation [7]. The important issues here are affinity for blood components such as albumin or other plasma proteins (plasma protein binding) and local blood flow [7]. Vasodilatation enhances blood flow and may promote systemic distribution of a topically administered medication. Of note—some medications may have vasodilating properties—for example, transdermal nitroglycerin (a venodilator) acts within minutes and may be a temporary measure to provide sustained nitroglycerin blood concentrations before intravenous (IV) line insertion can be done to administer an IV nitroglycerin infusion. The converse should also be noted—some medications have vasoconstrictive effects (such as corticosteroids) and may inhibit systemic absorption. In addition to skin surfaces, drugs or chemicals may be applied to (or otherwise be in contact with) mucosal surfaces such as the eyes or nose—the nose has a highly vascular mucosa that almost guarantees systemic absorption.

Thus, there is potential for *systemic toxicity* from topical administration. As exposure from use of ophthalmic drops is to both the eye and surrounding skin, ophthalmic beta-blockers have caused bronchospasm, congestive heart failure and pulmonary edema, bradyarrhythmias and sinus arrest, CNS toxicity, impotence, and dyslipidemias [43–45]. Ophthalmic sulfonamides have induced Stevens-Johnson syndrome [46]. Topical corticosteroids have caused systemic side effects including HPA-axis suppression and adrenal insufficiency, Cushing's syndrome, and hypertension [43]. Topical salicylates have caused a refractory hypoglycemia [47] by increasing glucose metabolism and reducing gluconeogenesis [43]. Significant systemic absorption of topical salicylates has resulted in systemic salicylate toxicity: tinnitus, hearing loss, blurred vision, sweating, tachypnea, diarrhea, nausea/vomiting, weakness, etc. [43]. Topical minoxidil 2% applied to the scalp may have caused cardiovascular adverse effects including palpitations, dizziness, hypotension, tachycardia, paroxysmal atrial fibrillation, and sinus arrhythmia [43]. There are many other drugs and chemicals applied topically, which may have increased systemic toxicity as skin barrier properties change.

Inadvertent systemic toxicity from cosmeceuticals and other products have occurred, for example, phenol can be cardiotoxic: a phenol and croton oil solution used in deep chemical peels caused cardiac arrhythmias including atrial and ventricular tachycardia, premature ventricular beats and bigeminy; people with diabetes mellitus, hypertension, and depression may be at higher risk [43]. There is also concern about mercury-containing skin care products (such as skin-lightening creams and soaps and local antiseptics) and their potential to cause neurotoxicity or nephrotoxicity with enough systemic absorption [43]. Arsenic is another toxic metal that is used (or is a contaminant) in cosmetics, medications, pigments, and natural health products that when applied onto skin over time or in sufficient amounts can result in systemic toxicity effects including psychoses, seizures, multi-organ failure, and death [43].

Be cognizant that *any* drug or chemical that touches the skin has the potential for percutaneous absorption that may result in systemic distribution and possible systemic toxicity.

How, If at All, Does Exfoliation Affect Topical Absorption?

Exfoliation is part of a natural skin cell renewal process: keratinocytes begin as boxlike basal cells at the base of the epidermis and then migrate up toward the skin surface, flattening out to become a layer of overlapping corneocytes, which have no nuclei—thus termed dead skin cells—which are then "sloughed off," that is, exfoliated. Drugs or chemicals bound to skin cells could either be *lost by the exfoliation process* or be *absorbed deeper into the dermis*; thus, exfoliation can affect drug bioavailability after topical administration. Urea, which is minimally absorbed topically, can be used as an exfoliation marker [48].

Does Washing Affect Topical Absorption?

There are two opposing *wash effects* that can affect topical absorption of drugs and chemicals. Loss by exfoliation can be enhanced by washing [2] even hours after application [48] if there is drug remaining in the stratum corneum, and this would be a "*washing-off*" effect. Note that for highly lipid-soluble drugs or chemicals (e.g., pesticides), washing with soap and water may not be sufficiently effective in removing them [49].

In fact, the opposite may happen: washing the site of application in between doses may actually enhance topical absorption/penetration, and this would be a "*wash-in*" effect [50–52] (see also section "Does rubbing or massaging affect topical absorption?" below). Be aware that washing may promote drug or chemical penetrance through the skin leading to toxicity—for example with insect repellents [50–52]. Care should be taken when insect repellents are used, especially in children. The US Environmental Protection Agency (EPA) recommends that instructions on the label be followed [5] for insect repellent products, and they should be used according to the time of day when mosquitoes are most active—which may vary for the species and type of diseases transmitted [5]. Care should also be taken in the work environment if there is occupational exposure to chemicals: workers should be counselled to wear protective clothing and use protective equipment and warned about the "wash-in" phenomenon [5]. They should be aware that the mechanical friction from handwashing may increase percutaneous absorption in particular of inorganic compounds [50].

Does Rubbing or Massaging Affect Topical Absorption?

There are two important concepts here: *rub enhancement* and *rub resistance,* both of which occur with rubbing/massaging. One example of *rub enhancement* relates to sunscreen application and washing: the mechanical stress of skin washing can massage the sunscreen deeper into the hair follicle [53], and this washing/massaging may enhance transfollicular sunscreen absorption [50]. Massaging may also increase the follicular penetration depth of liposomes (used as drug carriers) [54, 55]. Massaging/rubbing reduces skin barrier function to facilitate penetration [55]. However, this effect differs between hydrophilic and lipophilic substances—lipophilic/organic substances are less affected, if at all.

With regard to *rub resistance,* this is a term used to describe whether a substance applied topically will still be effective after being rubbed with a textile (clothing, towel, etc.). Rub resistance would be an important factor for a sunscreen or a topical medication to possess, and a rub resistance factor (RRF) can be calculated to allow comparisons between products of the same class (e.g., sunscreens) [56]. Parameters that influence RRF include rubbing pressure, rubbing duration, rubbing speed, and the textile (composition, thickness, etc.) [56]. Obviously, the higher the RRF, the greater the amount of drug or chemical remaining on the skin and the greater the likelihood for percutaneous absorption.

Can Medications or Chemicals Be Transferred from One Person to Another Through Skin Contact, Clothing, or Contact with an Inanimate Surface?

Yes. As briefly mentioned in section "What effects do the conditions of drug exposure (Dose, duration, surface area, and frequency of exposure) have on drug absorption?" above, inadvertent drug or chemical exposure can occur via transfer from one person to another—such as a mother wearing sunscreen and holding her baby with bare arms. Drug transfer can sometimes have serious consequences: a father who used testosterone cream without routine handwashing after application transferred enough testosterone over time to his infant son to cause precocious puberty—pronounced virilization in a 2-year-old boy [57]. The skin-to-skin contact time need not be lengthy: a controlled 15-min ventral forearm to ventral forearm rub/contact time transferred sufficient estradiol from donor volunteers to recipient volunteers for estradiol to be detected in the recipients' urine [58]. There was also enough estradiol left on the sleeve of the donors for the possibility of transfer from clothing to occur [58]. Using a hair follicle drug screening test, a Department of Human Services detected methamphetamine in newborns and young children—postulating that "sweat glands glom onto meth which can then be transferred through skin-to-skin contact, like coddling an infant [59]." However, besides sweat, other possibilities were children picking it up "from the environment, from the smoke or residue" [59]. Other examples include additional controlled studies confirming that skin-to-skin drug transfers exist [60, 61]. Skin-to-skin transfer can also occur in the same individual [61].

Practically, what does this mean? Anytime that a topical medication or chemical substance is used, we should be aware that transfer may occur from one person to another, including to infants who may be at greater risk of systemic toxicity—unless the substance is inert. Obviously, the other factors of percutaneous absorption would also apply to the transferred drug or chemical, and those factors would ultimately determine the clinical significance of the drug or chemical transfer.

How Is Topical Absorption Affected If a Drug or Chemical Is Volatile?

Volatility means that a substance has the ability to spontaneously vaporize into the air, or, in the case of a topical agent applied on skin, to evaporate from skin over time. Medications or chemicals applied to skin are often in product formulations that are a mixture of active and inactive ingredients, some of which may be volatile while others are not. For volatile substances, the degree of volatility may vary from substance to substance and may be affected by other factors such as formulation (pH, etc.), environment (humidity, temperature, etc.), and skin characteristics (pH, hydration, skin temperature, etc.). Some substances may be volatile only when certain conditions are met. For example, methamphetamine HCl (a basic drug with a pKa of 9.9) in aqueous solution can change from a nonvolatile salt to a volatile free base when the pH of the solution exceeds 4 or 5 [62].

What implications does volatility of a drug or chemical have on percutaneous absorption? Important issues include the following: (a) For a multi-ingredient product, the contents of what is left behind may alter the function of the applied product, which may have implications for efficacy and safety [63]. (b) If the vehicle and not the active ingredient is volatile, over time, there will be a concentrating effect as more and more of the vehicle evaporates, potentially increasing the potency and/or toxicity of the active ingredient. This is important as volatile solvents are commonly used in drug and other formulations (cosmetic, patch test [64], etc.), for example, an acetone-based benzoyl peroxide product or an acetone-based patch test chemical [64]. (c) Skin patch testing detects contact irritants and allergens, and volatility can lead to false positives and false negatives—test vehicle evaporation leading to too high a test chemical concentration causing a false-positive result [64] and test chemical evaporation leading to too low a test chemical concentration causing a false-negative result [64, 65]. For example, fragrance chemicals are usually volatile substances and are common contact allergens often patch tested as "Fragrance mix 1" and "Fragrance mix 2." A study of two radiolabelled fragrance chemicals (geraniol and citronellol) detected that, due to evaporation, within 40 min geraniol lost up to 39% of its dose and citronellol up to 26% of its dose [65]. (d) Rapid volatilization reduces the dose and prevents oversaturation of skin's absorptive capacity. This allows for a direct relationship between dose and percutaneous absorption of volatile substances that is calculable (i.e., predictable). Two equations have been developed to correlate the relationship between volatilization and absorption for a small dose versus a large dose [66]. These equations may be useful in assessing the risk of topical products and their pharmacokinetics/pharmacodynamics/toxicities. An in-depth discussion of these equations is beyond the scope of this paper, and the interested reader should review the reference indicated [66].

Volatility is important in other ways. Mosquito repellents depend on volatility for their effects, and volatility remains a limiting efficacy factor (i.e., in providing sufficient biting protection from mosquitos). Traditional contact repellents such as *N,N*-diethyl-*meta*-toluamide (DEET) applied on human skin require frequent reapplication and may carry a risk of systemic absorption [67]. However, spatial repellents may prevent mosquito entry into particular areas or into a home and may be particularly useful in mosquito-borne disease endemic areas [67]. For example, metofluthrin-impregnated latticework plastic strips were capable of preventing the resting of *Aedes Aegypti* (L.) within residences in Vietnam for a minimum of 8 weeks after they were introduced [67, 68].

Does Metabolic Transformation Occur During Topical Absorption and If So, How and What? Does Cutaneous Metabolism Occur?

Depending on the drug or chemical, *metabolic transformation* can occur in skin prior to systemic absorption, since there are metabolizing enzymes in skin. Both phase I (e.g., CYP450 enzymes) and phase II (e.g., N-acetyltransferase) enzymes have been found in skin—the mRNA and protein being detected more often than the quantified enzyme activity (being much lower than in the liver and often at the limit of detection) [69]. Sometimes, UV light is required for transformation (see section "Does photochemical transformation occur during topical absorption and if so, how and what"). Biotransformation changes the drug or chemical. This change can be in the drug's physicochemical properties or in its pharmacodynamic activity, or it may be both. This can result in the following: (a) active agent becoming inactive (a degradation process); (b) inactive agent becoming active (an activation process for a pro-drug); (c) a lipophilic agent becoming more water soluble (via various metabolic pathways, e.g., oxidation, hydroxylation, and acetylation). These changes can affect the drug's penetration through skin. For example, highly lipophilic compounds, often large, do not penetrate through skin well—(a good thing). However, the highly lipophilic preservative butylparaben (one example) can be metabolized to p-hydroxybenzoic acid in skin—this metabolite is less lipophilic thus more readily penetrates through skin [2, 70]. Cutaneous metabolism of endogenous substrates such as vitamin A and vitamin D also occurs [2].

Does Photochemical Transformation Occur During Topical Absorption and If So, How and What?

Similarly to section "Does metabolic transformation occur during topical absorption and if so, how and what? Does cutaneous metabolism occur?", the effect of UV light on a drug or chemical applied to the skin can cause a *photochemical transformation* (degradation or activation, etc.) In particular, photochemical changes to a drug or chemical can induce a phototoxic or photoallergic reaction. A *phototoxic* reaction is caused by a drug or chemical absorbing UVA and causing direct damage to sun-exposed skin, whereas a *photoallergic* reaction requires the drug or chemical to be changed by UVA into an allergen—with skin damage occasionally spreading beyond the sun-exposed skin areas. *Photosensitivity*—an adverse cutaneous response to normally harmless doses of UV radiation—is a property related to the drug chemistry and can be seen with topical or systemic administration. Examples of phototoxic agents include amiodarone, tetracyclines (e.g., doxycycline), coal tar, psoralens, and sulfonamides. Examples of photoallergic agents include sulfonamides, sulfonylureas, thiazides, chloroquine, carbamazepine, etc. Practically, if a drug or chemical is known to cause photosensitivity, sun protection is recommended if used during the day; application/dosing at night rather than in more sunlit hours may minimize photosensitivity.

How Does Metabolism Affect Excretion Kinetics of the Drug or Chemical? And How Does Excretion Kinetics Relate to Topical Absorption?

A drug or chemical can be excreted from the body unchanged, or it may undergo metabolic changes before excretion. Thus, the discussions in sections "Does metabolic transformation occur during topical absorption and if so, how and what? Does cutaneous metabolism occur?" and "Does photochemical transformation occur during topical absorption and if so, how and what?" regarding biotransformation in the skin will affect excretion kinetics. For example, a highly lipophilic drug or chemical that is biotransformed into a more water-soluble metabolite will not only be more easily absorbed through the skin; it will also be more easily excreted in the urine. Water-soluble drugs often do not require metabolic changes for urinary excretion, and a greater proportion of the administered dose may be excreted unchanged.

Metabolism and excretion are two mechanisms for elimination of drug or chemical, which can be affected by numerous factors [7]. Note that metabolism and excretion pharmacokinetics can differ greatly between structurally similar drugs or chemicals. Thus, depending on the substance, elimination (i.e., *drug clearance*) may or may not be in proportion to the dose absorbed. For researchers conducting in vivo studies, the clearance rate of the drug or chemical must be considered when estimating percutaneous absorption from blood or tissue samples [7].

How Does Lateral Spread Affect Percutaneous Absorption?

Lateral spread is the ability of a topical agent to spread beyond the site of application, that is, the drug or chemical "flows" laterally on the skin surface from the application area to outside of it [71]. (Note that lateral spread is also more commonly used in describing earthquake phenomena.) Lateral spread of a topically applied drug or chemical is a competitive process to drug or chemical penetration into the stratum corneum [71, 72]. The spreading can reduce the amount of drug substance within the area of application, which can modify the desirable effect expected in the treated area [71]. *Time* is a factor: for example, a 10% urea in water solution applied to skin provided a 90.4% recovery rate at the site of application after 1 h versus a 79.6% recovery rate after 6 h [71]. Why is there less urea remaining at the site of application after 6 h than after 1 h? The cause is lateral spread and not percutaneous absorption as less than 1% of urea penetrates in vivo in man [73]. Thus, lateral spread is time dependent. Furthermore, *skin surface topography* can affect the degree of lateral spread: primary furrow networks such as fingerprints and palm prints can function as pathways for lateral spreading [72], whereas follicles and wrinkles can be reservoirs for drugs or chemicals, and little is known about lateral spread in these areas. Although there is no difference in lateral spread between forearm and back [72], little is known about other anatomical sites. Practically, we should be aware that lateral spread happens, and the lengthier the time from the time of application, the greater the effect of lateral spread, resulting in less and less drug or chemical remaining at the site of application for percutaneous absorption.

For Investigators, Does the Method of Determining Percutaneous Absorption Influence the Results and the Interpretation of Study Results?

Based on what has been discussed from the 19 factors above, many issues can influence percutaneous absorption and, if not controlled for, can be confounders to study results. In particular, in vivo studies would be subject to many more confounding variables than in vitro studies. In vitro experiments can sometimes be better controlled than in vivo studies. Also, differences in experimental parameters such as animal species, anatomical site, vehicle, preparation of skin samples (in vitro studies), and other exposure conditions may affect the interpretation of and comparison between studies [2]. Furthermore, there are limits of quantification and limits of detection, which must be kept in mind when interpreting study results.

Summary

In summary, percutaneous absorption is complex and requires more thought than just simply applying a topical formulation on the skin and assuming that it works. Many factors—at least the 20 that have been discussed here (Table 1.1)—need to be considered as they may affect the efficacy and/or toxicity of the medications and hence patient outcome.

Table 1.1 Twenty clinically pertinent factors of percutaneous absorption

1	Relevant physicochemical properties (particle size/molecular weight, lipophilicity, pH, pKa, and partition coefficient)
2	Vehicle/formulation
3	Conditions of drug exposure (dose, duration, surface area, and exposure frequency)
4	Skin appendages (hair follicles and glands) as sub-anatomical pathways
5	Skin application sites (regional variation in penetration)
6	Population variability (prematurity, infants, and aged)
7	Skin surface conditions (hydration, temperature, and pH)
8	Skin health and integrity (trauma and skin diseases)
9	Substantivity and binding to different skin components
10	Systemic distribution and systemic toxicity
11	Exfoliation
12	Washing-off and washing-in
13	Rubbing/massaging
14	Transfer to others (from human to human and hard surface to human)
15	Volatility
16	Metabolic biotransformation/cutaneous metabolism
17	Photochemical transformation and photosensitivity
18	Excretion kinetics
19	Lateral spread
20	Chemical method of determining percutaneous absorption

Acknowledgments This chapter was originally published in the American Journal of Clinical Dermatology (2020), Vol 21, No. 1, pp. 85–95. It has been reprinted with permission.

References

1. Wester RC, Maibach HI. Cutaneous pharmacokinetics: 10 steps to percutaneous absorption. Drug Metab Rev. 1983;14(2):169–205.
2. Ngo MA, Maibach HI. Chapter 6: 15 factors of percutaneous penetration of pesticides, ACS symposium series. American Chemical Society; 2012. p. 67–86.

3. Hui X, Lamel S, Qiao P, Maibach HI. Isolated human/animal stratum corneum as a partial model for 15 steps in percutaneous absorption: emphasizing decontamination, Part I. J Appl Toxicol. 2013;33:157–72.
4. Hui X, Lamel S, Qiao P, Maibach HI. Isolated human and animal stratum corneum as a partial model for the 15 steps in percutaneous absorption: emphasizing decontamination, part II. J Appl Toxicol. 2013;33:173–82.
5. Li BS, Ngo MA, Maibach HI. Clinical relevance of complex factors of percutaneous penetration in man. Curr Top Pharmacol. 2017;21:85–107. Available at: http://www.researchtrends.net/tia/title_issue.asp?id=11&in=0&vn=21
6. Keurentjes AJ, Maibach HI. Percutaneous penetration of drugs applied in transdermal delivery systems: an in vivo based approach for evaluating computer generated penetration models. Regul Toxicol Pharmacol. 2019 Jul;18:104428.
7. Burton ME, Schentag JJ, Shaw LM, Evans WE. Applied pharmacokinetics and pharmacodynamics: principles of therapeutic drug monitoring. 4th ed. Lippincott, Williams, and Wilkins; 2006.
8. Marechal Y. The water molecule in (bio)macromolecules. In: The hydrogen bond and the water molecule: the physics and chemistry of water, aqueous and bio media. Elsevier; 2007. p. 249–75. https://doi.org/10.1016/B978-044451957-3.50011-1. ISBN 9780444519573, 0444519572;.
9. Wester RC, Noonan PK, Maibach HI. Frequency of application on percutaneous absorption of hydrocortisone. Arch Dermatol. 1977;113:620–2.
10. Berardesca E, Mariano M, Cameli N. Biophysical properties of ethnic skin. In: Vashi NA, Maibach HI, editors. Dermatoanthropology of ethnic skin and hair. Cham: Springer Nature, Springer International Publishing AG; 2017.
11. Berardesca E, Maibach HI. Racial differences in sodium lauryl sulfate induced cutaneous irritation: black and white. Contact Derm. 1988;18:65–70.
12. Berardesca E, Maibach HI. Sodium-lauryl-sulfate-induced cutaneous irritation. Comparison of white and Hispanic subjects. Contact Derm. 1988;19:136–40.
13. Roskos KV, Maibach HI, Guy RH. The effect of aging on percutaneous absorption in man. J Pharmacokinet Biopharm. 1989;17(6):617–30.
14. Hoath SB, Maibach HI. Neonatal skin: structure and function. 2nd ed. CRC Press; 2003.
15. Mauro TM, Behne MJ. Chapter 3: Acid mantle. In: Hoath SB, Maibach HI, editors. Neonatal skin: structure and function. 2nd ed. CRC Press; 2003.
16. Nikolovski J, Stamatas GN, Kollias N, et al. Barrier function and water-holding and transport properties of infant stratum corneum are different from adult and continue to develop through the first year of life. J Invest Dermatol. 2008;128:1728–36.

17. Oranges T, Dini V, Romanelli M. Skin physiology of the neonate and infant: clinical implications. Adv Wound Care. 2015;4(10):587–95.
18. Hoeger PH, Enzmann CC. Skin physiology of the neonate and young infant: a prospective study of functional skin parameters during early infancy. Pediatr Dermatol. 2002;19:256–62.
19. Visscher MO, Chatterjee R, Munson KA, et al. Changes in diapered and non-diapered infant skin over the first month of life. Pediatr Dermatol. 2000;17:45–51.
20. Saijo S, Tagami HJ. Dry skin of newborn infants: functional analysis of the stratum corneum. Pediatr Dermatol. 1991;8:155–9.
21. Brayer C, Micheau P, Bony C, et al. Neonatal accidental burn by isopropyl alcohol. Arch Pediatr. 2004;11(8):932–5.
22. DeBellonia RR, Marcus S, Shih R, et al. Curanderismo: consequences of folk medicine. Pediatr Emerg Care. 2008;24(4):228–9.
23. George AJ. Toxicity of boric acid through skin and mucous membranes. Food Cosmet Toxicol. 1965;3:99–101.
24. Martin-Bouyer G, Toga M, Lebreton R, et al. Outbreak of accidental hexachlorophene poisoning in France. Lancet Public Health. 1982;319(8263):91–5.
25. Mullick FG. Hexachlorophene toxicity—human experience at the Armed Forces Institute of Pathology. Pediatrics. 1973;51(2):395.
26. Li BS, Cary JH, Maibach HI. Should we instruct patients to rub topical agents into skin? The evidence. J Dermatolog Treat. 2018;30:1–5.
27. Evans NJ, Rutter N, Hadgraft J, et al. Percutaneous administration of theophylline in the preterm infant. J Pediatr. 1985;107(2):307–11.
28. Zhai H, Maibach HI. Effects of skin occlusion on percutaneous absorption: an overview. Skin Pharmacol Appl Ski Physiol. 2001;14(1):1–10.
29. Shomaker TS, Zhang J, Ashburn MA. A pilot study assessing the impact of heat on the transdermal delivery of testosterone. J Clin Pharmacol. 2001;41(6):677–82.
30. Aly R, Shirley C, Cunico B, Maibach HI. Effect of prolonged occlusion on the microbial flora, pH, carbon dioxide and transepidermal water loss on human skin. J Invest Dermatol. 1978;71(6):378–81.
31. Gattu S, Maibach HI. Modest but increased penetration through damaged skin: an overview of the in vivo human model. Skin Pharmacol Physiol. 2011;24(1):2–9. (Published Dec 2010)
32. Gattu S, Maibach HI. Enhanced absorption through damaged skin: an overview of the in vitro human model. Skin Pharmacol Physiol. 2010;23:171–6.
33. Morgan CJ, Renwick AG, Friedmann PS. The role of stratum corneum and dermal microvascular perfusion in penetration and tissue levels of water-soluble drugs investigated by microdialysis. Br J Dermatol. 2003;148:434–43.

34. Jakasa I, Verberk MM, Bunge AL, et al. Increased permeability for polyethylene glycols through skin compromised by sodium lauryl sulfate. Exp Dermatol. 2006;15:801–7.
35. Jacob SE. Percutaneous absorption risks in atopic dermatitis. Br J Dermatol. 2017;177:11–2.
36. Halling-Overgaard AS, Kezic S, Jakasa I, et al. Skin absorption through atopic dermatitis skin: a systematic review. Br J Dermatol. 2017;177(1):84–106.
37. Garcia OP, Hansen SH, Shah VP, et al. Impact of adult atopic dermatitis on topical drug absorption: assessment by cutaneous microdialysis and tape strippimg. Acta Derm Venereol. 2009;89:33–8.
38. Tauber M, Balica S, Hsu CY, et al. Staphylococcus aureus density on lesional and nonlesional skin is strongly associated with disease severity in atopic dermatitis. J Allergy Clin Immunol. 2016;137:1272–1274, e1–e3.
39. Jakasa I, de Jongh CM, Verberk MM, et al. Percutaneous penetration of sodium lauryl sulfate is increased in uninvolved skin of patients with atopic dermatitis compared with control subjects. Br J Dermatol. 2006;155:104–9.
40. Jakasa I, Verbek MM, Esposito M, et al. Altered penetration of polyethylene glycols into uninvolved skin of atopic dermatitis patients. J Invest Dermatol. 2007;127:129–34.
41. Hata M, Tokura Y, Takigawa M, et al. Assessment of epidermal barrier function by photoacoustic spectrometry in relation to its importance in the pathogenesis of atopic dermatitis. Lab Investig. 2002;82:1451–61.
42. Mochizuki J, Tadaki H, Takami S, et al. Evaluation of out-in skin transparency using a colorimeter and food dye in patients with atopic dermatitis. Br J Dermatol. 2009;160:972–9.
43. Alikhan FS, Maibach HI. Topical absorption and systemic toxicity. Cutan Ocul Toxicol. 2011;30(3):175–86.
44. Lewis PR, Phillips TG, Sassani JW. Topical therapies for glaucoma: what family physicians need to know. Am Fam Phys. 1882;1999(59):1871–9.
45. Goldberg I, Moloney G, McCluskey P. Topical ophthalmic medications: what potential for systemic side effects and interactions with other medications? Med J Aust. 2008;189:356–7.
46. Rubin Z. Ophthalmic sulfonamide-induced Stevens-Johnson syndrome. Arch Dermatol. 1977;113:235–6.
47. Raschke R, Arnold-Capell PA, Richeson R, et al. Refractory hypoglycemia secondary to topical salicylate intoxication. Arch Intern Med. 1991;151:591–3.
48. Zheng Y, Vieille-Petit A, Chodoutard S, Maibach HI. Dislodgeable stratum corneum exfoliation: role in percutaneous penetration? Cutan Ocul Toxicol. 2011;30(3):198–204.
49. Suny XX, Maibach HI. Skin decontamination. Heidelberg: Springer; 2019. (in press)

50. Rodriguez J, Maibach HI. Percutaneous penetration and pharmacodynamics: wash-in and wash-off of sunscreen and insect repellent. J Dermatolog Treat. 2016;27:11.
51. Moody RP. Letter to the editor: the safety of diethyltoluamide insect repellents. JAMA. 1989;262:28–9.
52. Moody RP, Benoit FM, Riedel R, Ritter L. Dermal absorption of the insect repellent DEET (N,N-diethyl-m-toluamide) in rats and monkeys: effect of anatomical site and multiple exposure. J Toxicol Environ Health. 1989;26:137–47.
53. Lademann J, Patzelt A, Schanzer S, et al. *In vivo* laser scanning microscopic investigation of the decontamination of hazardous substances from the human skin. Laser Phys Lett. 2010;7:884–8.
54. Trauer S, Richter H, Kuntsche J, et al. Influence of massage and occlusion on the ex vivo skin penetration of rigid liposomes and invasomes. Eur J Pharm Biopharm. 2014;86:301–6.
55. Phuong C, Maibach HI. Effect of massage on percutaneous penetration and skin decontamination: man and animal. Cutan Ocul Toxicol. 2016;35(2):153–6.
56. Delamour E, Miksa S, Lutz D, Guy C. How to prove 'rub-resistant' sun protection. Cosmetics & Toiletries Science Applied 2016. Available at: https://www.cosmeticsandtoiletries.com/testing/efficacyclaims/How-to-Prove-Rub-resistant-Sun-Protection-373779591.html. Accessed 12 Mar 2019.
57. Franklin SF, Geffner ME. Precocious puberty secondary to topical testosterone exposure. J Pediatr Endocr Metab. 2003;16:107–10.
58. Wester RC, Hui X, Maibach HI. *In vivo* human transfer of topical bioactive drug between individuals: estradiol. J Invest Dermatol. 2006;126:2190–3.
59. Linck M. Screens detect all: Mom, dad, kids, newborns all test positive for meth. Sioux City Journal, December 18, 2003. Available at: https://siouxcityjournal.com/news/screens-detect-all-mom-dad-kids-newborns-all-test-postive/article_5c9a48cf-4855-5308-ba83-c11bf1b44239.html. Accessed 13 Mar 13 2019.
60. Dmochowski RR, Newman DK, Sand PK, et al. Pharmacokinetics of oxybutynin chloride topical gel. Clin Drug Investig. 2011;31(8):559–71.
61. Isnardo D, Vidal J, Panyella D, Vilaplana J. Nickel Transfer by Fingers Actas Dermo-Sifiliográficas (English Edition) 2015:106(5). https://doi.org/10.1016/j.adengl.2015.04.011.
62. Salocks CB, Hui X, Lamel S, et al. Dermal exposure to methamphetamine hydrochloride contaminated residential surfaces: surface pH values, volatility, and *in vitro* human skin. Food Chem Toxicol. 2012;50(12):4426–40.
63. Rouse NC, Maibach HI. The effect of volatility on percutaneous absorption. J Dermatol Treat. 2016;27(1):5–10.

64. Bruze M. Thoughts on how to improve the quality of multicentre patch test studies. Contact Derm. 2016;74:168–74.
65. Gilpin SJ, Hui X, Maibach HI. Volatility of fragrance chemicals: patch testing implications. Dermatitis. 2009;20(40):200–7.
66. Kasting GB, Miller MA. Kinetics of finite dose absorption through skin 2: volatile compounds. J Pharm Sci. 2006;95:268–80.
67. Norris EJ, Coats JR. Current and future repellent technologies: the potential of spatial repellents and their place in mosquito-borne disease control. Int J Environ Res Public Health. 2017;14(2):124–68.
68. Kawada H, Temu EA, Minjas JN, et al. Field evaluation of field repellency of metofluthrin impregnated latticework plastic strips against *Aedes aegypti* (L.) and analysis of environmental factors affecting its efficacy in My Tho City, Tien Giang, Vietnam. Am J Trop Med Hyg. 2006;75:1153–7.
69. Kazem S, Linssen EC, Gibbs S. Skin metabolism phase I and phase II enzymes in native and reconstructed human skin: a short review. Drug Discovery Today June 2019 ePub ahead of print. Available at: https://www.sciencedirect.com/science/article/pii/S1359644618302198.
70. Bando H, Mohri S, Yamashita F, et al. Effects of skin metabolism on percutaneous penetration of lipophilic drugs. J Pharm Sci. 1997;86(6):759–61.
71. Vieille-Petit A, Blickenstaff N, Coman G, Maibach H. Metrics and clinical relevance of percutaneous penetration and lateral spreading. Skin Pharmacol Physiol. 2015;28:57–64.
72. Jacobi U, Schanzer S, Weigmann H-J, et al. Pathways of lateral spreading. Skin Pharmacol Physiol. 2011;24:231–7.
73. Feldman RJ, Maibach HI. Absorption of some organic compounds through the skin in man. J Invest Dermatol. 1970;54:399–404.

Pharmaceutical Compounding of Topical Dermatologic Treatments

2

Maggie Shukla, Heather Warren, and Stephen Coombs

Contents

M. Shukla · H. Warren
Compounding Wellness Sterile Lab, Mount Pearl, NL, Canada
e-mail: maggiec@mun.ca; heatherw@compoundingwellness.ca

S. Coombs (✉)
School of Pharmacy, Memorial University, St. John's, NL, Canada

Faculty of Medicine, Discipline of Family Medicine, Memorial University, St. John's, NL, Canada
e-mail: n45sdc@mun.ca

R. M. Law, H. I. Maibach (eds.), *Handbook of Topical Drug Treatment in Dermatology*,
https://doi.org/10.1007/978-3-031-93616-6_2

Introduction

Pharmaceutical compounding is an integral part of pharmacy, medicine, and the healthcare system. Compounding in dermatology contributes to current therapeutics by personalizing treatments, filing therapeutic gaps, aiding adherence, and providing treatments during medication shortages. It can be defined as the process of combining, mixing, or altering ingredients to create medication tailored to the needs of a patient [1].

Pharmaceutical compounding can carry significant risk. Compounded medications are indicated for off-label use and not approved by national regulatory bodies such as the US Food and Drug Administration (FDA) or Health Canada. However, when appropriate standards of practice are considered, the benefits of administering a compounded medication can be much greater than the associated risks. Standards of practice for pharmaceutical compounding have become more stringent to ensure patient safety while preserving patient access. They are adopted and enforced primarily by state or provincial regulatory bodies.

In North America, United States Pharmacopeia (USP) includes General Chapter 795 directly addressing pharmaceutical compounding of non-sterile preparations and the National Association of Pharmacy Regulatory Authorities (NAPRA) developed the model standards of non-sterile preparations along with a guidance document [1, 2]. In general, these standards cover requirements for compounding personnel, training and skills assessment, policies and procedures, equipment, facility layout, and quality assurance.

When referring to this chapter, it is important to be cognizant of the fact that each country has different regulations pertaining to what active pharmaceutical ingredients (APIs) or bulk drug substances can be used when compounding. For example, the 503A compounding pharmacies bulk list (i.e., active pharmaceutical ingredient list) and the difficult to compound list have been created by the FDA. Before compounding, all compounders have a responsibility to ensure they are following their local compounding standards and regulations [3, 4].

Availability of evidence-based medicine is imperative to healthcare professional decision-making. Pharmaceutical compounding is a form of personalized medicine and therefore is often informed by lower-level evidence, such as case reports and case series. Depending on the frequency of use of a compounded preparation for a specific off-label indication, randomized controlled trials, systematic reviews, and other higher-level evidence may be available. However, higher-level evidence oftentimes requires a financial commitment unattainable for such personalized medicine. Nonetheless, when any level of evidence is combined with patient specific factors to support the use of a compounded medication, this shared decision should be made between the compounder, patient, and prescriber. The ability to offer compounded preparation options to patients can be a great tool for all healthcare professionals.

This chapter aims to cover common questions that may arise when recommending or writing a compounded prescription, preparing a compounded preparation, or discussing compounding options with a patient. The contents of this chapter are not a limitation to what compounding options are available for dermatology as pharmaceutical compounding is constantly evolving.

Important Abbreviations

The following abbreviations are used throughout this chapter:

APIs: Active Pharmaceutical Ingredients

FDA: Food and Drug Administration

NAPRA: National Association of Pharmacy Regulatory Authorities
USP-NF: United States Pharmacopeia and the National Formulary
BUD: Beyond use date
IJPC: International Journal of Pharmaceutical Compounding

When to Compound

When considering whether a compounded topical preparation for a patient is appropriate and beneficial, circumstances where compounding is inappropriate must be avoided. Table 2.1 is a useful tool to help guide the compounding decision-making process.

Quality Assurance [1, 2]

As mentioned previously, compounding is not regulated by national regulatory bodies such as the US FDA or Health Canada. Quality assurance is a standard of practice in compounding, and these programs must be created and enforced by the compounders and their facilities. Quality assurance programs are additionally audited for compliance by state or provincial regulatory bodies.

A quality assurance program is developed and implemented to ensure processes are clearly defined, including application and verification of all activities, that affect the quality of the final compounded preparations. It also ensures protection of personnel who are compounding. Each verification step (carried out in accordance with the quality assurance program) should be documented. Quality assurance programs cover multiple components involved in the compounding process such as facility requirements, equipment used, personnel, the act of compounding itself, and final preparation verification. Within these components, there will be designated controls (e.g., skills assessment of personnel) and frequency at which reassessment or certification should be carried out (e.g., yearly).

Table 2.1 When compounding is appropriate or inappropriate [1, 2, 5, 6]

Appropriate	Inappropriate
Customizing a compounded preparation for a patient by: Adjusting the dosage of the API Choosing the most appropriate base for the condition being treated Combining APIs that work synergistically together	Compounding a product that is the same as a product that is currently available on the market (i.e., duplication of a manufactured product)
Providing pharmaceutical dosage forms that are not available commercially (e.g., preparing a topical solution of an API when only oral capsules are commercially available)	Compounding beyond the scope of practice; this refers to compounding without the appropriate knowledge, expertise and equipment/facilities required to provide a quality, safe, effective compounded product
Meeting the needs of a patient requiring products for rare disease states, also known as orphan diseases, for which the pharmaceutical industry is not currently developing products	Compounding without a developed formula or without appropriate references and supporting documentation to develop your own formula
Offering a different dosage strength than those available by manufacturers. Dosage adjustment may be needed to optimize the risk-benefit profile specific to the patient	Compounding a product that includes an API deemed ineffective or unsafe for human use or has been discontinued from the market after being found unsafe or ineffective
Providing a compounded alternative when a product is not currently available because of manufacturer shortage, or the product is withdrawn from the market (i.e. for reasons other than medication safety issues)	Compounding with an API that has been excluded for use in compounding by your specific regulatory body (e.g., FDA, Health Canada)
Altering the preparation such that application is conducive to adherence, either by modifying the physical properties of the formulation (e.g., change base from ointment to cream) or combining several active ingredients into a single formulation (e.g., combining an antifungal and a corticosteroid)	
Removing or exchanging excipients or bases due to allergy, intolerance, or a possible drug interaction	

Master Formula Creation [1, 2]

Compounders develop master formulas for each compounded preparation. These formulas are specific to each compounding facility and follow requirements described in compounding standards of practice and their quality assurance program. A literature search should be completed to gather all information available regarding a specific ingredient or compound and listed as references in the master formula. Likewise, there are multiple resources to aid in formula creation (e.g., USP-NF, Remington, Trissel's, The Merck Index, IJPC, and Compounding Today). There are also formulas created by compounding supply companies who have carried out the majority of the physiochemical research required and make up the bulk of a master formula.

General Compounding Techniques and Equipment

To prepare a topical dermatological preparation that is both pharmaceutically elegant and optimally formulated the compounder must employ specific techniques during the mixing process. This may include the use of compounding equipment that not only produces a product with more favorable characteristics (e.g., small particle size of APIs) but also makes the compounding process more efficient. Table 2.2 describes some of the most common compounding techniques used when preparing topical preparations. Table 2.3 outlines equipment that can be used.

Table 2.2 Commonly used techniques when compounding topical preparations [7, 8]

Technique	Definition	How is this achieved?
Geometric addition/ dilution	The standard procedure is used to achieve a homogenous blend when two or more components are mixed. This ensures active ingredients are evenly dispersed within a preparation	The compounder starts with ingredients of the smallest quantity and effectively "dilutes" it by adding an equal portion of another ingredient of the next smallest quantity. This is continued incrementally by doubling the portions mixed The procedure is repeated until all the ingredients are incorporated
Trituration/ milling	The act of reducing the particle size of a powder	Can be achieved by the continuous grinding or rubbing of the powder in a mortar with a pestle Trituration may be achieved by levigation or wetting May be achieved mechanically through the use of equipment (e.g., ointment mill)
Levigation	The process of decreasing the particle size of powders via trituration with a mortar and pestle and a small amount of liquid in which the substance is insoluble	The specific liquid used is called a levigating agent and is viscous in nature. It has a low surface tension to easily wet the solid particles. Such agents also act as a lubricant as they also allow a smoother incorporation of solids in the preparation
Pulverization by intervention	Used with hard crystalline powders that do not crush or triturate easily, or for gummy type substances	A solvent, such as alcohol or acetone, that will dissolve the compound is mixed in a mortar with the powder. The evaporation of the solvent is carried out afterward
Spatulation	The mixing of powders and semisolids (ointments, creams, etc.) using a spatula	A spatula is used to continuously heap the powders and/or solids together and then smoothing the mass out on a glass or paper slab This process does not reduce particle size, so this must be previously accomplished if required

Table 2.3 Commonly used equipment for compounding of topical preparations [2, 8, 9]

Equipment	Explanation
Mortar and pestle	A set of two simple tools used to prepare ingredients or substances by crushing and grinding them into a fine paste or powder The mortar is the bowl, and the pestle is the blunt, club shaped object Pharmaceutical mortar and pestles are typically made of either ceramic, glass, or a more porous porcelain. The correct mortar and pestle type should be chosen based on the ingredients to be grinded; harder ingredients may require a more porous mortar and pestle The ingredient to be ground, which may be wet or dry, is placed in the mortar where the pestle is pounded, pressed, and rotated into the substance until the desired texture is achieved
Ointment slab and spatula	Ointment slabs provide a clean, hard surface for the mixing of preparations Types of ointment slabs include reusable glass slabs or disposable parchment paper slabs that require less cleaning in between preparations Typically, a spatula is used to mix the preparation on the slab
Electronic mortar and pestle (EMP)	The device uses both horizontal and vertical mixing movements via mixing blades contained in a polypropylene jar to produce a homogeneous preparation The mixing blade rotates at speeds between 200 and 2500 rpm depending on the specific brand and engine size The shear force between the blade and side of the EMP jar results in some particle size reduction, although powders that are crystalline and granular may still need to be triturated before incorporation It provides time-efficient preparation It is more costly than the traditional mortar and pestle set and requires regular maintenance, as well as specialized blades and containers for use

(continued)

Table 2.3 (continued)

Equipment	Explanation
Ointment mill	Used for intensive trituration and dispersion of ointments, creams, pastes, gels, and suspensions A preparation is run through the mill where there are generally three rollers made either from a ceramic or aluminum oxide material The preparation is fed through the instrument on the roller furthest from the operator. The preparation passes through the two gaps formed between the three rollers. The shearing action of the rollers results in the reduction of particle size and dispersion of powders The range of function of ointment mills varies between brands Cost is a considerable factor when purchasing
Electronic balance	A requirement to participate in pharmaceutical compounding, used to accurately weigh material Replaces traditional torsion balances and weight systems The lowest amount of material that can be weighed accurately on a scale, as well as the scale's sensitivity, must be considered by compounders, as there is great variation between scale models

Compounding Bases

The quality and efficacy of topical compounded preparations is largely influenced by the base chosen. The compounder must consider if the selected base is appropriate for the indication and the patient and if it can properly deliver the APIs to the site of action. Commercial cosmetic creams tend to be a poor choice for compounding. Many times, they already contain a large number of ingredients and are not generally designed to hold additional APIs. Therefore, it is a good idea to use an innovative proprietary compounding base that has been designed specifically to deliver the APIs required. These proprietary bases are also commonly fragrance free, hypoallergenic, preservative-free, and alcohol-free. However, to ensure informed decision-making while compounding, these bases should be used by compounders that have access to their composition.

Numerous bases have been preformulated by compounding supply companies for specific conditions; examples include muco-adhesive gels that prolong contact time between an API and the area of treatment and bases containing excipients that work synergistically with the API.

Considerations When Choosing an Appropriate Compounding Base [1, 2, 10–12]

- Carrying capacity of the base
  - Does the active ingredient have a salt concentration that the base can support?
  - Is there more than one ingredient?
  - How much of the API can be incorporated into the base without the preparation breaking, rendering the compound unusable?
- Beyond use date (BUD)
  - Is the base anhydrous? This generally extends the BUD the compounder can give (e.g., USP 795 states in the absence of stability data, the BUD 6 months or not later than the time remaining until the earliest expiration date of any API, whichever is earlier).
  - Does the base contain water? This generally shortens the BUD the compounder can give (e.g., USP 795 states in the absence of stability data, the BUD is not later than 30 days).
- Site of action
  - Where will the cream be applied? (e.g., skin and mucosal)
  - Is the area covered in hair or a smooth surface?
  - What is the surface area to be covered?
  - Does the area contain thick or thin skin?
  - Is the preparation intended to sit on top of skin locally, or is deeper penetration required to be effective (i.e., topical or transdermal delivery)?

- Patient preference
  - Nongreasy preparation?
  - Gluten free, vegan, nonallergenic?
  - An easily spreadable preparation?
  - A lower-cost preparation?
- Intended use of the compounding preparation
  - Provide moisture while healing?
  - Act as an occlusive?
  - Decrease exudate and promote wound healing?
  - Act as an adhesive to hold drugs at site of action?
  - Deeply penetrate through various layers of skin?
- Chemical properties of the API(s)
  - Hydrophilic or hydrophobic (or both)?
  - Acidic or basic (i.e., pH)?
  - Crystalline, powder, or liquid?
  - Stability at different temperatures and in different bases?
  - Molecular weight?
  - Partition coefficient?
- Integrity of the skin
  - Is the skin barrier damaged (e.g., open wound)?
  - Is the skin red, irritated, or dry?
  - Is there an exudate being produced?
  - Is there scar tissue?
  - Is the skin considered thick (e.g., soles and palms) or thin (e.g., genital area and eyelids)?
  - What is the patient's age (e.g., very old, very young)?

Tables 2.4 and 2.5 outline the most commonly used compounding bases and provide supplemental information on each.

Table 2.4 Ointment bases [7, 10–12]

Ointments				
Ointment type	Properties	Uses	Levitating agents that can be used to incorporate solid API into base[a]	Examples
Oleaginous base	Anhydrous Do not absorb water Forms occlusive film on skin Not water washable	Protectant, emollient, drug carrier for hydrophobic API(s) only	Mineral oil	Petrolatum, wax, synthetic esters, white soft paraffin
Absorption base	Oleaginous base plus a water-in-oil emulsifier Can incorporate aqueous solution and/or alcohol Not easily water washable	Protectant, emollient, drug carrier	Mineral oil	Anhydrous lanolin, hydrophilic petrolatum USP
Water-in-oil emulsion base	Contains water Oleaginous base plus water-in-oil emulsifier plus water Allows easier incorporation of an aqueous solution Not easily water washable	Emollient, drug carrier	Mineral oil, glycerin, propylene glycol	Hydrous lanolin, cold cream USP

Ointment type	Properties	Uses	Levitating agents that can be used to incorporate solid API into base[a]	Examples
Oil-in-water emulsion base (also known as water removable base)	Contains water Oleaginous base plus oil-in-water emulsifier plus water Leaves a hydrophobic film on the surface of skin when the water evaporates Water washable Has a cream like appearance Can be further diluted with water Can absorb serous discharge caused by dermatological conditions	Emollient, drug carrier	Glycerin propylene glycol, polysorbate 80	Vanishing cream, hydrophilic ointment USP
Water-soluble base	Contains water Nongreasy Nonocclusive Lipid-free and water-soluble Water washable Has a cream like appearance Can be further diluted with water	Drug carrier	Glycerin Propylene glycol Polyethylene glycol	Polyethylene glycol ointment USP, Emollient cream

[a]Levigating agents included in this table are not exhaustive and are included only to provide suggestions

Table 2.5 Other types of bases [11–13]

Base type	Important points
Creams	A highly viscous emulsion base is commonly referred to as a cream A semisolid base that may contain one or more ingredients dissolved or dispersed Either a w/o (i.e., oily creams) or o/w (i.e., aqueous creams) emulsion base Water-soluble drugs are dispersed in aqueous creams Lipid-soluble drugs are dispersed in oily creams Creams are more fluid than ointments Creams are desirable for the patient because they have an elegant appearance, are more readily spread on the skin, and are less greasy, and they rub into the skin leaving little or no trace
Lotions	Low-to-medium viscosity topical preparation, usually applied to unbroken skin An insoluble fine powder drug can be suspended or dispersed into a lotion Is easily spreadable and therefore can be used in hair covered areas and large areas Has no emollient or skin protective properties
Gels	Semisolid base that consists of small or large molecules in an aqueous liquid vehicle. The aqueous vehicle has been thickened with a gelling agent Nongreasy, easy to apply and wash off Once on the skin, it changes from a semisolid state to a liquefied state and then dries to a nonocclusive film Easy to apply to hair covered areas and can be used in mucosal areas Has no emollient or skin protective properties Compounded gels can be useful in wound care, as they are easily applied over the affected area
Solutions	A nonaqueous, aqueous, or hydroalcoholic liquid, which contains solutes that are dissolved to the point of clarity Is very easily spreadable, oftentimes leading to messy applications Very simple to compound Solutions are commonly used when compounding preparations for dermatological conditions affecting the scalp and ears

Excipients

Active pharmaceutical ingredient is the term generally used to describe the substances in drugs that are responsible for the beneficial health effects experienced by patients [5]. Therefore, all other ingredients are referred to as either inactive, non-medicinal, or excipients. Excipients are important for the integrity of the compounded preparation, functioning as stabilizers and therapeutically enhancing the API in the final dosage form [14]. Excipients used in compounding should be of pharmaceutical grade (e.g., USP-NF). Table 2.6 outlines common excipients and possible functions. To note, colorants are also excipients but not listed in Table 2.6 as they are most often approved dyes.

Considerations when choosing specific excipients:

- Patient preference
- Drug properties (hydrophilic, lipophilic, pH, and solubility)
- Desired viscosity of final preparation
- Desired consistency of final preparation
- Patient specific sensitivities
- Area of application
- Site of action (e.g., topical, transdermal)
- Cosmeceutical elegance (e.g., color and odor)

Table 2.6 Excipients commonly used in topical compounded preparations [14–20]

Example excipients	Functional category	Details
Alpha hydroxyl acids (lactic acid) Glycerin Propylene glycol Sorbitol Urea	Humectant	Hygroscopic substances that promote water retention and prevent drying of preparations. May be helpful in enhancing active ingredient solubility and, thus, its ability to penetrate the skin Should be stored in tight, light-resistant containers
Propylene glycol monostearate Emulsifying wax Diethylene glycol monoethyl ether Polysorbate 20/80/60 Docusate sodium Poloxamer Sodium lauryl sulfate Sorbitan monopalmitate Acacia	Emulsifying/solubilizing agent Surfactant	Reduce interfacial tension resulting in stabilizing an emulsion. In hydrophobic materials, these agents enhance solubility and wetting Selection of an appropriate surfactant is important for establishing the hydrophilic lipophilic balance system.

Ethanol Isopropyl alcohol Propylene glycol (adjunct for synergism) Polyethylene glycol Isopropyl palmitate Isopropyl myristate Azone Dimethyl sulfoxide (DMSO) Limonene Menthol Urea Water	Permeation enhancer Penetration enhancer	Enhances diffusion or solubility in order to pass through the stratum corneum Should be nontoxic, nonirritating, and nonallergenic Menthol, urea, and DMSO have the highest irritation potential If larger amounts of alcohol-based enhancers are required in a particular formula, there is potential for excessive skin drying
Imidurea Sorbic acid Benzoid acid Boric acid Imidurea propyl paraben Benzalkonium chloride Methyl paraben	Preservative	Inhibits bacterial and fungal growth. However, these ingredients frequently cause allergic contact dermatitis and sensitive patients may need them removed

(continued)

Table 2.6 (continued)

Example excipients	Functional category	Details
Guar gum Xanthan gum Gelatin Carbomer Sodium carboxyl methyl cellulose Carrageenan Colloidal silicon dioxide Carboxymethylcellulose sodium Hydroxyethyl cellulose Hydroxypropyl cellulose Hydroxypropyl methylcellulose Methylcellulose	Thickening/gelling agent	Used to increase viscosity. Enables easier application of drugs to various parts of the body so they do not run off
Cetyl alcohol Cetyl esters wax Microcrystalline wax Paraffin Stearyl alcohol White wax Yellow wax	Stiffening agent	Used to increase thickness or hardness of a preparation, usually an ointment

Ethylene diamine tetraacetate	Chelating agent	Enhances stability by minimizing metal-catalyzed degradation
Butylated hydroxytoluene Butylated hydroxyanisole	Antioxidant	Decreases oxidative deterioration; oxidative deterioration may manifest as an unpleasant odor, discoloration, and even slight loss of activity During product formulation, antioxidants should be used in their lowest effective concentrations and incorporated early in the preparation process
Mineral oil Propylene glycol Glycerin	Levigating agent	Liquid used as an intervening agent to reduce the particle size of a powder by grinding

Active Pharmaceutical Ingredients

Compounding in dermatology contributes to current therapeutics by personalizing treatments, filing therapeutic gaps, aiding adherence, and serving as an adjunct to commercially available therapies to further meet specific patient needs. Therefore, a compounded preparation could be requested for any indication (Table 2.7).

- As mentioned previously, a compounder cannot compound a preparation that is identical to a commercially available product. For more information on when and when not to compound a preparation, see Table 2.1—When compounding is appropriate or inappropriate.
- The strengths included in this table are not all inclusive, and the upper range may not be appropriate for all patients or for all indications.
- Combining APIs can result in synergisms that serve to potentiate efficacy and reduce the toxicity of the APIs when they are used separately. However, not all APIs can be combined; assessment of physicochemical properties and other stability information or prior clinical experience at minimum would be required before combining ingredients for the first time.

Table 2.7 Examples of active pharmaceutical ingredients used in compounded topical dermatology preparations[a] [21–23]

API	APIs expanded if applicable	Commonly requested strengths	Requested indications	Other notes
Acid (hydroxy)	Glycolic acid (alpha hydroxy)	2–70%	Acne Pre-peel preparations, skin cleansers, skin bleaching/skin lightening	
	Lactic acid (alpha hydroxy)	2–12%	Facial peels, pre-peel preparations, Skin cleansers, Skin bleaching/skin lightening, Keratosis pilaris	
	Mandelic acid (alpha hydroxy)	2–10%	Pre-peel preparation Mild facial peel	
	Salicylic acid (beta hydroxy)	0.5–60%	Keratosis pilaris, skin cleansers, warts	
Acyclovir		2–5%	Warts	
Amitriptyline		2–5%	Shingles/post herpetic neuralgia	

(continued)

Table 2.7 (continued)

API	APIs expanded if applicable	Commonly requested strengths	Requested indications	Other notes
Antibiotic	Ciprofloxacin	2%	Wound care[b]	
	Clindamycin	1–2%	Acne	
	Erythromycin	2–4%	Acne	
	Gentamicin	0.2–0.5%	Wound care[b]	
	Metronidazole	0.75–1%	Rosacea, Wound care[b]	
	Mupirocin	2–5%	Wound care[b]	
	Tobramycin	5%	Wound care[b]	
Antifungal	Clotrimazole	1–2%	Fungal infection	
	Itraconazole	1–2%	Nail fungus, wound care[b]	
	Nystatin	100,000–200,000 units/gm	Fungal infection	
	Terbinafine	2–3%	Fungal infection Nail fungus	
	Ketoconazole	2%	Fungal infection Nail fungus	

Ascorbic acid		5–20%	Antiaging, Skin bleaching/skin lightening	
Azelaic acid		1.5–18%	Acne, Hair loss	
Azelastine		0.1–0.175%	Eczema, psoriasis, and allergic contact dermatitis	
Benzoyl peroxide		2.5–20%	Acne, Skin cleansers	
Calcineurin inhibitor	Tacrolimus	0.03–0.1%	Atopic dermatitis, eczema, lichen planus, geographic tongue, psoriasis	
	Sirolimus (rapamycin)	0.1–1%	Eczema, angiofibromas caused by tubular sclerosis complex	

(continued)

Table 2.7 (continued)

API	APIs expanded if applicable	Commonly requested strengths	Requested indications	Other notes
Caffeine		1–3%	Androgenetic alopecia, prevent rosacea and skin cancer. Improve skin circulation and contains antioxidants	
Camphor		0.25–3%	Counterirritant	
Capsaicin		0.25–0.75%	Post-herpetic neuralgia	
Cimetidine		10–15%	Warts	
Coal tar		1–5%	Eczema Psoriasis	Available as pure coal tar or liquor carbonis detergens (LCD) usually 20% coal tar
Cholestyramine		5–10%	Wound care[b]	

Corticosteroid	Betamethasone valerate	0.05–0.1%	Scars	
	Betamethasone dipropionate	0.05%	Scars	
	Clobetasol propionate	0.025–0.05%	Eczema Psoriasis	
	Desonide	0.05%	Eczema Psoriasis	
	Fluocinolone acetonide	0.01–0.025%	Skin bleaching/skin lightening	
	Hydrocortisone	0.05–2.5%	Wound care[b], anti-itch, anti-inflammatory	
	Mometasone	0.1%	Eczema Psoriasis	
	Triamcinolone	0.05–0.5%	Skin bleaching/skin lightening, scarring	
Cromolyn sodium		0.21–10%	Eczema	Adjunct to topical steroids

(continued)

Table 2.7 (continued)

API	APIs expanded if applicable	Commonly requested strengths	Requested indications	Other notes
Cyanocobalamin		0.07–1%	Eczema Psoriasis	A non-steroid option
Deoxy-D-glucose		0.2–2%	Warts	
Diclofenac		1–3%	Actinic keratosis	
Diltiazem		2%	Wound care[b]	
Dimethylethanolamine (DMAE)		2.28–5%	Skin firming Skin masks	
Diphenhydramine		1–2%	Eczema Psoriasis Scars, pruritus	
Diphenylcyclopropenone (DCPC)		0.0001–4%	Alopecia areata	
Estriol		0.01–0.2%	Antiaging	
Finasteride		0.05–0.1%	Androgenetic alopecia	
5-Fluorouracil		1–5%	Skin cancer, warts	
Gabapentin		2–10%	Shingles/post herpetic neuralgia	
Glycopyrrolate		0.25–2%	Hyperhidrosis	
Hyaluronic acid		0.1–0.5%	Antiaging	

Hydroquinone		2–10%	Melasma Skin bleaching/skin lightening	
Ichthammol		10–20%	Topical drawing salve used for minor skin infections and irritations. Also used to treat eczema, dermatitis, psoriasis	
Imiquimod		5%	Actinic keratosis Warts	
Insulin (topical)		0.1–10 units/cm	Wound care[b]	
Ivermectin		1%	Rosacea	
Ketoprofen		2–10%	Shingles Wound care[b]	
Ketotifen		0.05%	Eczema Psoriasis Rosacea	
Kojic acid		0.05–6%	Skin masks, skin lightening	

(continued)

Table 2.7 (continued)

API	APIs expanded if applicable	Commonly requested strengths	Requested indications	Other notes
Menthol		0.25–10%	Counterirritant	Maximum 1% in a transdermal base
Methotrexate		1%	Eczema Psoriasis	
Methoxsalen		0.1—1% 10 mg capsules	Atopic dermatitis, psoriasis, vitiligo	Capsules NOT oral, to be opened for PUVA therapy
Minoxidil		5–10%	Androgenetic alopecia	
Misoprostol		0.0024%	Ulcers, Wound care[b]	
Naltrexone (low dose)		0.1–0.2%	Eczema, pruritis Psoriasis Hailey-Hailey disease Neuropathic itch Vitiligo Warts Wound care[b]	Prolonged use (greater than 2 weeks) without cycling may exacerbate condition, frequent monitoring required
Niacinamide		2–5%	Acne Rosacea	

Nifedipine		0.2–5%	Reynauds Wound care[b]	
Pentoxifylline		0.3–1%	Burns Contractures	
Phenytoin		1–5%	Wound care[b]	
Pyrogallic acid		10–25%	Corns Warts	
Resorcinol		1–14%	Facial peel Antiaging	
Retinoid	Adapalene	0.1–0.3%	Acne	Ingredient as a commercially available cream only
	Tazarotene	0.045–0.1%	Acne	Ingredient as a commercially available cream only
	Tretinoin	0.025–0.1%	Acne Facial peels, hair loss Skin bleaching/skin lightening Warts	

(continued)

Table 2.7 (continued)

API	APIs expanded if applicable	Commonly requested strengths	Requested indications	Other notes
Sildenafil		1–5%	Reynauds Wound care[b]	
Silver sulfadiazine		1%	Wound care[b]	
Simvastatin/cholesterol		2%/2%	Porokeratosis	
Spironolactone		1–5%	Acne, androgenetic alopecia	
Sucralfate		4%	Wound care[b]	
Sulfur		2–10%	Skin cleanser Scabies Seborrheic dermatitis	Can also be used adjunctively in acne compounds
Tea tree oil (also known as melaleuca oil)		1–5%	Antibacterial use to treat warts, acne, nail fungus, topical fungal infections	Often used in in combination with other APIs
Tranexamic acid		3–10%	Epistaxis Melasma Wound care	
Tranilast		1%	Eczema psoriasis Scars	A non-steroid option

Tofacitinib		2%	Alopecia and vitiligo	JAK inhibitor
Topical anesthetics	Benzocaine	0.5–20%	Numbing agent	Toxicity may occur if higher strengths are used over large area and/or occluded
	Bupivacaine	0.25–2%	Numbing agent	
	Lidocaine	2–5%	Shingles Wound care[b]	
	Prilocaine	1–10%	Numbing agent	
	Tetracaine	0.5–4%	Numbing agent	
Trichloroacetic acid		7–20%	Facial peels, warts	
Urea		10–40%	Moisturizer	
Vitamin A palmitate		0.3%	Antiaging	
Vitamin E acetate		0.6–1%	Antiaging	
Zinc		2–25%	Wound care[b]	Different salts (oxide, sulfate) use different strength

[a]This table is not inclusive and is based primarily on formulas produced by compounding supply companies [22, 23] and the clinical experience of the authors and their peers. Performing a literature search will provide information on individual APIs or compounded preparations; however, referencing each API or compounded preparation is outside the scope of this chapter. The requested indications are used off-label when compounding and API efficacy and adverse effects will vary per person and per master formulation

[b]Superficial wound care is non-sterile, and deep wounds may require sterile preparations

Communication

Communication and shared decision-making are essential components of the patient care process. This involves identifying plausible treatment plans, working with patients to decide which plan is optimal for them, and following up regularly to address any barriers to implementation or adherence. When prescribing compounded preparations, there are additional elements to consider to optimize the ability to achieve goals of therapy. Maintaining open lines of communication between prescriber, patient, and pharmacist and frequent engagement within this triad will aid in the facilitation of high-quality health care [25]. Here are some examples of these considerations:

Prescriber/patient:

- When deciding on therapy, notify patients that the product being prescribed will need to be compounded. Given that not all pharmacies are equipped to be able to compound, as well as the fact that compounding takes time, this will help to establish realistic expectations.
- Patients should be consulted on topical product characteristics that are acceptable for their individual circumstances. For example, would the greasy appearance of an ointment base be suitable for multiple daily applications?

Prescriber/pharmacist [24, 25]:

- Constructive communication is imperative for ensuring and improving the quality of prescriptions for compounded preparations. If incompatibilities in prescription ingredients exist, or if there are compounding strategies that may offer greater benefits than what is prescribed, for example. Timely communication ensures quality patient care.
- In keeping with the above, getting to know local practitioners as well as the breadth of compounding services offered will facilitate enhanced collaboration and communication. Ultimately, this will allow for pre-emptive discovery and management of issues related to prescriptions for compounded preparations.

- Providing rationale for recommendations can be more productive than just providing an answer; therapeutic relationships may be strengthened through demonstration of critical thinking and reasoning skills.

Pharmacist/patient:

- Patient counselling and education is certainly not a foreign topic to pharmacists, and this holds true in the realm of compounding. As there is no manufacturer provided information for patients to refer to, it is essential that they are counselled on the appropriate use, storage, and expiry (beyond use date) of the preparations dispensed. National and state/provincial regulations should be consulted to ensure any verbal or written information provided is acceptable.
- To reiterate, explaining that a preparation is compounded can help to establish realistic expectations for prescription wait times and help to avoid misconceptions that may hinder the patient-pharmacist relationship.
- Educating patients about the potential adverse effects of compounded preparations, including how they can be managed, is paramount to optimizing adherence. This should occur at the time of dispensing, as well as on subsequent follow-up.
- Follow-up should be tailored to each individual patient's needs. Goals of follow-up should include assessing degree of efficacy, identifying adverse effects, reviewing application technique, and inquiring about factors that may contribute to noncompliance.

Considerations When Writing a Compounded Preparation Prescription

Ultimately, one of the tangible products of the communication between a prescriber and a pharmacist is a prescription for a compounded preparation. Although legal requirements vary between provinces/states and countries, there are best practices for compounding prescription writing that are universal:

- Identifying that the prescribed preparation is to be compounded (e.g., compounded mediation, to compound). This indicates to both the patient and the compounding pharmacist that this is indeed the expectation.
- Explicitly writing APIs with their desired final concentrations/strengths in the compound is important to avoid confusion, as well as potential dilution, if assuming commercially available products will be used in the compounding process instead of pharmaceutical grade powders.
- With regard to the compounding base, if a specific brand product is not desired, including the type of base, and/or the desired site of action may be appropriate (e.g., topical lotion and transdermal cream).
- Specifically identify the area of application (e.g., trunk and legs), the amount to apply (e.g., sparingly and liberally), and duration of therapy.
- If the compounded preparation is to be applied on an as needed basis, it is important to indicate the maximum total daily dose (i.e., maximum number of daily applications).
- It may be helpful to include brief instruction on how to manage some potential adverse effects (e.g., discontinue use if experiencing extreme irritation, redness, or burning).
- Diligently assess the quantity of compounded preparation that will be required to treat the affected area and appropriate duration of therapy to prevent product wastage, and excessive use and cost.
- BUDs should always be considered when prescribing durations of therapy and quantities to dispense.

References

1. USP. General Chapter 795 Pharmaceutical Compounding Non Sterile Preparations. The United States Pharmacopeial Convention. 2022. https://www.usp.org/compounding/general-chapter-795. Accessed 15 Jan 2022.
2. NAPRA. Model Standards for Pharmacy Compounding of Non-Sterile preparations. https://napra.ca/general-practice-resources/model-standards-pharmacy-compounding-non-sterile-preparations. The National Association of Pharmacy Regulatory Authorities. 2018. Accessed 15 Jan 2022.

3. FDA. Bulk Drug Substances Used in Compounding. U.S. Food and Drug Administration. 2021. https://www.fda.gov/drugs/human-drug-compounding/bulk-drug-substances-used-compounding. Accessed 20 Jan 2022.
4. FDA. Drug products that present demonstrable difficulties for compounding Under the Federal Food, Drug, and Cosmetic Act. U.S. Food and Drug Administration. 2017. https://www.federalregister.gov/documents/2017/07/28/2017-15900/drug-products-that-present-demonstrable-difficulties-for-compounding-under-the-federal-food-drug-and. Accessed 22 Jan 2022.
5. Health Canada. Policy on manufacturing and compounding drug products in Canada (POL-0051). January 2009. https://www.canada.ca/en/health-canada/services/drugs-health-products/compliance-enforcement/good-manufacturing-practices/guidance-documents/policy-manufacturing-compounding-drug-products.html. Accessed 20 Jan 2022.
6. Sánchez-Regana M, Llambí-Mateos F, Salleras-Redonnet M, Iglesias Sancho M, Collgros Totosaus H, Umbert-Millet P. Compounding as a current therapeutic option in dermatology, vol. 104. Spain: Actas Dermo-Sifiliográficas; 2013. p. 738–56.
7. Nagel K, Ali F, Al-Khudari S, Patel A, Patel N, Desai P. Extemporaneous compounding of medicated ointments. IJPC. 2010;14(6):472–8.
8. Nguyen T, Ullmann P. Compounding from basics to modern technology. Medisca. 2018. https://www.medisca.com.au/Pages/Education/Files/AJP%20Oct%202018%20-%20Practice%20Update%20-%20Basic%20Skills%20to%20Modern%20Technology.pdf. Accessed 20 Jan 2022.
9. PCCA. Gako Unguator Electronic Mortar & Pestles. 2019. Available from: https://www.pccarx.com/Documents/C-Files/95002_emp.pdf. Accessed 20 Jan 2022.
10. Campbell E, Elston D, Straughan C. A review of the clinical indications, general principles and techniques related to compounding. J Am Acad Dermatol. 2020;83(1):179–83.
11. Weiss S. Conventional topical delivery systems. Dermatol Ther. 2011;24:471–6.
12. Conway J, Brown M. A flowchart for selecting an Ointment Base. Am J Pharm Educ. 2014;78(1):16.
13. Fiorillo L, Romano G. Gels in medicine and surgery: current trends and future perspectives. Gels. 2020;6(4):48.
14. Allen LV. Excipients used in nonsterile compounding, part 1. IJPC. 2019;23:305–11.
15. Allen LV. Excipients used in nonsterile compounding, part 8: humectants. IJPC. 2021;25:126–8.
16. Allen LV. Excipients used in nonsterile compounding, part 7: compounding with surfactants. IJPC. 2020;24:388–95.
17. Allen LV. Excipients used in nonsterile compounding, part 3: preservatives. IJPC. 2019;23:472–7.

18. Allen LV. Excipients used in nonsterile compounding, part 4: antioxidants and chelating agents. IJPC. 2020;24:38–43.
19. Newton SJ. Chemical penetration enhancers. IJPC. 2013;17:370–4.
20. Allen LV. Excipients used in nonsterile compounding, part 6: compounding with viscosity-increasing agents. IJPC. 2020;24:206–12.
21. The National Academies of Sciences, Engineering, and Medicine, et al. Compounded topical pain creams: review of select ingredients for safety, effectiveness and use. The National Academies Press. 2020; https://doi.org/10.17226/25689. Accessed 30 Jan 2022.
22. Medisca formulation support. Medisca, Canada. 2022. https://www.medisca.ca/compounding-services/dashboard. Accessed 26 Jan 2022.
23. PCCA formula search. PCCA, Canada. 2022. https://www.pccarx.com/Search/Formula. Accessed 26 Jan 2022.
24. Salzmann S, Salzmann M, Staubach P. Compounded preparations in dermatology – analysis of prescribing habits in everyday clinical practice in Germany. J Dtsch Dermatol Ges. 2020;18(4):334–40.
25. Cormier M. Bedside manner: not just for doctors anymore. IJPC. 2015;19(2):115–8.

Pharmacogenomics

3

Le Hanh Dung Do, Rebecca M. Law, and Howard I. Maibach

Contents

L. H. D. Do (✉)
Roger Williams Medical Center, Providence, RI, USA
e-mail: dolehanhdung@gmail.com

R. M. Law
School of Pharmacy and Faculty of Medicine (Discipline of Family Medicine), Memorial University of Newfoundland, St. John's, NL, Canada
e-mail: rlaw@mun.ca; rlawUCSF@gmail.com

H. I. Maibach
Department of Dermatology, University of California San Francisco (UCSF), San Francisco, CA, USA
e-mail: howard.maibach@ucsf.edu

R. M. Law, H. I. Maibach (eds.), *Handbook of Topical Drug Treatment in Dermatology*,
https://doi.org/10.1007/978-3-031-93616-6_3

Introduction

Pharmacogenomics is rapidly becoming a clinically useful and sometimes necessary consideration in the selection of appropriate pharmacotherapy. This includes the use of drug treatments in dermatology, both topical and systemic. This chapter provides a general discussion about pharmacogenomics (definition, the aims, and limitations of pharmacogenomics) and provides the currently available databases and resources on pharmacogenomics and FDA-approved pharmacogenomic tests and biomarkers of dermatologic drugs, for topical and/or systemic use. The goal is for clinicians to gain an understanding of how and when to use pharmacogenomic tests for various dermatologic conditions.

Key Concepts

- Pharmacogenomics is a science that can help to predict drug effects—both efficacious or adverse drug effects—in the human body. The predictions are based on variations in the patients' genetic makeup. These may relate to metabolic enzymes/enzymatic activity differences or HLA markers for increased risk for a particular adverse drug reaction, such as a severe cutaneous adverse reaction (SCAR). Thus, pharmacogenomics may help clinicians select the drugs and doses suited for a particular patient.
- Pharmacogenomic tests are selectively approved by the FDA, but not all are covered by insurance.
- Clinicians need to acknowledge the aim and limitations of those tests to effectively use them in clinical decision-making.

History and Definition of Pharmacogenomics

Since the 1950s, various authors have theorized that there is individual genetic susceptibility/variability in response to certain agents. Friedrich Vogel first used the terminology "pharmacogenetics" to describe drug response across patients and populations

[1]. In 1962, Pare et al. reported on the similarity in antidepressant response among first-degree relatives [2]. In 1994, O-Reily et al. also found familial tendency to respond to certain antidepressants [3]. Beyond psychiatry, Smith et al. found a binomial distribution in various subjects' responses to an antihypertensive drug and suggested that its metabolism was controlled by an autosomal gene [4]. However, the lack of true genetic data led to difficulties in proving these seemingly genetically linked hypotheses.

In April 2003, the National Human Genome Research Institute proclaimed the completion of the Human Genome Project, which enabled researchers to accelerate studies on gene-drug interactions [5]. This became the foundation on which many studies on gene-disease associations and gene-drug interactions have been built. Based on a quick search of the keyword "pharmacogenomics" on PubMed, one can see a great acceleration on this topic since 2004.

The National Institutes of Health (NIH) defined pharmacogenomics as a field that studies how a person's genes affect their response to drugs, thus helping clinicians choose appropriate drugs and doses for their patients [6]. Therefore, healthcare providers should be aware of the available pharmacogenomic databases and their interpretations.

Current Databases

Do and Maibach [7] provided a comprehensive summary of US-based available databases, where clinicians can look up drug-gene interactions. Table 3.1 was reproduced with permission from their publication, with recently expanded additional sources.

FDA's Table of Pharmacogenomic Biomarkers in Drug Labels lists FDA-approved therapeutic products with pharmacogenomic information found in the drug labeling [8]. Biomarkers in the table include germline or somatic gene variants, functional deficiencies with a genetic etiology, and gene expression differences. This guides clinicians with decisions regarding clinical response variability, genotype-specific dosing, and risk for adverse events. This list has expanded from 100 medications in 2007 [9] to more than 260 in 2018 and currently to 483 in 2021.

Table 3.1 Online resources with drug-gene associations

Online resources	Goals of site	Dosing guidelines	Lab test recommendation
FDA's table of pharmacogenomic biomarkers in drug labels	Official recommendations for clinicians practicing in the United States	Yes	Yes
CPIC	Evidence-based recommendations for clinicians	Yes	Yes
PharmGKB	Clinical implementation	Yes	Yes
eMERGE-PGX	Develop and validate electronic phenotyping algorithms for large-scale, high-throughput genomics research Assess health impact, cost effectiveness, and ethical, legal, and social implications of reporting genetic variants on a broader population scale	No	No
DGIdb	Research	No	No
UK Biobank			Yes

In 2000, the NIH founded the Pharmacogenomics Research Network (PGRN) and their products: Clinical Pharmacogenomics Implementation (CPIC), Pharmacogenomics Knowledge Base (PharmGKB), Pharmacogenomics iPSC Library & Services (PiLS), Functionalization of Variants in Clinically Actionable Pharmacogenes (F-CAP), and the Drug–Gene Interaction Database (DGIdb, www.dgidb.org), all of which aimed to amass discoveries worldwide, thus organizing and providing the hub for all clinicians and researchers.

Until 11/2021, CPIC had curated 443 peer-reviewed gene-drug clinical practice guidelines in one place, along with their lab test recommendations [10]. PharmGKB provides more comprehensive variant-drug phenotype summaries based on peer-reviewed publications, including associations that may not yet reach the requirement for an implementation guideline. Their clinical guideline annotations included 733 annotated drugs from not just CPIC but also the Royal Dutch Association for the Advancement of Pharmacy-Pharmacogenetics Working Group (DPWG), the Canadian Pharmacogenomics Network for Drug Safety (CPNDS), and other professional societies including the French National Network of Pharmacogenetics (RNPGx), the Cystic Fibrosis Foundation, and the American College of Rheumatology [11]. DGIdb organizes drug-gene interactions and potential protein-protein interactions under drug effects on an even larger scale, as it includes 30 sources and 56,309 interaction claims, which may or may not be relevant to clinical practice [12].

The eMERGE-PGx project was a US-based multicenter pilot of adopting pharmacogenetic sequencing to clinical practice. This project concluded its Phase III in 2019, with the goal to develop and validate electronic phenotyping algorithms while assessing health impact, cost-effectiveness, ethical, and legal implications of reporting genetic variants [13]. SPHINX is a searchable website of observed inherited variants among eMERGE-PGx project's 33,966 subjects [14].

UK Biobank provides one of the largest pharmacogenomic data based on around 500,000 European volunteers. In a 2021 study, McInnes et al. found that 99.5% of participants have at least one pharmacogenomic variant, leading to about 12 drugs among the 14 tested drugs that needed to be changed or alternate dosage [15]. Therefore, understanding pharmacogenetics and interpreting related tests is essential to optimizing prescribing practices.

Regulations

Similar to other genetic tests, results about patients' pharmacogenomics are protected under the Genetic Information Nondiscrimination Act (GINA), passed in 2008, to prevent employers from using genetic information to make career decisions [16]. Note that, although GINA applies to health insurance, it does not apply to life, disability, or long-term care insurance. Having this understanding may help physicians and patients make informed decisions when ordering these tests.

Table 3.2 in this chapter consolidates dermatologic drugs, their biomarkers, and indications from FDA's Table of Pharmacogenomic Biomarkers in Drug Labeling, CPIC, and PharmGKB, along with their PGx levels from PharmGKB: testing required, testing recommended, actionable PGx, and Informative PGx. Further definitions of these levels can be found on the PharmGKB website [30].

Table 3.2 FDA-approved pharmacogenomic biomarkers of dermatologic drugs, their PGx levels, and indications (updated 2022)

Biomarkers	Drugs and their PGx levels	FDA approved indications in dermatology	Off-label use in dermatology
BRAF	Binimetinib	Melanoma, with BRAF V600E, BRAF V600K, or NRAS mutation Non-small cell lung cancer with BRAF V6000E mutation	
	Cobimetinib	Histiocytic neoplasms Melanoma	
	Dabrafenib	Melanoma, with BRAF V600E or BRAF V600K mutation Non-small cell lung cancer, solid tumors, and anaplastic thyroid cancer with BRAF V6000E mutation	
	Encorafenib	Colorectal cancer, melanoma, or non-small cell lung cancer with BRAF V600E mutation Melanoma with BRAF V600K mutation	
	Nivolumab	Colorectal cancer (microsatellite instability-high or mismatch repair deficient) Eophageal cancer (adrenocarcinoma or squamous cell carcinoma) or	

(continued)

Table 3.2 (continued)

		gastroesophageal junction cancer or gastric cancer Head and neck cancer (squamous cell carcinoma) Hepatocellular carcinoma Hodgkin lymphoma (classical) Malignant pleural mesothelioma Melanoma Merkel cell carcinoma Non-small cell lung cancer Renal cell carcinoma Urothelial carcinoma	
	Trametinib	Melanoma, with BRAF V600E or BRAF V600K mutation Non-small cell lung cancer, solid tumors, and anaplastic thyroid cancer with BRAF V6000E mutation Ovarian carcinoma	
	Vemurafenib Testing required	Erdheim-Chester Disease with BRAF V600 mutation	Unresectable or metastatic melanoma with BRAF V600E mutation [31]
CYP2 C19	Drospirenone and Ethinyl Estradiol Informative PGx	Contraception	Acne vulgaris [32]; pyoderma gangrenosum [33]
CYP2 D6	Cevimeline Actionable PGx	Xerostomia in Sjögren's syndrome [34]	Limited information
	Terbinafine Informative PGx	Tinea pedis, tinea cruris, tinea corporis	Limited information

(continued)

Table 3.2 (continued)

	Pimozide Testing required	None in dermatology	Delusions of parasitosis, body dysmorphic disorder, metastatic melanoma, trichotillomania, and trigeminal and postherpetic neuralgia [35]
	Propranolol Informative PGx	None in dermatology	Infantile hemangiomas [36] Decrease recurrence and death in patients with thick cutaneous melanoma [37]
CYP2 D6, CYP2 C19	Doxepin Actionable PGx	Atopic dermatitis or lichen simplex chronicus	Urticaria [38]
DPYD	Fluorouracil Actionable PGx	Multiple actinic or solar keratoses, superficial basal cell carcinomas when conventional methods are impractical, (multiple lesions or difficult treatment sites)	Keloids and Hypertrophic Scars [39]
G6PD	Articaine and Epinephrine	Dental, gum	
	Bupivacaine	Local analgesia/anesthesia	
	Chloroquine Actionable PGx	None in dermatology	Lupus erythematosus, dermatomyositis, polymorphous light eruption, granuloma annulare [40]
	Dapsone Actionable PGx	Oral: dermatitis herpetiformis, leprosy 5% Gel: topical treatment of acne vulgaris.	Chronic inflammatory dermatoses; used as an adjunctive treatment modality [41]
	Lidocaine Actionable PGx	Local anesthetic	
	Mepivacaine	Dental anesthesia	

(continued)

Table 3.2 (continued)

		Local or regional anesthesia	
	Oxymetazoline and Tetracaine	Persistent facial erythema associated with rosacea in adults	
	Ropivacaine	Surgical anesthesia (nerve block or field block)	
HLA-B	Abacavir Testing recommended	HIV-1 treatment, used in combination with other medications as part of highly active antiretroviral therapy	Limited information
IL12A, IL12B, IL23A	Ustekinumab	Hidradenitis suppurativa Plaque psoriasis Psoriatic arthritis	
MS4A1	Rituximab Informative PGx	None in dermatology	Autoimmune bullous disorders, pemphigus foliaceus, mucous membrane pemphigoid, epidermolysis bullosa acquisita; chronic Graft-Versus-Host-Disease, dermatomyositis [42]
PML-RARA	Tretinoin (topical)	Acne vulgaris Palliation of fine wrinkles, mottled hyperpigmentation, and tactile roughness of facial skin	
TPMT	Azathioprine Testing recommended	None in dermatology	Immunosuppressant, used in severe atopic dermatitis, bullous pemphigoid, parthenium dermatitis, chronic actinic dermatitis, leprosy type 1 reactions, cutaneous vasculitis, vitiligo [43]
	Mercaptopurine Testing recommended		

(continued)

Clinical Use Examples

Biomarker screening is recommended by the Food and Drug Administration (FDA) and by Health Canada in drug selection to minimize the risk of severe cutaneous adverse reactions (SCARs) in patients being prescribed an anticonvulsant (carbamazepine or phenytoin). Some of the examples are HLA-B*15:02AQ4, HLA-A*31:01, HLA-B*15:11 for carbamazepine, and HLA-B*15:02 and CYP2C9 genotypes for phenytoin [31, 32]. The HLA-B*15:02 variant is common to both carbamazepine and phenytoin and more often found in people of Southeast Asian descent; these individuals are at higher risk of SCARs such as SJS/TEN. Allopurinol is another example where HLA biomarkers may predict a higher risk of developing a SCAR in susceptible populations.

Challenges to Test Utilization

Clinicians can use the aforementioned databases to discuss with their patients and order FDA- approved biomarkers. Factors that affect the utilization of the results may include insurance coverage, clinicians' and patients' knowledge, and the presentation of test results from laboratories [33].

Insurance Coverage

Many studies have been published on cost-effectiveness and improved health outcomes, two important criteria for insurance coverage. In 2017, Verbelen et al. provided a review of pharmacoeconomic studies of PGx-guided treatment [34]. Among the 137 available associations in the FDA table at that time, only ~18% (57% of 44 evaluations) favored PGx testing. One example is a systematic testing for HLA-B*57 when prescribing abacavir, by Ruiz-Iruela et al. in Spain [35]. The same conclusion in testing for HLA-B*1502 was found by Dong et al. in Singapore [36].

However, Rosenblat et al. found cost-effectiveness of pharmacogenomics, as well as the demonstration of improved health outcomes, is not yet supported with replicated evidence [37].

In 2016, Marshall et al. published results from an online survey on the willingness to pay out of pocket for PGx tests [38]. People with older age and higher income are associated with willingness to pay, but this association declined with more exposure to testing details and higher cost.

Clinicians and Patients' Knowledge

Clinicians need to understand the aim and limitations of these tests to effectively utilize them and discuss them with their patients. Pharmacogenomic tests are dependent on the pharmacokinetic aspects of the drug (how the human body affects a drug), which predicts drug absorption, distribution, metabolism, and elimination, hence affecting drug accumulation in the body. For example, the CYP2C9 gene, responsible for phenytoin metabolism, is highly polymorphic with over 50 known alleles. This variation is likely contributing to the pharmacogenetic variability in phenytoin metabolism. For the specific HLA markers, for example, Phenytoin Therapy and HLA-B*15:02 and CYP2C9 Genotypes with HLA-B*15:02 being strongly associated with phenytoin or carbamazepine-induced SJS/TEN as discussed above, testing for HLA-B*15:02 is recommended for all patients with ancestry in populations with increased frequency of HLA-B*15:02 (such as Southeast Asian) prior to drug use (FDA).

Secondly, pharmacogenomic tests aim for genotypes, not phenotypes. This means they will not provide information whether the tested genes are expressed in the patients. Furthermore, even if that information is known now, there is no guarantee that these genes will keep their expressions in the future.

Thirdly, even if a gene's expression is known both now and later, there are still uncertainties about its relation with other genes/genes' expressions. The human body is complex with many interactions on many levels.

Currently, in the United States, there are at least 34 laboratories that provided pharmacogenomic tests approved by the FDA [39]. A DNA sample (blood/saliva/cheek swab) is collected from the patient, and the results will be available in a few days or within 2–3 weeks.

In 2014, Brewer et al. found that women were interested in genomic testing, and many believed that extensive tamoxifen metabolizers had better breast cancer prognosis [40, 41]. This observation was consistent with previous studies by Tzeng et al. and O'Neill et al. [42, 43]. Note that these studies were conducted on female subjects; thus, they may or may not be applicable to the general population (i.e., males may rarely develop breast cancer).

Test Result Presentation

Since pharmacogenomic testing is novel and not widely used, the laboratories should provide the results in a way that accommodates the comprehension of clinicians and patients. One way is to use infographics [44]. Haga found many laboratories used a tricolor system to categorize medications as high risk, moderate risk, and normal in their results. They also used symbols, such as "X," flags, or checkmarks to inform the level of urgency/risk.

Conclusion

Since the completion of the Human Genome Project in 2003, pharmacogenomics has been extensively studied to aid drug and dosing choices. The FDA-approved biomarkers and other policies have brought pharmacologic tests to clinical settings, thus requiring clinicians and patients' knowledge to fully utilize these tools.

References

1. Pirmohamed M. Pharmacogenetics: past, present and future. Drug Discov Today. 2011;16(19–20):852–61. https://doi.org/10.1016/j.drudis.2011.08.006.
2. Pare CM, Rees L, Sainsbury MJ. Differentiation of two genetically specific types of depression by the response to anti-depressants. Lancet. 1962;2(7270):1340–3. https://doi.org/10.1016/s0140-6736(62)91019-x.
3. O'Reilly RL, Bogue L, Singh SM. Pharmacogenetic response to antidepressants in a multicase family with affective disorder. Biol Psychiatry. 1994;36(7):467–71. https://doi.org/10.1016/0006-3223(94)90642-4.
4. Mahgoub A, Idle JR, Dring LG, Lancaster R, Smith RL. Polymorphic hydroxylation of debrisoquine in man. Lancet. 1977;2(8038):584–6. https://doi.org/10.1016/s0140-6736(77)91430-1.
5. The Human Genome Project. 22 December 2020. https://www.genome.gov/human-genome-project. Accessed 31 Oct 2021.
6. Pharmacogenomics. https://www.nigms.nih.gov/education/fact-sheets/Pages/pharmacogenomics.aspx. Accessed 31 Oct 2021.
7. Do LHD, Maibach H. Pharmacogenomics/updated for precision medicine in dermatology. Journal of Dermatological Treatment, 2018;30(4):410–413. https://doi.org/10.1080/09546634.2018.1527434.
8. Table of Pharmacogenomic Biomarkers in Drug Labeling | FDA. 20 August 2021. https://www.fda.gov/drugs/science-and-research-drugs/table-pharmacogenomic-biomarkers-drug-labeling. Accessed 3 Jan 2022.
9. Drozda K, Müller DJ, Bishop JR. Pharmacogenomic testing for neuropsychiatric drugs: current status of drug labeling, guidelines for using genetic information, and test options. Pharmacotherapy. 2014;34(2):166–84. http://doi.org.ucsf.idm.oclc.org/10.1002/phar.1398
10. CPIC. https://cpicpgx.org/. Accessed 1 Jan 2022.
11. Clinical Guideline Annotations – PharmGKB. https://www.pharmgkb.org/guidelineAnnotations. Accessed 1 Jan 2022.
12. Cotto KC, Wagner AH, Feng Y-Y, et al. DGIdb 3.0: a redesign and expansion of the drug–gene interaction database. Nucleic Acids Res. 2018;46(Database issue):D1068–73. https://doi.org/10.1093/nar/gkx1143.
13. Electronic Medical Records and Genomics (eMERGE) Network. 23 February 2020, https://www.genome.gov/Funded-Programs-Projects/Electronic-Medical-Records-and-Genomics-Network-eMERGE. Accessed 3 Jan 2022.
14. SPHINX. https://www.emergesphinx.org/. Accessed 3 Jan 2022.
15. Pharmacogenetics at Scale: An Analysis of the UK Biobank – PubMed. https://pubmed.ncbi.nlm.nih.gov/33237584/. Accessed 3 Jan 2022.

16. Public Law 110–233 110th Congress An Act – Govinfo.gov. 21 May 2008, https://www.govinfo.gov/link/plaw/110/public/233. Accessed 1 Jan 2022.
17. Roos WP, Quiros S, Krumm A, et al. B-Raf inhibitor vemurafenib in combination with temozolomide and fotemustine in the killing response of malignant melanoma cells. Oncotarget. 2014;5(24):12607–20.
18. Trivedi MK, Shinkai K, Murase JE. A review of hormone-based therapies to treat adult acne vulgaris in women. Int J Women's Dermatol. 2017;3(1):44–52. https://doi.org/10.1016/j.ijwd.2017.02.018.
19. Jourabchi N, Rhee SM, Lazarus GS. Premenstrual flares of pyoderma gangrenosum controlled with use of a combined oral contraceptive and antiandrogen (ethinyl estradiol/drospirenone). Br J Dermatol. 2016;174(5):1096–7. https://doi.org/10.1111/bjd.14332.
20. Greenfield NP, Maibach H. Pharmacogenomic biomarkers in dermatologic drugs. J Dermatolog Treat. 2013;24(6):408–10. https://doi.org/10.3109/09546634.2012.697989.
21. Lorenzo CR, Koo J. Pimozide in dermatologic practice: a comprehensive review. Am J Clin Dermatol. 2004;5(5):339–49.
22. Hagen R, Ghareeb E, Jalali O, Zinn Z. Infantile hemangiomas: what have we learned from propranolol? Curr Opin Pediatr. 2018;30:499. https://doi.org/10.1097/MOP.0000000000000650.
23. De Giorgi V, Grazzini M, Benemei S, Marchionni N, Botteri E, Pennacchioli E, Geppetti P, Gandini S. Propranolol for off-label treatment of patients with melanoma: results from a cohort study. JAMA Oncol. 2018;4(2):e172908. https://doi.org/10.1001/jamaoncol.2017.2908.
24. Gupta MA, Gupta AK. Antidepressant drugs in dermatology. Skin Therapy Lett. 2001;6(8):3–5.
25. Shah VV, Aldahan AS, Mlacker S, Alsaidan M, Samarkandy S, Nouri K. 5-fluorouracil in the treatment of keloids and hypertrophic Scars: a comprehensive review of the literature. Dermatol Ther (Heidelb). 2016;6(2):169–83. https://doi.org/10.1007/s13555-016-0118-5.
26. Callen JP. Safe use of systemic agents in dermatology – Chicagoderm.
27. Wozel G, Blasum C. Dapsone in dermatology and beyond. Arch Dermatol Res. 2014;306(2):103–24. https://doi.org/10.1007/s00403-013-1409-7.
28. Gleghorn K, Wilson J, Wilkerson M. Rituximab: uses in dermatology. Skin Therapy Lett. 2016;21(5):5–7.
29. Schram ME, Borgonjen RJ, Bik CMJM, et al. Off-label use of azathioprine in dermatology: a systematic review. Arch Dermatol. 2011;147(4):474–88. https://doi.org/10.1001/archdermatol.2011.79.
30. Drug Label Information and Legend – PharmGKB. https://www.pharmgkb.org/page/drugLabelLegend. Accessed 4 Jan 2022.
31. Dean L. Carbamazepine therapy and HLA genotype. 2015 Oct 14 [Updated 2018 Aug 1]. In: Pratt VM, Scott SA, Pirmohamed M, et al.,

editors. Medical genetics summaries [Internet]. Bethesda: National Center for Biotechnology Information (US); 2012. Available from: https://www.ncbi.nlm.nih.gov/books/NBK321445/.

32. Dean L, Kane M. Phenytoin therapy and HLA-B*15:02 and CYP2C9 genotype. 2016 Sep 22 [updated 2021 Apr 7]. In: Pratt VM, Scott SA, Pirmohamed M, Esquivel B, Kattman BL, Malheiro AJ, editors. Medical genetics summaries [Internet]. Bethesda: National Center for Biotechnology Information (US); 2012. PMID: 28520374.
33. Integrating pharmacogenetic testing into primary care – NCBI. 3 November 2017, https://www.ncbi.nlm.nih.gov/pmc/articles/PMC6919655/. Accessed 3 Jan 2022.
34. Verbelen M, Weale ME, Lewis CM. Cost-effectiveness of pharmacogenetic-guided treatment: are we there yet? Pharmacogenomics J. 2017;17(5):395–402. https://doi.org/10.1038/tpj.2017.21.
35. HLA-B*57: 01 genotyping in the prevention of hypersensitivit…. https://www.x-mol.com/paperRedirect/1212907309917609986. Accessed 14 Jan 2022.
36. Dong D, Sung C, Finkelstein EA. Cost-effectiveness of HLA-B*1502 genotyping in adult patients with newly diagnosed epilepsy in Singapore. Neurology. 2012;79(12):1259–67. https://doi.org/10.1212/WNL.0b013e31826aac73.
37. Rosenblat JD, Lee Y, McIntyre RS. Does Pharmacogenomic testing improve clinical outcomes for major depressive disorder? A systematic review of clinical trials and cost-effectiveness studies. J Clin Psychiatry. 2017;78(6):720–9. https://doi.org/10.4088/JCP.15r10583.
38. Marshall DA, Gonzalez JM, Johnson FR, MacDonald KV, Pugh A, Douglas MP, Phillips KA. What are people willing to pay for whole-genome sequencing information, and who decides what they receive? Genet Med. 2016;18(12):1295–302. https://doi.org/10.1038/gim.2016.61.
39. Haga SB. Educating patients and providers through comprehensive pharmacogenetic test reports. Pharmacogenomics. 2017;18(11):1047–50. https://doi.org/10.2217/pgs-2017-0088.
40. N.T. Brewer, J.T. DeFrank, W.K. Chiu, J.G. Ibrahim, C.M. Walko, P. Rubin, O.A. Olajide, S.G. Moore, R.E. Raab, D.R. Carrizosa, S.W. Corso, G. Schwartz, J.M. Peppercorn, H.L. McLeod, L.A. Carey, W.J. Irvin Jr.; Patients' Understanding of how genotype variation affects benefits of tamoxifen therapy for breast cancer. Public Health Genomics 2014; 17 (1): 43–47. https://doi.org/10.1159/000356565.
41. Lautenbach DM, Christensen KD, Sparks JA, Green RC. Communicating genetic risk information for common disorders in the era of genomic medicine. Annu Rev Genomics Hum Genet. 2013;14:491–513. https://doi.org/10.1146/annurev-genom-092010-110722.

42. Tzeng JP, Mayer D, Richman AR, Lipkus I, Han PK, Valle CG, Carey LA, Brewer NT. Women's experiences with genomic testing for breast cancer recurrence risk. Cancer. 2010;116(8):1992–2000. https://doi.org/10.1002/cncr.24990.
43. O'Neill SC, Brewer NT, Lillie SE, Morrill EF, Dees EC, Carey LA, Rimer BK. Women's interest in gene expression analysis for breast cancer recurrence risk. J Clin Oncol. 2007;25(29):4628–34. https://doi.org/10.1200/JCO.2006.09.6255.
44. McCrorie AD, Donnelly C, McGlade KJ. Infographics: healthcare communication for the digital age. Ulster Med J. 2016;85(2):71–5.

Clinical Pharmacology of Dermatology Products in Pediatric Drug Development

4

Gilbert J. Burckart, Elimika Pfuma Fletcher, and Chinmay Shukla

Contents

Disclaimer: The opinions expressed are those of the authors and may not reflect the position of the US Food and Drug Administration.

G. J. Burckart (✉) · E. P. Fletcher · C. Shukla
Office of Clinical Pharmacology, Office of Translational Sciences, Center for Drug Evaluation and Research, US Food and Drug Administration, Silver Spring, MD, USA
e-mail: gilbert.burckart@fda.hhs.gov; elimika.fletcher@fda.hhs.gov; Chinmay.Shukla@fda.hhs.gov

R. M. Law, H. I. Maibach (eds.), *Handbook of Topical Drug Treatment in Dermatology*,
https://doi.org/10.1007/978-3-031-93616-6_4

Introduction

Pediatric dermatology is a relatively young medical specialty in spite of the fact that a significant percentage of pediatric medical and emergency room visits are related to dermatologic diseases or dermatologic manifestations of a disease. The subspecialty of pediatric dermatology was only certified as a subspecialty in 2000 [1], which was about the time that pediatric patients were just starting to be included in pediatric drug development studies. Therefore, the understanding of the specific aspects of pediatric drug development (determining the pediatric dose, proving efficacy, and assuring safety) was evolving as the specialty of pediatric dermatology was evolving. Twenty years later, the clinical pharmacology aspects of pediatric drug development have built a knowledge base for many therapeutic areas, including dermatology, that has allowed for a high success rate for pediatric therapeutic trials. The following narrative provides (a) the lessons learned from pediatric drug development studies and (b) their application to clinical pharmacology studies of therapy for pediatric dermatologic diseases in drug development.

Lessons Learned from Pediatric Drug Development Studies

Although pediatric patients were very much involved in some of the early incidents that produced federal legislation related to drug development, such as the elixir of sulfanilamide tragedy of 1937 that led to the 1938 Food Drug and Cosmetic Act, there was no requirement to include children in drug development studies through the twentieth century [2]. Therefore, children were "therapeutic orphans," and physicians had to rely on off-label use of drugs to treat pediatric patients.

Off-label drug use for pediatric patients was common practice in all therapeutic areas until recently. Approximately 80% of all drugs were not labeled for pediatric use from initial assessments in 1973 through the year 2000 [3]. Even when focusing only on new molecular entities, 71% of new molecular entities were without pediatric drug labeling by the US Food and Drug Administration in the period of 1991–1994. Without adequate drug development trials, the efficacy of off-label drug use is in question, and the poor safety record of off-label drug use has been established.

Off-label drug use is well known in dermatology practice both for pediatric patients and adults [4]. The off-label use of botulinum toxin, topical calcineurin inhibitors, and topical vitamin D analogues is particularly common. A 2002 report that surveyed dermatologic prescribing from 1990 to 1997 found that 73% of prescriptions for rosacea and 52% of prescriptions for actinic keratosis were off-label [5]. With the availability of more potent systemic therapies available for dermatologic diseases, off-label drug use carries a substantial safety risk, especially in pediatric patients.

The drug development system for pediatric patients started to change in 1997 with the Food and Drug Administration Modernization Act (FDAMA) of 1997. In this update to the Food Drug and Cosmetic Act, an additional 6 months of patent exclusivity was provided for sponsors who performed pediatric studies that were requested by the FDA under a formal Written Request. This section of FDAMA had a 5-year sunset and was renewed in 2002 under the Best Pharmaceuticals for Children Act (BPCA). At about the same time, the US Department of Health and Human Services and the US Congress worked together to create an act, which would require pediatric studies when the disease indication intended by the sponsor for adult patients also occurred in pediatric patients. This law was called the Pediatric Research Equity Act (PREA) and was passed into law in December 2003. Both BPCA and PREA were renewed in 2007 and eventually made permanent under the FDA Safety and Innovation Act of 2012. BPCA and PREA have worked together over the last two decades to study the pediatric use of almost 900 products.

A separate route of pediatric drug approval comes from the 1982 Orphan Drug Act. If a disease affects less than 200,000 patients in the United States, a drug to treat this disease can get orphan drug status, which carries with it some drug development incentives. An orphan drug is exempt from PREA studies, so this is considered a separate route for pediatric drug approval.

Multiple indicators appeared during the 1997–2007 period to demonstrate that there were serious problems in undertaking pediatric drug development. Pediatric drug development was a new science, but considerable work had been performed during the prior three decades to prepare for the pediatric drug development endeavor. The ethics of including children in drug studies had been worked out in the 1970s through the cooperation of the American Academy of Pediatrics and the National Institutes of Health with the US FDA [2]. Also, basic studies of drug pharmacokinetics and metabolism were conducted by investigators such as Dr. Sumner Yaffe and by the Pediatric Pharmacology Research Units supported by the NIH. Even so, the failure rate for these early studies (inability to label for pediatric use) was an unacceptable 42% for products already shown to be effective in adults [6].

Over the past decade, many of the problems that have plagued pediatric drug development, in terms of understanding trial design, pediatric dosing, and the application of modeling and simulation to pediatric drug development, have been worked out. The following discussion focuses on those trial design, dosing, and application of modeling in pediatrics and provides examples of pediatric dermatology drug development programs.

Pediatric and Dermatology Trial Design Elements

Trial Endpoints The choice of a primary endpoint in a pediatric drug development trial has a significant impact on the success of the trial in demonstrating efficacy. Green et al. examined 9 years of pediatric trials from 2007 to 2016 and recorded the primary endpoints of trials and their success in obtaining pediatric labeling for the use of the drug [7]. Sixty percent of the 234 trials examined utilized the same primary endpoint in both the pediatric and the adult efficacy trial. When the trial used the same endpoint in the pediatric trial as it did in the adult trial, the trial was significantly more successful in obtaining pediatric labeling.

The reason for this is most likely that adult endpoints have been validated as fit-for-purpose over multiple trials. New endpoints specific to pediatric patients are less likely to have long-term experience in drug development. Table 4.1 lists three products used in pediatric dermatology drug development that were studied with subjective, objective, and both types of endpoints [7]. All of the endpoints are clinical and did not use surrogate endpoints [8]. All three products were successful in obtaining pediatric labeling for these products.

Combined Pediatric and Adult Efficacy Trials In the early programs in pediatric drug development, a long lag time was observed between the adult approval and pediatric labeling for the drug's use. These lag times averaged more than 9 years and sometimes stretched to 15–20 years. One of the methods to decrease this lag time was to include pediatric patients in adult phase 3 trials whenever possible. The US FDA now routinely encourages this when the pediatric disease and response to therapy is expected to be or considered the same in adults and in at least some subgroup of pediatric patients. Adolescent patients are the most commonly

Table 4.1 Pediatric dermatology examples of successful trials using subjective, objective, and both endpoints

Indication	Primary endpoints	Subjective/ objective/both
Chronic idiopathic urticaria	Change from baseline to week 12 in weekly itch severity score	Subjective
Head lice	The proportion within each treatment group of index patients who are lice free (without live lice) on day 15	Objective
Tinea pedis	Complete cure at day 43, which is 2 weeks post treatment and is defined as score of 0 on all signs and symptoms and negative KOH and negative culture	Both

chosen group of pediatric patients to be included in phase 3 adult drug development trials.

Tanaudommongkon et al. examined these combined pediatric and adult trials from 2012 to 2018 [9]. They identified 72 products with 156 combined and adult trials studied under both BPCA/PREA and under the Orphan Drug Act. The majority of products and trials under BPCA/PREA combined only the adolescents (12–18 years old) with the adults, but the majority of products and trials under the Orphan Drug Act utilized the entire pediatric age group.

This review found that 23 dermatology drug products were included in this review under BPCA/PREA. Of those products, four (17%) included pediatric patients in the drug development trials. Considering the overlap between dermatology and allergy treatment guidelines [10], four biological products in the products studied under BPCA/PREA for allergy were identified and one included both adult and pediatric patients.

Under the Orphan Drug Act, the Tanaudommongkon et al. study [9] identified 25 biological orphan drug products that treated allergy. Only one of the 25 products had combined adult and pediatric drug development trials.

Placebo-Controlled Trials The choice of a control group is a critically important design consideration for a drug development trial, and a placebo-controlled trial is the gold standard for most drug development programs. Considering the ethical challenges associated with pediatric placebo-controlled trials, the design of such a trial is an important consideration [11].

In the discussion of the ethical considerations with pediatric placebo-controlled trials in drug development, Momper et al. [11] identified 96 placebo-controlled trials in pediatric patients for 67 unique products. The report listed three pediatric dermatology products with placebo-controlled trials in pediatric patients: adapalene and benzoyl alcohol for acne in patients aged 9–11 years, etanercept for chronic severe plaque psoriasis in 4–17 years of age, and ustekinumab for moderate to severe plaque psoriasis in pediatric patients aged 12 years and older. None of these products used the agent as an add-on medication, and no use of rescue medication was designed into the protocols.

The placebo response rate between pediatric patients and adults is always an important consideration in study design. If the pediatric placebo response rate is much greater in pediatric patients than in adults, it may be difficult to identify a significant therapeutic effect of the drug. For drugs with pediatric placebo-controlled trials having an identical study design and endpoint, etanercept in plaque psoriasis serves as an example with a pediatric placebo response rate of 11.4% (12/105 patients) in comparison to the adult response rate of 4% (6/168 patients). For products with an identical study design but different pediatric and adult endpoints, ustekinumab serves as an example and has almost identical physician's global assessment (PGA) score: 5.4% in pediatric patients and 4–5% in adult patients. When separate pediatric placebo-controlled trials for adapalene and benzoyl alcohol for acne were developed with the same endpoint as adult trials, the results for the placebo response rate were quite different. For example, for the changes in non-inflammatory counts from baseline to week 12, the pediatric placebo response rate was 2.3%, whereas the adult placebo response rate was 23–27%.

So while identical study designs and endpoints should produce similar placebo response rates in adults and pediatric patients, the placebo response rate in prior dermatologic trials has been unpredictable. This fact reinforces the need for a pediatric study control group whenever possible to have reliable study results and to make decisions about product efficacy.

Enrichment of the Patient Study Population Enrichment of the study population to assure that it represents the patient population of interest and represents the patient population most likely to respond to the drug is another important aspect of drug development trial design. The strategies are typically broken into three categories including practical, prognostic, and predictive enrichment strategies. An extensive guidance document from the US FDA is available to read more about these approaches to enriching the patient population [12]. Pharmacogenomic information in FDA labels is also part of enrichment criteria, do pertain to pediatric products, and include dermatologic products [13].

Green et al. investigated the enrichment strategies in pediatric drug development by examining 112 efficacy studies conducted from 2012 to 2016 [14]. Overall, if the trial utilized all three enrichment strategies in trial design, the success rate for pediatric labeling was 87.5%, whereas programs that used no enrichment strategies had a 65.4% rate of success for pediatric labeling. Therefore, proper enrichment strategies are considered crucial for developing pediatric efficacy trials that will successfully lead to pediatric labeling for use.

Included in this analysis [14] were four pediatric dermatologic trials for three products. All three of these products were successfully labeled for pediatric use. However, the use of enrichment criteria in these studies was quite narrow, with only two prognostic strategies used in these trials.

Exposure-Response and Modeling and Simulation An exposure-response (E-R) analysis is not always conducted during drug development but can be a powerful tool for dose-finding and in comparing the adult and the pediatric responsiveness to a drug in a given disease state. When using another tool that facilitates pediatric drug development, or efficacy extrapolation from adults to pediatric patients, an E-R analysis can help to assure that the response to the drug or biological agent is similar between adults and pediatric patients.

Zhang et al. examined 313 pediatric drug development programs from 2007 to 2018 and found that 84 programs contained an E-R analysis [15]. In 48 of those programs, the E-R analysis was determined to support decision-making related to dosing, extrapolation and trial design, or assessment of a new formulation or dosing regimen. In the two dermatology examples provided in the E-R assessments, both programs used E-R analysis to perform dose selection. The two examples were omalizumab in chronic idiopathic urticaria and terbinafine in tinea capitis. Infliximab is approved to treat plaque psoriasis in adults, and a standard dose results in enough of a wide range of concentrations to perform an E-R analysis [16].

The relationship between plasma concentrations and effect in dermatology may be different from many other therapeutic areas. While the examples provided above do represent situations in which the plasma concentration of systemic therapy may be related to the response in pediatric dermatology, plasma concentrations after the topical application of a drug are generally used in the safety analysis. The goal of topical drug therapy is often to minimize systemic absorption, and consequently low concentrations of drug would be expected systemically. However, the use of refined techniques such as microdialysis have been used to characterize the transfer process between plasma and skin and may be useful in preclinical and clinical studies during drug development [17].

Biological products make up an increasing part of the pharmacologic armamentarium for severe pediatric dermatologic diseases. Monoclonal antibodies and Fc-fusion proteins have a very different pharmacokinetic profile than do small molecule drugs, but it is still possible to perform an E-R analysis. Liu et al. found that 12 of 20 pediatric drug development programs used E-R analysis as part of their development programs [12].

Modeling and simulation (M&S) play an increasing part in pediatric drug development programs. The use of M&S allows for the optimal use of all data available, thereby decreasing the number of pediatric patients who have to be enrolled in a clinical study. This is not only an ethical imperative but also allows the extension of indications in FDA labeling for pediatric age groups who may not have been studied but are expected to have the same response as other pediatric populations.

Bi et al. have reviewed the applications of M&S to pediatric drug development and reviewed the use of M&S in approvals of 105 pediatric indications from 2017 to 2019 [18]. They found that 9.5% of programs used topical therapy, but did not use M&S. This study points to one of the critical problems in pediatric dermatology and drug development, which is the alternate way that plasma drug concentrations are used to make adequate predictions. As mentioned above, more intensive preclinical and clinical studies of drug transfer between skin and plasma [17] may assist in this process.

Summary

Drug development studies in pediatric patients have evolved in about the same time frame as the medical specialty of pediatric dermatology. Over this 20-year period, drug development studies of pediatric dermatology products have been complicated by a number of factors. While the efficacy trial design has a number of elements that have to be carefully planned, such as endpoints and enrichment of the study population, drug dosing and drug safety are the most critical factors to be addressed in pediatric dermatology drug development studies. The maximal use study is a critical part of the pediatric safety assessment. The observed higher systemic exposure observed in pediatric patients after topical application and its implications on safety have to be carefully considered at the time of drug approval, and products must be appropriately labeled with the available systemic exposure data to inform the prescribing clinicians. The use of more potent systemic therapies for pediatric dermatologic diseases suggests that other techniques such as exposure-response analyses may be necessary going forward. Studies of HPA axis suppression are necessary when appropriate and should be refined to provide more interpretable safety information. Studies of pediatric growth remain an essential part of the evaluation of corticosteroid products. Overall, the clinical pharmacology of drug development studies in pediatrics and pediatric dermatology have advanced considerably over the past 20 years, and this knowledge must be applied to future drug development studies in pediatric dermatology.

References

1. Prindaville B, Antaya RJ, Siegfried EC. Pediatric dermatology: past, present, and future. Pediatr Dermatol. 2015;32:1–12.
2. Burckart GJ, Kim C. The revolution in pediatric drug development and drug use: therapeutic orphans no more. J Pediatr Pharmacol Ther. 2020;25:565–73.
3. Wilson JT. An update on the therapeutic orphan. Pediatrics. 1999;104:585–90.

4. Franca K, Litewka S. Controversies in off-label prescriptions in dermatology: the perspective of the patient, the physician, and the pharmaceutical companies. Int J Dermatol. 2019;58:788–94.
5. Sugarman JH, Fleischer AB Jr, Feldman SR. Off-label prescribing in the treatment of dermatologic disease. J Am Acad Dermatol. 2002;47:217–23.
6. Wharton GT, Murphy MD, Avant D, et al. Impact of pediatric exclusivity on drug labeling and demonstrations of efficacy. Pediatrics. 2014;134:e512–8.
7. Green DJ, Burnham JM, Schuette P, et al. Primary endpoints in pediatric efficacy trials submitted to the US FDA. J Clin Pharmacol. 2018;58:885–90.
8. Green DJ, Sun H, Burnham J, et al. Surrogate endpoints in pediatric studies submitted to the US FDA. Clin Pharmacol Ther. 2019;105:555–7.
9. Tanaudommongkon I, John Miyagi S, Green DJ, et al. Combined Pediatric and Adult Trials Submitted to the US Food and Drug Administration 2012–2018. Clin Pharmacol Ther. 2020;108:1018–25.
10. Mohan GC, Lio PA. Comparison of dermatology and allergy guidelines for atopic dermatitis management. JAMA Dermatol. 2015;151:1009–13.
11. Momper JD, Green DJ, Park K, Burckart GJ, Snyder DL. Ethical considerations for pediatric placebo-controlled trials: FDA outcomes and perspectives. Ther Innov Regul Sci. 2021;55:282–303.
12. Liu XI, Dallmann A, Wang YM, et al. Monoclonal antibodies and fc-fusion proteins for pediatric use: dosing, immunogenicity, and modeling and simulation in data submitted to the US Food and Drug Administration. J Clin Pharmacol. 2019;59:1130–43.
13. Green DJ, Mummaneni P, Kim IW, Oh JM, Pacanowski M, Burckart GJ. Pharmacogenomic information in FDA-approved drug labels: application to pediatric patients. Clin Pharmacol Ther. 2016;99:622–32.
14. Green DJ, Liu XI, Hua T, et al. Enrichment strategies in pediatric drug development: an analysis of trials submitted to the US Food and Drug Administration. Clin Pharmacol Ther. 2018;104:983–8.
15. Zhang Y, Wang Y, Khurana M, et al. Exposure-response assessment in pediatric drug development studies submitted to the US Food and Drug Administration. Clin Pharmacol Ther. 2020;108:90–8.
16. Zhang Q, Travis J, Rothwell R, et al. Applying the noninferiority paradigm to assess exposure-response similarity and dose between pediatric and adult patients. J Clin Pharmacol. 2021;61(Suppl 1):S165–74.
17. Shukla C, Patel V, Juluru R, Stagni G. Quantification and prediction of skin pharmacokinetics of amoxicillin and cefuroxime. Biopharm Drug Dispos. 2009;30:281–93.
18. Bi Y, Liu J, Li L, et al. Role of model-informed drug development in pediatric drug development, regulatory evaluation, and labeling. J Clin Pharmacol. 2019;59(Suppl 1):S104–11.

Clinical Pharmacology of Topical Therapy in Pediatrics

5

Chinmay Shukla, Aaron Park, Elimika Pfuma Fletcher, and Gilbert J. Burckart

Contents

Disclaimer: The opinions expressed are those of the authors and may not reflect the position of the US Food and Drug Administration.

C. Shukla · E. P. Fletcher · G. J. Burckart (✉)
Office of Clinical Pharmacology, Office of Translational Sciences, Center for Drug Evaluation and Research, US Food and Drug Administration, Silver Spring, MD, USA
e-mail: Chinmay.Shukla@fda.hhs.gov; elimika.fletcher@fda.hhs.gov; gilbert.burckart@fda.hhs.gov

A. Park
Acelyrin Inc., McLean, Virginia, USA

R. M. Law, H. I. Maibach (eds.), *Handbook of Topical Drug Treatment in Dermatology*,
https://doi.org/10.1007/978-3-031-93616-6_5

Introduction

The previous introductory chapter introduced the current scenario of pediatric drug development for dermatological products. This chapter will look into the need for pharmacokinetic (PK) assessment in pediatric subjects and will delve into the details of the clinical pharmacology study design of topical products in pediatric subjects. In particular, this chapter focuses on the several design elements that create the building blocks of the maximal usage trial (MUsT), and some of these individual components are supported by examples to enhance the understanding of these concepts. The MUsT study is the primary clinical pharmacology study for topical dermatological products.

Pediatric Dosing and Ontogeny Developmental, anatomical, and physiological differences in pediatric patients and adults or across pediatric ages increase the complexity of dose selection for pediatric patients. Many drugs are initially developed in adults, and data from adults is used to inform dosing for pediatric studies. The most common strategy for selecting initial doses to be studied in pediatric patients reported by Green et al. [1], for drugs submitted for pediatric indications between 2012 and 2020 was previous experience with the product, followed by allometric scaling (19%) and exposure matching with adults (15%). The most common pivotal support for doses approved for pediatric patients was based on titration to target response (33%), pharmacokinetic (PK) or pharmacodynamic data (30%), and exposure matching (20%). The use of PK or exposure matching approaches are not applicable for topical dermatology products for which the exposure at the site of action is more relevant and systemic exposure may be minimal or not directly related to efficacy.

Ontogeny in the skin (larger surface to body volume, skin differences in water loss, and thinner stratum corium) can result in differences in systemic absorption of a topical product in pediatrics compared to adults or among pediatrics of varying ages and sizes [2]. For any systemic absorption that occurs, ontogeny in drug metabolism, transport, and excretion (e.g., renal function) may result in differences in elimination of the drug product in pediatrics. In addition to potential differences in the systemic exposure (PK), the susceptibility to adverse events resulting from systemic absorption may differ in pediatric patients.

Pediatric Dosing of Topical products in Dermatology Vinueza et al. reported that for locally acting drugs with pediatric indications approved since 2002 (about a third were dermatological products), 75% were labeled at the same dose as adults [3]. Topical dermatological product dosing is usually the same as adult dosing in terms of the specific number of times the drug is recommended to apply (e.g., apply to affected area twice a day). However, the dosing for most topical dermatology products is not precise (does not specify a mg, ml, or specific amount or thickness). A few drugs attempt to add some specificity to their recommendations (e.g. use thin layer, use pea-sized amount, do not exceed a percentage of total body surface area, and do not exceed a certain amount in a week), but the clinical application of such instructions may not be precise or interpreted in a consistent manner. Even if in most cases the instructions for use (dosing) are the same for pediatric and adult dosing, the amount of drug an individual applies may differ based on the skin surface area affected and other factors.

Considering the lack of precision in the dosing for most topical products and the ontogeny in skin and PK, a labeled dose and instructions for use that is similar to adults can result in differences in overall exposure on the skin and systemically. In addition, some indications may involve a greater portion of the body (more affected area) compared to adults (e.g., eczema). For these reasons, pediatric assessments related to PK, safety, and in some cases efficacy are needed in drug development [4].

A drug development program in pediatric dermatology may rely on the efficacy results from the sponsor's trials but may also require additional PK and/or safety studies in pediatrics both for local adverse events and systemic absorption and effects. In some situations, pharmacodynamic and efficacy studies in pediatrics are performed. The PK component of a pediatric topical drug development program is generally performed in a Maximal

Usage Trial (MUsT) to assess potential for systemic exposure, as detailed in the next section. In general, when topical product has more than one indication, the MUsT study may be performed in the indication/population for which highest potential for dermal absorption is expected. For example, PK assessment under maximal use conditions for the indication of eczema may support the localized indication of hand eczema without a separate PK assessment. However, if PK labeling of specific products related to the indication is desired due to a lower anticipated lower systemic exposure, a separate PK study under maximal use conditions would be desired. If there is a plan to extrapolate systemic exposure between different diseases, then that extrapolation plan should be discussed and agreed upon with the FDA. Differences in the formulation can impact the absorption of a drug and is an important consideration in choosing the formulation to study or the need for additional MUsT studies [4]. Pivotal MUsT studies are recommended to be conducted with the to-be-marketed formulation.

In addition to ontogeny that can result in differences in the PK, safety, and efficacy of a topical product in pediatrics compared to adults, some particular circumstances can be of greater concern or interest in pediatric assessments. Characteristics of the disease such as the extent the skin barrier is damaged can increase the chances of systemic exposure. Another consideration is whether a drug is dosed chronically versus acutely or as needed (topical antibiotic for minor scrapes). The risk of drug accumulation with more chronic treatment is a concern, and safety evaluations during drug development may be useful. Concerns related to chronic use highlight the utility of well-designed maximal use trials to inform the risk. The risk of systemic absorption as well is of particular interest including for agents such as corticosteroids for which additional safety assessments such as HPA axis effect are performed to assess the risk of any systemic exposure.

Dosing considerations of topical dermatologic products in pediatrics are important in drug development to ensure efficacy and safety. Dosing of these products also has clinical implications beyond safety and efficacy. The dosing informs the quantity needed to be prescribed to a patient. As mentioned, the amount of drug applied can differ, and quantifying specific amounts that may be needed by a patient can be challenging especially for chronic use. Nelson et al. and others have proposed rules or BSA estimates to estimate quantities needed for topical agents such as methods based on BSA in an individual or average BSA by age and gender [5]. Some have argued that quantities prescribed could affect the amount a person decides to apply (over or under dosing) based on the perception of available drug for application in a time period.

Pediatric Maximal Use Trial

The purpose of MUsT is to assess the systemic exposure of a topical product applied under maximal usage conditions with the aim of informing the systemic safety of such products. While the concepts and the purpose of MUsT do not change, the nature of disease manifestation will dictate the design of pediatric maximal usage trials, and this could make pediatric study design different from adult study design in certain instances. For example, atopic dermatitis is more common in pediatric patients compared to adults; hence, the minimum body surface area (BSA) that a drug is applied to in MUsT is larger in pediatric subjects compared to adults. Conversely, some diseases like psoriasis and onychomycosis usually manifest the opposite way with lower BSA involvement in pediatric subjects compared to adults. Hence, MUsT design of pediatric subjects in such diseases needs lesser % BSA involvement compared to adults. Such factors are considered to inform the design of a pediatric MUsT, and FDA encourages sponsors to discuss the MUsT study design with them prior to initiating the study. In diseases that are uncommon in pediatric subjects, such as, actinic keratosis, pediatric MUsT assessment is generally not needed.

In general, MUsT study design involves assessment of the systemic exposure at steady state following the application of the to-be-marketed formulation. The goal is to maximize drug absorption with the goal of capturing the worst-case scenario by designing the study to incorporate elements such as upper range of disease severity, % BSA in the upper range, frequency, and duration of dosing that would be recommended in the approved labeling, amount of dose applied within the upper range, and the use of highest proposed strength if multiple strengths of the product are going to be marketed [6]. The PK information from adult subjects could be used to inform the sampling scheme in pediatric subjects, and generally sparse PK assessment especially in younger pediatric subjects would be acceptable in lieu of serial PK sampling. If waiver of PK assessment in pediatric subjects is desired, then a formal request should be submitted to the FDA for review and concurrence.

Pediatric MUsT study could be conducted as a separate study or can be assessed in a subgroup of subjects within the Phase 3 trials. If a separate study is conducted, then the study's therapy should generally be continued despite the PK assessment completion in pediatric subjects. The goal of PK assessment only for a topical product is not generally considered a reasonable ethical approach for pediatric patients due to the lack of any potential clinical benefit for the enrolled pediatric subjects.

It is critical to assess PK of the topical product under maximal usage conditions in pediatric subjects within the upper range of disease severity. Exposing healthy pediatric subjects is not justifiable ethically and scientifically as disease skin is expected to have different drug permeation potential compared to healthy skin. In an example to illustrate the difference in the systemic exposure between healthy and disease skin, the systemic exposure of luliconazole cream is shown in Fig. 5.1 [7]. As illustrated in Fig. 5.1, the systemic exposure of luliconazole in subjects with tinea cruris is approximately more than fourfold higher compared to that observed following application to the healthy skin. It should be noted that the systemic exposure in healthy subjects was lower in spite of applying to larger body surface area and using approximately more than threefold higher dose than the dose used in patients with tinea cruris. This example illustrates the importance of assessing the systemic exposure in subjects with disease in the MUsT instead of healthy subjects in both adult and pediatric subjects as drug permeation properties of diseased skin could be different from healthy skin.

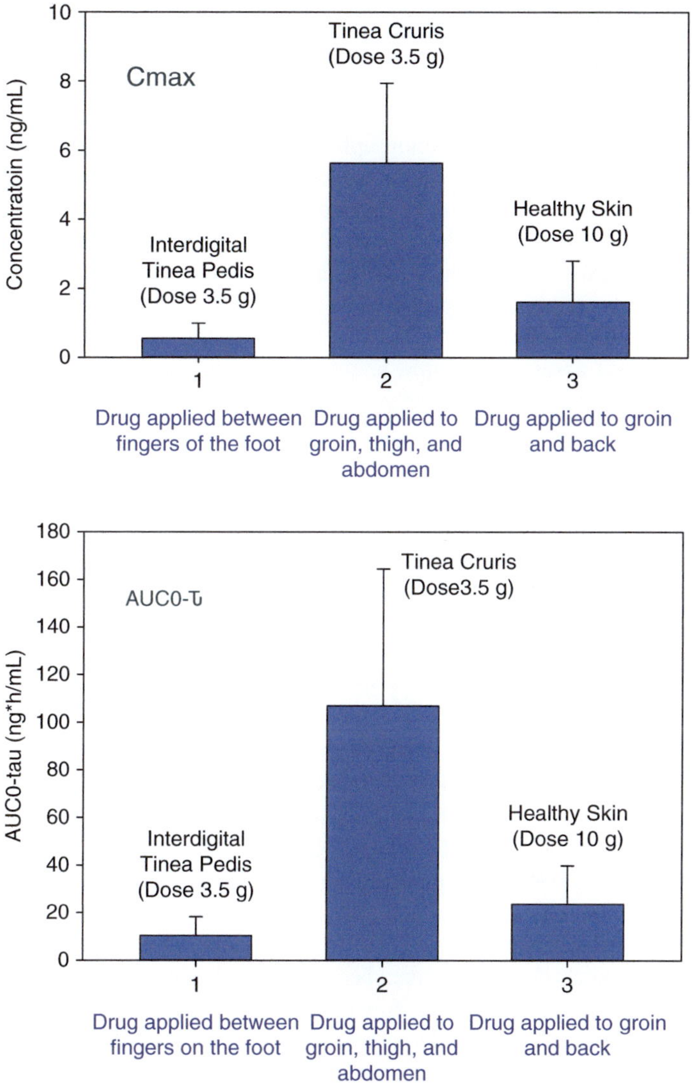

Fig. 5.1 Systemic exposure of luliconazole cream, 1% in healthy adult subjects and in adult patients with tinea cruris and tinea pedis [7]

Sunscreen

Sunscreens are marketed in a wide variety of formulations, and the active moieties for sunscreens are usually regulated under the monograph pathway. Monograph approval is for the active moiety, which when used under the conditions specified under the monograph could be marketed in a variety of formulations without the need for FDA approval of an individual formulation. In contrast, the NDA pathway is for a specific formulation, and the sponsor would need separate FDA approval to market each of the different formulations.

MUsT assessment is now an integral part of generally regarded as safe and effective (GRASE) determination under a monograph. For sunscreen products, initial MUsT assessment is recommended to be conducted in adults only by applying the product to at least 75% BSA [4]. The need for pediatric assessment should be considered only if substantial systemic exposure is observed in adult subjects, and this determination should be made in collaboration with FDA.

Pediatric Dermatology Safety Assessment: Corticosteroids

For several dermatological diseases like atopic dermatitis, psoriasis, and acne vulgaris, topical corticosteroids usually are the first line of therapy, unless the disease severity calls for systemic intervention. Hypothalamic pituitary adrenal (HPA) axis suppression is one of the serious adverse effects of corticosteroids. It becomes critical to monitor and assess HPA axis function especially in pediatric subjects during treatment because, in addition to other adverse effects, it impacts growth. Since HPA axis suppression is a systemic adverse effect, when assessed under maximal usage conditions, it has been used as a surrogate for systemic exposure in the times when bioanalytical technology had its limitations toward quantification due to lack of sensitivity. Today, with advancing bioanalytical capabilities, it is now increasingly possible to quantify systemic concentrations of topically applied corticosteroids.

The US FDA has been inconsistent in providing guidance related to conducting HPA axis suppression studies in adults and in pediatric patients. Burnham et al. have documented the HPA axis studies submitted to the FDA from 2002 to 2018 [8]. At one point, seven separate FDA Guidances for Industry were active, but several guidances have now been withdrawn. The active guidance related to pediatric patients is titled "Guidance for Industry: Orally Inhaled and Intranasal Corticosteroids: Evaluation of the Effects on Growth in Children" and is dated March 2007 [9]. Burnham et al. [8] found that of 83 corticosteroid product studies conducted in pediatric patients, 37 conducted HPA axis suppression studies, and 46 did not. Five different methods were used to assess HPA axis suppression in corticosteroid safety studies. The primary approach used in dermatology drug development studies has been ACTH stimulation tests.

There are several examples of topical corticosteroids where higher HPA axis suppression rates were observed in pediatric subjects compared to adults, and also, an increase in the incidence of the rate of HPA axis suppression has been observed with a decrease in age. Although it is a huge challenge to tease out which intrinsic or extrinsic factor (e.g., ontogenetic difference, dose, disease severity, and % BSA exposed) actually contributed to an increase in the incidence of HPA axis suppression, the available data suggests that HPA axis suppression should ideally be assessed in pediatric subjects to inform the safety of the topical corticosteroid product.

Diprolene AF Cream (betamethasone), 0.05%, is approved for the treatment of corticosteroid-responsive dermatoses in subjects 13 years of age and older, and the rate of HPA axis suppression is shown in Table 5.1. The data suggests an increase in the HPA axis suppression rate with decrease in age. Although the goal of this

Table 5.1 Rate of HPA axis suppression for Diprolene AF (betamethasone) cream [15, 16]

Age group	3 months to 1 year	2–5 years	6–8 years	9–12 years
% subjects with HPA axis suppression	50	38	32	17

chapter is to not provide an exhaustive list of products showing differences in the rate of HPA axis suppression in adults and pediatric subjects, another example is Clobex (clobetasol) lotion, which showed a 64% HPA axis suppression rate in adolescent subjects 12–17 years old with atopic dermatitis following 2 weeks of drug application compared to a rate of 56% in adults. Due to unfavorable benefit-risk, topical corticosteroids with a high incidence of HPA axis suppression are usually not approved for use in the pediatric population, or they could be approved only in older pediatric subjects (i.e., adolescent) and not younger ones [10].

Sometimes, pediatric studies of topical corticosteroids are conducted in a stepwise manner starting from adolescent subjects and then going down in age sequentially. The rate of HPA axis suppression determined in the older pediatric cohort would inform the progression of the study in the next lower age cohort. The study progression would be stopped if the rate of HPA axis suppression is high in the older pediatric cohort with the aim of lowering the risk to the younger age study participants.

One example that supports this strategy is Topicort (desoximetasone) Spray where the HPA axis suppression potential was assessed via cosyntropin stimulation testing at baseline and following 4 weeks of twice daily dosing in an open-label, sequential cohort, safety trial in 100 subjects 2–17 years of age with moderate to severe plaque psoriasis with at least 10% of their body surface area involved. The results indicated that, overall, 36% of pediatric subjects 2–17 years of age demonstrated HPA axis suppression defined as a serum cortisol level ≤ 18 mcg/dL 30-min post cosyntropin stimulation. The proportion of subjects demonstrating HPA axis suppression was 35% in Cohort 1 (12–17 years of age) and 43% in Cohort 2 (6 years to less than 12 years of age). Due to the high incidence of HPA axis suppression observed in subjects 6–17 years of age, trial enrollment in the youngest cohort (2–5 years of age) was discontinued early [11].

There are several topical retinoid and retinoid like products (e.g., TAZORAC (tazarotene) gel and cream, AVAGE (tazarotene) cream, and ARAZLO (tazarotene) lotion) approved for the treatment of several dermatological diseases like acne vulgaris, plaque psoriasis, and hyper- and hypopigmentation. Products of this class carry the risk of teratogenicity and the PK assessment in adult and pediatric subjects under maximal usage conditions are used to assess safety margins based on animal toxicity data. A MUsT study in 24 subjects (18 adolescent +6 adult) 12 years of age and older was a pivotal study to support the prescription (Rx) to over-the-counter (OTC) switch of Differin (adapalene) Gel, 0.1% for the treatment of acne vulgaris. The systemic exposure observed in the MUsT was used to assess the safety margin based on animal toxicity data and the wide margin of safety (at least 70-fold) supported the Rx to OTC switch of Differin Gel, 0.1% making the first retinoid like product to be available OTC [12].

To enhance the favorability of benefit-risk, the systemic exposure information in both adult and pediatric subjects could be used to inform the % BSA and dosing limitation in the drug product labeling. Ruxolitinib cream is the first topical JAK inhibitor class of product to be approved for the treatment of mild to moderate atopic dermatitis [13]. Based on the systemic exposure from MUsT in both adults and adolescent subjects, the approved labeling has a % BSA limitation of up to 20% and dosing limitation to not use more than 60 g per week. With additional data in younger pediatric subjects, the % BSA and dosing limitation would need to be revisited to ensure a favorable benefit-risk in the younger pediatric population.

Another example is abametapir lotion, a pediculicide product approved for the treatment of head lice infestation [14]. This product showed that the systemic exposure in subjects less than 1 year of age was approximately between three- to fourfold higher compared to the systemic exposure in subjects 3–17 years of age following application of the product to the entire scalp and hair and rinsing it off after 10 min (Table 5.2). This example suggests that ontogenetic differences, especially surface area-to-volume ratio, could be the reason for the increased systemic exposure in younger pediatric subjects. This suggests that obtaining PK under maximal usage conditions in pediatric subjects of all age ranges would be essential to inform systemic safety and labeling of the product, and extrapolating from older age cohorts would be very challenging.

Table 5.2 Abametapir PK parameters in pediatric subjects with headlice infestation from trials B and C [14]

Study	Age group	*n*	C_{max} (ng/mL) mean (%CV)	$AUC_{0\text{-}8h}$ (ng*h/mL) mean (%CV)
B	6 months to <1 year	1	418	1057
C		5	228 (50%)	688 (43%)
B	1 year to <2 years	3	209 (62%)	446 (65%)
C		8	147 (49%)	406 (37%)
B	2 years to <3 years	6	206 (66%)	633 (57%)
C		8	160 (48%)	602 (51%)
B	3 years to 17 years	12	121 (60%)	330 (49%)
C		7	52 (45%)	194 (39%)

The few examples presented here suggest that assessment of PK in pediatric subjects would be needed not only for assessment of systemic safety but also to inform labeling to ensure safety of the patients. Although some of the products approved in pediatric subjects have shown higher systemic exposure than adults, one should not interpret this as the approved product being unsafe in the pediatric population compared to adults. The observed higher systemic exposure and its implications on safety were carefully considered at the time of drug approval and products are appropriately labeled with the available systemic exposure data to inform the prescribing physician.

Educating the Caregiver

For topical dermatological products, the target site is the skin, and the drug is administered directly at the target site. Systemic absorption, though not desired, does occur, and this leads to the need to address the systemic safety of these products. Pediatric subjects should not be considered as miniature adults as in several cases, we have observed higher systemic exposure in pediatric patients compared to adults following topical application of dermatological products.

Educating the caregiver to the correct use of the product as well as making sure they comprehend the label to understand the limitation of use in terms of % BSA, dosing, approved indications, approved age range, etc. is critical, especially in case of younger pediatric patients who are not old enough to self-administer the medication correctly.

Summary

The need for clinical pharmacology studies for topical dermatologic agents in pediatric subjects has been met with some criticism. However, several examples discussed in this chapter do suggest that there is significant value in pediatric MUsT studies related to support for drug approval, safety, and dosing instructions in terms of limitations of % BSA and amount applied. The pediatric population is vulnerable to multiple adverse effects, and the risks of extrapolation of safety and/or efficacy from the adult population are well known. Product labeling claims for the pediatric use of topical dermatologic products that are supported by data inform the safe use of the product and do guide health-care providers toward not only prescribing the optimal treatment but also educate the caregiver. Hence, conducting adequately designed MUsT studies in pediatric patients pre-approval does support the safe use of the topical dermatological products, and the FDA encourages sponsors to discuss the MUsT study design prior to initiating this study. The ultimate mission of the FDA is to protect and promote the health and well-being of the American people, and this goal in pediatric dermatology can be achieved through the performance of controlled clinical trials especially in the pediatric patient population.

References

1. Green FG, Park K, Burckart GJ. Methods used for pediatric dose selection in drug development programs submitted to the US FDA 2012–2020. J Clin Pharmacol. 2021;61(Suppl 1):S28–35.
2. Nikolovski J, Stamatas GN, Kollias N, Wiegand BC. Barrier function and water-holding and transport properties of infant Stratum Corneum are different from adult and continue to develop through the first year of life. J Invest Dermatol. 2008;128:1728–36.

3. Vinueza G, Ramamoorthy A, Burckart GJ, Madabushi R, Zineh I, Pfuma Fletcher E. Deriving pediatric doses for locally-acting drugs: a US Food & Drug Administration evaluation. In: American Association of Colleges of Pharmacy Annual Meeting; 2021.
4. US Food and Drug Administration: Guidance for Industry: Maximal Usage Trials for Topically Applied Active Ingredients Being Considered for Inclusion in an Over-The – Counter Monograph: Study Elements and Considerations. 2019. Access at: https://www.fda.gov/media/125080/download. Accessed 26 Nov 2021.
5. Nelson AA, Miller AD, Fleischer AB, Balkrishnan R, Feldman SR. How much of a topical agent should be prescribed for children of different sizes? J Dermatolog Treat. 2006;17:224–8.
6. Bashaw ED, Tran DC, Shukla CG, Liu X. Maximal usage trial: an overview of the Design of Systemic Bioavailability Trial for topical dermatological products. Ther Innov Regul Sci. 2015;49:108–15.
7. US Food and Drug Administration: Clinical Pharmacology Review: Luliconazole cream 1%. 2012. Access at: https://www.accessdata.fda.gov/drugsatfda_docs/nda/2013/204153Orig1s000ClinPharmR.pdf Accessed 26 Nov 2021.
8. Burnham JM, Green DJ, Ray A, et al. Hypothalamic-pituitary-adrenal Axis pediatric safety studies submitted to the FDA. Ther Innov Regul Sci. 2021;55:622–30.
9. US Food and Drug Administration: Guidance for Industry: Orally Inhaled and Intranasal Corticosteroids: Evaluation of the Effects on Growth in Children. 2007. Access at: https://www.fda.gov/media/71624/download. Accessed 27 Nov 2021.
10. US Food and Drug Administration: CLOBEX (clobetasol propionate) Lotion. 2012. Access at: https://www.accessdata.fda.gov/drugsatfda_docs/label/2012/021535Orig1s003,%20021644Orig1s003lbl.pdf. Accessed 27 Nov 2021.
11. US Food and Drug Administration: TOPICORT (desoximetasone) topical spray. 2021. Access at: https://www.accessdata.fda.gov/drugsatfda_docs/label/2021/204141s009lbl.pdf. Accessed 27 Nov 2021.
12. US Food and Drug Administration: Nonprescription Drugs Advisory Committee Meeting, April 15, 2016: Consideration of adapalene gel 0.1% for over-the-counter use for the treatment of acne in consumers 12 years and older. 2016. Access at: https://www.fda.gov/media/96934/download. Accessed 27 Nov 2021.
13. US Food and Drug Admnistration: OPZELURA (ruxolitinib phosphate). 2021. Access at: https://www.accessdata.fda.gov/scripts/cder/daf/index.cfm?event=overview.process&ApplNo=215309. Accessed 27 Nov 2021.
14. US Food and Drug Administration: XEGLYZE (abametapir). 2020. Access at: https://www.accessdata.fda.gov/drugsatfda_docs/label/2020/206966lbl.pdf. Accessed 27 Nov 2021.

15. US Food and Dug Aministration: DIPROLENE AF (augmented betamthasone diproprionate) cream. 2019. Access at: https://www.accessdata.fda.gov/drugsatfda_docs/label/2019/019555s035lbl.pdf. Accessed 27 Nov 2021.
16. US Food and Drug Administration: Joint Meeting of the Dermatologic and Ophthalmic Drugs Advisory Committee and the Nonprescription Drugs Advisory Committee; Notice of Meeting: Adapted from presentation by Denise Cook, MD. 2005. Access at: https://www.federalregister.gov/documents/2005/02/17/05-3055/joint-meeting-of-the-dermatologic-and-ophthalmic-drugs-advisory-committee-and-the-nonprescription. Accessed 27 Nov 2021.

Topical Drug Use in the Elderly

6

Rebecca M. Law and Meghan T. Greene

Contents

Factors Relating to Topical Drug Absorption in the Elderly

1. Skin

   Skin changes due to aging can significantly affect topical absorption of drugs and chemicals.

R. M. Law (✉)
School of Pharmacy and Faculty of Medicine (Discipline of Family Medicine), Memorial University of Newfoundland, St. John's, NL, Canada
e-mail: rlaw@mun.ca; rlawUCSF@gmail.com

M. T. Greene
Faculty of Medicine, Memorial University of Newfoundland, St. John's, NL, Canada
e-mail: meghan.greene@mun.ca

R. M. Law, H. I. Maibach (eds.), *Handbook of Topical Drug Treatment in Dermatology*,
https://doi.org/10.1007/978-3-031-93616-6_6

Aged skin is drier with less skin surface lipids [1, 2]. It is also thinner and more friable—skin aging is associated with progressive dermal atrophy. This includes atrophy of the skin's capillary network, resulting in a gradual reduction of blood supply to the skin [1, 2]. All of these changes may potentially affect topical absorption.

Overall, it paradoxically appears that the permeability barrier function of the skin is increased as we age. In particular, percutaneous absorption of less lipophilic substances (e.g., hydrocortisone, benzoic acid, acetylsalicylic acid, and caffeine) is reduced, while more lipophilic substances (e.g., testosterone and estradiol) are not [1, 2].

However, increased friability may result in broken skin, resulting in the loss of permeability barrier function and increased percutaneous absorption. There may be significant systemic drug concentration to result in systemic pharmacologic effect and/or adverse effect from topical drug application (refer to Chap. 1: Factors Affecting Percutaneous Penetration: Twenty clinically pertinent factors/observations for percutaneous absorption in humans for more information).

Moisture-associated skin damage occurs in the elderly population secondary to prolonged exposure to moisture in an occluded environment (e.g., if incontinence products are used). This damage results in disruption of skin barrier function.

2. Renal Function

   Age-related renal impairment may have an effect on excretion of drugs applied on skin, if significant systemic absorption occurs. This is specific to each drug and the amount of drug absorbed systemically may be different based on drug formulation and the physicochemical properties of the drug and other factors [2]. Please refer to specific drug monographs for more information.

   Age-related renal impairment may potentially also have an effect on topical absorption of drugs if significant hypoalbuminemia is present. See Chap. 7: Systemic Considerations Relating to Topical Drug Treatment for More Information.

3. Hepatic Function

   Age-related hepatic dysfunction may have an effect on metabolism of drugs applied on skin, if significant systemic absorption occurs and if the drug is metabolized by the liver. Metabolism also occurs in the skin [2] for some drugs, and many drugs may not be metabolized at all.

   Thus, the impact of age-related changes in hepatic function is specific to each drug. Furthermore, the amount of drug absorbed systemically may be different based on drug formulation and the physicochemical properties of the drug and other factors [2]. In addition, patients with severe liver disease may develop the hepato-renal syndrome: even if the drug is metabolized, renal excretion may be impaired. Please refer to specific drug monographs for more information.

Disease States (Chronic Diseases) in the Elderly That May Affect Topical Drug Efficacy and Toxicity

1. Xerosis and Pruritus

   Xerosis or dry skin is caused by diminished natural moisturizing factors, sebum, and lipid production [3]. As we age sebaceous gland function decreases, particularly on the extremities, leading to less endogenous emolliation. Xerosis often occurs on the arms, legs and trunk [4]. Comorbid conditions and medications can also contribute to xerosis and pruritus. Hypothyroidism, renal or hepatic insufficiency, and peripheral neuropathies can be associated with xerosis. The chronic state of inflammation or associated excoriations due to xerosis may affect topical drug efficacy.
2. Frailty

   Patients with moderate to severe frailty due to physical and/or cognitive deficits may have difficulty applying topical medications adequately or appropriately, thus impacting their use. Decreased dexterity or impaired vision may impact the patient's ability to apply topical medications.

3. Weakened Immune Response

   A weakened immune system can alter skin barrier function. Without the appropriate immune response, the skin barrier of elderly patients may allow more microorganisms to penetrate the skin causing more frequent bacterial, viral, or fungal infections [3]. These disruptions to the skin barrier function could impact the efficacy of topical drugs in the older adult population.

4. Socioeconomic Factors

   Compliance or accessibility to topical medications can be impacted by socioeconomic factors such as cost of medication or availability of home care to assist with medication application.

References

1. Roskos KV, Maibach HI, Guy RH. The effect of aging on percutaneous absorption in man. J Pharmacokinet Biopharm. 1989;17(6):617–30.
2. Law RM, Ngo MA, Maibach HI. Twenty clinically pertinent factors/observations for percutaneous absorption in humans. Am J Clin Dermatol. 2020;21(1):85–95.
3. Humbert P, Dreno B, Krutmann J, et al. Recommendations for managing cutaneous disorders associated with advancing age. Clin Interv Aging. 2016;11:141–8.
4. Chang ALS, Wong JW, Endo JO, Norma RA. Geriatric dermatology review: major changes in skin function in older patients and their contribution to common clinical challenges. J Am Med Dir Assoc. 8:110.

Systemic Considerations Relating to Topical Drug Treatment

7

Amanda Tzenov and Rebecca M. Law

Contents

A. Tzenov (✉)
Faculty of Medicine, Memorial University of Newfoundland, St. John's, NL, Canada
e-mail: Amanda.Tzenov@mun.ca

R. M. Law (✉)
School of Pharmacy and Faculty of Medicine (Discipline of Family Medicine), Memorial University of Newfoundland, St. John's, NL, Canada
e-mail: rlaw@mun.ca; rlawUCSF@gmail.com

R. M. Law, H. I. Maibach (eds.), *Handbook of Topical Drug Treatment in Dermatology*,
https://doi.org/10.1007/978-3-031-93616-6_7

Introduction

There are numerous factors that affect percutaneous absorption after topical application of a drug. Twenty factors have been discussed in Chap. 1 [1]. With significant percutaneous absorption, systemic drug concentrations leading to systemic pharmacologic effects and adverse effects may be seen. This is drug and sometimes formulation specific and is discussed in more detail in individual drug monographs in this textbook.

Systemic considerations include potential issues relevant to pregnancy, lactation, renal dysfunction, hepatic dysfunction, potential drug interaction, and altered physiologic states such as hypoalbuminemia.

Pregnancy

Physiologic Changes in Pregnancy

The body undergoes a tremendous number of physiologic changes during pregnancy, which include things like increased total body water, decreased plasma protein, physiologic anemia due to maternal blood volume increasing more so than red blood cell increase, increased blood flow to the kidneys, and decreased gastric emptying, to name a few [2]. There are particular cutaneous changes that occur during pregnancy as well, which can contribute to the absorption and therefore the systemic effects of a variety of topical medications [3]. Pigment changes, striae, increased telangiectasias, and telogen effluvium are common, as is increased hair growth and nail changes [4]. Preexisting skin changes may also be exacerbated or improved during pregnancy, and it is often difficult to determine the course during pregnancy. For example, psoriasis improves for some patients during pregnancy but might worsen for others and in fact might vary from one pregnancy to the next in the same patient [5]. The treatment of these preexisting skin conditions also warrants more careful consideration during pregnancy due to the above noted changes.

Systemic Absorption in Pregnancy

Because of the changes noted above, systemic absorption can be altered for topical drug treatments in pregnancy (either increased or decreased, depending on numerous factors discussed in Chap. 1). This section will look at specific topical dermatologic drugs in pregnancy and their unique systemic absorption during pregnancy. It will also review the effects of this systemic absorption on the patient as well as potential teratogenicity [6, 7].

Drugs with significant systemic absorption after topical administration (and effects of same including potential teratogenicity):

Acne vulgaris is often worsened during pregnancy, and one of the treatments often asked about in practice is topical retinoids [8]. Oral retinoids are very effective in treating acne vulgaris but are contraindicated in pregnancy due to their teratogenicity including neurological and cardiovascular sequelae (among others) [9]. **Topical retinoids** carry with them the same concerns. For example, tazarotene is contraindicated in pregnancy due to the above noted risks. Other topical retinoids include adapalene, isotretinoin, tretinoin, and trifarotene. A systematic review by Kaplan et al. [8] noted that while inadvertent exposure may not increase rates of major malformations, the study was not powered to justify their use in pregnancy. Refer to Chap. 23: Retinoids for their drug monographs.

Treatment of acne during pregnancy has been summarized [10]. Some other topical acne treatments to be mindful of in pregnancy include **salicylic acid** and **glycolic acid,** which are keratolytic agents. While animal studies have shown teratogenicity with systemic salicylic acid [11], the recommendation for topical salicylic acid is to limit duration of use and to a small area, and to avoid occlusion, which can increase systemic absorption [7]. Topical antibiotics (i.e., erythromycin and clindamycin) are safer to use in pregnancy [7], classified as a Category B by the US FDA (in the former Pregnancy Risk classification scheme).

Topical Corticosteroids (TCS) are used for a large number of skin conditions, including those that can first appear or worsen during pregnancy (including eczema, lupus, and atopic eruptions during pregnancy). An updated Cochrane Review from 2015 concluded that there is no association between TCS exposure (regardless of potency) in pregnancy and pregnancy outcomes [12]. There was a "probable" association between low birth weight and use of potent to very potent corticosteroids if the cumulative dosage was very large [12]. That said, there are guidelines published in the British Journal of Dermatology that review the appropriate use of TCS in pregnancy [13]. They note that whenever possible, mild/moderate TCS should be used in preference to more potent corticosteroids. These more potent TCS should be reserved for second-line therapy for as short a time as possible. The theoretical risk of adverse events is increased in areas of high absorption (i.e., genitals, eyelids, and flexures). Refer to Chap. 17: Corticosteroids for a potency table for TCS.

5-Fluorouricil (5-FU) is a topical cream used in the treatment of actinic keratoses, basal cell carcinomas, and squamous cell carcinomas of the skin. Since it is an antineoplastic agent and interferes with DNA synthesis, there is a risk of fetal harm, and therefore, its use is contraindicated in pregnancy [6]. A number of studies have demonstrated fetal harm when 5-FU is used inadvertently during pregnancy [14]. Refer to Chap. 13: Antineoplastic Agents for its drug monograph.

Given that melasma is a common dermatological condition in pregnancy, it is worthwhile to mention the use of *hydroquinone* topically. Hydroquinone is a first-line agent for melasma and is a bleaching agent [15]. There have been teratogenic and carcinogenic effects following oral administration in animal studies, and since it is readily absorbed cutaneously, it is not recommended for use in pregnancy [15]. Resolution of melasma can occur without treatment but may be slow, and sun avoidance or use of barriers (i.e., physical sunscreen) is also key [16]. Topical retinoids have also been used for melasma, but as discussed above, their use in pregnancy should be avoided [8, 9]. Refer to Chap. 20: Pigmenting and Depigmenting Agents for the hydroquinone drug monograph.

Musculoskeletal (MSK) aches and pains are common in pregnancy. *Topical non-steroidal anti-inflammatory drugs (NSAIDS)* are used in nonpregnant adults to treat musculoskeletal pain; however, evidence in pregnant patients is lacking. Health Canada has recommended avoidance of oral NSAIDS at 20 weeks or later in pregnancy unless advised otherwise by a healthcare professional [17]. A recent systematic review examined the available evidence and safety of topical NSAIDs for the treatment of MSK issues in pregnancy and found that there is no evidence [18].

Tacrolimus is a calcineurin inhibitor and therefore an immunosuppressant agent. It is used for a number of skin conditions, including atopic and allergic dermatitis, lichen planus, psoriasis, pyoderma gangrenosum, and vitiligo [19]. While there are no studies of topical tacrolimus in pregnancy, manufacturers advise avoidance of topical calcineurin inhibitors during pregnancy. Given that the absorption of topical calcineurin inhibitors is quite low [20], topical tacrolimus is generally considered safe in pregnancy, if used on small areas for short durations [21]. Refer to Chap. 17 Atopic Dermatitis: Topical Agents for Drug Monographs on Tacrolimus and Pimecrolimus

Dermatologic Conditions in Pregnancy

There are some dermatologic conditions that commonly occur in pregnancy. Pruritus occurs more commonly in pregnancy. It affects up to 20% of pregnant women. Consequences may include affecting the woman's sleep and quality of life, as well as the pruritus being associated with either inconsequential or a more serious medical condition [22, 23]. Several pruritic skin disorders are unique to pregnancy. These include intrahepatic cholestasis of pregnancy (ICP), pruritic urticarial papules and plaques of pregnancy (PUPPP), pemphigoid gestationis (PG), and atopic eruption of pregnancy [22]. ICP has been associated with adverse fetal outcomes including preterm labor and fetal death [22, 23].

Other dermatologic conditions or changes in pregnancy include melasma, striae, and hyperpigmentation (linea nigra, acanthosis nigricans, darkened areolas, and darkened skin folds). The hyperpigmentation is suspected to be due to melanocyte sensitivity to hormones that increase during pregnancy (including estrogen and progesterone) [3]. Increased androgens lead to worsening of acne vulgaris [10]. Increased hair growth (thickness/diameter, anagen/telogen ratio, and growth rate) is related to the effects of estrogen, progesterone, prolactin, and growth factors on the hair follicles [24]. With the increase in plasma volume, as well as the effects of the gravid uterus on venous return, both venous stasis and varicose veins can become more problematic [25].

Systemic Metabolism and Excretion of Drugs

Metabolism and excretion are two mechanisms for elimination of drugs or chemicals, which can be affected by numerous factors. Metabolism and excretion pharmacokinetics can differ greatly between structurally similar drugs or chemicals. Thus, depending on the substance, elimination (i.e., drug clearance) may or may not be in proportion to the dose absorbed. Even for researchers conducting in vivo studies, the clearance rate of the drug or chemical must be considered when estimating percutaneous absorption from blood or tissue samples [1, 26].

Renal Dysfunction

The major organ for drug excretion from the body is the kidneys. If enough drug is absorbed systemically after topical administration, elimination and renal clearance would be needed, and the significance of renal impairment would need to be considered. This differs between drugs—some drugs may be extensively metabolized prior to drug excretion, while other drugs may be minimally metabolized (if at all) and be 99–100% cleared from the kidneys unchanged.

Furthermore, drug metabolism often changes a drug into a more hydrophilic metabolite, which is then excreted by the kidneys. In renal dysfunction, the metabolite may accumulate and—if it is an active metabolite, that is, it has pharmacologic activity—may add to the original drug's pharmacologic effects and/or adverse effects [26].

Thus, whether the original drug is excreted unchanged or is metabolized, renal dysfunction may be a concern. How drug usage is affected by renal dysfunction is further discussed in each drug monograph.

Hepatic Dysfunction

The liver is the major organ for metabolism of drugs and chemicals. However, metabolism can occur in other organs including the skin [1]. Similarly to drug excretion, metabolism is drug specific: the degree of metabolism differs from one drug to another, and some drugs may not be metabolized at all.

For drugs that are extensively metabolized by the liver, significant hepatic dysfunction may reduce the amount of drug metabolized, resulting in potential for increased pharmacologic effect and/or toxic effects.

Furthermore, cirrhosis of the liver—or even acute hepatic injury—may result in hepatorenal syndrome, causing functional renal failure [27]. Thus, even drugs that are not metabolized by the liver but are excreted unchanged by the kidneys may be affected by acute or chronic liver injury.

Potential Drug Interactions of Topical Drugs with Systemic Drug Treatment

Obviously, the use of two topical drugs may result in a potential drug interaction. With enough drug through percutaneous absorption, a topical drug may also interact with a systemic drug, resulting in a clinically significant drug interaction.

Topical Miconazole and Warfarin

Warnings by USFDA and Health Canada about this drug interaction were first raised in 2001, when case reports surfaced (two in the United States and one in Canada) about *vaginal* miconazole increasing INR resulting in associated bleeding tendencies (bruising, gingival bleeding, and nosebleeds) [28].

Subsequently, other similar case reports appeared. A potentially life-threatening case involved a patient using a tube of miconazole oral gel, which he purchased on his own from a community pharmacy two weeks prior to the interaction being discovered. The patient was on warfarin for atrial fibrillation, and his INR had previously been well controlled within the 2–3 range. In this instance, the patient's INR was found to be 8 then increased to 15, and he had presented with hematuria [29, 30].

Topical Econazole and Warfarin

Other topical azoles have been reported to interact with warfarin as well. Topical econazole cream prescribed twice daily for at least one week beyond clearing or a minimum of two weeks, (for a *Candida* infection on the scrotum and inner thighs), led to a marked increase in bruising within the first week of use, a large ecchymosis on the hip from a trivial injury, and a bleed for over 24 h from a small superficial cut on the hand. The patient's INR had increased from 2.2 to 12 while using topical econazole [31]. Previous to this, the patient's INR had been within a stable range (1.8–3) for three years on the same dose of warfarin [31].

The case report further noted that this patient had previously used topical miconazole without a similar effect [31].

Hypoalbuminemia Effects on Drug-Binding Interactions

Serum albumin is a plasma protein, which binds to acidic or neutral drugs and other substances, keeping them in the systemic circulation but not actively producing an effect. In states of hypoalbuminemia (such as malnutrition and chronic kidney disease), if a drug is highly bound to serum albumin, there will be less binding, thus releasing more free drug into the circulation, potentially enhancing pharmacologic effect and toxicities including drug interactions [26]. Warfarin, for example, is a drug highly bound to serum albumin. Thus, in states of hypoalbuminemia, there is a greater potential for increased INR and potential drug-bind interactions. Other drugs with high binding to serum albumin include salicylates, phenytoin, and many more.

Systemic Toxicity from Topical Drug Treatment

In summary, it is possible for topical drug treatments to have systemic toxicity (Table 7.1). The risk varies from drug to drug and may be formulation dependent as well as dependent on many other factors affecting percutaneous absorption as discussed, including patient-specific factors such as renal and hepatic dysfunction. Skin-to-skin transfer of a topical drug can result in systemic toxicity in another person. A father using testosterone

Table 7.1 Some examples of systemic toxicity from topical drug treatments

Topical drug	Systemic adverse effect
Clindamycin	Pseudomembranous colitis [33, 34]
Corticosteroids	HPA-axis suppression, adrenal insufficiency, Cushing's syndrome, hypertension [1, 35]
EMLA cream (prilocaine and lidocaine)	Methemoglobinemia [31]
Minoxidil	Palpitations, hypotension, tachycardia, paroxysmal atrial fibrillation, sinus arrhythmia [1, 35]
Salicylates	Refractory hypoglycemia, tinnitus, hearing loss, blurred vision, sweating [1, 35]
Ophthalmic sulfonamides	Stevens-Johnson syndrome [1, 35]
Testosterone	Hyperandrogenic effects, including acne, hirsutism, menstrual irregularities [31], and precocious puberty upon skin transfer [32]

cream without routine handwashing after application transferred enough testosterone over time to his infant son to cause precocious puberty—pronounced virilization in a 2-year-old boy [32].

The use of topical drugs in pregnancy must include considerations of potential risks to the fetus as discussed above. Please refer to each drug monograph for more specific discussion.

References

1. Law RM, Ngo MA, Maibach HI. Twenty clinically pertinent factors/observations for percutaneous absorption in humans. Am J Clin Dermatol. 2020;21(1):85–95.
2. Constantine M. Physiologic and pharmacokinetic changes in pregnancy. Front Pharmacol. 2014;5:1–5.
3. Panicker VV, Riyaz N, Balachandran PK. A clinical study of cutaneous changes in pregnancy. J Epidemiol Glob Health. 2017;7(1):63–70. https://doi.org/10.1016/j.jegh.2016.10.002. Epub 2016 Nov 19. PMID: 27870929; PMCID: PMC7320517.
4. Motosko CC, Bieber AK, Pomeranz MK, Stein JA, Maritires KJ. Physiologic changes of pregnancy: a review of the literature. Int J Women's Dermatol. 2017;3(4):219–24.
5. Simionescu AA, Danciu BM, Stanescu AMA. State-of-the-art review of pregnancy-related Psoriasis. Medicina. 2021;57:804. https://doi.org/10.3390/medicina57080804.
6. Patel V, Schwartz RA, Lambert WC. Safety of topical dermatologic medications in pregnancy. J Drugs Dermatol. 2016;15(7)
7. Putra IB, Jusuf NK, Dewi NK. Skin changes and safety profile of topical products during pregnancy. J Clin Aesthet Dermatol. 2022;15(2):49–57. PMID: 35309882; PMCID: PMC8884185
8. Kaplan YC, Ozsarfati J, Etwel F, Nickel C, Nulman I, Koren G. Pregnancy outcomes following first-trimester exposure to topical retinoids: a systematic review and meta-analysis. Br J Dermatol. 2015;173(5):1132–41. https://doi.org/10.1111/bjd.14053.
9. Choi JS, Koren G, Nulman I. Pregnancy and isotretinoin therapy. CMAJ. 2013;185(5):411–3. https://doi.org/10.1503/cmaj.120729.
10. Kong YL, Tey HL. Treatment of acne vulgaris during pregnancy and lactation. Drugs. 2013;73(8):779–87. Retrieved from https://qe2a-proxy.mun.ca/login?url=https://www.proquest.com/scholarly-journals/treatment-acne-vulgaris-during-pregnancy/docview/1466259872/se-2.
11. Akhavan A, Bershad S. Topical acne drugs: review of clinical properties, systemic exposure, and safety. Am J Clin Dermatol. 2003;4(7):473–92. https://doi.org/10.2165/00128071-200304070-00004. PMID: 12814337

12. Chi C, Wang S, Wojnarowska F, Kirtschig G, Davies E, Bennett C. Safety of topical corticosteroids in pregnancy. Cochrane Database Syst Rev. 2015, Issue 10. Art. No.: CD007346; https://doi.org/10.1002/14651858.CD007346.pub3.
13. Chi C, Kirtschig G, Aberer W, Gabbud JP, Lipozencic J, Karpati S, Haustein UF, Zuberbier T, Wojnarowska F. Evidence-based (S3) guideline on topical corticosteroids in pregnancy. Br J Dermatol. 2011;165(5):943–52.
14. Efudex (Fluorouracil) product monograph. (2014). Valeant Canada LP. 2150 St Elzear Blvd West. Laval, Quebec. H7L 4A8. Canada. Retrieved from https://pdf.hres.ca/dpd_pm/00026974.PDF.
15. Bio LL, Cies JJ. Lack of pregnancy warnings on over-the-counter dermatologic products containing potentially harmful hydroquinone. J Perinatol. 2017;37:778–81.
16. Handel AC, Miot LDB, Miot HA. Melasma: a clinical and epidemiological review. An Bras Dermatol. 2014;89(5):771–82.
17. Health Canada Advisory (Oct 30, 2020). RA-74239. Use of Non-Steroidal Anti-Inflammatory Drugs (NSAIDs) beyond 20 weeks of pregnancy and risk of kidney damage in unborn babies, leading to low amniotic fluid. Retrieved from https://recalls-rappels.canada.ca/en/alert-recall/use-non-steroidal-anti-inflammatory-drugs-nsaids-beyond-20-weeks-pregnancy-and-risk on October 24, 2023.
18. Shi C, et al. Multidisciplinary guidelines for the rational use of topical non-steroidal anti-inflammatory drugs for musculoskeletal pain. J Clin Med. 2023;12(4):1544.
19. Tacrolimus (topical): Drug Information. UpToDate. Wolters Kluwer. Retrieved from https://www.uptodate.com/contents/tacrolimus-topical-drug-information?search=tacrolimus&source=panel_search_result&selectedTitle=1~145&usage_type=panel&showDrugLabel=true&display_rank=1 on October 24, 2023.
20. Undre NA, Moloney FJ, Ahmadi S, Stevenson P, Murphy GM. Skin and systemic pharmacokinetics of tacrolimus following topical application of tacrolimus ointment in adults with moderate to severe atopic dermatitis. Br J Dermatol. 2009;160(3):665–9. https://doi.org/10.1111/j.1365-2133.2008.08974.x. Epub 2008 Dec 12. PMID: 19076975.
21. Heilskov S, Deleuran M, Vestergaard C. Immunosuppressive and immunomodulating therapy for atopic dermatitis in pregnancy: an appraisal of the literature. Dermatol Ther (Heidelb). 2020;10(6):1215–28.
22. Law RM, Law DTS, Maibach HI. Chapter e-121: Dermatologic drug reactions, contact dermatitis, and common skin conditions. In: DiPiro's pharmacotherapy: a pathophysiologic approach. 12th ed. McGraw-Hill Medical; 2023. p. 1693.
23. Bergman H, Melamed N, Koren G. Pruritus in pregnancy: treatment of dermatoses unique to pregnancy. Can Fam Phy. 2013;59(12):1290–4.
24. Grymowicz M, Rudnicka E, Podfigurna A, Napierala P, Smolarczyk R, Smolarczyk K, Meczekalski B. Hormonal effects on hair follicles. Int J

Mol Sci. 2020;21(15):5342. https://doi.org/10.3390/ijms21155342. PMID: 32731328; PMCID: PMC7432488.
25. Goulart VB, Cabral ACV, Reis ZS, et al. Anatomical and physiological changes in the venous system of lower limbs in pregnant women and findings associated with the symptomatology. Arch Gynecol Obstet. 2013;288:73–8. https://doi-org.qe2a-proxy.mun.ca/10.1007/s00404-013-2728-9
26. Burton ME, Schentag JJ, Shaw LM, Evans WE. Applied pharmacokinetics and pharmacodynamics: principles of therapeutic drug monitoring. 4th ed. Lippincott, Williams, and Wilkins; 2006.
27. Ranasinghe IR, Sharma B, Bashir K. Hepatorenal syndrome. NIH National Library of Medicine StatPearls. Last update Aug 8, 2023. https://www.ncbi.nlm.nih.gov/books/NBK430856/#:~:text=Hepatorenal%20syndrome%20(HRS)%20is%20a%20multiorgan%20condition%20affecting%20the%20kidneys,observed%20in%20the%20late%201800s. Accessed 4 Dec 2023.
28. O'Reilly M. Drug advisory: the interaction between warfarin and vaginal miconazole. JAMC. 2001;165(7):938.
29. Filmer S. Warfarin and oral miconazole: a major interaction overlooked in practice. Pharm J. 2012;288:527.
30. Miki A, Ohtani H, Sawada Y. Warfarin and miconazole oral gel interactions: analysis and therapy recommendations based on clinical data and a pharmacokinetic model. J Clin Pharm Ther. 2011;36:642–50.
31. Lang PG, LeClercq AH. Increase in anticoagulant effect of warfarin in a patient using econazole cream. J Am Acad Dermatol. 2005;55(5 Supplement):S117–9.
32. Franklin SF, Geffner ME. Precocious puberty secondary to topical testosterone exposure. J Pediatr Endocr Metab. 2003;16:107–10.
33. Trexler M, Fraser T, Jones M. Fulminant psedomembranous colitis caused by clindamycin phosphate vaginal cream. Am J Gastroenterol. 1997;92:2112–3.
34. Parry MF, Rha CK. Pseudomembranous colitis caused by topical clindamycin phosphate. Arch Dermatol. 1986;122:583–4.
35. Alikhan FS, Maibach HI. Topical absorption and systemic toxicity. Cutan Ocul Toxicol. 2011;30(3):175–86.

Part II

Drug Monographs

8 Topical Drug Treatments for Acne

Brian W. Connor, Jason Ya, and Lisa E. Maier

Contents

Introduction

Acne vulgaris is a common inflammatory disorder primarily affecting the sebaceous follicles of face, chest and back. Although acne can affect any age, it is more common in adolescence and

B. W. Connor
Schweiger Dermatology Group, New York, NY, USA
e-mail: bwconnor@uw.edu

J. Ya
Department of Dermatology, Stanford University School of Medicine, Redwood City, CA, USA
e-mail: jasonya@uw.edu

L. E. Maier (✉)
Department of Dermatology, UW Medicine, Seattle, WA, USA
e-mail: lemaier@uw.edu

R. M. Law, H. I. Maibach (eds.), *Handbook of Topical Drug Treatment in Dermatology*,
https://doi.org/10.1007/978-3-031-93616-6_8

early adulthood. Various clinical features can be seen in acne including comedones, inflammatory lesions (papules, pustules, and nodules), scars, and dyspigmentation. Acne pathogenesis is complex, but there appear to be several key pathogenic steps that contribute to the development of acne. These include abnormal follicular keratinization resulting in follicular hyperkeratosis, overabundant sebum production, follicular colonization by the skin flora resident bacteria *Cutibacterium acnes* and subsequent inflammatory response surrounding the sebaceous follicle. The microcomedone, characterized by follicular hyperkeratosis and sebum, is considered the precursor lesion for comedones, papules, pustules, and nodules. Microcomedones progress to comedones or inflammatory lesions as they become increasingly filled with sebum, keratin, and *C. acnes* and other bacteria. Rupture of the distended sebaceous follicle aggravates the inflammatory response and results more severe inflammatory lesions and nodules [1].

Androgen hormones are thought to play an important role in the development of acne by driving sebum production and contributing to follicular hyperkeratosis. Other factors such as decreased linoleic acid and increased IL-1-α and FGFR-2 signaling may also contribute to microcomedone development. *C. acnes* contributes to follicular inflammation, by activating the innate and adaptive immune responses. Some of the possible mechanisms by which this occurs includes *C. acnes* ability to break down sebum to inflammatory free fatty acids, the production of production of enzymes that trigger rupture of comedones, activating the expression of Toll-like receptors and activating of NOD-like receptor protein 3 of inflammasomes in neutrophils and monocytes. *C. acnes* contributes to a Th1/Th17 adaptive immune response [2].

Currently available topical acne treatments are not curative but aim to reduce acne lesions and subsequently minimize scarring and dyspigmentation. Treatment choice is based on the types of lesions present, the location, and extent of involvement. Topical-only therapy is generally appropriate for milder and more limited forms of acne. Various topical agents may be combined to achieve greater control of acne and to limit the development of bacterial resistance—topical antibiotic monotherapy should be avoided to prevent development of bacterial resistance. When combining therapies, special attention should be given to overlapping or potentiating adverse effects, such as skin irritation. In more severe or widespread presentations of acne, topical can be combined with oral therapies (e.g., oral antibiotics, spironolactone, and oral contraceptives).

Topical medications that improve comedonal acne include topical retinoids, azelaic acid, benzoyl peroxide, sulfur, salicylic acid, and clascoterone. Most of these work by decreasing follicular hyperkeratosis. Medications that treat inflammatory lesions include benzoyl peroxide, sodium sulfacetamide-sulfur, clascoterone, and topical antibiotics such as erythromycin, clindamycin, minocycline, and dapsone. These typically work by reducing inflammation and decreasing bacteria in the sebaceous follicle [3]. Because microcomedone formation is a key step in acne pathogenesis, it is often recommended to use a product that reduces follicular hyperkeratosis even in the management of primarily inflammatory acne. Some products such as benzoyl peroxide and clascoterone improve both comedonal and inflammatory acne equally.

Commercially available combination topical therapies combining a retinoid and antibiotic such as benzoyl peroxide + clindamycin gel and tretinoin + clindamycin gel can target both inflammatory and comedonal acne and help limit bacterial resistance to the antibiotic component [3]. Although these combination products are often easier for patients to use, depending on availability, cost, tolerability, and clinical presentation, the practitioner can combine more than one individual topical agent in the patient's daily treatment regimen (e.g., benzoyl peroxide wash qam and tretinoin 0.025% cream qhs). Data regarding comparative efficacy of different topical medications is limited, although one recent meta-analysis suggested that topical treatments with antibiotics were not more effective than those that did not contain antibiotics. This study did not include all topical therapies, notably omitting topical dapsone, topical minocycline, clascoterone, and some topical retinoids (trifarotene and tazarotene) [4].

There are a variety of topical agents such as resorcinol and tea tree oil that are used in over-the-counter products worldwide but for which supporting evidence for efficacy is minimal. We have briefly included these medications in this chapter given their common use.

Drug Monographs

Adapalene

Classification and Mode of Action

- Retinoic acid derivative: Adapalene is a retinoid-like substance that modulates cellular differentiation, keratinization, and inflammation. Topical adapalene may normalize the differentiation of follicular epithelial cells resulting in decreased microcomedone formation. Adapalene is better than tretinoin or tazarotene in reducing inflammatory acne lesions and total lesion count and causes less irritation.

Indications and Dermatological Uses

- *Clinical indications (FDA)*: Acne vulgaris
- *Off-label common uses*: Rosacea

Formulations/Presentation

- US: 0.1% gel, 0.1% cream, 0.1% lotion, 0.1% pad, 0.1% solution
- Canada: 0.1% cream, 0,1% gel

Dosages and Suggested Regimens

- Apply once daily before bedtime
- No suggested dosage adjustment for renal or hepatic impairment due to low systemic absorption

Baseline Investigations and Considerations

- None

Pharmacokinetics

- Minimal topical absorption, even after chronic use (trace amounts measured in serum). Elimination half-life between 7 and 51 h (gel). Excreted in bile.
- Onset of effect: between 8 and 12 weeks.

Use in Special Populations

Pediatrics:

- Approved for use in children. May cause mild hyperglycemia, which is more common in children. Avoid internal use.

Pregnancy and Lactation:

- Listed as FDA pregnancy classification C (former classification system).
- Unknown whether adapalene is present in breast milk.

Renal Insufficiency:

- Not evaluated; dose adjustment is not expected to be needed.

Hepatic Insufficiency:

- Not evaluated; dose adjustment is not expected to be needed.

Monitoring

- Skin irritation/dryness
- Initial acne flare
- Severe skin reactions (exfoliation and desquamation)
- Allergy (angioedema, lip swelling, facial edema—reported postmarketing with gel)

Contraindications and Cautions

- Accidental ingestion especially of large amounts of products containing propylene glycol may result in toxicity (metabolic acidosis/lactic acidosis, hyperosmolality, respiratory depression, and seizures). Fatalities have been reported in neonates given large amounts of propylene glycol internally (po or IV).

Important Drug Interactions

- Other topical medications, which may cause skin irritation, will potentially exacerbate the skin irritation. (e.g., benzoyl peroxide, medicated soaps, and cleansers).
- Other topical medications (or cosmetics) containing alcohol, acetone, or astringents may exacerbate adapalene's drying effect.
- Adapalene may increase the levels/effects of aminolevulinic acid (topical or systemic). Avoid concomitant use.
- Levels/effects of adapalene may be increased by concomitant use of multivitamins with minerals (i.e., ADEK, folate, or iron).

Adverse Effects and Their Management

- Skin irritation can occur. Less skin irritation than other retinoids, that is, tretinoin. Erythema, stinging/burning, dryness, or pruritus may occur especially during the initial 2–4 weeks of use. These may lessen with continued use.
- May cause initial exacerbation of acne.
- May cause increased sensitivity to UV rays. Use sunscreen and avoid sunlamp use.
- Hypersensitivity reactions including facial and eyelid edema and swelling have been reported. Use must be discontinued immediately as anaphylactoid/anaphylactic reactions may occur.

Carcinogenicity

- Unknown. Carcinogenicity studies conducted in mice at topical doses of 0.3, 0.9, and 2.6 mg/kg/day and in rats at oral doses of 0.15, 0.5, and 1.5 mg/kg/day (approximately 4–75 times the maximal daily human topical dose). In the oral study, positive linear trends were observed in the incidence of follicular cell adenomas and carcinomas in the thyroid glands of female rats and in the incidence of benign and malignant pheochromocytomas in the adrenal medullas of male rats.
- No photocarcinogenicity studies were conducted. Animal studies have shown an increased tumorigenic risk with similar drugs (e.g., retinoids). Although the significance of these studies to human use is not clear, patients should be advised to avoid or minimize exposure to either sunlight or artificial UV irradiation sources.

Patch Test Concentration

- 0.1% and 0.01% pet

Essential Patient Information

- Avoid contact with broken, sunburned, eczematous, or abraded skin.
- Avoid contact with eyes, lips, or other mucous membranes (e.g., inside nose).

- Avoid using products including cosmetics which contain alpha hydroxyl or glycolic acid, as they may further irritate the skin.
- Do not ingest. For external use only.
- Use sun protection. Apply sunscreen with SPF 30 daily. If there is a sunburn, discontinue use until sunburn has healed.

Benzoyl Peroxide

Classification and Mode of Action

- Releases oxygen free radicals that both break down keratin (comedolytic) and result in a bactericidal effect on pathogenic skin bacteria.

Indications and Dermatological Uses

- *Clinical indications (FDA)*: Acne vulgaris, inflammatory rosacea, folliculitis, pseudofolliculitis barbae
- *Off-label common uses*: N/A

Formulations/Presentations

US: Many prescription brands, generic, and OTC products exist. Multiple different formulations exist including cleansing bars, creams, gels, foams, liquid washes, foaming cloths, masks, and shaving creams. Some representative brands and strengths are listed below. Microencapsulated benzoyl peroxide is a novel prescription-only formulation in which benzoyl peroxide is encapsulated by silica microcapsules. This is used alone as a 5% cream for rosacea or in a combination product with tretinoin.

- Cream: 10% (Clearskin)
- Cream: Microencapsulated benzoyl peroxide 5% cream (Epsolay)
- Gel: 2.5% 5%, 10% (BP Gel, Acne-Clear, Acne Medication, Persa-Gel)
- Foam: 5.2%, 5.5%, 5.3%, 9.8% (BenzePro, Riax)
- Liquid Wash: 2.5%, 3.5%, 4%, 5%, 5.25%, 6%, 7%, 10% (Panoxyl, Neutrogena Clear Pore, Benzac, BenzePrO, Benziq Wash, BP Wash, PR Benzoyl peroxide wash)

- Liquid extended release Wash: 4.4% (Advanced Acne Wash)
- Lotion: 5%, 8%, 10% (Acne Medication 5, Acne Medication 10, Zaclir Cleansing)
- Foaming cloths: 6% (BenzePrO, BPO foaming cloths)
- Cleansing bar: 5%,10% (Panoxyl)
- Masks: 2.5% (Rapid Clear Daily leave on mask)
- Shaving creams: 5%, 10% (BenzaShave)

Canada: Numerous prescription and OTC products similar to the United States

Dosages and Suggested Regimens: Adult

Topical formulations:

- Apply sparingly once daily. Can increase to twice daily if necessary. Decrease application frequency or active ingredient strength for skin dryness/irritation.

Topical cleansers:

- Wash affected areas once to twice daily. Decrease application frequency and/or active ingredient strength for skin dryness/irritation.

Baseline Investigations and Considerations

- None

Pharmacokinetics

- Absorption: Approximately 5% through the skin. Gel-based products are more penetrating.
- Metabolism: Converted to benzoic acid in the skin. Cleared renally.

Use in Special Populations

Pregnancy:

- Safety studies have not been conducted in human or animal models. In general, topical agents are preferred in treating acne in pregnant patients. Among the topical options, benzoyl peroxide is a preferred agent [17, 25].

Lactation:

- While the manufacturer recommends caution in using benzoyl peroxide in breastfeeding patients, the World Health Organization considers use of the topical medication compatible with breastfeeding [27]. As above, topical agents are preferable to systemic acne medications in breastfeeding patients, and benzoyl peroxide is a preferred agent [17, 25].

Renal insufficiency:

- There are no dosing adjustments provided on the manufacturer's label.

Hepatic insufficiency:

- There are no dosing adjustments provided on the manufacturer's label.

Monitoring

- No specific monitoring guidelines

Contraindications and Cautions

- Hypersensitivity to benzoyl peroxide or any component of the product's formulation. Consult product label for comprehensive ingredient list, as inactive ingredients can vary significantly between products.
- Benzoyl peroxide can bleach or discolor hair and fabrics.
- Hypersensitivity reactions: Rare but potential life-threatening allergic reactions have been reported with over-the-counter benzoyl peroxide products. Allergic reactions can occur to active ingredients (benzoyl peroxide), inactive ingredients, or both. Treatment should be discontinued in the setting of urticaria or significant skin pain/irritation. Patients should seek emergency medical assistance in the setting of anaphylaxis. The FDA recommends spot treatment (one to two areas) with small amount of product for the first few applications to mitigate this risk.
- Skin irritation/erythema
- Only for external use: do not apply to eyes, lips, or other mucosal surfaces.
- Avoid use of benzoyl peroxide containing products in neonates.

Important Drug Interactions

The frequency of the following potential drug interactions is not defined.

- Dapsone (topical): Concurrent use may cause temporary discoloration (yellow-orange) of face/hair.
- Sodium sulfacetamide-sulfur: Concurrent use may cause temporary discoloration (yellow-orange) of face/hair
- Tretinoin (topical): Concurrent application of non-microencapsulated formulations of benzoyl peroxide may decrease effectiveness of tretinoin. Do not apply both medications at the same time. Generally, it is recommended to apply benzoyl peroxide products in the morning and topical retinoid products at night (as the latter can cause some photosensitivity).
- Topical anesthetics (benzocaine, tetracaine, procaine, pramoxine, prilocaine, and lidocaine): Concurrent use may decrease effectiveness of anesthetic.

Adverse Effects and Their Management

- Bleaching of hair and clothing may occur.
- Dry skin, desquamation, burning, or stinging (irritant dermatitis). This can be minimized by decreasing concentration or frequency of benzoyl peroxide use. Additionally, this is often soothed and improved by using a light non-comedogenic moisturizer. Discontinue if significant discomfort develops. Use with caution in patients with dry skin and atopic dermatitis.
- Allergic contact dermatitis. Patch testing may be indicated for diagnosis.
- Photosensitivity/rare phototoxicity

Essential Patient information

- Bleaching and staining of fabrics may occur. Cotton fabrics appear to be more affected than synthetic fabrics. Washing fabrics within 8 h of contact with benzoyl peroxide may decrease staining. Wait until product is completely dry if

leave-on product, or make sure washed off completely (if short contact foam, cleansing wash/bar, shave cream) prior to putting on clothes.
- Discontinue if significant redness, scaling, and irritation develops. Let your clinician know if this occurs.
- Practice sun protection while using this medication including sunscreen when appropriate.
- Do not mix with other acne medications unless directed by your clinician.

Carcinogenicity
- In animal studies, benzoyl peroxide has been shown to promote tumor progression and to increase photocarcinogicity (including in over-the-counter combination products). In one study, BPO in acetone administered twice a week over 20 weeks induced squamous cell skin cancers. These studies have not been performed or replicated in humans, and the clinical significance remains unknown.

Patch Test Concentration
- 1.0% pet. (Chemotechnique, SmartPracticeEurope, SmartPracticeCanada); great risk of irritant reactions

Clascoterone

Classification and Mode of Action
- Topical acne medication; androgen receptor antagonist
- MOA: Competitive androgen receptor antagonist. By competing with dihydrotestosterone for androgen receptor binding, clascoterone limits downstream sebum production and curbs local inflammation.

Indications and Dermatological Uses
- *Clinical indications (FDA)*: Acne vulgaris (patients 12 years of age and older)
- *Off-label common uses*: N/A

Formulations/Presentation

- US: Cream 1% (Winlevi) clascoterone 1%; inactive ingredients

Dosages and Suggested Regimens: Adult

- Acne vulgaris: Gently cleanse acne prone area with mild soap and water. Gently dry skin, then apply thin, even layer to the affected area(s) twice daily, morning and evening.

Pharmacokinetics

- Absorption: Systemic absorption reaches steady state by day 5. In general, metabolites of clascoterone were below or near detectable levels in the serum (0.5 ng/mL) in patients >12 years of age.
- Elimination: Cortexolone is the possible primary metabolite. In vitro studies indicate at least partial hepatic metabolism.
- Excretion: Has not been characterized yet in human studies

Use in Special Populations

Pregnancy

- There are no data evaluating the safety of using Clascoterone cream in pregnant adults.
- There are animal studies suggesting fetal pregnancy complications and pregnancy loss attributed to dosing above maximal recommended dose. As such, it is most prudent to recommend against use in pregnancy.

Lactation:

- There are no data evaluating the safety of using topical Clascoterone in breastfeeding patients.
- The potential risks and benefits of androgen blockage and the risks and benefits of breastfeeding while using this medication should be discussed with each patient individually.
- Additionally, assessing lactating patients need for the medication while breastfeeding an infant should be addressed.

Pediatric use:

- Safety and efficacy have been reported with using topical Clascoterone in children age 12 and older for acne vulgaris.

- There are no safety/efficacy data available for children under 12 years of age.
- It is important to note that Hypothalamic-pituitary-adrenal (HPA) axis suppression was noted in 2/22 (9%) of adolescents. Both affected children had axis function return to normal one month after stopping the medication.

Geriatric use:
- To date, there is not sufficient data in the safe use of Clascoterone in patients older than 65.
- Recommend caution in starting geriatric patients on this medication, with consideration for lower dosing/frequency of application.

Renal and hepatic insufficiency
- There are no dosing adjustments provided on the manufacturer's label.

Monitoring
- No specific monitoring guidelines

Contraindications and Cautions
- HPA axis suppression observed.
- Hyperkalemia, caution when using in patient with underlying heart disease
- Caution with use in pregnant, lactating, pediatric and elderly patients
- Not approved for use in children under the age of 12
- Do not apply to open wounds or abraded, eczematous, or sunburned skin.

Important Drug Interactions
- No clinical studies evaluating drug-drug interactions have been completed to date.

Adverse Effects and Their Management
- Skin irritation: erythema, pruritus, scaling/dry texture (~7–12%), edema, and stinging/burning (>3%). In phase 3 clinical trials, these occurred with a similar frequency as the

vehicle control arm. If this occurs and is significant, consider decreasing frequency, medication holidays, and/or discontinuation.
- Less commonly observed local cutaneous side effects in the phase 3 clinical trials included striae rubrae (2.5%) and telangiectasia (1.2%). In phase 3 clinical trials, these occurred with a similar frequency as the vehicle control arm. A 9-month safety trial did not show increase in striae rubra, telangiectasia, or atrophy in subjects treated with topical Clascoterone. If new atrophy, striae, or telangiectasia is observed, discontinue use.
- In the long-term safety trial, one patient developed depigmented hair in the area treated with Clascoterone cream.
- HPA axis suppression was observed in PK studies (adult: 1/20 subjects, pediatric: 2/22). If symptoms of HPA axis suppression develop, discontinue medication. Risk of systemic Clascoterone absorption increases with occlusion, use on large body surface area, and prolonged use. Of note, clinical trials did not show systemic antiandrogen activity.

Essential Patient Information

- Do not apply to open wounds or abraded, eczematous, or sunburned skin.
- Do not apply to mucous membranes.
- Avoid concomitant use of potentially drying and irritating skin products (e.g., astringents, drying soaps, and cleansers)
- Notify clinician if symptoms of HPA-axis suppression occur including weakness, malaise, fatigue, nausea, abdominal pain, headache, and poor weight gain.

Carcinogenesis

- In a 2-year long rat study, daily application of Clascoterone cream (0.1%, 1%, 5%) was not carcinogenic. An Ames reverse mutation assay showed that Clascoterone was not mutagenic.

Patch Test Concentration

- N/A

Common Brand Names

- Winlevi

Clindamycin

Classification and Mode of Action

- Topical acne product; topical antibiotic, lincosamide
- Reversibly binds the bacterial 50S ribosomal subunit, preventing protein synthesis. This effect can be either bacteriostatic or bactericidal depending on the drug concentration used and organism targeted.

Indications and Dermatological Uses

- *Clinical indications (FDA)*: Inflammatory lesions of acne vulgaris
- *Off-label common uses*: Hidradenitis suppurativa, rosacea (inflammatory lesions), folliculitis

Formulations/Presentation (Vaginal Creams/ Suppositories Not Outlined)

US:

- Foam, 1% (Evoclin, Generic)
- Gel, 1% (Cleocin-T, Clindagel, Generic)
- Pledgets and Swab, 1% (Clindacin ETZ, Clindacin Pac—available in Kit with acne wash, Clindacin-P, Generic)
- Lotion, 1% (Cleocin-T, Generic)
- Solution, 1% (Cleocin-T, Generic)
- Foam, 1% (Evoclin)
- Generic: 1%

Canada:

- Solution, 1% (Clinda-T, Dalacin T, Generic)
- Gel, 1% (Biacna, Generic)

Dosages and Suggested Regimens

Acne vulgaris:

- Gel, pledgets, lotion, and solution: Apply a thin film to acne-prone areas twice daily
- Gel (Clindagel) and foam (Evoclin): Apply to acne-prone areas once daily

Hidradenitis suppurativa (off-label use):

- Solution: apply twice daily to affected area(s)

Rosacea (off-label use):

- Lotion: Apply twice daily to the face

Folliculitis (off-label use):

- Gel, lotion, solution: apply twice a day to affected area × 7–10 days

Pharmacokinetics

- Absorption: Topical solution, lotions, gels, or foams have minimal systemic absorption. As such, there is no relevant data on systemic metabolism, half-life, or time to peak serum concentration.
- Excretion: Urine (<0.2% with topical preparations)

Use in Special Populations

Pregnancy:

- Clindamycin crosses the placenta when administered through oral or parenteral routes. The amount of clindamycin present systemically is significantly less when administered topically.
- If antibiotic treatment for acne vulgaris is deemed necessary during pregnancy by patient and clinician, topical clindamycin is a reasonable option to consider. However, pregnant patients should avoid repetitive application inflamed or open skin and should not apply to large surface areas, just locally to affected skin.

Lactation:

- While clindamycin is present in breast milk following oral and IV dosing, it is not presently known if clindamycin is present in breast milk following topical application. In general, it is known that there is very minimal systemic absorption of topical clindamycin, which should minimize potential exposure to breastfeeding infant.

- Consider monitoring breastfeeding infants for diarrhea and hematochezia if clindamycin is indicated for a breastfeeding mother.
- To decrease level of systemic exposure, breastfeeding patients should avoid repetitive application to inflamed or open skin and should not apply to large surface areas.
- The manufacturer states the decision to continue or discontinue breastfeeding should be made after a discussion of the potential risks of exposure to the infant and potential benefits to the breastfeeding mother.

Pediatric use:

- Safety and efficacy in children under 12 years of age have not been established.

Renal insufficiency:

- There are no dosing adjustments provided on the manufacturer's label.

Hepatic insufficiency:

- There are no dosing adjustments provided on the manufacturer's label.

Monitoring

- No specific monitoring guidelines

Contraindications and Cautions

- Hypersensitivity to clindamycin, lincomycin, or any component of the product's formulation
- History of antibiotic-associated colitis
- Regional enteritis
- Ulcerative colitis
- *Caution:* Given the risk of bacterial resistance, it is recommended clindamycin be used in combination with other agents, such as topical benzoyl peroxide, topical retinoids, and/or systemic antibiotics.

Important Drug Interactions

The frequency of the following potential drug interactions is not defined.

- Erythromycin (systemic): May reduce the therapeutic effect of topical clindamycin. Avoid concurrent use in treating acne vulgaris.
- Erythromycin (topical): May reduce the therapeutic effect of topical clindamycin. Avoid concurrent use (especially at the same application site) in treating acne vulgaris.
- Neuromuscular-blocking agents: Topical clindamycin may enhance the effect of neuromuscular-blocking agents.

Adverse Effects and Their Management

- Local skin irritation (itching, burning, dryness, redness, and peeling/desquamation). Discontinue if this occurs. This may occur with any of the formulations but may be less frequent with the foam when used in acne vulgaris.
- Oily skin
- Hypersensitivity: Allergic contact dermatitis or urticaria. Discontinue therapy if this occurs.
- Rare diarrhea, bloody diarrhea, nausea, and abdominal discomfort. Discontinue if this occurs. *C. difficile* colitis has rarely been reported with topical clindamycin.
- Gram-negative folliculitis. If suspected, discontinue clindamycin, culture skin pustule if possible, and start therapy for gram-negative folliculitis.

Essential Patient Information

- Topical clindamycin should be used whenever possible with other topical acne treatments such as benzoyl peroxide or topical retinoids to minimize bacterial resistance.
- Foam is flammable and should not be used around open fire, flame, or smoking.
- Let your clinician know if you have worsening acne despite treatment with topical clindamycin. In some cases, this may indicate gram-negative folliculitis, which requires a different approach to treatment.

Carcinogenicity

- Daily application of topical clindamycin at 3–15 times higher doses than commercially available resulted in no significant increase in tumors in animal studies.

Patch Test Concentration

- Phosphate, 10.0% pet. (Chemotechnique)

Common Brand Names

Cleocin; Cleocin-T; Clindacin ETZ; Clindacin Pac; Clindacin-P; Clindagel; Clindesse; Evoclin: Clinda-T; Dalacin T [DSC]; Dalacin Vaginal; TARO-Clindamycin

Dapsone

Classification and Mode of Action

- Sulfone, unknown but thought to work as an anti-inflammatory agent.

Indications and Dermatological Uses

- *Clinical indications (FDA)*: topical treatment of acne vulgaris
- *Off-label common uses*: none

Formulations/Presentation

- US: Acne 5% or 7.5% gel (Aczone, generic)
- Canada: 5% gel (Aczone)

Dosages and Suggested Regimens

- Acne vulgaris: apply approximately a pea-sized amount of gel in a thin layer to the entire face once daily. A thin layer can also be applied to other affected areas.

Baseline Investigations and Considerations

- None

Pharmacokinetics

Absorption:

- The systemic exposure from dapsone gel, 7.5% is expected to be about 1% of that from a 100 mg oral dose.

Use in Special Populations

Pregnancy:

- There are no available data on dapsone use in pregnant women to inform risk for adverse developmental outcomes.
- In animal studies on rats, maternal toxicity and developmental effects were seen at a dapsone dose of 30 mg/kg/day (approximately 563 times the systemic exposure with maximum recommended human dose of dapsone gel, 7.5%).

Lactation:

- There is no information regarding the presence of topical dapsone in breastmilk, the effects on the breastfed infant, or the effects on milk production.
- Orally administered dapsone appears in human milk and could result in hemolytic anemia and hyperbilirubinemia, especially in infants with G6PD deficiency.
- The manufacturer states that the decision to use dapsone should include a discussion of the developmental and health benefits of breastfeeding, along with the mother's clinical need for treatment, and any potential adverse effects on the child from dapsone or the underlying maternal condition.

Pediatric use:

- Dapsone gel, 7.5%, is safe to use for the topical treatment of acne vulgaris in patients 9 years of age or older.
- Safety and effectiveness of dapsone gel, 7.5%, have not been established in patients below age 9 years.

Renal insufficiency: There are no dosing adjustments provided on the manufacturer's label.

Hepatic insufficiency: There are no dosing adjustments provided on the manufacturer's label.

Monitoring

- No specific monitoring guidelines

Contraindications and Cautions

- No contraindications
- Temporary yellow or orange discoloration of the skin and facial hair may be seen when benzoyl peroxide is applied after dapsone.
- *Caution:* Cases of methemoglobinemia have been reported with twice daily dapsone gel, 5%, treatment. Patients with G6PD deficiency or congenital or idiopathic methemoglobinemia are more susceptible. Avoid use in these patients.
- *Caution:* Dose-related hemolysis and hemolytic anemia have been seen with oral dapsone treatment. There was no evidence of clinically relevant hemolysis or hemolytic anemia in clinical trials with topical dapsone, but some subjects with G6PD deficiency using dapsone gel, 5%, twice daily did show laboratory changes suggestive of hemolysis. Avoid use in patients who are taking oral dapsone or antimalarials due to potential for hemolytic reactions. Additionally, combination of dapsone gel, 7.5%, with trimethoprim/sulfamethoxazole (TMP/SMX) may increase the likelihood of hemolysis in patients with G6PD deficiency.

Important Drug Interactions

- No formal drug-drug interaction studies have been conducted with dapsone gel, 7.5%.
- Trimethoprim-sulfamethoxazole (TMP/SMX): When combined with double strength (160 mg/800 mg) TMP/SMX, levels of dapsone and its metabolites were increased. However, the systemic exposure with dapsone gel, 7.5%, is still expected to be about 1% of that from the 100 mg oral dose when administered with TMP/SMX.
- Drugs that induce methemoglobinemia: The risk for developing methemoglobinemia may be increased when administered with drugs that induce methemoglobinemia, such as sulfonamides, acetaminophen, phenytoin, and others.

Adverse Effects and Their Management

- Skin irritation, peeling, dryness, erythema, pruritus, dermatitis, and swelling of the face, lips, and eyes. If this occurs and is severe or intolerable, discontinue therapy.
- Methemoglobinemia. May present initially as cyanosis of mucous membranes, lips, and nail beds. Discontinue topical dapsone if this occurs.
- Respiratory: Nasopharyngitis, sinusitis, and cough were reported in less than 5% of subjects in the Aczone 5% clinical trials. Unclear if these symptoms are truly related to the topical dapsone. If it occurs, consider discontinuing. If not severe, can consider retrial topical dapsone once symptoms resolve.
- Headache was also noted in 4% of patients in the Aczone clinical trials. Unclear if these symptoms are truly related to the topical dapsone. If it occurs, consider discontinuing. If not severe, can consider retrial topical dapsone once symptoms resolve.
- In clinical trials of Aczone 5% the following severe adverse events were reported: suicide attempt, tonic clonic movements, abdominal pain, severe vomiting, and pancreatitis. This was not reported in the Aczone 7.5%.
- Orally administered dapsone has been associated with hemolytic anemia, agranulocytosis, motor peripheral neuropathy, and severe cutaneous drug reactions. These were not observed in clinical trials of topical dapsone.

Carcinogenicity

- No carcinogenesis observed when rats were exposed to systemic dapsone in doses up to 340 times the systemic exposure observed in humans as a result of the use of the maximum recommended human dose of Aczone gel, 7.5%. Dermal studies in Tg.AC transgenic mice showed no induction of carcinogenesis with topically applied dapsone 3%, 5% and 10%.
- Ames test of Dapsone did not show mutagenesis; however, it did induce structural chromosomal aberrations in Chinese hamster ovary cells.

Patch Test Concentration

- N/A

Essential Patient Information

- Seek immediate medical attention if cyanosis develops while using this medication.

Erythromycin

Classification and Mode of Action

- Topical acne product; topical antibiotic, macrolide
- MOA: Reversibly binds the bacterial 50S ribosomal subunit, preventing protein synthesis. Alcohol component can be quite drying.

Indications and Dermatological Uses

- *Clinical indications (FDA)*: Acne vulgaris
- Note: The AAD recommends against use as monotherapy given risk for bacterial resistance (AAD [48]).
- *Off-label common uses*: Rosacea, perioral dermatitis

Formulations/Presentation (Vaginal Creams/ Suppositories Not Outlined)

US:

- Gel: 2% (Erygel, Generic)
- Swab: 2% (Generic)
- Solution: 2% (Erythra-Derm, Generic)

Canada:

- Gel: 3% with 5% benzoyl peroxide (Benzamycin)

Dosages and Suggested Regimens

Prior to treatment, wash affected areas with soap and water and rinse and pat dry. Avoid contact with mucous membranes.

- Gel: Apply thin film to acne-prone areas once to twice daily. May take 6–8 weeks before effect is appreciated. Discontinue if no improvement after 6–8 weeks.

- Pads: Rub pad over acne prone areas twice daily. More than one pad can be used, if necessary.
- Solution: Apply to the affected area twice daily. Frequency of application may be limited by skin dryness.

Baseline Investigations and Considerations

- None

Pharmacokinetics

- Absorption: Topical formulations have minimal systemic absorption. As such, there is no relevant data on systemic metabolism, half-life, or time to peak serum concentration.

Use in Special Populations

Pregnancy:

- The amount of erythromycin available systemically after being applied topically is exceedingly low. Systemic absorption is required for the medication to cross the placenta.
- Because the risk to the fetus is low, antibiotic treatment for acne vulgaris with topical erythromycin is a reasonable option to consider.

Lactation:

- Currently, it is not known if erythromycin is present in breast milk after topical application. As above, amount of erythromycin systemically available after topical application is exceedingly low and is thus considered generally compatible to use in lactating patients.

Pediatric use:

- Safety and efficacy in patients less than 12 years of age have not been established.

Renal insufficiency:

- There are no dosing adjustments provided on the manufacturer's label.

Hepatic insufficiency:

- There are no dosing adjustments provided on the manufacturer's label.

Monitoring

No specific monitoring guidelines

Contraindications and Cautions

- Hypersensitivity to erythromycin, macrolide antibiotics, or any component of its formulation
- Pseudomembranous colitis. Discontinue if patient develops diarrhea, abdominal pain, hematochezia, or melena
- Given the risk of bacterial resistance, it is recommended clindamycin be used in combination with other agents, such as topical benzoyl peroxide, topical retinoids, and/or systemic antibiotics.
- Topical gel may be flammable.
- May cause significant skin dryness and/or redness when used in combination with other topical acne products.
- Keep away from broken/damaged skin. Do not apply to any mucous membranes, including eyes, nose, mouth, etc.

Important Drug Interactions

The frequency of the following potential drug interactions is not defined.

- Clindamycin (topical): May reduce the therapeutic effect of topical clindamycin. Avoid concurrent use in treating acne vulgaris.
- Isotretinoin (topical): May enhance the adverse effects of topical erythromycin, see below.

Adverse Effects and Their Management

- Local skin effects: Skin peeling, xerosis, itching, burning, redness, irritation, and oily skin. Discontinue if symptoms are significant.
- May irritate eyes and mucosal surfaces if used on nearby skin or mucosal surface itself.
- Generalized urticaria and other hypersensitivity reactions have been reported. Discontinue if this occurs.
- Superinfection of skin by non-susceptible organisms may occur with the use of topical antibiotics. If this occurs, discontinue therapy and treat superinfection

Carcinogenesis

- No investigations into the carcinogenic potential of topical erythromycin have been performed. Studies of rats exposed to oral erythromycin (base) over 2 years did not show tumorigenicity.

Patch Test Concentration

- 2% pet. (SmartPractice Canada, SmartPracticeEurope), 1% pet. (SmartPracticeCanada), 10.0% pet (Chemotechnique). 1% may sometimes be too low.

Common Brand Names

- Erygel

Minocycline

Classification and Mode of Action

- Tetracycline class antibiotic. Bacteriostatic medication that suppresses bacterial protein synthesis. Antibiotic effect against skin flora including some strains of *Cutibacterium acnes*.
- Minocycline also has anti-inflammatory effects, which may help improve acne. Some proposed anti-inflammatory mechanisms include inhibition of matrix metalloproteinases, suppression of neutrophil chemotaxis, and downregulation of inflammatory cytokines.

Indications and Dermatological Uses

- *Clinical indications (FDA)*: Inflammatory lesions of rosacea and acne
- *Off-label common uses*: N/A

Formulations/Presentation

- US:
  - Rosacea: Topical foam 1.5%, 15 mg minocycline/gram (Zilxi)
  - Acne: foam 4%, 40 mg minocycline/gram (Amzeeq)

Dosages and Suggested Regimens

- Acne: Shake can before use. Apply a "cherry-sized" amount of foam once a day to affected areas of face at least 1 h before bedtime. Additional amount of foam can be used to other acne affected areas (e.g., chest, back, neck, shoulders, and arms).
- Rosacea: Shake can before use. Apply a "cherry-sized" amount of foam once a day to affected areas of face at least 1 h before bedtime. Additional amount of foam can be used if needed to cover the entire affected area.

Baseline Investigations and Considerations

- None

Pharmacokinetics

Absorption:

- Minocycline 4% foam (Amzeeq): Following application once daily for 21 days, systemic minocycline exposure was 730–765 times lower than minocycline administered orally.
- Minocycline 1.5% foam (Zilxi): When 2 g applied to the whole face, a very low amount absorbed in plasma (day 1: Cmax 1.30 ng/mL and day 14: 0.75 ng/mL). Systemic accumulation was not observed.

Use in Special Populations

Pregnancy:

- Safety in pregnant women has not been established, but systemic absorption of topical minocycline foam is low. Administration of oral minocycline can result in skeletal defects, permanent discoloration of teeth and bone growth inhibition.

Lactation:

- Safety in lactation has not been established. Accumulation of minocycline in breast milk after topical application has not been studied. Recommend avoidance in lactation.

Pediatric use:

- Safety has not been established in children younger than 9 years old. Recommend avoiding use in this age group given risks of permanent tooth discoloration, tooth enamel hypoplasia, and potential bone growth abnormalities with oral administration of tetracycline antibiotics.

Renal: No dose adjustments have been recommended by the manufacturer.

Hepatic: No dose adjustments have been recommended by the manufacturer.

Monitoring

- Skin sensitivity
- Photosensitivity
- Diarrhea
- Headache with visual changes
- Skin discoloration

Contraindications and Cautions

- The propellant used in the can is flammable. Advise patients during and immediately after application to avoid open flames and smoking.

Important Drug Interactions

- Anticoagulants. Tetracycline class antibiotics can reduce prothrombin activity. Patients on tetracycline class antibiotics and anticoagulants may require a decrease in the dose of their anticoagulant.
- Penicillin. Avoid concomitant use. Tetracycline class antibiotics can affect penicillin bactericidal activity.
- Benzoyl peroxide. If applied together, benzoyl peroxide can inactivate minocycline foam.

Adverse Effects and Their Management

- May cause application site discomfort, skin dryness, and erythema. Discontinue if significant.
- Headache was the most common side effect with minocycline 4% foam in the clinical studies affecting 3% of subjects com-

pared to 2% of vehicle treated patients. If persistent or "unusual" headaches (particularly if associated with changes in vision) develop, the medication should be discontinued.

- May cause temporary yellow tint of skin and nails that can be washed off with soap and water. Wait at least 1 h after application before washing off.
- May discolor fabrics.
- Orally administered minocycline has been associated with multiple adverse reactions. These have not been demonstrated with topical application; however, patients and prescribers should be aware of these side effects. If they occur, the topical minocycline foam should be discontinued. These side effects include: *Clostridioides difficile* associated diarrhea, hepatotoxicity, autoimmune syndromes (fevers, arthralgia, malaise, and rash), central nervous system effects, intracranial hypertension, hyperpigmentation of scars, skin, teeth and gums, superinfection by non-susceptible organisms, and hypersensitivity reactions (e.g., anaphylaxis, Stevens-Johnson syndrome, drug reaction with eosinophilia, and other serious cutaneous eruptions).
- May increase the risk of superinfection by minocycline non-susceptible microbes and fungi. Discontinue topical minocycline if this occurs and start therapy for the superinfection.
- Possible photosensitivity. Orally administered minocycline is associated with photosensitivity; however, studies of minocycline foam application under ultraviolet light did not show development of phototoxicity or photoallergy.

Carcinogenicity

- Carcinogenicity studies are available in rats. One study showed that orally administered minocycline in doses up to 200 mg/kg/day for 104 weeks was associated with follicular cell tumors (adenomas and carcinomas) of the thyroid gland in both male and female rats. Another study that administered oral minocycline up to 150 mg/kg/day for 104 weeks showed no increase in neoplasms.

Patch Test Concentration

- N/A

Essential Patient Information

- Patients should be advised to practice diligent sun protection and minimize exposure to natural or artificial ultraviolet light. Discontinue minocycline foam if sunburn occurs.
- Avoid open flames and smoking during and immediately after application.
- At home, store at temperatures below 25 °C (77 °F) for 90 days. Do not store in refrigerator. Do not expose to temperatures above 49 °C (120 °F). Do not store near flame.
- Foam should be applied at approximately the same time each day. Avoid bathing, swimming, or showering for at least 1 h after application.
- Don't use on mucous membranes or ocular mucosa.
- May take up to 3 months to see full benefit of minocycline 1.5% foam.
- Wait at least 8 h between application of minocycline foam and any benzoyl peroxide product.
- Avoid use in children under 9 years old.

Resorcinol

Classification and Mode of Action

- Isomer of hydroquinone.
- Reducing agent with antibacterial and keratolytic properties by disrupting hydrogen bonds of keratin.

Indications and Dermatological Uses

- *Clinical indications (FDA):* Topical treatment of acne vulgaris and seborrheic dermatitis
- *Off-label common uses:* Post-inflammatory hyperpigmentation/erythema, acne scarring, and analgesia

Formulations/Presentation

- US: There are a variety of over-the-counter formulations. Examples include Resorcinol 2% ointment (Resinol) or 2% cream with 2%, 5%, or 8% sulfur (Rezamid, Acnomel, and other generic).
- Resorcinol is also used in a variety of chemical peels.

Dosages and Suggested Regimens

- Acne vulgaris:
  - 2% ointment: apply to affected area not more than three to four times daily
  - 2% cream: cover the entire affected area with a thin layer one to three times a day

Pharmacokinetics

Absorption:

- Dermal absorption appears to be low (<1%) when applied on intact skin.

Use in Special Populations

Pregnancy:

- Contraindicated in pregnancy due to lack of study data.

Lactation:

- No data available.

Pediatric use:

- Safety and effectiveness of topical resorcinol in pediatric patients have not been established.

Renal insufficiency: There are no dosing adjustments provided on the manufacturer's label.

Hepatic insufficiency: There are no dosing adjustments provided on the manufacturer's label.

Monitoring

- No specific monitoring guidelines.

Contraindications and Cautions

- *Contraindications:* Pregnancy and skin type VI, due to lack of data regarding complications.
- Resorcinol should not be applied to large areas of the body, for prolonged periods, or in high concentrations due to potential for interference with thyroid function or production of methemoglobinemia.
- May produce hyperpigmentation and darken lighter hair colors.

Important Drug Interactions

- There have been no formal studies of the interaction of topical resorcinol with other drugs.

Adverse Effects and Their Management

- No manufacturer studies of adverse effects available.
- Adverse effects that have been reported include hyperpigmentation, burning sensations, and paresthesias.

Carcinogenicity

- In studies of oral administration to male and female rats at doses of 50 mg/kg or greater, there was no evidence of carcinogenic activity.

Patch Test Concentration

- 1% pet. (Chemotechnique, SmartPracticeCanada), 2% pet (SmartPracticeEurope, SmartPracticeCanada)

Essential Patient Information

- N/A

Retinoids

See under Chap. 22: Retinoids

Salicylic Acid

See under Chap. 21: Psoriasis

Sulfur and Sulfacetamide

Classification and Mode of Action

- Sulfur is a chemical element thought to have antibacterial effects by conversion of sulfur to pentathionic acid.

- May suppress C. acnes proliferation in sebaceous follicle.
- Also thought to possess keratolytic action when reduced via direct interaction with keratinocytes to form hydrogen sulfide.
- May also have effect on decreasing facial demodex counts.

- Sodium sulfacetamide is a sulfonamide that has a bacteriostatic effect by restricting synthesis of folic acid through competition with para-aminobenzoic acid.

Indications and Dermatological Uses

- *Clinical indications (FDA)*: Acne vulgaris, rosacea (inflammatory papules and pustules), seborrheic dermatitis
- *Off-label common uses*: perioral dermatitis, scabies, superficial fungal infections, secondary bacterial infections due to organisms susceptible to sulfonamides

Formulations/Presentation

- Available products include combination sulfur and sulfacetamide, sulfacetamide-only and sulfur-only in a variety of formulations. Some formulations contain additional ingredients such as salicylic acid, resorcinol, sunscreen, tints, bakuchiol, and urea.
- US:
  - Sulfur and sulfacetamide sodium products:
    - Cleanser, topical:
      - Sulfur 5% and sulfacetamide sodium 10%: AVAR, Clenia, Prascion, Rosanil. Generic formulations available
      - Sulfur 2% and sulfacetamide sodium 10%; AVAR LS, Generic formulations available
      - Sulfur 4.8% and sulfacetamide sodium 9.8%; Prascion cleanser. Generic formulations available.
    - Cream, topical:
      - Sulfur 5% and sodium sulfacetamide 10% : AVAR-e, AVAR-e Green (corrective cream), Clenia, SSS, Virti-sulf. Generic formulations available.
      - Sulfur 2% and sulfacetamide sodium 10%: AVAR-e LS, Generic formulations available.

    - Sulfur 4.8% and sulfacetamide sodium 9.8%: Generic formulations available.
  - Foam, topical:
    - Sulfur 5% and sulfacetamide sodium 10%: SSS. Generic formulations available.
    - Sulfur 5% and sulfacetamide sodium 9.5%: AVAR
    - Sulfur 2% and sulfacetamide sodium 10%: AVAR LS
  - Lotion, topical:
    - Sulfur 4.8% and sulfacetamide sodium 9.8%; Generic.
  - Gel, topical:
    - Sulfur 5%, sodium sulfacetamide 10% and urea 10%; Rosula, Generic.
  - Cleansing cloth:
    - Sulfur 5% and sulfacetamide sodium 10%; Rosula.
    - Sulfur 4.8% and sulfacetamide sodium 9.8%; Generic.
    - Sulfur 4% and sulfacetamide sodium 10%; Sumaxin, Generic.
  - Suspension, topical:
    - Sulfur 4% and sulfacetamide sodium 8%; SulfaCleanse 8/4, Sumaxin TS, Generic.
  - Wash:
    - Sulfur 1% and sulfacetamide sodium 10%: BP 10-1, Sulfamez wash, Generic.
    - Sulfur 4% and sulfacetamide sodum 10%: BP cleansing Wash
    - Sulfur 4.5% and sulfacetamide sodium 10%: Rosula wash
    - Sulfur 4.5% and sulfacetamide sodium 9%: Sumadan, Sumadan XLT
    - Sulfur 4% and sulfacetamide sodium 9%: Sumaxin, Generic.
- Sodium sulfacetamide only products:
  - Lotion, external:
    - 10% sulfacetamide sodium: Klaron, Generic (indicated for acne)
    - 9.8% sulfacetamide sodium: Ovace Plus

    - Liquid:
      - 10% sulfacetamide sodium: Ovace Plus Wash, Ovace Wash, Seb-Prev Wash, Generic.
      - Combination therapy of sodium sulfacetamide 10% -Bakuchiol: APOP gel.
    - Cream, external
      - 10% sodium sulfacetamide: Ovace Plus (indicated for seborrheic dermatitis/scaling dermatoses and bacteria infections)
    - Foam, external
      - 9.8% sodium sulfacetamide: Ovace Plus
    - Wash/cleansing gel, external (indicated for seborrheic dermatitis):
      - 10% sodium sulfacetamide: Ovace Plus Wash cleansing gel, SEB-Prev, Generic.
    - Shampoo:
      - 10% sodium sulfacetamide: Ovace Plus
      - 9.8% sodium sulfacetamide: Generic.
  - Sulfur products (also comes with salicylic acid for seborrheic dermatitis):
    - Sulfur is found in many over-the-counter formulations such as bar soaps, cleansers, creams, lotions and masks.
    - Precipitated sulfur can be compounded as a 2–9% topical gel, cream, body wash and lotion for treatment of acne, seborrheic dermatitis, scabies.
    - Many additional over-the-counter formulations of sulfur or sodium sulfacetamide available.
    - Combination sodium sulfacetamide-sulfur is typically only found in prescription products.
- Canada:
  - Sulfur products (also comes with salicylic acid for seborrheic dermatitis):
    - Sulfur is found in many over-the-counter formulations such as bar soaps, cleansers, creams, lotions, and masks.
    - Precipitated sulfur can be compounded as a 2–9% topical gel, cream, body wash, and lotion for treatment of acne, seborrheic dermatitis, and scabies.

    - Many additional over-the-counter formulations of sulfur or sodium sulfacetamide available.
    - Combination sodium sulfacetamide-sulfur is typically only found in prescription products

Dosages and Suggested Regimens

- Different products have different regimens, so it is important to read the package insert before applying.
- Acne/rosacea:
  - Sodium sulfacetamide-sulfur lotion and cream: apply one to three times daily to affected skin after cleansing.
  - Sodium sulfacetamide-sulfur cleansing cloth: use one to two times a day. Moisten cloth with water, massage skin for 10–20 s then rinse skin completely.
  - Sodium sulfacetamide-sulfur washes, cleansers, and suspensions: Use to wash affected areas one to two times a day.
  - Sodium sulfacetamide-sulfur foam:
    - SSS foam: Apply one or two times a day after washing affected areas. May use in a wash-off application (product washed off after 1–2 min) or as a leave-on application (product is not washed off).
    - Avar foam: Apply one to three times a day. After washing skin, apply product to affected area and wait 10 min. Rinse off with water.
  - Sodium sulfacetamide lotion: Apply a thin film to affected areas twice daily.
- Seborrheic dermatitis:
  - Sodium sulfacetamide lotion, foam, and cream: Apply a thin film to affected areas twice daily.

Pharmacokinetics

Absorption:

- After topical application, approximately 1% of sulfur is systematically absorbed. Systemic absorption of sulfacetamide after topical administration is unknown.

Use in Special Populations

Pregnancy:

- There have not been any animal reproductive studies for topical sulfur or sulfacetamide. The manufacturer recommends administration to a pregnant woman only if clearly needed.

Lactation:

- Systemically administered sulfonamides are capable of producing kernicterus in infants of lactating women. Excretion in human milk following topical use of sulfur sulfacetamide is unknown.

Pediatric use:

- Safety in children under 12 years is unknown.
- Some formulations contain benzyl alcohol which can cause fatal "gasping syndrome" in neonates.

Renal insufficiency: There are no dosing adjustments provided on the manufacturer's label.

Hepatic insufficiency: There are no dosing adjustments provided on the manufacturer's label.

Monitoring

- No specific monitoring guidelines.

Contraindications and Cautions

- *Contraindications:* Hypersensitivity to sulfonamides, sulfur, or any other component of the preparation.
- *Caution:* Sulfonamide class mediations have been associated with severe reactions including Stevens-Johnson syndrome, toxic epidermal necrolysis, fulminant hepatic necrosis, agranulocytosis, aplastic anemia, and other blood dyscrasias. Sensitivity reactions have been reported in individuals with no prior history of sulfonamide hypersensitivity. Discontinue use at the first sign of any such reactions.
- *Caution:* Klaron lotion contains sodium metabisulfite, which may cause anaphylactic symptoms and life-threatening asthmatic episodes in susceptible persons.

Important Drug Interactions

- Concomitant use of benzoyl peroxide and sulfacetamide can result in orange-brown staining on skin or clothing.
- Do not concomitantly use with preparations containing silver.
- There have been no formal studies of the interaction of topical sulfur/sulfacetamide with other drugs.

Adverse Effects and Their Management

- Rare local side effects reported including pruritus, dryness, and erythema. If irritation develops, stop the use of medication.
- Use around the eyes may irritate conjunctiva.
- Case reports of Stevens-Johnson syndrome and erythema multiforme following ophthalmic use of sodium sulfacetamide.
- May stain clothes and skin if used together with benzoyl peroxide. Use at a separate time from benzoyl peroxide application.

Carcinogenicity

- Long-term studies in animals have not been performed to evaluate carcinogenic potential.

Patch Test Concentration

- Sulfacetamide: 5% pet.

Tea Tree Oil

Classification and Mode of Action

- Tea tree oil is derived by distillation of leaves from the tea tree.
- This distillate contains over 100 monoterpenoid, sesquiterpenoid, and alcohol compounds. Up to 90% is composed of terpinene-4-ol, 1,8-cineole, alpha-terpineol, terpinolene, and alpha- and gamma-terpinene.
- The primary component is terpinene-4-ol, and some products are standardized to this component.
- Tea tree oil has been found to have activity against *C. acnes*.

Indications and Dermatological Uses

- *Clinical indications (FDA):* none
- *Off-label common uses:* acne, onychomycosis, tinea pedis, oral candidiasis, molluscum contagiosum, and seborrheic dermatitis

Formulations/Presentation

- US: Tea tree oil is available over the counter as a natural health product in numerous formats, including as undiluted product, gel, shampoo, body wash, mouth rinse, spray, or cream at varying concentrations from 5% to 50%. It is marketed both alone and in combination with other topical acne treatments.

Dosages and Suggested Regimens

- Acne vulgaris: various concentrations of different vehicle: typically applied twice daily (left on or washed off) for 8 weeks

Pharmacokinetics

- There is insufficient reliable information to comment on the pharmacokinetics of tea tree oil.

Use in Special Populations

Pregnancy:

- Possibly safe when used topically and appropriately.

Lactation:

- Possibly safe when used topically and appropriately.

Pediatric use:

- Possibly safe when used topically and appropriately.

Renal insufficiency: There are no dosing adjustments provided on the manufacturer's label.

Hepatic insufficiency: There are no dosing adjustments provided on the manufacturer's label.

Monitoring

- No specific monitoring guidelines.

Contraindications and Cautions

- Contraindications: None reported.
- Tea tree oil can be potentially toxic if ingested.
- Multiple dermatologic conditions including skin irritation, allergic contact dermatitis, systemic contact dermatitis, linear IgA disease, erythema multiforme-like reactions, and systemic hypersensitivity reactions have been reported to parallel increased levels of tea tree oil use.
- In particular, there is substantial literature to support tea tree oil as a known cause of allergic contact dermatitis.

Important Drug Interactions

- There have been no formal studies of the interaction of topical tea tree oil with other drugs.

Adverse Effects and Their Management

- No manufacturer studies of adverse effects available. The most commonly reported adverse effects include allergic reactions, burning, dryness, irritation, pruritus, redness, and stinging.

Carcinogenicity

- There is no available data in the literature on carcinogenic potential of tea tree oil.

Patch Test Concentration

- N/A

Essential Patient Information

- Do not consume this medication orally.

Common Brand Names

- N/A

Acne Combination Products

Classification and Mode of Action

- Topical combination acne medications.
- In general, there are three main classes of topical combination acne products. For the products listed below, see individual drug monographs outlining each active ingredient for more detailed information, including mechanism of action, indications, contraindications/cautions, drug-drug interactions, considerations in special populations, and pharmacokinetic properties. See combination product label for specific application instructions.

The five main classes of topical combination acne medications are as follows:

- Benzoyl peroxide (BPO) and topical antibiotic (clindamycin or erythromycin)
- Adapalene and benzoyl peroxide (BPO)
- Clindamycin and tretinoin
- Tretinoin and microencapsulated benzoyl peroxide
- Clindamycin, adapalene, and benzoyl peroxide

Indications and Dermatological Uses

- *Clinical indications (FDA)*: Acne vulgaris
- *Off-label common uses*: Combination clindamycin and benzoyl peroxide has been used off-label for rosacea

Formulations/Presentation

- Many formulations with differing vehicles exist. Some formulations report to have better tolerability.

Clindamycin and Benzoyl Peroxide
US:

- Clindamycin phosphate 1.2% and benzoyl peroxide 2.5% gel (Acanya, generic)
- Clindamycin phosphate 1% and benzoyl peroxide 5% gel (BenzaClin, pump dispenser available, generic)
- Clindamycin phosphate 1.2% and benzoyl peroxide 5% gel (Neuac, Duac, generic)

- Clindamycin phosphate 1.2% and benzoyl peroxide 3.75% gel (Onexton)
- Generic formulations of clindamycin phosphate 1% and BPO 5% gel, clindamycin 1.2% and BPO 2.5%, and clindamycin phosphate 1.2% and BPO 5% are available
- Neuac: Clindamycin phosphate 1.2% and benzoyl peroxide 5% kit

Canada:

- Clindamycin phosphate 1% and benzoyl peroxide 5% gel (BenzaClin, Clindoxyl, Generic)
- Clindamycin phosphate 1% and benzoyl peroxide 3% gel (Clindoxyl ADV)

Erythromycin and benzoyl peroxide

US:

- Erythromycin 3% and benzoyl peroxide 5% gel (Benzamycin, Generic)

Canada:

- Erythromycin 3% and benzoyl peroxide 5% gel (Benzamycin)

Adapalene and benzoyl peroxide

US:

- Adapalene 0.1% and benzoyl peroxide 2.5% gel (Epiduo)
- Adapalene 0.3% and benzoyl peroxide 2.5% gel (Epiduo Forte)

Canada:

- Adapalene 0.1% and benzoyl peroxide 2.5% gel (Taro-Adapalene/Benzoyl Peroxide)
- Adapalene 0.3% and benzoyl peroxide 2.5% gel (Taro-Adapalene/Benzoyl Peroxide Forte)

Clindamycin and Tretinoin

US:

- Clindamycin phosphate 1% and tretinoin 0.025% gel (Ziana, Generic)

Canada:

- Clindamycin phosphate 1% and tretinoin 0.025% gel (Biacna)

Tretinoin and microencapsulated benzoyl peroxide
US and Canada:

- Tretinoin 0.1% and microencapsulated benzoyl peroxide 3% cream (Twyneo)

Clindamycin, adapalene, and benzoyl peroxide
US and Canada:

- Clindamycin phosphate 1.2%, adapalene 0.15%, benzoyl peroxide 3.1% gel (Cabtreo)

Dosages and Suggested Regimens

Acne:

- Clindamycin and benzoyl peroxide (BPO) Gel:
  - Clindamycin 1.2% and BPO 2.5% & 3.75%: Apply to affected area(s) once daily. Avoid contact with eyes or mucous membranes.
  - Clindamycin 1.2% and BPO 5%: Apply to the affected area(s) once daily at night. Avoid contact with eyes and mucous membranes.
  - Clindamycin 1% and BPO 5% (BenzaClin): Apply to affected area(s) twice daily. Avoid contact with eyes or mucous membranes.
- Erythromycin and BPO Gel: Apply thin layer twice daily. Avoid contact with eyes or mucous membranes.
- Adapalene and BPO: Apply a thin layer to affected area (face and/or body) once daily after washing. Avoid eyes and mucous membranes.
- Clindamycin and tretinoin: Apply pea-sized amount QHS at bedtime. Do not apply to eyes or mucous membranes.
- Clindamycin, adapalene, and benzoyl peroxide: Apply a thin layer to affected area once a day. Avoid the eyes, mucous membranes, nasal creases, and areas of damaged skin or areas affected by eczema or sunburn.

Rosacea (off-label use):

- Clindamycin 1% and BPO 5%: Apply to affected area(s) once daily Avoid contact with eyes and mucous membranes.
- Erythromycin and BPO Gel: Apply thin layer twice daily. Avoid contact with eyes or mucous membranes

Use in Special Populations

Pregnancy:

- No adequate studies of these products in pregnant women
- Manufacturer recommend only to consider if potential benefit justifies potential fetal risk
- Extrapolating from mouse data for topical retinoids, the theoretical risk of topical retinoids in pregnancy generally outweighs potential benefits

Lactation:

- There are no robust data on the presence of topical retinoids, benzoyl peroxide or topical antibiotic metabolites in human breast mild, the effects on breastfed infants or effects on mild production

Pediatric use:

- Safety and efficacy of benzoyl peroxide (BPO) and topical antibiotics (clindamycin or erythromycin) have not been established in children less than 12 years of age.
- Safety and efficacy of adapalene and BPO has not been established in children less than 9 years of age.
- Safety and efficacy of clindamycin and tretinoin have not been established in children less than 9 years of age.

Renal: No dose modifications are mentioned in the manufacturer's prescribing information.

Hepatic: No dose modifications are mentioned in the manufacturer's prescribing information.

Monitoring

- Hypersensitivity
- Skin irritation
- Photosensitivity

Contraindications and Cautions*

- All benzoyl peroxide-containing products may have a bleaching effect on hair/fabric
- Use of benzoyl peroxide with topical sulfone products may cause yellow-orange discoloration at the application site(s)
- Benzoyl peroxide-containing products may enhance the adverse/toxic effects of dapsone and diminish the therapeutic effects of topical isotretinoin.
- Diarrhea may result with the use of topical clindamycin. Topical clindamycin should be discontinued if diarrhea occurs.
- Erythromycin may diminish the therapeutic effect of clindamycin. Do not use together in combination.
- Avoid/limit UV-exposure after application of topical retinoids (adapalene/tretinoin). Nighttime application is one strategy to achieve this goal. Wear SPF 30+ sunscreen when exposure cannot be completely avoided
- Ziana (along with any clindamycin-containing topical medication) is contraindicated in patients with regional enteritis, ulcerative colitis, or history of antibiotic-associated colitis.
- Ziana has also been reported to cause nasopharyngitis, pharyngolaryngeal pain, cough, and sinusitis in >1% of patients.
- Skin irritation, dermatitis, dryness, erythema, and burning sensations are all possible side effect of the aforementioned combination products.
- Avoid all medications to which patients have known hypersensitivity reactions, including topical medications.

*See individual drug monographs for comprehensive listing of contraindications/cautions

Carcinogenicity

Clindamycin/benzoyl peroxide:

In one study of mice treated with clindamycin phosphate and benzoyl peroxide gel 1.2%/5% at up to 16 times the highest recommended human dose for two years, no increase in skin tumors was observed. A 2-year study in rats treated with a different formulation of 1% clindamycin and 5% benzoyl peroxide demonstrated dose dependent increase in keratoacanthoma incidence in males. A study of hairless mice exposed to chronic concurrent topical treatment with clindamycin and benzoyl peroxide gel 1.2%/5% and ultraviolet radiation showed a decrease in the median time to onset of skin tumor formation and number of tumors per mouse increased.

Patch Test Concentration

- See individual ingredients

Common Brand Names

Clindamycin and Benzoyl Peroxide:
- Acanya, BenzaClin, Neuac, Onexton, Clindoxyl, Clindoxyl ADV

Erythromycin and Benzoyl Peroxide:
- Benzamycin

Adapalene and Benzoyl Peroxide:
- Epiduo Forte

Clindamycin and Tretinoin:
- Ziana

References

1. Goh C, Cheng C, Agak G, Zaenglein AL, Graber EM, Thiboutot DM, Kim J. Acne Vulgaris. In: Kang S, Amagai M, Bruckner AL, Enk AH, Margolis DJ, McMichael AJ, Orringer JS, editors. Fitzpatrick's Dermatology, 9e. McGraw Hill; 2019. Accessed 06 Mar 2022.
2. Kistowska M, et al. Propionibacterium acne Promotes Th17 and Th17/Th1 responses in Acne Patient. J Investig Dermatol. 2015;135(1):110–8.
3. Eichenfield DZ, Sprague J, Eichenfield LF. Management of Acne Vulgaris: a review. JAMA. 2021;326(20):2055–67.
4. Stuart B, et al. Topical preparations for the treatment of mild-to-moderate acne vulgaris: systematic review and network meta-analysis. Br J Dermatol. 2021;185(3):512–525
5. Barbieri JS, Drucker AM. The need for comparative effectiveness data to guide management of acne vulgaris. Br J Dermatol. 2021;185(3):476–7.

Drug Monographs: Adapalene

6. FDA drug monograph (Adapalene). Available from https://www.accessdata.fda.gov/drugsatfda_docs/label/2007/020380s004lbl.pdf. Accessed 12 Aug 2023.
7. LexiComp drug monograph (Adapalene). Available from: LexiComp Online at online.Lexi.com. Copyright 2023 UptoDate, Inc.
8. Brogden R, Goa K. Adapalene: a review of its pharmacological properties and clinical potential in the management of mild to moderate acne. Drugs. 1997;53(3):511–9.
9. Altinyazar HC, Koca R, Tekin NS, et al. Adapalene vs metronidazole gel for the treatment of rosacea. Int J Dermatol. 2005;44(3):252–5.
10. Autret E, Berjot M, Jonville-Bera AP, et al. Anophthalmia and agenesis of optic chiasma associated with adapalene gel in early pregnancy. Lancet. 1997;350(9074):339.
11. Shehab N, Lewis CL, Streetman DD, et al. Exposure to the pharmaceutical excipients benzoyl alcohol and propylene glycol among critically ill neonates. Pediatr Crit Care Med. 2009;10(2):256–9.
12. Kong YL, Tey HL. Treatment of acne volgaris during pregnancy and lactation. Drugs. 2013;73(8):779–87.
13. Eichenfield LF, Krakowski AC, Piggott C, et al. Evidence-based recommendations for the diagnosis and treatment of pediatric acne. Pediatrics. 2013;131(Suppl 3):S163–86.
14. Asai Y, Baibergenova A, Dutil M, et al. Management of acne: Canadian clinical practice guideline. CMAJ 2016.
15. Maguiness S. Acne. 5-minute video available from the Society for Pediatric Dermatology Website at https://tinyurl.com/saa9t4s. Accessed 12 Aug 2023.

Drug Monographs: Benzoyl Peroxide

16. Burkhart CG, Burkhart CN. Decreased efficacy of topical anesthetic creams in presence of benzoyl peroxide. Dermatol Surg. 2005;31(11 Pt 1):1479–80.
17. Chien AL, Qi J, Rainer B, Sachs DL, Helfrich YR. Treatment of acne in pregnancy. J Am Board Fam Med. 2016;29(2):254–62.
18. deGroots AC. Chapter 3: Monographs of topical drugs that have caused contact allergy/allergic contact dermatitis. In: Monographs in contact allergy, volume 3. Topical drugs. CRC Press; 2021.
19. Del Rosso J, Sugarman J, Green L, Lain T, Levy-Hacham O, Mizrahi R, Gold LS. Efficacy and safety of microencapsulated benzoyl peroxide and microencapsulated tretinoin for the treatment of acne vulgaris: results

from two phase 3 double-blind, randomized, vehicle-controlled studies. J Am Acad Dermatol. 2023;89(4):719–27.
20. Edwards T, Cardwell LA, Patel N, Feldman SR. Benzoyl peroxide gel stains synthetic fabrics less than they stain cotton. J Am Acad Dermatol. 2021;85(2):481–2.
21. FDA Drug Safety Communication. http://www.fda.gov/downloads/Drugs/DrugSafety/UCM402663.pdf. 26957383
22. FDA drug monograph Epsolay. Available at: https://www.accessdata.fda.gov/drugsatfda_docs/nda/2023/214510Orig1s000lbl.pdf. Accessed 11 Mar 2025.
23. Foti C, Romita P, Borghi A, Angelini G, Bonamonte D, Corazza M. Contact dermatitis to topical acne drugs: a review of the literature. Dermatol Ther. 2015;28(5):323–9.
24. Kong YL, Tey HL. Treatment of acne vulgaris during pregnancy and lactation. Drugs. 2013;73(8):779–87.
25. Leachman SA, Reed BR. The use of dermatologic drugs in pregnancy and lactation. Dermatol Clin. 2006;24(2):167–97.
26. LexiComp drug monograph Benzoyl peroxide. Available from: LexiComp Online at online.lexi.com. Copyright 2023 UpToDate, Inc.
27. World Health Organization (WHO). Breastfeeding and maternal medication, recommendations for drugs in the Eleventh WHO Model List of Essential Drugs. Breastfeeding and maternal medication (who.int). https://www.who.int/publications/i/item/55732 (2002 Feb 25). Accessed 8 Aug 2023.

Drug Monographs: Clascoterone

28. FDA drug monograph Clascoterone. Available from: https://www.accessdata.fda.gov/drugsatfda_docs/label/2020/213433s000lbl.pdf. Accessed 8 Aug 2023.
29. Eichenfield L, Hebert A, Gold LS, Cartwright M, Fragasso E, Moro L, Mazzetti A. Open-label, long-term extension study to evaluate the safety of clascoterone (CB-03-01) cream, 1% twice daily, in patients with acne vulgaris. J Am Acad Dermatol. 2020;83(2):477–85.
30. Hebert A, Thiboutot D, Stein Gold L, Cartwright M, Gerloni M, Fragasso E, Mazzetti A. Efficacy and safety of topical Clascoterone cream, 1%, for treatment in patients with facial Acne: Two Phase 3 randomized clinical trials. JAMA Dermatol. 2020;156(6):621–30.

Drug Monographs: Clindamycin

31. deGroots AC. Chapter 3: Monographs of topical drugs that have caused contact allergy/allergic contact dermatitis. In: Monographs in contact allergy, volume 3. Topical drugs. CRC Press; 2021.
32. FDA drug monograph Cleocin-T and clindamycin phosphate gel. Available from: https://www.accessdata.fda.gov/drugsatfda_docs/label/2019/050537s040,050600s017,050615s018lbl.pdf and https://www.accessdata.fda.gov/drugsatfda_docs/label/2001/50782lbl.pdf. Accessed 8 Aug 2023.
33. FDA drug monograph EVOCLIN foam. Available from: https://www.accessdata.fda.gov/drugsatfda_docs/label/2012/050801s015lbl.pdf. Accessed 8 Aug 2023.
34. LexiComp drug monograph Clindamycin. Available from: LexiComp Online at online.lexi.com. Copyright 2023 UpToDate, Inc.
35. Barza M, Goldstein JA, Kane A, et al. Systemic absorption of Clindamycin hydrochloride after topical application. J Am Acad Dermatol. 1982;7(2):208–14.
36. Rehmus W. Folliculitis. Merk Manual Professional Version. Kenilworth, NJ. https://www.merckmanuals.com/professional/dermatologic-disorders/bacterial-skin-infections/folliculitis#. Accessed 8 Aug 2023.
37. World Health Organization (WHO). Breastfeeding and maternal medication, recommendations for drugs in the Eleventh WHO Model List of Essential Drugs. Breastfeeding and maternal medication (who.int). https://www.who.int/publications/i/item/55732 (2002 Feb 25). Accessed 8 Aug 2023.
38. Zaenglein AL, Pathy AL, Schlosser BJ, et al. Guidelines of care for the management of acne vulgaris. J Am Acad Dermatol. 2016;74(5):945–973.e33.

Drug Monographs: Dapsone

39. FDA drug monograph ACZONE (dapsone) gel. Available from: https://www.accessdata.fda.gov/drugsatfda_docs/label/2018/021794s016lbl.pdf and https://www.accessdata.fda.gov/drugsatfda_docs/label/2016/207154s000lbl.pdf. Accessed 8 Aug 2023.
40. LexiComp drug monograph Dapsone (topical). Available from: LexiComp Online at online.lexi.com. Copyright 2022 UpToDate, Inc. Accessed 3 Mar 2022.
41. Nickles MA, Lake E. Topical dapsone in the treatment of acne: a systematic review. Int J Dermatol. 2022; https://doi.org/10.1111/ijd.16074. Epub ahead of print. PMID: 35132625.

42. Zaenglein AL, Pathy AL, Schlosser BJ, et al. Guidelines of care for the management of acne vulgaris. J Am Acad Dermatol. 2016;74(5):945–73. e33. https://doi.org/10.1016/j.jaad.2015.12.037. Epub 2016 Feb 17. Erratum in: J Am Acad Dermatol. 2020 Jun;82(6):1576. PMID: 26897386.

Drug Monographs: Erythromycin

43. Akhavan A, Bershad S. Topical Acne drugs: review of clinical properties, systemic exposure, and safety. Am J Clin Dermatol. 2003;4(7):473–92.
44. deGroots AC. Chapter 3: Monographs of topical drugs that have caused contact allergy/allergic contact dermatitis. In: Monographs in contact allergy, Volume 3. Topical drugs. CRC Press; 2021.
45. FDA Monograph ERYGEL. Available at: https://www.accessdata.fda.gov/drugsatfda_docs/anda/97/64184ap.pdf. Accessed 17 Mar 2022.
46. FDA Monograph ERYTHROMYCIN PLEDGETS USP 2%. Available at: https://www.accessdata.fda.gov/drugsatfda_docs/anda/96/064126ap.pdf. Accessed 17 Mar 2022.
47. Manders SM, Lucky AW. Perioral dermatitis in childhood. J Am Acad Dermatol. 1992;27(5 pt 1):688–92.
48. Zaenglein AL, Pathy AL, Schlosser BJ, et al. Guidelines of care for the management of acne vulgaris. J Am Acad Dermatol. 2016;74(5):945–73.

Drug Monographs: Minocycline

49. FDA drug monograph. AMZEEQ. Available from: https://www.accessdata.fda.gov/drugsatfda_docs/label/2019/212379s000lbl.pdf. Accessed 11 Aug 2023.
50. FDA drug monograph. ZILXI. Available from: https://www.accessdata.fda.gov/drugsatfda_docs/label/2020/213690s000lbl.pdf. Accessed 11 Aug 2023.
51. Dosik J, Ellman H, Stuart I. Topical minocycline foam 4%: results of four phase 1 studies evaluating the potential for phototoxicity, photoallergy, sensitization, and cumulative irritation. J Immunotoxicol. 2019;16(1):133–9.
52. Gold LS, Del Rosso JQ, Kircik L, Bhatia ND, Hooper D, Nahm WK, Stuart I. Minocycline 1.5% foam for the topical treatment of moderate to severe papulopustular rosacea: results of 2 phase 3, randomized, clinical trials. J Am Acad Dermatol. 2020;82(5):1166–73.
53. Jones TM, Ellman H, deVries T. Pharmacokinetic comparison of once-daily topical minocycline foam 4% vs oral minocycline for moderate-to-severe acne. J Drugs Dermatol. 2017;16:1022–8.

54. Jones TM, Stuart I. Safety and pharmacokinetics of FMX103 (1.5% Minocycline topical foam) in subjects with moderate-to-severe Papulopustular Rosacea under maximum-use treatment conditions. J Clin Aesthet Dermatol. 2021;14(3):E53–7.
55. Onge ES, Mobley WC. Minocycline topical foam: a new drug for the treatment of Acne. Ann Pharmacother. 2021;55(1):105–10.
56. Stein Gold L, Del Rosso JQ, Kircik L, et al. Open-label extension study evaluating long-term safety and efficacy of FMX103 1.5% Minocycline topical foam for the treatment of moderate-to-severe papulopustular Rosacea. J Clin Aesthet Dermatol. 2020;13(11):44–9.

Drug Monographs: Resorcinol

57. deGroots AC. Chapter 3: Monographs of topical drugs that have caused contact allergy/allergic contact dermatitis. In: Monographs in contact allergy, volume 3. Topical drugs. CRC Press; 2021.
58. Martindale resorcinol monograph. Accessed 3/3/2022.
59. Alikhan A, Maibach HI. Keratolytic treatment of acne. In: Textbook of cosmetic dermatology. Essay. CRC Press; 2017.
60. Resinol label information. Available from: https://resical.com/resinol-medicated-ointment/label-information/. Accessed 3/3/2022.
61. Tinted acne treatment – resorcinol 2.00% sulfur 8.00% cream. Available from: https://dailymed.nlm.nih.gov/dailymed/getFile.cfm?setid=30e7d8f7-ca10-436a-8cce-25f97a7163a9&type=pdf. Accessed 3/3/2022
62. Substance evaluation conclusion – Resorcinol. Finland. Available from: https://s3-us-west-2.amazonaws.com/drugbank/cite_this/attachments/files/000/000/062/original/SEV-203-585-2-1_conclusion_and_report_public_5148_en.pdf?1526062531. Accessed 3/3/2022.
63. National Toxicology Program. Toxicology and Carcinogenesis Studies of Resorcinol (CAS No. 108-46-3) in F344 Rats and B6C3F1 Mice (Gavage Studies). Natl Toxicol Program Tech Rep Ser. 1992;403:1–234. PMID: 12621515

Drug Monographs: Sulfur and Sulfacetamide

64. deGroots AC. Chapter 3: Monographs of topical drugs that have caused contact allergy/allergic contact dermatitis. In: Monographs in contact allergy, volume 3. Topical drugs. CRC Press; 2021.
65. FDA drug monograph Klaron. Available from: https://www.accessdata.fda.gov/drugsatfda_docs/label/2010/019931s019lbl.pdf. Accessed 8/11/2023.

66. Sarac G. A comparison of the efficacy and tolerability of topical agents used in facial Demodex treatment. J Cosmet Dermatol. 2019;18(6):1784–7.
67. Liu H, Yu H, Xia J, Liu L, Liu GJ, Sang H, Peinemann F. Topical azelaic acid, salicylic acid, nicotinamide, sulphur, zinc and fruit acid (alpha-hydroxy acid) for acne. Cochrane Database Syst Rev. 2020;5(5):CD011368.
68. Ovace Plus Wash. Available from: https://ovace.com/wp-content/uploads/2020/10/Ovace-Combined-PI.pdf. Accessed 11 Aug 2023.
69. Natural medicines monograph sulfur. Available from: https://naturalmedicines.therapeuticresearch.com/. Accessed 3/3/2022.
70. Martindale sulfur monograph. Available from: https://about.medicinescomplete.com/publication/martindale-the-complete-drug-reference/. Accessed 3/3/2022.
71. LexiComp drug monograph Sulfur and Sulfacetamide. Available from: LexiComp Online at online.lexi.com. Copyright 2022 UpToDate, Inc. Accessed 3/3/2022.
72. AVAR Cleanser. Available from: https://avarinfo.com/wp-content/uploads/2020/10/AVAR_PI_R2016.pdf. Accessed 11 Aug 2023.
73. Dubina M, Fleischer AB. Interaction of topical sulfacetamide and topical dapsone with benzoyl peroxide. Arch Dermatol. 2009;145(9):1027–9.
74. Wolf K, Silapunt S. The use of sodium sulfacetamide in dermatology. Cutis. 2015;96(2):128–30. PMID: 26367751
75. Sodium sulfacetamide 10% and Sulfur 5% emollient foam- sulfacetamide sodium and sulfur aerosol, foam. Acella Pharmaceuticals, LLC. Available from: https://dailymed.nlm.nih.gov/dailymed/fda/fdaDrugXsl.cfm?setid=79ffd6f1-f3ad-4b4b-bc23-abd9295c5f2d&type=display. Accessed 11 Aug 2023.
76. Yuen MV, Gianturco SL, Pavlech LL, et al. Precipitated Sulfur: summary report. 2020. Available from: https://archive.hshsl.umaryland.edu/bitstream/handle/10713/12274/Precipitated%20sulfur_Final_2020_02.pdf?sequence=6. Accessed 11 Aug 2023.

Drug Monographs: Tea Tree Oil

77. Natural medicines monograph Tea tree oil. Available from: https://naturalmedicines.therapeuticresearch.com/
78. Hammer KA. Treatment of acne with tea tree oil (melaleuca) products: a review of efficacy, tolerability and potential modes of action. Int J Antimicrob Agents. 2015;45(2):106–10. https://doi.org/10.1016/j.ijantimicag.2014.10.011. Epub 2014 Nov 13. PMID: 25465857.

79. Pazyar N, Yaghoobi R, Bagherani N, Kazerouni A. A review of applications of tea tree oil in dermatology. Int J Dermatol. 2013;52(7):784–90. https://doi.org/10.1111/j.1365-4632.2012.05654.x. Epub 2012 Sep 24. PMID: 22998411.
80. de Groot AC, Schmidt E. Tea tree oil: contact allergy and chemical composition. Contact Dermat. 2016;75(3):129–43. https://doi.org/10.1111/cod.12591. Epub 2016 May 13. PMID: 27173437.
81. Bergfeld WF, Belsito DV, Cohen DE, et al. Safety assessment of Melaleuca alternifolia (Tea Tree)-derived ingredients as used in cosmetics. Available from: https://www.cir-safety.org/sites/default/files/Tea%20Tree_0.pdf. Accessed 11 Aug 2023.
82. Tea tree oil. National Center for Complementary and Integrative Health. Available from: https://www.nccih.nih.gov/health/tea-tree-oil. Accessed 11 Aug 2023.

Drug Monographs: Acne Combination Products

83. Breneman D, Savin R, VandePol C, Vamvakias G, Levy S, Leyden J. Double-blind, randomized, vehicle-controlled clinical trial of once-daily benzoyl peroxide/clindamycin topical gel in the treatment of patients with moderate to severe rosacea. Int J Dermatol. 2004;43(5):381–7.
84. FDA drug monograph Epiduo Forte (adapalene and benzoyl peroxide). Available from: https://www.accessdata.fda.gov/drugsatfda_docs/label/2015/207917Orig1s000lbl.pdf Accessed 12 Aug 2023.
85. FDA drug monograph Ziana (clindamycin phosphate 1.2% and tretinoin 0.025%). Available from: https://www.accessdata.fda.gov/drugsatfda_docs/label/2006/050802lbl.pdf Accessed 12 Aug 2023.
86. FDA drug monograph Neuac. Available at https://www.medimetriks.com/sites/default/files/pi-files/Neuac_pi_website.pdf. Accessed 13 Aug 2023.
87. FDA drug monograph Twyneo. Available at https://www.accessdata.fda.gov/drugsatfda_docs/label/2021/214902s000lbl.pdf
88. FDA drug monograph Cabtreo. Available at https://www.accessdata.fda.gov/drugsatfda_docs/label/2023/216632s000lbl.pdf. Accessed 11 Mar 2025.
89. LexiComp drug monograph Clindamycin and benzoyl peroxide. Available from: LexiComp Online at online.lexi.com. Copyright 2023 UpToDate, Inc.
90. LexiComp drug monograph Erythromycin and benzoyl peroxide. Available from: LexiComp Online at online.lexi.com. Copyright 2023 UpToDate, Inc.

91. Leyden JJ, Thiboutot D, Shalita A. Photographic review of results from a clinical study comparing benzoyl peroxide 5%/clindamycin 1% topical gel with vehicle in the treatment of rosacea. Cutis. 2004;73((6)(suppl)):11–7. [PubMed 15228129]
92. Oztürkcan S, Ermertcan AT, Sahin MT, Afşar FS. Efficiency of benzoyl peroxide-erythromycin gel in comparison with metronidazole gel in the treatment of acne rosacea. J Dermatol. 2004;31(8):610–7.

Rosacea and Topical Drug Treatments

9

Lisa E. Maier, Brian W. Connor, and Jason Ya

Contents

L. E. Maier (✉)
Department of Dermatology, UW Medicine, Seattle, WA, USA
e-mail: lemaier@uw.edu

B. W. Connor
Schweiger Dermatology Group, New York, NY, USA
e-mail: bwconnor@uw.edu

J. Ya
Department of Dermatology, Stanford University School of Medicine, Redwood City, CA, USA
e-mail: jasonya@uw.edu

R. M. Law, H. I. Maibach (eds.), *Handbook of Topical Drug Treatment in Dermatology*,
https://doi.org/10.1007/978-3-031-93616-6_9

Rosacea is a common chronic inflammatory condition with multiple clinical features that typically affects the skin of the face. It may also affect the eyes, but this is beyond the scope of this handbook. The etiology of rosacea is unknown, but aberrant immune and neurovascular responses to various external triggers such as microbes, ultraviolet light, and extremes of temperature in genetically susceptible individuals are thought to be contributory [1].

As outlined by National Rosacea Society Expert Committee in 2017, diagnostic features for rosacea include (1) fixed centrofacial erythema that may wax and wane in intensity or (2) phymatous changes (often characterized by thickened and irregularly textured skin, patulous follicles, and nodular hyperplasia). Patients should have one or both of these features to be diagnosed with rosacea. Other major features that may be present with these diagnostic features include papules and pustules, flushing, and telangiectasia. Patients with rosacea may also have secondary features of edema, rough and scaly texture, and symptoms of burning or stinging. Various rosacea clinical features may be present in different combinations in different individuals [2].

Available rosacea treatments are not curative but aim to manage specific rosacea clinical features—most commonly fixed erythema and papules and pustules. Telangiectasia, phymatous changes, and flushing typically are unaffected by topical treatment. Topical vasoconstrictors such as topical brimonidine and oxymetazoline specifically target fixed erythema. Reduction of the inflammatory lesions (papules and pustules) is typically achieved with the use of topical antimicrobials and anti-inflammatories including metronidazole, azelaic acid, ivermectin, topical minocycline, and microencapsulated benzoyl peroxide [4]. Secondary features of rosacea such as edema, burning and stinging, and dry texture may improve as treatment of the inflammatory lesions and transient erythema improve. To control various clinical features of rosacea, more than one topical therapy may be used, or they may be combined with systemic rosacea treatments and/or laser/light devices [3].

Topical Treatments for Non-transient Erythema of Rosacea
- Brimonidine
- Oxymetazoline

Topical Treatments for Inflammatory Lesions of Rosacea
- Metronidazole
- Azelaic acid
- Ivermectin
- Topical minocycline*
- Sodium sulfacetamide and sulfur*
- Microencapsulated benzoyl peroxide*
- Less commonly used antimicrobials and antiparasitic agents:
  - Clindamycin*
  - Erythromycin*
  - Dapsone*
  - Benzoyl peroxide*
  - Permethrin**

*Drug monograph for this agent is in the acne section of this chapter.

**Drug monograph for this agent is in the parasitic agents chapter.

Brimonidine

Classification and Mode of Action

- Selective alpha-2 adrenergic receptor
- Temporary reduction in non-transient erythema occurs due to vasoconstrictive effects
- The greatest reduction in erythema is observed around 3–6 h, and there is a diminishment of effect by 12 h.

Indications and Dermatological Uses

- *Clinical indications (FDA)*: Treatment of fixed centrofacial erythema associated with rosacea in adults (18 years or older)
- *Off-label common uses*: N/A

Formulations/Presentation

- US: MIRVASO (brimonidine) topical gel, 0.33%
- Canada: ONRELTEA (brimonidine) topical gel, 0.33%
- Europe: MIRVASO (as above)

Dosages and Suggested Regimens

- Apply pea size amount in a thin layer to the face (forehead, bilateral cheeks, nose, and chin) once a day. Typically, this is applied in the morning.

Baseline Investigations and Considerations

- None

Pharmacokinetics

- Absorption: A very small amount of topical absorption is noted with use topically to the cutaneous face (non-mucosal surfaces). Absorption is less than noted with ocular administration of brimonidine. No drug accumulation was noted in plasma.
- In a clinical trial, 1 g of brimonidine 0.33% topical gel was applied to the entire face of 24 adult subjects with rosacea associated facial erythema for 29 days. Pharmacokinetic assessments performed on day 1, day 15, and day 29 demonstrated the greatest mean plasma concentration (Cmax) and area under the

concentration-time curve (AUC) on day 15 (Cmax 46 ± 62 pg/mL and AUC 417 ± 264 pg.hr/mL). At day 29, the systemic drug exposure was lower, suggesting that there was no further drug accumulation. Topical application to the face was compared to a single day of ocular application of 0.2% ophthalmic drops (applied every 8 h for three doses). Day 15 topical brimonidine gel Cmax and AUC were approximately twofold lower than those found with single day ocular use.

- Metabolism: hepatically metabolized
- Excretion: Urinary excretion.

Use in Special Populations

- Pregnancy:
  - No adequate studies of use in pregnant women.
  - Manufacturer recommends only to use if potential benefit justifies potential fetal risk.
  - Ocular administration of brimonidine is considered first line for the treatment of glaucoma but is typically discontinued late in the third trimester due to potential for induction of newborn central nervous system. Effect of topical administration is unknown.
- Lactation:
  - Unknown if excreted in breast milk.
  - Manufacturer recommends avoidance during breastfeeding.
- Pediatric use:
  - Not indicated for use in children under the age of 18; ONRELTEA gel is contraindicated in children under 2 years of age.
  - Concerns for possible systemic absorption of brimonidine gel in 2–12 years old age group.
  - In a clinical trial, two young children who accidentally ingested MIRVASO gel experienced serious adverse reactions including respiratory distress requiring intubation, sinus bradycardia, lethargy, and confusion.

- Renal: No dose modifications are mentioned in the manufacturer's prescribing information.
- Hepatic: No dose modifications are mentioned in the manufacturer's prescribing information.

Monitoring

- Skin irritation
- Worsening of erythema and flushing
- Allergic contact dermatitis
- Undesirable pallor
- Symptoms of low blood pressure (e.g., dizziness or lightheadedness, fatigue, fainting, and blurred vision)

Contraindications and Cautions

- Hypersensitivity: Avoid use in patients with known hypersensitivity to brimonidine or the components of the gel.
- Vascular insufficiency: Due to potential to potentiate vascular insufficiency, use with caution in patients with cerebral or coronary insufficiency, scleroderma, Raynaud phenomenon, thromboangiitis obliterans, depression, and Sjögren syndrome.
- Cardiovascular disease: Due to potential to decrease blood pressure, use with caution in patients with cardiovascular disease that is unstable, uncontrolled or severe.
- Keep out of reach of children and avoid ingestion as this can result in serious side effects (difficulty breathing, bradycardia, confusion, fatigue, restlessness, muscle spasms, or twitching).

Important Drug Interactions

- *Anti-hypertensives and cardiac glycosides*: As a class, Alpha-2 agonists can reduce blood pressure. Patients on beta-blockers, other anti-hypertensives, and/or cardiac glycosides should be monitored while using Mirvaso.

- *CNS depressants:* Drug-drug interactions studies have not been conducted with MIRVASO topical gel, but consideration of possibility of additive or potentiating effects with CNS depressants (alcohol, opiates, sedatives, anesthetics, and barbituates) has been advised.
- *Monoamine oxidase inhibitors monoamine oxidase (MAO) inhibitors*: Theoretically, MAO inhibitors may interfere with brimonidine metabolism. This could result in increased systemic side effects such as low blood pressure and potentially result in an increased systemic side effect such as hypotension.

Adverse Effects and Their Management

- Worsening of facial erythema compared to baseline may occur in an estimated 20% of patients. This may occur within 3–6 h of application, also known as "paradoxical erythema," or present as redness that is greater than baseline after the medication fully wears off. Typically, this resolves with discontinuation of therapy, although some patients may be able to "treat through" and eventually tolerate the medication. Occasionally, more profound or prolonged redness, edema, warmth, pruritus, burning, and stinging can occur. In these cases, cool compresses, aspirin, or other NSAID can be used to manage discomfort. Antihistamines may help with pruritus and edema.
- More frequent or new onset flushing may also occur during therapy (30 min to hours). Typically resolves with discontinuation of therapy.
- Patients may experience temporary cosmetically undesirable facial pallor after application.
- Allergic contact dermatitis to both the active ingredient, brimonidine, and the inactive ingredients has been reported. Additionally, angioedema, throat tightening, tongue swelling, and urticaria may also rarely occur. Discontinue use if significant hypersensitivity reactions occur.

Patch Test Concentration

- 1%, 5%, and 10% pet.

Essential Patient Information

- Erythema reduction is temporary with brimonidine gel. Studies demonstrate recurrence of erythema within 8–12 h of initial application.
- Redness reduction is temporary and not curative.
- Brimonidine gel will not treat inflammatory lesions (papules and pustules) or phymatous changes associated with rosacea. Any inflammatory lesions if not treated by other methods may temporarily appear accentuated due to the reduction of surrounding erythema.
- Worsening redness, more frequent or new onset flushing may occur during therapy. If prolonged redness, burning, stinging, or warmth occurs, patients should contact their prescribing clinician.
- Do not use on broken skin or mucous membranes.

Oxymetazoline

Classification and Mode of Action

- a $_{1A}$-adrenergic receptor agonist.
- Temporary reduction in non-transient erythema reduction occurs due to vasoconstrictive effects.
- Greatest reduction in erythema is observed around 6–9 h, and there is a diminishment of effect by 12 h.
- Based on available study data, use of topical oxymetazoline appears to produce less “rebound erythema” (worsening of baseline erythema or flushing) than topical brimonidine.
- Best results may come from daily, long-term, continued use of oxymetazoline over weeks to months rather than intermittent use.

Indications and Dermatological Uses

- *Clinical indications (FDA)*: Topical treatment of rosacea related non-transient facial erythema
- *Off-label common uses*: N/A

Formulations/Presentation

- US: RHOFADE.
- Each gram of Rhofade contains 10 mg of oxymetazoline hydrochloride, equivalent to 8. 8 mg of oxymetazoline-free base.

Dosages and Suggested Regimens

- Oxymetazoline 1% cream. Apply a pea-sized amount to face (forehead, nose, bilateral cheeks, and chin) once daily. Avoid eyes and lips.

Baseline Investigations and Considerations

- None

Pharmacokinetics

- Absorption: A very small amount of percutaneous absorption occurs with use of oxymetazoline 1% cream when applied to the face to treat rosacea associated facial erythema. Specifically, when 0.3 g was applied to the face of adult rosacea patients, the mean concentration (Cmax) after first dose application was 60.5 ± 53.9 pg/mL.
- The mean area under the concentration-time curves from time 0–24 h ($AUC_{0-24\ h}$) after first dose was 895 ± 798 pg*h/mL. After 28 days of daily applications, the mean Cmax and

$AUC_{0-24\,h}$ were 66.4 ± 67.1 pg/mL and 1050 ± 992 pg*h/mL, respectively. Researchers also evaluated twice daily applications for 28 days and found that the mean Cmax and $AUC_{0-24\,h}$ were 68.8 ± 61.1 pg/mL and 1530 ± 922 pg*h/mL, respectively.
- Distribution: Approximately 57% is bound to plasma protein.
- Metabolism: Minimally metabolized.
- Excretion: Has not been characterized in humans.

Use in Special Populations

- Pregnancy:
  - There is no available data on use in pregnant women. Intranasal use of oxymetazoline in the second trimester may be potentially associated with renal collecting system anomalies. No adverse developmental effects noted in pregnant rats and rabbits when exposed to oral oxymetazoline up to three times and 73 times the maximum recommended human dose.
- Lactation:
  - No available data on the effects of topical oxymetazoline cream on lactation or its presence in human breast milk. Oxymetazoline has been found in the milk of lactating rats.
- Pediatric use:
  - Safety and effectiveness of oxymetazoline cream has not been studied in pediatric patients.
- Renal insufficiency:
  - No dose modifications are mentioned in the manufacturer's prescribing information.
- Hepatic insufficiency:
  - No dose modifications are mentioned in the manufacturer's prescribing information.

Monitoring

- None

Contraindications and Cautions

- Hypersensitivity: Avoid use in patients with known hypersensitivity to oxymetazoline or the components of the cream.
- Vascular insufficiency: Due to potential to potentiate vascular insufficiency, use with caution in patients with cerebral or coronary insufficiency, scleroderma, Raynaud phenomenon, thromboangiitis obliterans, depression, and Sjögren syndrome.
- Cardiovascular disease: Due to potential to decrease blood pressure, use with caution in patients with cardiovascular disease that is unstable, uncontrolled, or severe.
- Narrow angle glaucoma: Angle closure may occur with use of oxymetazoline.

Important Drug Interactions

- MAO inhibitors. May potentiate vasoconstrictive effects.
- Antihypertensives/cardiac glycosides. May affect blood pressure.

Adverse Effects and Their Management

- Local application site adverse effects may occur including application site dermatitis, erythema, pruritus, pain, worsening of inflammatory lesions, and photosensitivity. This typically resolves with treatment discontinuation. May require treatment of persistent dermatitis with topical steroid or topical calcineurin inhibitor. Worsening of inflammatory lesions of rosacea may require therapy with topical or oral therapies that target inflammatory lesions.
- Worsening of facial erythema and flushing during treatment or when the medication effect wears off. One 52-week open-label study of daily oxymetazoline cream observed this phenomenon in less than 1% of patients.

Patch Test Concentration

- N/A

Essential Patient Information

- Avoid ocular exposure. Wash hands immediately after applying cream to prevent inadvertent ocular exposure.
- Redness reduction is temporary and not curative.
- Oxymetazoline cream will not treat inflammatory lesions (papules and pustules) or phymatous changes associated with rosacea. Any inflammatory lesions if not treated by other methods may temporarily appear accentuated due to the reduction of surrounding erythema.
- Worsening redness, more frequent or new onset flushing may occur during therapy. If prolonged redness, burning, stinging, or warmth occurs, patients should contact their prescribing clinician.
- Do not use on broken skin or mucous membranes.
- At initial use, priming of a new RHOFADE dispenser is required. To do this, pump the dispenser three times and discard the product. Product can be used normally thereafter.
- Keep away from children.

Metronidazole

Classification and Mode of Action

- Metronidazole is an antibiotic with effects against anerobic bacteria and protozoa. Mechanism of action in the treatment of rosacea is unknown. Effects may be related to anti-inflammatory, antioxidant, and/or antimicrobial properties.
- Often used as a first-line topical treatment for papulopustular rosacea.
- Less irritating than azelaic acid in the treatment of rosacea, with equal to slightly lower effectiveness as azelaic acid.

- Less effective than topical ivermectin in the treatment of moderate to severe inflammatory rosacea.
- Onset of effect within 2–4 weeks, but greatest results are noted after 8 weeks of treatment.

Indications and Dermatological Uses

- *Clinical indications (FDA)*: Rosacea (topical), bacterial vaginosis (intravaginal), trichomoniasis (intravaginal)
- *Off-label common uses*: Periorificial dermatitis (topical)

Formulations/Presentation

- US:
  - External: 0.75% gel, 0.75% lotion, 0.75% cream, 1% cream, 1% gel (Metrogel, Metrocream, Metrolotion, Noritate cream, generic)
  - Vaginal: 0.75% vaginal gel, 1.3% vaginal gel
- Canada:
  - External: 0.75% gel, 1% gel and cream (Metrocream, Metrogel, Noritate)
  - Vaginal: 0.75% gel, 10% cream
- Europe:
  - External: 0.75% topical gel and cream (UK: Metrogel, Acea, Rozex)
  - Vaginal: 0.75% vaginal gel (UK: Zidoval)

Dosages and Suggested Regimens

Rosacea:

- External 0.75% gel, cream or lotion: apply a thin film to the affected area twice a day. Apply in the morning and evening.
- External 1% gel or cream: apply a thin film to the affected area once a day

Periorificial dermatitis (off label):

Adult:

- External 0.75% gel, cream, or lotion: apply a thin film to the affected area twice a day. Apply in the morning and evening.
- External 1% gel or cream: apply a thin film to the affected area once a day

Pediatric (6 months or older):

- Safety and effectiveness in pediatric patients have not been established. In clinical practice, this has been used to manage pediatric rosacea and perioral dermatitis.

Baseline Investigations and Considerations

- None

Pharmacokinetics

Absorption:

- Topical (external) administration of metronidazole is absorbed systemically in negligible amounts. Administration of a 1 g dose of metronidazole 1% gel resulted in absorption of less than 1% of a 250 mg oral dose. Maximum plasma concentration occurred 6–10 h after application.

Metabolism: Hepatic (30–60%)

Excretion: Urine (unchanged (20%) and metabolites (40–60%), feces (6–15%)

Use in Special Populations

Pregnancy:

- Topical use for the treatment of rosacea is considered compatible with pregnancy. Although metronidazole has been found to cross the placenta with oral administration, there is less absorption systemically with topical application. Based on available studies, there has not been an increased risk of adverse events to the fetus following maternal use of metronidazole.

Lactation:

- Topical use for the treatment of rosacea is considered compatible with lactation. Metronidazole has been found in breast milk after oral administration; however, there is less absorption with topical application.

Pediatric use:

- Safety data is limited; however, several studies support its use in this population.

Renal insufficiency:

- No adjustments recommended.

Hepatic insufficiency:

- No adjustment recommended; however, use with caution in severe liver impairment.

Monitoring

- Skin irritation (scaling, itching, burning, stinging, and dryness)
- Eye irritation
- Contact dermatitis (identified post-marketing); may cross react with imidazoles such as clotrimazole and tioconazole

Contraindications and Cautions (Topical Non-Vaginal Metronidazole)

- Contact with ocular mucosa should be avoided, as topical metronidazole can cause tearing and conjunctivitis of the eyes.
- Per manufacturer, topical metronidazole should be used with caution in patients with a history of, or active blood dyscrasia. Likelihood of worsening blood cell dyscrasia is low due to low systemic absorption.

- Use caution in patients with underlying neurologic disorders. Peripheral neuropathy can occur with systemic metronidazole use and has been reported rarely with topical use in the post-approval period.
- Use caution in patients with severe liver impairment.
- Oral metronidazole has a black box warning due to potential carcinogenesis demonstrated with high dose, long-term use in mice and rats. Carcinogenesis has not been demonstrated in humans. Black box warning has not been assigned to the topical and vaginal forms of metronidazole. No definitive carcinogenic effect has been noted with long term real-life clinical use of topical metronidazole.

Important Drug Interactions

- Although drug interactions are less likely with topical administration due to less systemic absorption, metronidazole may interact with the following:
- Coumarin and warfarin: may potentiate the anticoagulant effect
- Alcohol: disulfuram-like reaction

Adverse Effects and Their Management

- Skin irritation
- Allergic contact dermatitis
- Eye irritation
- Post marketing adverse effects reported include tingling or numbness of extremities, metallic taste, headache, nausea, and constipation.

Patch Test Concentration

- 1% pet

Essential Patient Information

- Avoid contact with the eyes.
- Gently cleanse affected area(s) before applying.
- Do not ingest. For external use only.
- Inflammatory lesions of rosacea can re-occur with discontinuation of treatment; thus, chronic treatment may be needed to control the condition.

Ivermectin

Classification and Mode of Action

- Postulated to have antiparasitic effect against Demodex mites and anti-inflammatory actions.
- Antiparasitic effect via binding to glutamate-gated chloride channels in invertebrate muscle and nerves. *For more information about use as a ectoparasiticide, please refer to Chap. 19: Ectoparasiticides, Invermectin monograph.*
- More effective than metronidazole in reducing inflammatory lesions of moderate to severe papulopustular rosacea.

Indications and Dermatological Uses

- *Clinical indications (FDA)*: Rosacea, head lice
- *Off-label common uses*: N/A

Formulations/Presentation

- US: Rosacea: 1% cream (Soolantra, Generic)
  Head lice: 0.5% lotion (Sklice, Generic)
- Canada: Rosacea: 1% cream (Rosiver)
- Europe: 1% cream (Efacti, Soolantra)

Dosages and Suggested Regimens for Rosacea

- Once a day application to the affected area of the face. Avoid eyes and lips.

Baseline Investigations and Considerations

- None

Pharmacokinetics

Absorption:

- Low transepidermal absorption when used topically on the face for rosacea. Steady state of a low systemic level was achieved by 2 weeks. Over 52 weeks of use, there was no additional plasma accumulation. After a 10 min exposure in 6 months to 3 years old, ivermectin lotion absorption was very low compared to oral administration.

Metabolism: Hepatic, metabolized by CYP3A4

Excretion: Fecal

Use in Special Populations

Pregnancy:

- Insufficient information about safety in pregnant people. Animal studies have demonstrated the potential for adverse developmental effects with oral administration of ivermectin.

Lactation:

- Insufficient information about safety of topical ivermectin in lactation. Orally administered ivermectin is found in low concentrations in human breast milk. Rat studies demonstrated potential for neonatal toxicity when ivermectin is absorbed during nursing.

Pediatric use: Insufficient information about safety of ivermectin in pediatric patients

Renal insufficiency: No alterations in dosing recommended in renal insufficiency

Hepatic insufficiency: No alterations in dosing recommended in hepatic insufficiency

Monitoring

- N/A

Contraindications and Cautions

- None

Important Drug Interactions

- None described

Adverse Effects and Their Management

- A localized burning sensation may occur with application. Rosacea patients in general may be sensitive to topical medications application to the skin. To minimize this possibility, make sure to wait at least 30 min after washing prior to applying the topical cream.
- Dry skin has been reported. Consider addition of light emollient cream if this occurs.
- Eye irritation and conjunctivitis may occur. Recommend avoiding using near the eyes.
- Irritant and allergic contact dermatitis has been reported.

Patch Test Concentration

- N/A

Essential Patient Information

- Do not ingest.
- Avoid contact with eyes and lips.
- Not for vaginal use.

Azelaic Acid

Classification and Mode of Action

- Dicarboxylic acid
- Possible anti-inflammatory and antioxidative effects
  - Inhibits serine protease kallikrein-5 involved in the production of cathelicidin, a pro-inflammatory antimicrobial peptide involved in rosacea pathogenesis
  - Activation of PPARγ resulting in anti-inflammatory activity
  - Inhibition of Il-1, IL-6 and TNF-a expression
  - Decreasing reactive oxygen species
- Antimicrobial activity against *Staphylococcus epidermidis* and *Cutibacterium acnes*
- Comparative efficacy in rosacea
  - Available studies have shown equal or greater efficacy compared to topical metronidazole.
  - Azelaic acid gel is more likely to be irritating to the skin compared to topical metronidazole and topical ivermectin.
  - Azelaic acid 15% foam may be better tolerated than metronidazole cream and gel.
- Comparative efficacy in acne vulgaris:
  - Azelaic acid 20% cream twice a day was less effective than once daily application combination benzoyl peroxide 3% plus clindamycin 1%.

Indications and Dermatological Uses

- *Clinical indications (FDA)*: Inflammatory lesions of rosacea, inflammatory lesions of acne vulgaris
- *Off-label common uses*: Melasma, hyperpigmentation, perioral dermatitis

Formulations/Presentation

- US: Rosacea: 15% gel (Finacea, generic) or foam (Finacea foam), acne: 20% cream or lotion (Azelex, generic); also available in OTC products up to 10%
  - Finacea gel: 0.15 gm azelaic acid per gram of gel.
  - Finacea foam: 1 g of Finacea Foam contains 0.15 g of azelaic acid.
  - Azelex cream: 0.2 g (azelaic acid) per gram of cream.
- Canada: 15% gel (Finacea)
- Europe: 15% gel (Finacea), 20% cream (Skinoren)

Dosages and Suggested Regimens

- Rosacea: apply gel or foam to affected areas twice a day (morning and evening)
- Acne vulgaris: apply thin film to affected areas twice daily (morning and evening)

Baseline Investigations and Considerations

- None

Pharmacokinetics

Absorption:

- Approximately 4% of topically applied azelaic acid 20% cream. Studies of the use of azelaic acid 15% gel did not show an increase plasma azelaic acid concentration beyond the normal range.

Metabolism:

- Negligible cutaneous metabolism occurs after topical application.

Excretion:

- Mainly excreted unchanged in the urine but undergoes some β-oxidation to shorter chain dicarboxylic acids.

Use in Special Populations

Pregnancy:

- There are no adequate and well-controlled studies in pregnant women. The manufacturer recommends use during pregnancy only if clearly needed. However, because less than 4% is absorbed systemically, exposure to fetus is thought to be minimal. Azelaic acid is typically considered by the dermatologic community to be a low-risk treatment option for acne vulgaris and rosacea in pregnant people.

Lactation:

- Passage of drug into maternal milk may occur. However, as less than 4% of a topical dose is systemically absorbed, this is not expected to cause a significant change in baseline azelaic acid levels in the milk.
- The manufacturer recommends caution when administering to nursing mothers.

Pediatric use:

- Safety and effectiveness of topical azelaic acid in pediatric patients has not been established. However, based on available studies and guidelines, it is likely safe in children aged 12 and older with same dosing as in adults.

Renal insufficiency: No dosing adjustments are provided on the manufacturer's label.

Hepatic insufficiency: No dosing adjustments are provided on the manufacturer's label.

Monitoring

- No specific monitoring guidelines.

Contraindications and Cautions

- *Contraindications*: Hypersensitivity to any of its components.
- This product is not well studied in patients with dark complexion. Monitor these patients for early signs of hypopigmentation as there have been isolated reports of hypopigmentation after use of azelaic acid.
- Temporary skin irritation may occur when applied to broken or inflamed skin, usually at the start of treatment. This typically subsides if treatment is continued. If it continues, reduce to once daily use or stop treatment until these effects have subsided.
- The propellant in Finacea foam is flammable. Avoid fire, flame, and smoking during and immediately following application.

Important Drug Interactions

- There have been no formal studies of the interaction of topical azelaic acid with other drugs.

Adverse Effects and Their Management

- Skin erythema, dryness, peeling, stinging, pruritus, and pain at application site. Patients may tolerate foam better than gel formulation.
- Eye irritation—avoid contact with eyes and periorbital skin.
- Post marketing rash, hypersensitivity and worsening of asthma has been reported. If this occurs discontinue therapy.
- Rare cases of hypopigmentation and vitiligo.

- Rare hypertrichosis.
- Rare exacerbation of recurrent herpes labialis.
- Foam only: avoid flames/fire and smoking during and immediately after application.

Patch Test Concentration

- N/A

Essential Patient Information

- To minimize irritation to skin, avoid alcohol containing toners, astringents, and cleansers. Also avoid abrasive cleansers.
- Avoid concomitant use of other topical acid containing products and peels such as glycolic acid, lactic acid, salicylic acid, alpha-hydroxy acids, and beta-hydroxy acids unless directed by clinician. Combining use may increase the risk of skin irritation.
- Concomitant use with topical retinoids may increase the risk of skin irritation.

Additional Rosacea Topical Therapies

FDA approved: Topical Minocycline—see section on Acne

Other: Sulfur and sulfacetamide, dapsone, clindamycin, erythromycin—see section on Acne; Topical Permethrin—see section on Parasitic treatment

References

1. Buddenkotte J, Steinhoff M. Recent advances in understanding and managing rosacea. F1000 Research. 2018;7(F1000 Faculty Rev-1885) https://doi.org/10.12688/f1000research.16537.
2. Gallo RL, Granstein RD, Kang S, Mannis M, Steinhoff M, Tan J, Thiboutot D. Standard classification and pathophysiology of rosacea: the 2017 update by the National Rosacea Society Expert Committee. J Am Acad Dermatol. 2018;78(1):148–55.

3. Thiboutot D, Anderson R, Cook-Bolden F, Draelos Z, Gallo RL, Granstein RD, Kang S, Macsai M, Gold LS, Tan J. Standard management options for rosacea: the 2019 update by the National Rosacea Society Expert Committee. J Am Acad Dermatol. 2020;82(6):1501–10.
4. Desai SR, Baldwin H, Del Rosso JQ, Gallo RL, Bhatia N, Harper JC, York JP, Gold LS. Microencapsulated Benzoyl Peroxide for Rosacea in context: a review of the current treatment landscape. Drugs. 2024;84(3):275–84.

Brimonidine

5. FDA drug monograph. Mirvaso. Available from: http://www.accessdata.fda.gov/drugsatfda_docs/label/2013/204708lbl.pdf. Accessed 1/2/2022.
6. Anton C. de Groot – Monographs in contact allergy volume 3: topical drugs. Chapter 3.
7. Onreltea product monograph. Galderma Canada. Available at https://www.galderma.com/sites/default/files/inline-files/Onreltea%20English%20PM.pdf. Accessed 1/2/2022.
8. Okwundu N, Cline A, Feldman SR. Difference in vasoconstrictors: oxymetazoline vs. brimonidine. J Dermatolog Treat. 2021;32(2):137–43.
9. Sethi HS, Naik M, Gupta VS. Management of glaucoma in pregnancy: risks or choices, a dilemma? Int J Ophthalmol. 2016;9(11):1684–90.
10. Tanghetti EA, Jackson JM, Belasco KT, Friedrichs A, Hougier F, Johnson SM, Kerdel FA, Palceski D, Hong HC, Hinek A, Cadena MJ. Optimizing the use of topical brimonidine in rosacea management: panel recommendations. J Drugs Dermatol. 2015;14(1):33–40.

Oxymetazoline

11. FDA drug monograph RHOFADE. https://www.accessdata.fda.gov/drugsatfda_docs/label/2017/208552s000lbl.pdf. Accessed 1/2/2022.
12. LexiComp drug monograph (name of monograph). Available from: LexiComp Online at online.Lexi.com. Copyright 2021 UptoDate, Inc.
13. Draelos ZD, Gold MH, Weiss RA, et al. Efficacy and safety of oxymetazoline cream 1.0% for treatment of persistent facial erythema associated with rosacea: findings from the 52- week open label REVEAL trial. J Am Acad Dermatol. 2018;78:1156–63.
14. Okwundu N, Cline A, Feldman SR. Difference in vasoconstrictors: oxymetazoline vs. brimonidine. J Dermatolog Treat. 2021;32(2):137–43.

Metronidazole

15. deGroots AC. Chapter 3: Monographs of topical drugs that have caused contact allergy/allergic contact dermatitis. In: Monographs in contact allergy, volume 3. Topical drugs. CRC Press; 2021.
16. FDA drug monograph METROGEL 1%. Available from: https://www.accessdata.fda.gov/drugsatfda_docs/label/2005/021789lbl.pdf. Accessed 12 Aug 2023.
17. FDA drug monograph Metrogel 0.75%. Available from: https://www.galderma.com/sites/default/files/inline-files/METROGEL-PM-E-Feb-22-2018.pdf. Accessed 12 Aug 2023.
18. FDA drug monograph MetroLotion 0.75%. Available from: https://www.accessdata.fda.gov/drugsatfda_docs/label/1998/20901lbl.pdf. Accessed 12 Aug 2023.
19. FDA monograph NORITATE cream 1%. Available from: https://www.accessdata.fda.gov/drugsatfda_docs/label/2003/020743s002lbl.pdf. Accessed 12 Aug 2023.
20. LexiComp drug monographs (metronidazole – topical and systemic). Available from: LexiComp Online at online.Lexi.com. Copyright 2023 UptoDate, Inc.
21. Hernández Ceruelos A, Romero-Quezada LC, Ruvalcaba Ledezma JC, López Contreras L. Therapeutic uses of metronidazole and its side effects: an update. Eur Rev Med Pharmacol Sci. 2019;23(1):397–401.
22. Jarmuda S, O'Reilly N, Żaba R, Jakubowicz O, Szkaradkiewicz A, Kavanagh K. Potential role of Demodex mites and bacteria in the induction of rosacea. J Med Microbiol. 2012;61(Pt 11):1504–10.
23. Kellen R, Silverberg NB. Pediatric periorificial dermatitis. Cutis. 2017;100(6):385–8.
24. Kroshinsky D, Glick SA. Pediatric rosacea. Dermatol Ther. 2006;19(4):196–201.
25. Mostafa FF, El Harras MA, Gomaa SM, et al. Comparative study of some treatment modalities of rosacea. J Eur Acad Dermatol Venereol. 2009;23:22.
26. Miyachi Y. Potential antioxidant mechanism of action for metronidazole: implications for rosacea management. Adv Ther. 2001;18:237.
27. Murase JE, Heller MM, Butler DC. Safety of dermatologic medications in pregnancy and lactation: Part I. Pregnancy. J Am Acad Dermatol. 2014;70(3):401.
28. Taieb A, Ortonne JP, Ruzicka T, Roszkiewicz J, Berth-Jones J, Peirone MH, Jacovella J. Ivermectin Phase III study group. Superiority of ivermectin 1% cream over metronidazole 0·75% cream in treating inflammatory lesions of rosacea: a randomized, investigator-blinded trial. Br J Dermatol. 2015;172(4):1103–10.
29. Wolf JE Jr, Kerrouche N, Arsonnaud S. Efficacy and safety of once-daily metronidazole 1% gel compared with twice-daily azelaic acid 15% gel in the treatment of rosacea. Cutis. 2006;77:3.

30. Ziel K, Yelverton CB, Balkrishnan R, Feldman SR. Cumulative irritation potential of metronidazole gel compared to azelaic acid gel after repeated applications to healthy skin. J Drugs Dermatol. 2005;4:727.

Ivermectin

31. FDA drug monograph SOOLANTRA cream. Available from https://www.accessdata.fda.gov/drugsatfda_docs/label/2014/206255lbl.pdf. Accessed 12 Aug 2023.
32. FDA drug monograph SKLICE lotion. Available from https://www.accessdata.fda.gov/drugsatfda_docs/label/2017/202736s003lbl.pdf. Accessed 12 Aug 2023.
33. https://www.ema.europa.eu/en/documents/psusa/ivermectin-topical-use-list-nationally-authorised-medicinal-products-psusa/00010376/201610_en.pdf. Accessed 12 Aug 2023.
34. LexiComp drug monograph (Ivermectin). Available from: LexiComp Online at online.Lexi.com. Copyright 2023 UptoDate, Inc.
35. Benkali K, Rony F, Graeber M, Jacovella J, Chappuis JP, Peirone MH, Poncet M, Delage S, Bouer R, Wagner N. Clinical pharmacokinetics profile of ivermectin 1% cream after dermal applications on the face. World J Dermatol. 2016;5(1):57–64.
36. González Canga A, Sahagún Prieto AM, Diez Liébana MJ, Fernández Martínez N, Sierra Vega M, García Vieitez JJ. The pharmacokinetics and interactions of ivermectin in humans–a mini-review. AAPS J. 2008;10(1):42–6.
37. Schaller M, Gonser L, Belge K, et al. Dual anti-inflammatory and anti-parasitic action of topical ivermectin 1% in papulopustular rosacea. J Eur Acad Dermatol Venereol. 2017;31:1907–11.
38. Taieb A, Ortonne JP, Ruzicka T, et al. Superiority of ivermectin 1% cream over metronidazole 0·75% cream in treating inflammatory lesions of rosacea: a randomized, investigator-blinded trial. Br J Dermatol. 2015;172:1103.

Azelaic Acid

39. FDA drug monograph FINACEA gel, 15%. Available from: https://www.accessdata.fda.gov/drugsatfda_docs/label/2010/021470s005lbl.pdf. Accessed 12 Aug 2023.
40. FDA drug monograph FINACEA foam. Available from: https://www.accessdata.fda.gov/drugsatfda_docs/label/2015/207071s000lbl.pdf. Accessed 12 Aug 2023.

41. FDA drug monograph AZELEX (azelaic acid cream). Available from: https://www.accessdata.fda.gov/drugsatfda_docs/label/2003/20428slr016_azelex_lbl.pdf. Accessed 12 Aug 2023.
42. Afarideh M, Rodriguez Baisi KE, Davis DMR, Hand JL, Tollefson MM. Trends in utilization of non-first-line topical acne medications among children, adolescents, and adults in the United States, 2012–2016. Pediatr Dermatol. 2021;38(5):1066–73.
43. Coda AB, Hata T, Miller J, et al. Cathelicidin, kallikrein 5, and serine protease activity is inhibited during treatment of rosacea with azelaic acid 15% gel. J Am Acad Dermatol. 2013;69(4):570–7.
44. Koh YP, Tian EA, Oon HH. New changes in pregnancy and lactation labelling: review of dermatologic drugs. Int J Womens Dermatol. 2019;5(4):216–26.
45. Jansen T, Melnik BC, Schadendorf D. Steroid-induced periorificial dermatitis in children-clinical features and response to azelaic acid. Pediatr Dermatol. 2010;27(2):137–42.
46. Mastrofrancesco A, Ottaviani M, Aspite N, Cardinali G, Izzo E, Graupe K, Zouboulis CC, Camera E, Picardo M. Azelaic acid modulates the inflammatory response in normal human keratinocytes through PPARgamma activation. Exp Dermatol. 2010;19(9):813–20.
47. Schaller M, Sebastian M, Ress C, et al. A multicentre, randomized, single-blind, parallel-group study comparing the efficacy and tolerability of benzoyl peroxide 3%/clindamycin 1% with azelaic acid 20% in the topical treatment of mild-to-moderate acne vulgaris. J Eur Acad Dermatol Venereol. 2016;30(6):966–73.
48. Schulte BC, Wu W, Rosen T. Azelaic acid: evidence-based update on mechanism of action and clinical application. J Drugs Dermatol. 2015;14(9):964–8.
49. Täuber U, Weiss C, Matthes H. Percutaneous absorption of azelaic acid in humans. Exp Dermatol. 1992;1(4):176–9.
50. Williamson T, LaRose A, Cameron J, et al. Rosacea treatment satisfaction: matching adjusted indirect treatment comparison analysis of metronidazole gel or cream vs azelaic acid foam. J Drugs Dermatol. 2020;19(3):295–304.
51. Zaenglein AL, Pathy AL, Schlosser BJ, et al. Guidelines of care for the management of acne vulgaris. J Am Acad Dermatol. 2016;74(5):945–73.e33. https://doi.org/10.1016/j.jaad.2015.12.037. Epub 2016 Feb 17. Erratum in: J Am Acad Dermatol. 2020 Jun;82(6):1576.

Topical Drug Treatment in Actinic Keratosis

10

Chavy Chiang and Anuk Burli

Contents

Treatment options for actinic keratosis include topical aminolevulinic acid in conjunction with photodynamic therapy or fluorouracil (covered under antineoplastics). Ingenol mebutate was previously approved and marketed as Picato gel for treatment of actinic keratosis but was withdrawn by its manufacturer LEO Pharma in October 2020 after studies showed a potential increased

C. Chiang (✉)
Department of Dermatology, University of Rochester Medical Center, Rochester, NY, USA
e-mail: chavyz@gmail.com

A. Burli
Department of Dermatology, Stanford University School of Medicine, Redwood City, CA, USA
e-mail: anukb@stanford.edu

R. M. Law, H. I. Maibach (eds.), *Handbook of Topical Drug Treatment in Dermatology*,
https://doi.org/10.1007/978-3-031-93616-6_10

risk of nonmelanoma skin cancer. Topical tirbanibulin, a first-in-class microtubule inhibitor, was approved by the FDA in 2020 for treatment of actinic keratosis.

Aminolevulinic Acid

Classification and Mode of Action

- Photosensitizing agent. Following topical application, aminolevulinic acid is metabolized to photosensitizer protoporphyrin IX (PpIX), which accumulates in the skin. Light exposure of proper wavelength and energy excites PpIX and generates cytotoxic reactive oxygen species (AMELUZ: combine with red light from BF-RhodoLED® lamp at a dose of 37 J/cm^2; LEVULAN KERASTICK: combine with blue light from BLU-U Blue Light Photodynamic Therapy Illuminator at a dose of 10 J/cm^2).

Indications and Dermatological Uses

- *Clinical indications (FDA)*: Actinic keratosis
- *Off-label common uses*: Actinic cheilitis (level of evidence: C), basal cell skin cancer, superficial, low risk (level of evidence: G), squamous cell skin cancer in situ, low risk (Bowen disease; level of evidence: G)

Formulations/Presentation

- US: 10% gel (AMELUZ), 20% solution (LEVULAN KERASTICK)
- Canada: 20% solution (LEVULAN KERASTICK)
- Europe: 7.8% gel (AMELUZ)

Dosages and Suggested Regimens

- Gel: Apply gel, amounting 1 mm in thickness, to cover lesion(s) and 5 mm of surrounding skin. Application area and amount should not exceed 20 cm^2 and 2 g, respectively. Allow gel to dry for 10 min and then use light-blocking, occlusive dressing to cover the application area for 3 h. Remove dressing and wipe off remaining gel afterward and treat with red light illumination. Lamp head should be positioned 5–8 cm from the skin surface. Lesions may be retreated if they have not completely resolved in 3 months following initial treatment.
- Solution: Apply to lesion and uniformly wet the surface, including edges without excess running or dipping. Do not apply solution to surrounding healthy skin. For face or scalp lesions, repeat application once more after initial application as dried. Administer blue light treatment 14–18 h afterward. For upper extremity lesions, occlude upper extremity with low-density polyethylene plastic wrap and secure wrap with an elastic net dressing. After 3 h, remove dressing, rinse with water, pat dry, and treat with blue light. Lesions may be retreated once if they have not completely resolved in 8 weeks following initial treatment.
- Significant drug interactions exist, which may require dose/frequency adjustment or avoidance. Consult drug interactions database for guidance/information.

Baseline Investigations and Considerations

Pharmacokinetics (Percutaneous Absorption, Distribution, Metabolism, Excretion) as Relevant

- Two grams of AMELUZ applied under occlusion over 20 cm^2 for 3 h in 12 adults with subsequent photodynamic therapy yielded a mean ± SD area under the concentration time curve and maximum concentration of 142.83 ± 75.50 ng/mL and 27.19 ± 20.02 ng/mL, respectively, for baseline-corrected aminolevulinic acid. Mean ± SD baseline plasma levels measured 20.16 ± 16.53 ng/mL. The median time to reach maximum concentration (Tmax) was 3 h.

Use in Special Populations

- No lactation or pediatric data.
- Unknown risk of fetal exposure upon maternal use.
- *Renal insufficiency*: No data.
- *Hepatic insufficiency*: No data.

Monitoring

- Educate patients on proper post-treatment care.

Contraindications and Cautions

- Skin photosensitivity to light
- Known hypersensitivity to porphyrins
- Porphyria

Important Drug Interactions

- No formal studies conducted.
- Use of other known photosensitizing agents, such as St. John's wort, griseofulvin, thiazide diuretics, sulfonylureas, phenothiazines, quinolones, and tetracyclines may enhance phototoxic reaction to photodynamic therapy.

Adverse Effects and Their Management

- Erythema, edema, stinging/burning, scaling/crusting, itching, erosion, hypo/hyperpigmentation, oozing/vesiculation/crusting, scaling, and dryness.

Patch Test Concentration

- 20% water; a concentration of 10% in petrolatum causes irritant reactions.

Essential Patient Information

- Avoid exposing treated skin to sun and prolonged or intense light for 48 h after treatment.
- Avoid medications that may enhance phototoxic reaction.

Tirbanibulin

Classification and Mode of Action

- Microtubule inhibitor. Blocks polymerization of tubulin.

Indications and Dermatological Uses

- *Clinical indications (FDA)*: Actinic keratosis (of face and scalp)
- *Off-label common uses*: None

Formulations/Presentation

- US: 1% ointment (KLISYRI)

Dosages and Suggested Regimens

- Apply evenly to cover up to 25 cm^2 of affected area once daily for five consecutive days, using one single-dose packet per application.

Baseline Investigations and Considerations

Pharmacokinetics (Percutaneous Absorption, Distribution, Metabolism, Excretion) as Relevant

- Topical application of a mean daily dose of 138 mg (range: 54–295 mg) of KLISYRI to 25 cm^2 of facial skin or balding scalp once daily for five consecutive days achieved steady state concentration by 72 h, with a mean±SD trough concentration (C_{trough}) of 0.11 ± 0.08 ng/mL. Low systemic exposure was demonstrated on Day 5, with mean ± SD maximum plasma concentration (C_{max}) measuring 0.34 ± 0.30 ng/mL and 0.18 ± 0.10 ng/mL. Mean±SD area under the plasma concentration from time zero to 24 h (AUC_{24}) measured 5.0 ± 3.9 h*ng/mL and 3.2 ± 1.9 h*ng/mL in facial- and scalp-treated subjects, respectively. Median time to reach C_{max} (T_{max}) was about 7 h.
- Plasma protein binding measures 88% and is unaffected by concentrations within the range of 0.01–10 μg/mL.
- Topical treatment to adult subjects with actinic keratosis induced detectable levels of two pharmacologically inactive metabolites, KX2-5036 and KX2-5163, with respective maximum plasma concentrations measuring 0.09 ng/mL and 0.12 ng/mL. In vitro data indicate that when 1 or 10 μM tirbanibulin are incubated with hepatocytes, KX2-5036, KX-5163, and other unidentified metabolites are generated. In vitro, tirbanibulin is largely metabolized by CYP3A4, with a smaller contribution by CYP2C8.
- Excretion data not fully characterized in humans.

Use in Special Populations

- No human pregnancy, human lactation, or pediatric data available.
- *Renal insufficiency*: not evaluated.
- *Hepatic insufficiency*: not evaluated.

Monitoring

- Local skin reactions
- Ophthalmic reactions

Contraindications and Cautions

- None.

Important Drug Interactions

- No data.

Adverse Effects amd Their Management

- Local skin reactions can occur, including erythema, flaking/scaling, crusting, swelling, vesiculation/pustulation, erosions/ulcerations.

Patch Test Concentration

- N/A

Essential Patient Information

- Apply to skin only.
- Do not use more than needed to cover treatment area.
- Do not apply in, around, or near eyes, mouth, or lips.

Fluorouracil (5-FU)

Classification and Mode of Action

- Antineoplastic. Fluorouracil prevents methylation of deoxyuridylic acid to thymidylic acid to block DNA and, to a lesser extent, RNA synthesis, particularly so in rapidly growing cells.

Indications and Dermatological Uses

- *Clinical indications (FDA)*: Actinic keratosis. Basal cell carcinoma, superficial.
- *Off-label common uses*: Penile carcinoma in situ (level of evidence: C). Squamous cell carcinoma in situ (Bowen disease; level of evidence: C)

Formulations/Presentation

- US: 0.5% cream (Carac or generic), 1% cream (Fluoroplex or generic), 4% cream (Tolak—contains peanut oil), 5% cream (Efudex or generic), 2% solution (generic), 5% solution (generic)
- Canada: 4% cream (Tolak—contains peanut oil), 5% cream (Efudex)
- Europe: Not on LexiComp

Dosages and Suggested Regimens

- Actinic keratosis:
  - 0.5% cream: apply thin film once daily to lesions for up to 4 weeks, as tolerated
  - 1% cream: apply twice daily to lesions for 2–6 weeks
  - 4% cream: apply once daily to lesions for 4 weeks as tolerated

  - 5% cream, 2% or 5% solution: apply sufficiently to cover lesions twice daily for 2–4 weeks, until the inflammatory response reaches the erosion stage, then stop. Complete healing may take 1–2 months post-treatment cessation to be evident.
- Basal cell carcinoma:
  - 5% cream or solution: Apply sufficiently to cover lesions twice daily for at least 3–6 weeks; treatment can be extended up to 10–12 weeks.
- Penile carcinoma in situ (off-label):
  - 5% cream: Apply to and leave on lesion for 12 h every 48 h for 28 days
- Squamous cell carcinoma in situ (Bowen disease; off-label):
  - 5% cream: Apply twice daily to lesion for 9 weeks

Baseline Investigations and Considerations

Pharmacokinetics (Percutaneous Absorption, Distribution, Metabolism, Excretion) as Relevant

- Approximately 6% absorbed systemically for 5% cream, with a time to peak of about 1 h.
- After bolus intravenous injection, fluorouracil distributes throughout the body in sites including the intestinal mucosa, bone marrow, liver, cerebrospinal fluid, and brain tissue following bolus injection.
- After bolus intravenous injection, 5–20% of parent drug is excreted unchanged in the urine in 6 h, while the remaining is metabolized primarily by the liver. Metabolites of 5-FU, such as urea and α-fluoro-ß-alanine, are excreted in urine over 3–4 h.

Use in Special Populations

- Unknown if excreted in human milk; decision to discontinue nursing or use of drug should be made.

- May cause fetal harm when used by pregnant women. Miscarriages, ventricular septal defects, and cleft lips and palates have been reported when pregnant women were topically or parenterally exposed.
- No safety or efficacy data in children.
- *Renal insufficiency*: No data.
- *Hepatic insufficiency*: No data.

Monitoring

- Dihydropyrimidine dehydrogenase enzyme deficiency
- Hypersensitivity or local skin reactions

Contraindications and Cautions

- Not to be used in pregnant women or women planning to become pregnant.
- Not to be used in patients with dihydropyrimidine dehydrogenase enzyme deficiency, as fluorouracil is largely metabolized by this enzyme and life-threatening toxicity has been reported.

Important Drug Interactions

- Brivudine (not approved by FDA): May enhance 5-FU toxicity.

Adverse Effects and Their Management

- Burning, crusting, allergic contact dermatitis, erosions, erythema, hyperpigmentation, irritation, pain, photosensitivity, pruritus, scarring, rash, soreness, and ulceration.
- Ulcerations, other local reactions, cases of miscarriage, and a birth defect (ventricular septal defect) have been reported when Efudex was applied to mucous membrane areas.

- Leukocytosis is most frequent hematological side effect.
- Other adverse reactions: emotional upset, insomnia, irritability, medicinal taste, stomatitis, eosinophilia, thrombocytopenia, toxic granulation, alopecia, blistering, bullous pemphigoid, discomfort, ichthyosis, scaling, suppuration, swelling, telangiectasia, tenderness, urticaria, skin rash, conjunctival reaction, corneal reaction, lacrimation, nasal irritation, herpes simplex.

Patch Test Concentration

- Commercial 5% cream "as is"; 5-FU 50 mg/mL (5%) and 10 mg/mL (1%) in saline or 5% pet; if negative and contact allergy is strongly suspected, or with 7+ patch tests, perform intradermal tests with 5-FU 10 mg/mL (1%) saline with reading at Day 2.

Essential Patient Information

- Do not apply to eyelids, into eyes, nose, or mouth. Miscarriage and birth defects have been reported following mucous membrane application during pregnancy.
- Wash hands immediately after if using fingers to apply the medication.
- Use by pregnant women may cause harm to fetus. Contraception use advised in females of reproductive potential during and for one month following last dose of medication.
- Four percent cream contains peanut oil and can cause hypersensitivity reactions as well as ophthalmic reactions.
- Avoid sun exposure, sun lamps, and tanning beds during and immediately following treatment since ultraviolet rays can increase reaction intensity.
- Skin reaction caused by treatment may be unsightly during treatment and for several weeks upon completion of therapy.

Diclofenac (Alternate Agent)

Refer to *Chap. 11: Analgesics* for the Diclofenac drug monograph.

References

Aminolevulinic Acid

1. https://www.ema.europa.eu/en/documents/product-information/ameluz-epar-product-information_en.pdf.
2. https://www.accessdata.fda.gov/drugsatfda_docs/label/2018/020965s015lbl.pdf.
3. https://www.accessdata.fda.gov/drugsatfda_docs/label/2016/208081s000lbl.pdf.
4. Lexicomp: Aminolevulinic acid. Available from: LexiComp Online at online.Lexi.com. Copyright 2024 UptoDate, Inc.
5. De Groot AC. Patch testing. 3rd edition. Volume 3 Chapter 3
6. De Groot AC. Patch testing, 4th edition: update 2018–2022. Wapserveen: Acdegroot Publishing, 2022 (37 pages). ISBN/EAN 978-90-813233-7-6.

Tirbanibulin

7. Lexicomp: Tirbanibulin LexiComp drug monograph (name of monograph). Available from: LexiComp Online at online.Lexi.com. Copyright 2024 UptoDate, Inc.
8. Kempers S, DuBois J, Forman S, et al. Tirbanibulin Ointment 1% as a novel treatment for actinic keratosis: Phase 1 and 2 results. J Drugs Dermatol. 2020;19(11):1093–100. https://doi.org/10.36849/JDD.2020.5576.

Fluorouracil (5-FU)

9. https://www.accessdata.fda.gov/drugsatfda_docs/label/2016/012209s040lbl.pdf.
10. LexiComp drug monograph Fluorouracil. Available from: LexiComp Online at online.Lexi.com. Copyright 2024 UptoDate, Inc.
11. De Groot AC. Patch testing. 3rd edition. Volume 3 Chapter 3
12. De Groot AC. Patch testing, 4th edition: update 2018–2022. Wapserveen: Acdegroot Publishing, 2022 (37 pages). ISBN/EAN 978-90-813233-7-6.

11 Topical Analgesics

Sheeva Shahinfar, Rebecca M. Law, and Howard I. Maibach

Contents

S. Shahinfar (✉)
Texas A&M University College of Medicine, Bryan, TX, USA
e-mail: sheeva.shahinfar@tamu.edu

R. M. Law (✉)
School of Pharmacy and Faculty of Medicine (Discipline of Family Medicine), Memorial University of Newfoundland, St. John's, NL, Canada
e-mail: rlaw@mun.ca; rlawUCSF@gmail.com

H. I. Maibach
Department of Dermatology, University of California San Francisco (UCSF), San Francisco, CA, USA
e-mail: howard.maibach@ucsf.edu

R. M. Law, H. I. Maibach (eds.), *Handbook of Topical Drug Treatment in Dermatology*,
https://doi.org/10.1007/978-3-031-93616-6_11

Capsaicin

Classification and Mode of Action

- A compound originally discovered in chili peppers.
- Initially recognized in its ability to produce pain with its burning and irritant effects. Over time, capsaicin's analgesic properties have also been recognized.
- Mechanism of action: not entirely understood. It is believed that a high or repeated dose of capsaicin induces a refractory state in TRPV1 receptors.
  - TRPV1 receptors are ion channels part of the transient receptor potential (TRP) family and implicated in nociception along pain pathways.
  - Capsaicin-induced refraction leads to desensitization and eventual inhibition of receptor function. Part of this process includes a decrease in nociceptive peptides (e.g., Substance P) on nerves that express TRPV1.
  - It has been hypothesized that initial stimulation with capsaicin produces pain via antagonism of TRPV1 receptors. Repeated stimulation with capsaicin causes a refractory state in TRPV1 receptors and depletes neurons of substance P, leading to the desensitization and analgesic effect.

Indications and Dermatological Uses

- *Clinical indications (FDA)*: neuropathic pain (post-herpetic)
- *Off-label common uses*: psoriasis pain, intractable pruritus, neuropathic post-surgical pain, notalgia paresthetica, apocrine chromhidrosis, lipodermatosclerosis, prurigo nodularis, lichen simplex chronicus, aquagenic pruritus, alopecia areata
  - Level of evidence for psoriasis: B
  - Level of evidence for intractable pruritis: B

Formulations/Presentation

- US: Qutenza® 8% patch (available as cream, gel, liquid, lotion, patch for non-dermatologic clinical indications).
- Canada: Cream (0.025%, 0.05%, 0.075%), gel (0.025%), patch (0.025%). Note: Capsaicin (Qutenza®) is not approved for use in post-herpetic neuralgia in Canada.
- Europe: Qutenza® 8% patch (available as cream, gel, liquid, lotion, patch for non-dermatologic clinical indications).

Dosages and Suggested Regimens

- Qutenza®: Health professional should apply patch in-office to most painful areas for 60 min. A maximum of four patches can be applied at once. Repeat treatment every 3 months as needed for pain. Do not apply sooner than 3 months after application.
- Cream for off-label use: Apply a thin film of substance to the affected area three to four times a day for pain.

Baseline Investigations and Considerations

Pharmacokinetics (Percutaneous Absorption, Distribution, Metabolism, Excretion) as Relevant

- Qutenza® patch showed low and transient systemic absorption (<5 ng/mL) in one out of three patients when evaluated after 60 min of application. Most patients with higher concentrations had a noticeable drop in concentration (below the quantifiable limit) at 3–6 h after a 60-min application cycle.
- Half-life seen at 1.64 h.
- Onset of action at 1 week after application. Cream's onset of action seen with 2–4 weeks of regular, directed application.

Use in Special Populations

- Pregnancy: Systemic absorption is limited after topical application. Fetal exposure is not anticipated with maternal use of topical medication. Plasma concentration is below quantifiable level at 3–6 h after 60-min patch application.
- Lactation: Systemic absorption is limited after topical application. Exposure to infant via breast milk is not anticipated. According to manufacturer, breastfeeding decision while using topical therapy should consider risks of infant exposure, benefits of infant breastfeeding, and benefits of topical treatment for mother. Avoid application to the nipple or surrounding areas to decrease infant exposure.
- Children: Qutenza® 8% patch is not approved for us in children.
  - Off-label lotion (0.025%) use: children 8+ years old may apply to affected area three to four times per day.
  - Off-label patch (0.0375%) use: children 8+ years old may apply 1 patch to affected area, maximum use of three patches/day.
  - Off-label patch (0.03%) use: children 8+ years old may apply one patch to affected area for <8 h, maximum use of four patches/day, do not use more than five consecutive days.
  - Off-label patch (0.0225%) use: children 8+ years old may apply one patch to affected area for <8 h, maximum use of three patches/day.
  - Off-label patch (0.0375%) use: children 8+ years old may apply one patch to affected area, maximum use of three patches/day
  - Off-label patch (0.025%) use: children 8+ years old may apply one patch to affected area for <8 h, maximum use of three patches/day
  - Off-label patch (0.05%) use: Adolescents 16+ years may apply one patch to affected area, maximum use of two patches/day
- Renal insufficiency: No dose adjustments listed on manufacturer's labeling
- Hepatic insufficiency: No dose adjustments listed on manufacturer's labeling

Monitoring

- Monitor blood pressure periodically during treatments.
- Severe irritation to the eyes, respiratory tract, skin, or mucous membranes may occur from unintended product exposure. Refer to "Adverse effects & their management" for further information.
- Sensory function (thermal, harmful stimuli) may be decreased with patch use. These are typically temporary and minor. Continue to monitor and reevaluate patients for worsening sensory deficits.
- Serious burns may occur and may need hospitalization. Discontinue use if signs of burn are present.
- Remove patches slowly and gently to decrease exposure through aerosols. Inhalation may induce coughing or sneezing.

Contraindications and Cautions

- Use with caution in patients with a history of cardiovascular events or uncontrolled hypertension. Temporary increases in blood pressure may occur due to pain during and after product application. Monitor blood pressure throughout application period.
- Use with caution in patients with history of cerebrovascular events. Temporary increases in blood pressure may occur due to pain during and after product application.
- Contraindicated in patients with hypersensitivity to capsaicin, menthol, or any vehicles or parts of the formulation.
- Contraindicated for use on wounds, open skin, irritated skin, or into skin folds.

Important Drug Interactions

- No known significant drug interactions

Adverse Effects and Their Management

- Serious burns may occur and may need hospitalization. Discontinue use if signs of burns are present. Treat burn or pursue hospitalization for serious burns.
- CNS depression may occur after application; patients should be cautioned about performing activities such as operating heavy machinery or driving.
- Severe irritation to the eyes, respiratory tract, skin, or mucous membranes may occur from unintended product exposure. If irritation to eyes or mucous membranes occurs, remove the patient from the treatment area and flush affected areas with cool water. If irritation to respiratory tract occurs, remove the patient from the treatment area and provide symptomatic care if shortness of breath ensues. If irritation worsens or does not improve, do not expose patient to capsaicin. Ensure that proper protective measures (gloves, ventilation, face mask, and glasses) are used during product application. If skin not intended for the use of capsaicin is exposed to product, use cleansing gel on exposed area for 1 min and remove with dry gauze. Wash with soap and water. Pain from exposure can be treated with ice packs and analgesics.
- Sensory function (thermal, harmful stimuli) may be decreased with patch use. These are typically temporary and minor. Continue to monitor and reevaluate patients for worsening sensory deficits.
- Blood pressure should be monitored in patients with history of cardiovascular events, uncontrolled hypertension, or history of cerebrovascular events. Discontinue use if blood pressure is not maintained.
- Some forms of capsaicin include benzyl alcohol. Benzyl alcohol has been implicated in fatal neonatal toxicity known as "gasping syndrome." Signs and symptoms include CNS dysfunction, gasping respirations, respiratory distress, hypotension, cardiovascular failure, and metabolic acidosis. Avoid use in neonates.

Carcinogenicity

- No published studies on carcinogenicity

Patch Test Concentration

- *N/A*

Essential Patient Information

- Temporary burning may be present for several days after application.
- Qutenza® is directed for use under direct supervision and placement by a healthcare provider in-office. It should not be used by patient at home.
- Off-label cream use should not be used on wounds, open skin, damaged skin, irritated skin, or into skin folds. Do not cover area with bandage. Do not use simultaneously with other topical analgesics.
- Use caution while operating heavy machinery or driving after application.
- Do not use before or after showering, tanning, heavy exercise, swimming, or other heat/sun exposure.
- Consult your healthcare provider if you notice excessive redness, blistering, irritation, burning, or worsening symptoms.
- Seek immediate medical attention if you have difficulty breathing or swallowing. Do not touch contact lenses for 1 h after using capsaicin.

Diclofenac

Classification and Mode of Action

- Diclofenac is a topical non-steroidal anti-inflammatory drug (NSAID).

- Mechanism of action: inhibition of cyclooxygenase 1 and 2 (COX-1, COX-2), which produce prostaglandins and key inflammatory mediators. This inhibition decreases the number of circulating prostaglandins in the body and, in turn, decreases the inflammatory cascade.

Indications and Dermatological Uses

- *Clinical indications (FDA)*: Actinic Keratosis (alternate agent). Refer to *Chap. 10* for topical drug treatments for actinic keratosis.
- *Off-label common uses*: Acute musculoskeletal pain

Formulations/Presentation

- US: 3% Gel, 3% gel + 2.5% hyaluronic acid vehicle
- Canada: 3% Gel, 3% gel + 2.5% hyaluronic acid vehicle
- Europe: 3% Gel, 3% gel + 2.5% hyaluronic acid vehicle

Dosages and Suggested Regimens

- Apply gel to affected area twice a day for 60–90 days. It is typically recommended to use a 0.5 g amount on a 5 × 5 cm surface area.

Baseline Investigations and Considerations

Pharmacokinetics (Percutaneous Absorption, Distribution, Metabolism, Excretion) as Relevant

- 6–10% of applied product is systemically absorbed.
- >99% of absorbed product binds to albumin.
- Undergoes hepatic first-pass metabolism with formation of several metabolites. Most are phenolic metabolites, which are subsequently converted to glucuronide conjugates. Two phenolic metabolites are biologically active but much less than diclofenac, the effect of which is recognized as negligible.

- Peak concentration noted at 4.5 ± 8 h.
- Excretion through urine (~65%) and feces (~3.5%).

Use in Special Populations: Pregnancy (FDA Guidance), Lactation, Children, Renal Insufficiency, and Hepatic Insufficiency

- Unknown if diclofenac is present in breast milk after topical administration. Manufacturer states that the drug's systemic availability is much less with topical administration than oral administration. Breastfeeding decision should include consideration of infant's risk, benefits of breastfeeding infant, and benefits of treatment for mother.
- Concentration of diclofenac in systemic circulation is less when used topically, compared to orally. No studies have evaluated the use of topical diclofenac in pregnancy. NSAIDs have been shown to correlate with birth defects in some studies, including constriction of the ductus arteriosus, oligohydramnios, renal dysfunction, necrotizing enterocolitis, persistent pulmonary hypertension, and intracranial hemorrhage. Prolonged maternal use of NSAIDs increases the risk of renal dysfunction leading to oligohydramnios. This may be reversed with cessation of NSAID use. Persistent ductus arteriosus may be resistant to future medical management. Collectively, NSAIDs may be used with caution during the first two trimesters but not used in the third trimester.
- Actinic keratosis is not a condition seen in the pediatric population. Diclofenac 3% gel is not recommended for use in children.
- No dosing adjustments made by manufacturer for renal insufficiency, recommend avoidance of product in advanced renal disease.
- No dosing adjustments made by manufacturer for hepatic insufficiency, recommend proceeding with caution.

Monitoring

- Anaphylactoid reactions
- Adverse cardiovascular thrombotic events (e.g., MI and stroke)
- Adverse gastrointestinal side effects (e.g., inflammation, ulceration, bleeding, and perforation)
- DRESS syndrome
- Hematologic prolonged bleeding time
- Hyperkalemia
- Adverse skin events (e.g., Stevens-Johnsons syndrome, toxic epidermal necrolysis, and exfoliative dermatitis)

Contraindications and Cautions

- Hypersensitivity to diclofenac or vehicles used in formulation (history of urticaria, allergic reactions, or asthma after NSAID or aspirin use)
- Coronary artery bypass graft surgery: increased post-operative risk of MI and stroke
- Advanced renal disease
- Do not use on damaged or open skin (burns, wounds, eczema, infected skin lesions, and exudative dermatitis)
- Do not use before or after cardiac surgery
- Do not use on more than two body areas at the same time

Important Drug Interactions

Risk C: Monitor Therapy

- Alcohol: Alcohol may increase risk of GI bleed with use of topical NSAIDs.
- Angiotensin II receptor blockers: Topical NSAIDs may decrease the intended effect of ARBs.
- Angiotensin-converting enzyme inhibitors: Topical NSAIDs may decrease the intended effect of ACE inhibitors.
- Anticoagulants: Topical NSAIDs may increase the intended effect of anticoagulants.

- Beta-blockers: Topical NSAIDs may decrease the intended effect of beta blockers.
- Corticosteroids (systemic): Topical NSAIDs may increase the adverse effects of systemic corticosteroids. Increased risk of GI bleeding, perforation, and ulceration.
- Cyclosporine (systemic): Topical NSAIDs may increase the adverse effects of systemic cyclosporine. Increased risk of nephrotoxicity.
- Deferasirox: Topical NSAIDs may increase the adverse effects of Deferasirox. Increased risk of GI bleeding and ulceration.
- Digoxin: Topical NSAIDs may increase Digoxin's circulating serum concentration.
- Herbal anticoagulant/antiplatelet products: Topical NSAIDs may increase the intended effect of herbal anticoagulants/antiplatelets
- Lithium: Topical NSAIDs may increase lithium's circulating serum concentration.
- Loop diuretics: Topical NSAIDs may decrease the intended effect of loop diuretics.
- Methotrexate: Topical NSAIDs may increase methotrexate's circulating serum concentration.
- Selective serotonin reuptake inhibitors: SSRIs may increase the antiplatelet effect of topical NSAIDs.
- Serotonin/norepinephrine reuptake inhibitors: SNRIs may increase the antiplatelet effect of topical NSAIDs.
- Tacrolimus (systemic): Topical NSAIDs may increase adverse effects of tacrolimus, particularly nephrotoxicity.
- Tenofovir and thiazide-like diuretics: topical NSAIDs may increase adverse effects of Tenofovir, particularly nephrotoxicity.
- Voriconazole: Voriconazole may increase the circulating serum concentration of topical diclofenac.

Risk D: Consider therapy modification

- NSAIDs: Topical NSAIDs may increase the adverse effects of other NSAIDs. Increased risk of GI toxicity. Not recommended to co-administer systemic and topical NSAIDs.
- Salicylates: Topical NSAIDs may increase the adverse effects of salicylates. Increased risk of GI toxicity. Not recommended to co-administer systemic and topical NSAIDs.

Adverse Effects and Their Management

- Anaphylactoid reactions: Anaphylactoid reactions may occur in patients with no prior exposure. Patients with "aspirin triad" are at increased risk of anaphylactoid reaction.
- Cardiovascular effects: NSAIDs have been shown to increase risk of serious thrombotic events (e.g., MI and stroke). Patients with known CV disease or CV risk factors have a higher incidence of serious thrombotic events with the use of NSAIDs. Also linked to hypertension and exacerbation of existing hypertension. Monitor blood pressure, particularly in patients with existing hypertension. Should be used with caution in patients with edema, as NSAIDs may cause retention of sodium and fluid. Avoid use in patients with heart failure or recent MI.
- DRESS syndrome (drug reaction with eosinophilia and systemic symptoms): Monitor patients for signs and symptoms (eosinophilia, fever, lymphadenopathy, and rash). Discontinue therapy if symptoms point to DRESS.
- Gastrointestinal side effects: NSAIDs increase the risk of serious GI bleeds, ulceration, perforation, or inflammation. Greatest risk among patients with history of peptic ulcer disease, elderly patient, and patients with history of GI bleeds.

Carcinogenicity

- No studies have been performed to evaluate the carcinogenicity of NSAIDs.

Patch Test Concentration

- Sodium salt, 2.5% pet. (SmartPractice Canada, Smart PracticeEurope); sodium salt, 5% pet. (Chemotechnique, SmartPracticeCanada); sodium salt, 1% pet. (Chemotechnique)

Essential Patient Information

- Diclofenac is used for the treatment of actinic keratosis. Concurrently, sun avoidance should be followed (physical clothing covers, sitting in the shade, and wearing sunscreen regularly).
- Get medical help if these side effects persist: dizziness/headache, constipation, diarrhea, upset stomach, vomiting, gas, heartburn.
- Seek immediate medical condition if these side effects (although rare) are present:
  - Vomiting or coughing up blood. Brown "coffee-ground" appearing vomit
  - Black/red/tarry stools
  - Gum bleeding
  - Abnormal vaginal bleeding
  - Unstoppable bleeding
  - High blood pressure (persistent headache, dizziness, passing out, and vision changes)
  - Kidney problems (difficulty passing urine and blood in urine)
  - High potassium (abnormal heartbeat, confusion, weak, lightheadedness, dizziness, passing out, numbness/tingling, and shortness of breath)
  - Irritation of the skin (redness, blistering, and peeling)
  - Chest pain, chest pressure, increased heartbeat
  - Abnormal increase in weight, swelling in extremities
  - Weakness on one side of the body, difficulty speaking or thinking, changes in balance, drooping face
  - Fatigue, flu-like symptoms, muscle pain
  - Liver problems (dark urine, loss of appetite, abdominal pain, change in stool color, and yellow skin/eyes)
  - Allergic reaction (rash, hives, itching, wheezing, tight chest, and difficulty breathing or swallowing)
  - Abnormal burning, numbness, or tingling

- US Boxed Warnings:
  - Serious cardiovascular thrombotic events: "Nonsteroidal anti-inflammatory drugs (NSAIDs) cause an increased risk of serious cardiovascular thrombotic events, including myocardial infarction and stroke, which can be fatal. This risk may occur early in treatment and may increase with duration of use. Diclofenac gel is contraindicated in the setting of coronary artery bypass graft surgery [26]."
  - Serious GI bleeding, ulceration, and perforation: "NSAIDs cause an increased risk of serious GI adverse reactions, including bleeding, ulceration, and perforation of the stomach or intestines, which can be fatal. These reactions can occur at any time during use and without warning symptoms. Elderly patients and patients with a prior history of peptic ulcer disease and/or GI bleeding are at greater risk of serious GI events [26]."

References

Capsaicin

1. FDA drug monograph Qutenza® (capsaicin) patch. Available from https://www.accessdata.fda.gov/drugsatfda_docs/label/2020/022395s019lbl.pdf. Accessed 15 Jan 2023.
2. LexiComp drug monograph Capsaicin. Available from: LexiComp Online at online.Lexi.com. Copyright 2021 UptoDate, Inc.
3. Babbar S, Marier J-F, Mouksassi M-S, Beliveau M, Vanhove GF, Chanda S, Bley K. Pharmacokinetic analysis of capsaicin after topical administration of a high-concentration capsaicin patch to patients with peripheral neuropathic pain. Ther Drug Monit. 2009;31:502–10.
4. Backonja M, Wallace MS, Blonsky ER, Cutler BJ, Malan P, Rauck R, Tobias J. NGX-4010, a high-concentration capsaicin patch, for the treatment of postherpetic neuralgia: a randomised, double-blind study. Lancet Neurol. 2008;7:1106–12.
5. Bernstein JE, Korman NJ, Bickers DR, Dahl MV, Millikan LE. Topical capsaicin treatment of chronic postherpetic neuralgia. J Am Acad Dermatol. 1989;21:265–70.
6. Boyd K, Shea SM, Patterson JW. The role of capsaicin in dermatology. In: Capsaicin as a therapeutic molecule. Basel: Springer; 2014. p. 293–306.

7. Fattori V, Hohmann M, Rossaneis A, Pinho-Ribeiro F, Verri W. Capsaicin: current understanding of its mechanisms and therapy of pain and other pre-clinical and clinical uses. Molecules. 2016;21:844.
8. Guillet C, Steinmann S, Maul J-T, Kolm I. Primary localized cutaneous amyloidosis: a retrospective study of an uncommon skin disease in the largest tertiary care center in Switzerland. Dermatology. 2021;238:579–86.
9. Laude-Pagniez E, Leclerc J, Lok C, Chaby G, Arnault J-P. Capsaicin 8% patch as therapy for neuropathic chronic postsurgical pain after melanoma excision surgery: a single center case series. JAAD Case Rep. 2022;30:70–5.
10. Marks JG. Treatment of apocrine chromhidrosis with topical capsaicin. J Am Acad Dermatol. 1989;21:418–20.
11. Rumsfield JA, West DP. Topical capsaicin in dermatologic and peripheral pain disorders. DICP. 1991;25:381–7.
12. S; BSMC Capsaicin for acute or chronic non-cancer pain: A review of Clinical Effectiveness, safety, and cost-effectiveness [internet]. In: National Center for Biotechnology Information. https://pubmed.ncbi.nlm.nih.gov/33284564/. Accessed 16 Jan 2023.
13. Schäfer RC, Sohn A, Kersten A, Amr A, Held M, Wenger A. Quantification of dermal microcirculatory changes after topical administration of capsaicin: a randomized placebo-controlled study in 46 subjects. J Investig Surg. 2022;35:1673–8.
14. Zakaria A, Amerson E. Treatment modalities in Brachioradial pruritis: a systematic review. Dermatol Online J. 2022; https://doi.org/10.5070/d328458503.

Diclofenac

15. FDA drug monograph Solaraze® Gel. Available from https://www.accessdata.fda.gov/drugsatfda_docs/label/2000/21005lbl.pdf. Accessed 09 Jan 2023.
16. LexiComp drug monograph Diclofenac (Topical). Available from: LexiComp Online at online.Lexi.com. Copyright 2021 UptoDate, Inc.
17. De Groot AC. Patch testing. 3rd edition. Volume 3 Chapter 3.
18. Akarsu S, Aktan Ş, Atahan A, Koç P, Özkan Ş. Comparison of topical 3% diclofenac sodium gel and 5% imiquimod cream for the treatment of actinic keratoses. Clin Exp Dermatol. 2011;36:479–84.
19. Arisi M, Zane C, Polonioli M, et al. Effects of Mal-PDT, Ingenol Mebutate and diclofenac plus hyaluronate gel monitored by high-frequency ultrasound and digital dermoscopy in actinic keratosis – a randomized trial. J Eur Acad Dermatol Venereol. 2020;34:1225–32.

20. Bloor M, Paech M. Nonsteroidal anti-inflammatory drugs during pregnancy and the initiation of lactation. Anesthesia Analg. 2013;116:1063–75.
21. Bermas BL. Non-steroidal anti inflammatory drugs, glucocorticoids and disease modifying anti-rheumatic drugs for the management of rheumatoid arthritis before and during pregnancy. Curr Opin Rheum. 2014;26:334–40.
22. Cantisani C, Paolino G, Scarnò M, et al. Sequential methyl-aminolevulinate daylight photodynamic therapy and diclofenac plus hyaluronic acid gel treatment for multiple actinic keratosis evaluation. Dermatol Ther. 2018; https://doi.org/10.1111/dth.12710.
23. Çayirli M, Köse O, Demiriz M. Clinical, dermoscopic and immunohistochemical assessment of actinic keratoses and evaluation of the effectiveness of diclofenac therapy with immunohistochemical analysis. Arch Dermatol Res. 2013;305:389–95.
24. Dathe K, Hultzsch S, Pritchard LW, Schaefer C. Risk estimation of fetal adverse effects after short-term second trimester exposure to non-steroidal anti-inflammatory drugs: a literature review. Eur J Clin Pharmacol. 2019;75:1347–53.
25. Dianzani C, Conforti C, Giuffrida R, Corneli P, Meo N, Farinazzo E, Moret A, Magaton Rizzi G, Zalaudek I. Current therapies for actinic keratosis. Int J Dermatol. 2020;59:677–84.
26. Diclofenac gel: Package insert / prescribing information. In: Drugs.com. https://www.drugs.com/pro/diclofenac-gel.html. Accessed 11 Jan 2023.
27. Koch F, Salva KA, Wirtz M, Hadaschik E, Varaljai R, Schadendorf D, Roesch A. Efficacy of cold atmospheric plasma vs. Diclofenac 3% gel in patients with actinic keratoses: a prospective, randomized and rater-blinded study (ACTICAP). J Eur Acad Dermatol Venereol. 2020; https://doi.org/10.1111/jdv.16735.
28. Pflugfelder A, Welter A-K, Leiter U, Weide B, Held L, Eigentler TK, Dirschka T, Stockfleth E, Nashan D, Garbe C. Open label randomized study comparing 3 months vs. 6 months treatment of actinic keratoses with 3% diclofenac in 2.5% hyaluronic acid gel: a trial of the German Dermatologic Cooperative Oncology Group. J Eur Acad Dermatol Venereol. 2011;26:48–53.
29. Sammaritano LR, Bermas BL, Chakravarty EE, et al. 2020 American College of Rheumatology guideline for the management of reproductive health in rheumatic and musculoskeletal diseases. Arthritis Rheum. 2020;72:529–56.
30. Zane C, Facchinetti E, Rossi MT, Specchia C, Calzavara-Pinton PG. A randomized clinical trial of photodynamic therapy with methyl aminolaevulinate vs. Diclofenac 3% plus hyaluronic acid gel for the treatment of multiple actinic keratoses of the face and scalp. Br J Dermatol. 2014;170:1143–50.

Topical Antibiotics

12

Taylor Skinner, Parsa Abdi, Mahan Maazi, and Rebecca M. Law

Contents

T. Skinner · P. Abdi
Faculty of Medicine, Memorial University of Newfoundland, St. John's, NL, Canada
e-mail: pabedinzadeg@mun.ca; tcskinner@mun.ca

M. Maazi
Faculty of Medicine, University of British Columbia, Vancouver, BC, Canada
e-mail: maazi@student.ubc.edu

R. M. Law (✉)
School of Pharmacy and Faculty of Medicine (Discipline of Family Medicine), Memorial University of Newfoundland, St. John's, NL, Canada
e-mail: rlaw@mun.ca; rlawUCSF@gmail.com

R. M. Law, H. I. Maibach (eds.), *Handbook of Topical Drug Treatment in Dermatology*,
https://doi.org/10.1007/978-3-031-93616-6_12

Introduction

Taylor Skinner and Rebecca M. Law

Topical antibiotics are used to treat localized skin infections related to minor cuts, scrapes, and burns. There is a myriad of specific indications for various topical antibiotics, including blepharitis, conjunctivitis, rosacea keratitis, scleritis, episcleritis, iridocylitis, and otitis externa. Silver sulfadiazine is specifically indicated as an adjunct for the prevention and treatment of wound sepsis in patients with second- and third-degree burns. There are also combination products, for example, comprising an anti-infective agent plus a corticosteroid. This chapter is not meant to be a comprehensive compilation, and most monographs are single entity monographs. The product monographs included in this chapter are as follows:

Acetasol HC (Acetic Acid and Hydrocortisone)	1
Bacitracin	4
Gentamicin	7
Gramicidin	11
Mupirocin	13
Neomycin	16
Ozenoxacin	24
Polymyxin-B sulfate	26
Retapamulin	29
Silver sulfadiazine	34

Acetic Acid and Hydrocortisone (Acetasol HC)

Parsa Abdi

Classification and Mode of Action

- Acetasol HC is an otic solution, comprising a combination of a hydrocortisone and acetic acid, which is indicated for the management of otitis externa. Hydrocortisone exerts anti-inflammatory and antipruritic effects, whereas acetic acid exhibits antibacterial and antifungal properties.

Indications and Dermatological Uses

- *Clinical indications (FDA):* Otitis externa.
- *Off-label common uses:* N/A.

Formulations/Presentation

- US: Acetic acid 2%, propylene glycol diacetate 3%, and hydrocortisone 1% (10 mL). Solution, otic (drops).
- Canada:
- Europe:

Dosages and Suggested Regimens

- Place a saturated cotton wick, ensuring it is thoroughly wet, and maintain its moisture for 24 h by adding three to five drops of the solution every 4–6 h. After 24 h, remove the wick and instill five drops of the solution into the affected area three to four times a day, for as long as indicated.
- *Missed Dose:* In the event that a dose of acetasol HC is missed, it is recommended to apply the solution at earliest recollection and subsequently adhere to the appropriate time interval for

the next application. Do not apply two doses or use more than the recommended amount.

- *Overdosage:* While an overdose of acetasol HC is not typically considered dangerous, it is still important to seek emergency medical attention in the event of a suspected overdose.

Pharmacokinetics

- *Absorption:* As corticosteroids are absorbed through the aqueous humor, systemic absorption is minimal, if any, given that only low doses are administered.

Use in Special Populations

- Currently, there are no specific dosage recommendations for Gentamicin in special populations.
- *Pediatrics:* Approved for use in children. Safety and efficacy of acetasol HC has not established in children <3 years of age.
- *Geriatrics:* No dosage change is required. Clinical experience has not identified differences in response.
- *Hepatic insufficiency:* The manufacturer's labeling does not include any recommended dosage adjustments, and the need for such adjustments is unlikely due to the low systemic absorption of the medication.
- *Renal insufficiency:* The manufacturer's labeling does not include any recommended dosage adjustments, and the need for such adjustments is unlikely due to the low systemic absorption of the medication.
- *Pregnancy:* Listed as FDA pregnancy classification C.
- *Lactation:* It is unclear whether the topical application of corticosteroids could lead to enough systemic absorption to produce detectable amounts in breast milk. Caution if used in nursing women.

Monitoring

Contraindications and Cautions

- Individuals who have a known hypersensitivity to hydrocortisone, other corticosteroids, or any component present in the formulation should avoid using the product.
- The use of acetasol HC is contraindicated in individuals with a confirmed or suspected viral infection, such as herpes simplex virus, vaccinia, or varicella-zoster virus, of the external ear canal.
- The presence of fungal disease in the ear structures is a contraindication for the use of acetasol HC.
- The use of this product is contraindicated in cases of acute, untreated purulent infections of the ear.
- Patients with a perforated tympanic membrane should avoid using acetasol HC.
- To prevent the development of secondary infections, this product should not be used for more than ten consecutive days. If there is no improvement in the initial infection following seven to ten days of treatment, it is advisable to obtain cultures to assist in the determination of subsequent treatment measures.

Warnings and Precautions

- *Corticosteroid hypersensitivity:* Acetasol HC is contraindicated for individuals who have a known or suspected hypersensitivity to any of the product's ingredients, including those who are sensitive to hydrocortisone (i.e., corticosteroid hypersensitivity). If any signs of skin irritation or rash develop, discontinue the use of the product immediately.
- *Sulfite sensitivity:* Certain individuals who are susceptible may experience allergic-type reactions (such as anaphylaxis or life-threatening or mild asthmatic episodes) to sulfites, which may be present in certain otic preparations.
- *Local reaction:* When used for the first time in an inflamed ear, a temporary stinging or burning sensation may be experienced. If any signs of sensitization or irritation arise, discontinuation of the product is recommended.

Important Drug Interactions

- *Drug-drug interactions.*
  - *Aldesleukin:* The concurrent use of corticosteroids and Aldesleukin may result in a reduced antineoplastic effect of Aldesleukin. Risk X: should be avoided.
  - *Calcipotriene:* If hydrocortisone (topical) is used with calcipotriene, the therapeutic effect of calcipotriene may be reduced. To avoid this potential interaction, monitor for reduced calcipotriene efficacy and consider separating the administration of these agents by 10–12 h.
- *Drug-food interactions:* There is currently no evidence of any interactions between acetasol HC and food.

Adverse Effects and Their Management

- Headache, pruritus, and transient stinging or burning noticed in some patients.

Carcinogenicity

- There are no published carcinogenicity studies on acetasol HC.

Patch Test Concentration

- Patch testing information not available.

Essential Patient Information

- Some side effects of acetasol HC may include burning or stinging. Contact your doctor if these or other side effects persist.
- If you experience signs of irritation at the site of application or an allergic reaction such as rash, hives, itching, blistered or

peeling skin, wheezing, tightness in chest or throat, difficulty breathing, swallowing, or speaking, unusual hoarseness, swelling of mouth, face, lips, tongue or throat, seek immediate medical attention.

- Important to inform healthcare providers about any current or planned concomitant therapies, including prescription and over-the-counter medications, as well as any concurrent illnesses.
- Patients should be informed about other significant precautionary information (see monitoring).

Bacitracin

Taylor Skinner

Classification and Mode of Action

- Bacitracin inhibits bacterial cell wall synthesis by preventing the transfer of mucopeptides into the growing cell wall and thus preventing bacterial replication. Many gram-positive bacteria are susceptible to bacitracin, such as *Staphylococcus* spp. and *Streptococcus* spp. Some gram-negative bacteria are susceptible to bacitracin; however, most are resistant.
- In comparison to placebo, bacitracin ointment has been shown to reduce the occurrence of surgical site infections.

Indications

- *Clinical indications (FDA):* Short-term prevention and treatment of both acute and chronic localized skin infections in minor cuts, scrapes, or burns.
- *Off-label common uses.*

Formulations

- US: Ointment as Bacitracin Zinc (500 units/gram).
- Canada: Ointment (500 units/gram).
- Europe:

Dosages and Suggested Regimens

- Adults: apply one to three times daily.
- Infants, children, adolescents: apply a small amount one to three times daily. It is not recommended to exceed 7 days of therapy, unless directed by a healthcare professional.
- Do not use topical ointment in the eyes or over large areas of the body. Prior to application, the affected area should be cleansed gently with mild soap and water, if possible. Ointment may be applied directly on to the implicated wound or infected area, though enough should be used to cover the entire area.
- Missed dose: In the event that a dose of bacitracin ointment is missed, it is recommended to apply at the earliest recollection and continue as intended. Do not apply two doses or use more than the recommended amount.

Pharmacokinetics

- Absorption is limited following topical application as bacitracin displays poor absorption from mucous membranes and intact or denuded skin. A sterile dressing may be placed over the applied ointment to assist in absorption.

Use in Special Populations

- No dosage change is required for pediatric patients.
- No dosage change is required for geriatric patients.
- There is no available information to suggest dosing changes would be required in patients with hepatic or renal dysfunction.

- Pregnancy risk category C, though no large studies have been conducted with the use of topical bacitracin during pregnancy, and, to date, there is no evidence to suggest that there is an increased risk of adverse fetal effects with the use of topical bacitracin.
- To date, no large studies have been done with the use of topical bacitracin during lactation. However, the use of bacitracin while breastfeeding has not been associated with an increased risk of adverse effects in the infant.

Contraindications and Cautions

- Contraindicated in those with a hypersensitivity to bacitracin or to any component of the formulation of the available product. If signs of allergic reaction or rash occur, discontinue use immediately.
- Patients with a known hypersensitivity to neomycin may also be sensitive to bacitracin.
- Application of bacitracin on a wound from a viral or fungal infection may increase the risk of developing drug-resistant bacteria.
- There is no mention of toxicity with the use of topical bacitracin as a single agent ointment or as part of a triple therapy ointment.

Important Drug Interactions

- There are no significant drug-drug interactions with bacitracin.
- There are no significant drug-food interactions with bacitracin.

Adverse Effects and Management

- May cause allergic contact dermatitis upon application.

Carcinogenicity

- There are no carcinogenic studies of bacitracin; however, bacitracin ointment is not considered to be a carcinogenic agent according to the IARC, ACGIH, NTP, or OSHA.

Patch Test Concentration

- 5% in petrolatum or 20% in petrolatum. Patch test may become positive only at day 4.

Clinical Pearls

- 1 unit of ointment is equivalent to 0.026 mg bacitracin.

Essential Patient Information

- Bacitracin is available as an over the counter (OTC) medication.
- Bacitracin ointment should be stored at room temperature (15–30 °C).
- If symptoms worsen, bacitracin should be discontinued and a healthcare provider consulted.

Gentamicin Sulfate

Parsa Abdi

Classification and Mode of Action

- Gentamicin sulfate is an aminoglycoside antibiotic that blocks protein synthesis in susceptible bacteria by binding to the prokaryotic ribosome. It exhibits bactericidal activity against both gram-positive and gram-negative bacteria in vitro. Compared to mupirocin ointment, gentamicin sulfate has similar efficacy, however, a significantly faster onset of action in the treatment of impetigo.

Indications and Dermatological Uses

- *Clinical indications (FDA):* Skin and skin structure infections, including burn wound infection and necrotizing infections as well as minor skin infections, including impetigo, infected seborrheic dermatitis, folliculitis, furunculosis, sycosis barbae, eczema, pustular acne, pyoderma gangrenosum, infectious eczematoid dermatitis, infected contact dermatitis, pustular psoriasis, and infected excoriations.
- *Off-label common uses.*

Formulations/Presentation

- US: 0.1% (15 g, 30 g) cream, 0.1% (15 g, 30 g) ointment.
- Canada: 0.1% (15 g, 30 g) cream, 0.1% (15 g, 30 g) ointment.
- Europe:

Dosages and Suggested Regimens

- Apply gentamicin sulfate to the affected area three to four times per day.
- Gentamicin should only be used externally and is not indicated for ophthalmic use. Gently apply it to the affected area and consider covering it with gauze dressing. For impetigo contagiosa, remove any crust before applying.
- *Missed dose:* In the event that a dose of gentamicin sulfate is missed, it is recommended to apply the ointment/cream at earliest recollection and subsequently adhere to the appropriate time interval for the next application. Do not apply two doses or use more than the recommended amount.

- *Overdosage:* If an overdose to occurs, hemodialysis may be helpful in removing the drug from the blood, particularly if renal function is impaired. Peritoneal dialysis is less effective than hemodialysis at removing gentamicin sulfate from the body.

Pharmacokinetics

- *Absorption.*
  - Gentamicin sulfate is typically not absorbed through intact skin. However, it can be readily absorbed through denuded areas of skin, such as wounds, burns, or ulcers, as well as skin that has lost the keratin layer.
  - Gentamicin cream is more readily absorbed than gentamicin ointment.
  - Topical application to burn patients has been reported to result in systemic absorption.

Use in Special Populations

- Currently, there are no specific dosage recommendations for Gentamicin in special populations.
- *Pediatrics:* Approved for use in children. May cause irritation or allergic reaction. Do not administer orally, topical application only. Safety and efficacy not established in children <1 year of age.
- *Geriatrics:* No dosage change is required.
- *Hepatic insufficiency:* The manufacturer's labeling does not include any recommended dosage adjustments, and the need for such adjustments is unlikely due to the low systemic absorption of the medication.
- *Renal insufficiency:* The manufacturer's labeling does not include any recommended dosage adjustments, and the need for such adjustments is unlikely due to the low systemic absorption of the medication.
- *Pregnancy:* Listed as FDA pregnancy classification C.

- *Lactation:* It is uncertain whether gentamicin sulfate is excreted in breast milk after topical application. When administered systemically, known to be excreted in small amounts in breast milk. Nevertheless, the American Academy of Pediatrics (AAP) considers gentamicin sulfate to be compatible with breastfeeding.

Monitoring

Contraindications and Cautions

- Patients who have a known hypersensitivity to gentamicin sulfate or any ingredients in the formulation should not use topical gentamicin sulfate. Patients who are allergic to other topical antibiotics should be closely monitored during treatment with gentamicin sulfate. If any signs of irritation or hypersensitivity appear, the medication should be discontinued immediately. It should be noted that cross-allergenicity has been demonstrated among aminoglycosides, and patients who become sensitized to topical gentamicin sulfate may also be sensitive to other topical and systemic aminoglycosides. Therefore, caution should be exercised in these patients.

Warnings and Precautions

- *Sensitivity reactions:* Sensitization and photosensitivity have been reported in some cases following the use of topical gentamicin.
- *Superinfection:* Overgrowth and possible development of resistant bacteria or fungi. If superinfection arises, stop taking the medication and commence appropriate therapy.
- *Cross-hypersensitivity:* There is a risk of cross-allergenicity among aminoglycosides. Therefore, it's important to be aware that patients who develop sensitivity to topical gentamicin sulfate may also be sensitive to other types of topical and/or systemic aminoglycosides. If patients are known to be hypersensitive to other topical antibiotics, it is recommended to closely monitor them when using gentamicin sulfate. If any signs of irritation or hypersensitivity appear, it is advised to discontinue use.

- *Cumulative toxicity:* When topical aminoglycosides are used in combination with systemic aminoglycoside therapy and applied to large skin lesions or denuded areas, there is a risk of cumulative toxicity.

Important Drug Interactions

- *Drug-drug interactions:* There are currently no known clinically significant drug interactions with gentamicin sulfate use. No interactions of Risk Level A or greater identified.
- *Drug-food interactions:* There is currently no evidence of any interactions between gentamicin sulfate and food.

Adverse Effects and Their Management

- Application of gentamicin sulfate is generally considered to be relatively nontoxic, although it is possible to develop sensitization to the drug from its topical use.
- Commercially available preparations of Gentamicin often contain additional ingredients like parabens that could cause allergic contact dermatitis.
- Although infrequent, local irritation including erythema and pruritus may occur following topical administration.
- Several patients treated with topical gentamicin sulfate have reported photosensitivity reactions; however, it remains unclear whether the drug was the direct cause of these reactions.

Carcinogenicity, Mutagenesis, and Impairment of Fertility—If Known

- There are no published carcinogenicity studies on gentamicin sulfate. Aminoglycoside antibiotics have been found to be nonmutagenic.

Patch Test Concentration

- 20% in petrolatum. Late readings at days 6–8 are necessary to avoid possibly missing a positive patch test evolving after day 3 or 4.

Essential Patient Information

- It is crucial to discontinue gentamicin and initiate appropriate treatment if superinfection occurs.
- Topical gentamicin preparations are meant for external use only and should not be ingested or used in the eyes.
- Important to inform healthcare providers about any current or planned concomitant therapies, including prescription and over-the-counter medications, as well as any concurrent illnesses.
- Patients should be informed about other significant precautionary information (see monitoring).

Gramicidin

Mahan Maazi

Classification and Mode of Action

- Gramicidin a cyclic polypeptide antibiotic is a heterogenous mixture of antimicrobial linear polypeptides that have been extracted from tyrothricin through the growth and fermentation of *Brevibacillus brevis*. It causes bacterial cell wall disruption and permeabilization and works well against most gram-positive and some gram-negative bacteria. It is used topically for infections often in combination with other antibacterials neomycin, bacitracin, nystatin, and polymyxin B and corticosteroids.

Indications and Dermatological Uses

- *Clinical indications (FDA):* blepharitis, eczema (eyelid), conjunctivitis (allergic, infective, rosacea), rosacea keratitis, scleritis and epscleritis, iridocylitis, otitis externa, pruritus.
- *Off-label common uses:* other skin infections and surface wounds.

Formulations/Presentation

- US: 0.05 mg/g cream (multi-ingredient), 0.05 mg/g ointment (multi-ingredient), 0.025 mg per 1 mL eyedrops (multi-ingredient), 0.05 mg/g nasal spray (multi-ingredient).
- Canada: 0.25 mg/g, 0.05 mg/g cream (multi-ingredient), 0.25 mg/g, 0.05 mg/g cream ointment (multi-ingredient), 0.025 mg per 1 mL eye-drops (multi-ingredient), 0.25 mg/g, 0.05 mg nasal spray (multi-ingredient).
- Europe: 0.05 mg/g cream cream (multi-ingredient), 0.05 mg cream ointment (multi-ingredient), 0.025 mg per 1 mL eye-drops (multi-ingredient), 0.05 mg nasal spray (multi-ingredient).

Dosages and Suggested Regimens

- Cream/ointment (multi-ingredient): apply small quantity two to three times per day.
- Eyedrops (multi-ingredient): ophthalmic: one or two drops every 1–2 h for 2 or 3 days and then follow with one or two drops three to four times daily. Otic: two or three drops three or four times daily.
- Intransal (multi-ingredient): two sprays in each nostril every 4 h for 3–5 days.
- No suggested dosage adjustment for renal or hepatic impairment due to low dose topical use only.

Pharmacokinetics

- Only used on skin, with insignificant absorption, thus no relevant pharmacokinetics.

Use in Special Populations

- Approved for use in children.
- Listed as FDA pregnancy classification A. (former classification system).
- Unknown whether gramicidin is present in breast milk.
- Renal insufficiency: not evaluated; dose adjustment is not expected to be needed.
- Hepatic insufficiency: not evaluated; dose adjustment is not expected to be needed.

Monitoring

- Hypersensitivity reaction.
- Dermatologic conditions: dermatitis, pruritus, maculopapular rash, urticaria, vesicular eruption, burning sensations.

Contraindications and Cautions

- Hypersensitivity reactions.
- Accidental ingestion may cause hemolysis and can be toxic to the liver, kidney, meninges, and olfactory system.
- Other indications would be related to other drugs in the formulation.

Important Drug Interactions

- Risk/severity of bleeding increased when combined with Acenocoumarol.
- Risk/severity of methemoglobinemia increased with local anaesthetics (benzocaine, bupivacaine, buacaine, and chloroprocaine), capsaicin, butamben, and benzyl alcohol.

Adverse Effects and Their Management

- Skin atrophy, striae.
- Burning, itching, erythema.
- Dryness, hypertrichosis.
- Hypopigmentation folliculitis.
- Superinfection due to prolonged use.
- Discontinue use if local irritation/sensitization occurs.

Carcinogenicity

- Long-term studies in animals to evaluate carcinogenic or mutagenic potential with gramicidin have not been conducted.

Patch Test Concentration

- Patch testing unavailable.

Essential Patient Information

- Be aware of any signs of an allergic reaction and seek medical help as necessary.
- Do not use longer than indicated due to risk of second infection.
- Do not take by mouth. For use on skin only.

Mupirocin

Mahan Maazi

Classification and Mode of Action

- Also known as pseudomonic acid A. Natural crotonic acid derivative and antibiotic extracted from a strain of *Pseudomonas fluorescens*. It reversibly and selectively binds to bacterial isoleucyl tRNA synthase causing inhibition of bacterial protein synthesis. Most gram-positive aerobic bacteria are sensitive to mupirocin. Mupirocin is more effective than oral erythromycin, topical bacitracin, and oral cephalexin for impetigo and more effective than silver sulfadiazine, silver nitrate, mafenide acetate, and honey, for *S. aureus* acquired burn wounds.

Indications and Dermatological Uses

- *Clinical indications (FDA):* impetigo due to *Staphylococcus aureus* and *Streptococcus pyogenes,* secondary skin infection, *S. aureus* (including MSRA) decolonization.
- *Off-label common uses:* folliculitis, nasal vestibulitis, peritoneal dialysis catheter exit-site, or tunnel infection prophylaxis.

Formulations/Presentation

- US: 2% cream, 2% ointment containing polyethylene gycol (PEG), 2% ointment without PEG, 2% nasal ointment.
- Canada:
- Europe:

Dosages and Suggested Regimens

Adult

- Impetigo: ointment—apply to affected area two to three times daily for 5 days.
- Secondary skin infection: cream/ointment—apply to affected area two to three times daily, typically for 7–14 days; re-evaluate if no response after 3–5 days.
- Folliculitis (off-label): ointment—apply to affected area three times daily for 7 days.
- Nasal vestibulitis (off-label): intranasal ointment—apply to affected nostril twice daily for 5 days.
- Peritoneal dialysis catheter exit-site or tunnel infection prophylaxis (off-label): cream—apply once daily to catheter exit site.

- Recurrent *S. aureus* infection or preoperative decolonization: ointment/intranasal ointment—apply one-half of the ointment from single-use 1 g tube into each nostril twice daily for 5–10 days.

Pediatric

- Nasal MRSA decolonization: intranasal ointment—infants/children apply a small amount twice daily for 5–10 days, children 12 or older and adolescents apply 500 mg twice daily for 5–10 days.
- MRSA or impetigo; minor skin infection: cream/ointment—small amount three times daily for 5–10 days, re-evaluate for patients not showing a response after 5 days.

Pharmacokinetics

- Absorption: Topical ointment and cream penetrates outer layer of skin and has minimal systemic absorption. Intranasal has 3% absorption and adults and may be significant in neonates and premature infants.
- Has a protein binding of more than 97% and is metabolized to monic acid which is its inactive form.
- The half-life is 17–36 min and is excreted in the urine as monic acid.

Use in Special Populations

- Approved for use in children. Avoid high dosage use in neonates and internal use.
- Listed as FDA pregnancy classification B (former classification system).
- Unknown whether mupirocin is present in breast milk.
- Renal insufficiency: not evaluated; dose adjustment is not expected to be needed.
- Hepatic insufficiency: not evaluated; dose adjustment is not expected to be needed.

Monitoring

- Central nervous system: headache, localized burning, stinging sensation.
- Dermatologic issues: pruritus, skin rash.
- Gastrointestinal issues nausea, dysgeusia.
- Local pain.
- Respiratory: rhinitis, respiratory congestion, pharyngitis, cough.

Contraindications and Cautions

- Hypersensitivity including system reactions, sensitization, or local irritation.
- Superinfection due to prolonged use.
- Polyethylene glycol from percutaneous absorption in open wounds or burns may cause toxic effects especially in large quantities.
- Benzyl alcohol may cause fatal toxicity known as "gasping syndrome" in neonates which consists of metabolic acidosis, respiratory distress, gasping respirations, CNS dysfunction, hypotension, and cardiovascular collapse. Avoid or use benzyl alcohol containing dosage forms with caution.
- Large amounts in neonates, children, and adults may cause potentially fatal toxicities (metabolic acidosis, seizures, renal failure, respiratory depression, hyperosmolality, lactic acidosis, and CNS depression) through some forms containing propylene glycol.

Important Drug Interactions

- No known drug interactions.

Adverse Effects and Their Management

- Hypersensitivity reactions which include systemic allergic reactions (urticaria, angioedema, and generalized rash). Discontinue use if it occurs.
- Superinfection may result in bacterial or fungal infection (*C. difficile*-associated diarrhea (CDAD) and pseudomembranous colitis).
- May cause severe burning and tearing in eyes for intranasal ointments, which resolves within days to weeks after discontinuation.

Carcinogenicity

- Evaluation of carcinogenic potential for mupirocin in long-term studies in animals has not been conducted.

Patch Test Concentration

- 2% in petrolatum

Essential Patient Information

- Do not put it on skin that is damaged or has open wounds.
- Do not use in an area where drugs are given into a vein.
- Be aware of any signs of an allergic reaction, which include rash, hives, itchiness, redness, swelling, blistering, peeling skin with or without fever, wheezing, tightness in chest or throat, breathing difficulties, unusual hoarseness, or any angioedema (swelling).
- Be aware of any signs or symptoms of dizziness or fast/abnormal heartbeat.
- Be aware of any diarrhea symptoms, which can be a sign of CDAD.
- Use only on skin and keep out of mouth, nose, and eyes.
- For single use nose ointment, half into one nostril and the other half into the other nostril and spread into the nose.

Neomycin Sulfate

Parsa Abdi

Classification and Mode of Action

- Neomycin sulfate is classified as an aminoglycoside antibiotic and is primarily used for its bactericidal effects. Neomycin sulfate is believed to exert its antibacterial effect by binding irreversibly to the 30S ribosomal subunit of susceptible bacteria, disrupting protein synthesis. The use of neomycin sulfate has been evaluated in several clinical trials, which have demonstrated its effectiveness in treating a variety of bacterial infections. Notable trials include those examining its use in treating skin infections and urinary tract infections.

Indications and Dermatological Uses

- *Clinical indications (FDA):*
  - *Prevention of superficial bacterial skin infections associated with minor cuts, scrapes, or burns* (neomycin sulfate fixed combination with other anti-infectives).
  - *Treatment of corticosteroid-responsive dermatoses with secondary infection* (neomycin sulfate fixed combination with a corticosteroid with or without other anti-infectives).
  - *Prevention of bacteriuria and gram-negative septicemia associated with use of indwelling catheters* (fixed combination of neomycin and polymyxin B).
- *Off-label common uses:*
  - *Treatment of minor skin infections caused by susceptible bacteria* (neomycin sulfate fixed combination with other anti-infectives).
  - *Peritoneal instillation* (no longer recommended due to potential severe toxicity).
  - *Irrigation of wounds or surgical sites* (no longer recommended due to potential severe toxicity).

Formulations/Presentation

- US:
  - Neomycin and Polymyxin B Sulfates: Each mL contains 40 mg of neomycin sulfate and 200,000 units of polymyxin B sulfate (Urogenital—irrigation concentrate).
  - *Neomycin and polymyxin B sulfates and bacitracin zinc:* Each gram contains 3.5 mg of neomycin sulfate, 5000 units of polymyxin B sulfate, and 400 units of bacitracin zinc (topical—ointment).
  - *Neomycin and polymyxin B sulfates, bacitracin zinc, and hydrocortisone:* Each gram contains 3.5 mg of neomycin sulfate, 5000 units of polymyxin B sulfate, 400 units of bacitracin zinc, and 1% hydrocortisone (topical—ointment).
  - *Neomycin and polymyxin B sulfates and hydrocortisone acetate:* Each gram contains 3.5 mg of neomycin sulfate, 10,000 units of polymyxin B sulfate, and 5 mg of hydrocortisone acetate (topical—cream).
  - *Neomycin sulfate and fluocinolone acetonide:* Each gram contains 3.5 mg of neomycin sulfate and 0.25 mg of fluocinolone acetonide (topical—cream).
  - *Other neomycin sulfate combinations:* Each gram contains 3.5 mg of neomycin sulfate, 5000 units of polymyxin B sulfate, 400 units of bacitracin zinc, and 20 mg of lidocaine hydrochloride (topical—cream); each gram contains 3.5 mg of neomycin sulfate, 10,000 units of polymyxin B sulfate, and 10 mg of pramoxine hydrochloride (topical—cream); each gram contains 3.5 mg of neomycin sulfate, 5000 units of polymyxin B sulfate, 400 units of bacitracin zinc, and 40 mg of lidocaine (topical—ointment); each gram contains 3.5 mg of neomycin sulfate, 10,000 units of polymyxin B sulfate, 500 units of bacitracin zinc, and 10 mg of pramoxine hydrochloride (topical—ointment).

Dosages and Suggested Regimens

- Neomycin sulfate is available in cream and ointment forms that are applied topically to the skin. The recommended frequency of use is usually one to three times a day.
- The maximum duration of use for neomycin sulfate is typically one week, unless otherwise directed by a healthcare provider. To ensure safe and effective use of the medication, it is important to follow the directions on your prescription label carefully.
- Start by thoroughly cleaning the infected area and allowing it to dry. Gently rub the medication into the skin until most of it disappears, using only enough to cover the affected area. After application, be sure to wash your hands.
- It is important not to apply neomycin to a child's diaper area, especially if the skin is raw, unless directed to do so by a doctor. If directed to apply neomycin in this area, avoid using tightly fitting diapers or plastic pants, as they can increase the absorption of the drug, leading to harmful effects.
- When using neomycin on scrapes, cuts, burns, sores, and wounds, apply only small amounts and follow the recommended frequency of use.
- May cover affected areas with a sterile bandage.
- *Missed Dose:* In the event that a dose of neomycin sulfate is missed, it is recommended to apply the solution at earliest recollection and subsequently adhere to the appropriate time interval for the next application. Do not apply two doses or use more than the recommended amount.
- *Overdosage:* It is unlikely for an acute overdose to occur with neomycin sulfate due to its low absorption rate. However, prolonged use of the medication may lead to sufficient systemic drug levels that can result in neurotoxicity, ototoxicity, and/or nephrotoxicity. If you experience any symptoms of toxicity, such as hearing difficulties, dizziness, or kidney problems, seek medical attention immediately.

Pharmacokinetics

- *Absorption:*
  - Neomycin sulfate is not significantly absorbed through intact skin, but it can be absorbed through areas of skin that have been denuded or have lost the keratin layer, such as wounds, burns, or ulcers.
  - When used for bladder irrigation, systemic absorption of neomycin is not expected to be clinically significant if the bladder is intact and the duration of irrigation is less than or equal to 10 days. However, systemic absorption may occur if the bladder surface is denuded or inflamed.
  - In cases where neomycin sulfate is administered into the peritoneum, drainage sinuses, wounds, or surgical sites, it is rapidly absorbed into the systemic circulation.
  - When neomycin sulfate is topically applied to open wounds, burns, or granulating surfaces, the resulting plasma concentrations are similar to or greater than those achieved with oral or parenteral administration (parenteral preparation is no longer available in the US).

Use in Special Populations

- *Pediatrics:*
  - Topical: Certain manufacturers advise against using neomycin sulfate product in children under 2 years of age unless specifically instructed by a healthcare provider.
  - Topical (fixed combination of neomycin and fluocinolone): The manufacturer recommends utilizing the minimum effective dose when incorporating neomycin sulfate into a therapeutic regimen. In pediatric patients, due to their higher skin surface area-to-body weight ratio, they may be more vulnerable to experiencing hypothalamic-pituitary-adrenal (HPA) axis suppression and Cushing's syndrome resulting from topical corticosteroid use compared to older patients.

- Topical (fixed combination of neomycin, polymyxin B with or without bacitracin, and hydrocortisone): There is no established evidence regarding the safety and efficacy of using neomycin sulfate in pediatric patients. However, prolonged use of topical hydrocortisone in infants and children can lead to significant absorption of the drug through the skin, which may cause growth cessation and other manifestations of hyperadrenocorticism.
- Topical (fixed combination of neomycin, polymyxin B, bacitracin, and lidocaine): According to at least one manufacturer, neomycin sulfate should not be used in children under the age of 12 years unless specifically instructed to do so by a healthcare provider.
- Bladder irrigation (fixed combination of neomycin and polymyxin B): Safety and efficacy not established in pediatric patients.

• *Geriatrics:*
  - Topical (fixed combination of neomycin, polymyxin B with or without bacitracin, and hydrocortisone): The clinical trials did not enroll a significant number of patients aged 65 years and above to ascertain whether the geriatric population has a distinct response from younger patients; however, available anecdotal evidence from other clinical experiences has not identified any significant difference in response between the two groups.
  - Bladder irrigation (fixed combination of neomycin and polymyxin B): Geriatric patients who receive high doses of neomycin sulfate for an extended period are at an increased risk of toxicity.
• *Renal insufficiency:* Patients with renal impairment are at an increased risk of toxicity when using the fixed combination of neomycin and polymyxin B for bladder irrigation.
• *Pregnancy:*
  - Aminoglycosides can be harmful to a developing fetus if absorbed systemically in pregnant women. Neomycin sulfate can cross the placenta, and some children whose mothers received parenteral streptomycin during pregnancy have reported total, irreversible, bilateral, congenital deafness.

- When used in a fixed combination with a corticosteroid, with or without other anti-infectives, during pregnancy, it should only be used if the potential benefits justify the potential risks to the fetus. Topical corticosteroids have been found to be teratogenic in animals such as mice and rabbits.
- If the fixed combination of neomycin and polymyxin B is used during pregnancy, the patient should be informed about the potential hazard to the fetus.
- Listed as FDA pregnancy classification C in the former FDA pregnancy risk classification system.

- *Lactation:*
  - It is unclear whether the topical application of corticosteroids could lead to enough systemic absorption to produce detectable amounts in breast milk. Caution if used in nursing women. Small amounts of neomycin may pass into breast milk if it is absorbed systemically, but it is not considered clinically significant.
  - Caution should be exercised when using the topical fixed combination of neomycin and a corticosteroid with or without other anti-infectives in nursing women as systemic corticosteroids can be distributed into human milk.

Monitoring

Contraindications

- Topical (fixed combinations of neomycin and other anti-infectives with or without a topical anesthetic): Individuals with a known hypersensitivity to neomycin or any of the components in the formulation should avoid using this product.
- Topical (fixed combinations of neomycin and a corticosteroid with or without other anti-infectives): Should not be used by individuals who have a known hypersensitivity to any of the ingredients in the formulation. Contraindicated for use on skin lesions caused by tuberculosis, fungus, or viruses such as herpes simplex or varicella zoster. Should not be used in the eyes or in the external ear canal if the eardrum is perforated.

- Bladder irrigation (fixed combination of neomycin and polymyxin B): Individuals who have a known hypersensitivity to neomycin, polymyxins, or any of the ingredients in the formulation should avoid using this product. Due to the potential for cross-sensitivity among aminoglycosides, the product may also be contraindicated in individuals who have a history of hypersensitivity or serious toxic reactions to any aminoglycoside.

Warnings and Precautions

- *Sensitivity Reactions.*
  - Patients using topical preparations that contain neomycin sulfate should be advised to discontinue use and seek medical attention if they experience symptoms such as itching, burning, rash, or any other signs of sensitivity or allergic reaction.
  - Clinicians should consider that patients who are allergic to topical neomycin sulfate may develop cutaneous sensitivity reactions or anaphylactic reactions to the drug.
  - Cross-allergenicity can occur among aminoglycosides, and patients who become sensitized to topical neomycin may also be sensitive to other topical or systemic aminoglycosides.
  - Patients who are allergic to one fixed-combination topical preparation that contains neomycin sulfate should avoid using any products that contain any of the component drugs.
- *Topical Use.*
  - Use of this medication for more than one week should only be done under the direction of a clinician to avoid promoting bacterial resistance.
  - Prolonged use may lead to overgrowth of nonsusceptible organisms, including fungi.
  - There have been reports of ototoxicity, nephrotoxicity, and neuromuscular blockade following topical application of neomycin, particularly when used for peritoneal instilla-

tion, irrigation of wounds or surgical sites, or topical treatment of skin ulcers, granulating wounds, serious burns, or extensive areas of denuded skin, resulting in systemic absorption of the drug. Rare cases of death have also been reported.
  - Risk of systemic absorption and the possibility of toxicity such as ototoxicity, nephrotoxicity, and neuromuscular blockade, caution should be exercised when using neomycin topically for extensive burns, trophic ulceration, or other extensive dermatologic conditions where rapid absorption of the drug is possible. In patients with burns covering ≥20% of their body surface area, especially those with impaired renal function or who are receiving other aminoglycosides concurrently, topical neomycin should be applied no more than once daily.
- *Bladder Irrigation.*
  - The fixed combination of neomycin and polymyxin B should not be used as an irrigation solution if there is a possibility of systemic absorption. This solution is intended for continuous prophylactic bladder irrigation only in patients with an intact urinary bladder. To avoid toxicity and the risk of systemic absorption, it should not be used in patients with defects in bladder mucosa or bladder wall or in conjunction with operative procedures involving bladder wall. Patients with impaired renal function, infants, dehydrated patients, geriatric patients, and those receiving prolonged treatment with high doses are especially at risk for toxicity.
  - The safety and efficacy of bladder irrigation with the fixed combination solution have not been established in patients with recent lower urinary tract surgery.
  - Overgrowth of nonsusceptible organisms, including fungi, may occur during bladder irrigation, and appropriate measures should be taken if needed.
  - Urine specimens should be collected for urinalysis, culture, and susceptibility testing. In the event of isolation of uropathogens, in vitro susceptibility testing should be performed, and systemic anti-infective therapy should be initiated if appropriate.

- *Use of Fixed Combinations.*
  - When a fixed combination of neomycin with other topical anti-infectives, topical corticosteroids, or topical anesthetics are used, caution should be taken, and contraindications associated with each drug should be considered.
  - If a fixed combination of neomycin with corticosteroid is used, it should be kept in mind that topical corticosteroids used in fixed combination with topical anti-infectives may hide clinical signs of bacterial, fungal, or viral infections or suppress hypersensitivity reactions to the anti-infectives or other ingredients in the formulation.
  - The use of topical corticosteroids can result in signs and symptoms of exogenous hyperadrenocorticism, including adrenal suppression, and if applied to extensive body surface areas or with occlusive dressing, systemic absorption of the topically applied corticosteroids can be increased. If redness, irritation, swelling, or pain persists or increases, the use should be discontinued.

Important Drug Interactions

- *Drug-Drug Interactions.*
  - It is important to use caution when using neomycin sulfate along with other drugs that are neurotoxic or nephrotoxic as this could potentially increase the risk of nephrotoxicity or ototoxicity.
  - Similarly, caution should also be taken when using neomycin along with other aminoglycosides or polymyxins, as this may increase the risk of nephrotoxicity or ototoxicity and may also enhance neomycin's neuromuscular blocking effects.
- *Drug-Food Interactions:* There is currently no evidence of any interactions between neomycin sulfate and food.

Adverse Effects and Their Management

- *Topical:* Allergic contact dermatitis. May result in systemic absorption of the drug, leading to ototoxicity, nephrotoxicity, and neuromuscular blockade. This risk is especially significant when neomycin is used for peritoneal instillation, irrigation of wounds or surgical sites, or topical treatment of skin ulcers, granulating wounds, serious burns, or extensive areas of denuded skin.
- *Bladder irrigation:* Irritation of urinary bladder mucosa.

Carcinogenicity

- There have been no long-term animal studies conducted on neomycin sulfate to assess its potential for carcinogenicity or mutagenicity.

Patch Test Concentration

- 20% in petrolatum. It is recommended to read patch test at day 7 or day 8, as late positive reactions after day 4 are frequent.

Essential Patient Information

- Neomycin sulfate and other antibacterial medications should only be used to treat bacterial infections. They are not effective in treating viral infections.
- Neomycin-containing topical products are intended for external use only and should not be applied to the eyes. Additionally, patients should be advised to avoid using these products over large areas of the body.
- In topical preparations containing neomycin for self-medication to prevent infection in minor skin injuries like cuts, scrapes, and burns, patients should not be used for more than

one week unless directed by a clinician. Discontinue use and consult a clinician if the condition persists or worsens.
- Discontinue use of any topical preparation containing neomycin and consult a healthcare professional if any signs of sensitivity or allergic reaction, such as itching, burning, or rash, occur.
- Consult a clinician before using topical preparations containing neomycin for self-medication in cases of deep or puncture wounds, animal bites, or serious burns.
- Inform healthcare provider if you are pregnant, planning to become pregnant, or planning to breastfeed while using neomycin sulfate.

Ozenoxacin

Taylor Skinner

Classification and Mode of Action

- Ozenoxacin is a quinolone antimicrobial that inhibits the bacterial DNA replication enzymes; DNA gyrase A and topoisomerase IV.
- Ozenoxacin has been found to display potent activity against many common skin and soft tissue infections, including those displaying resistance to other common antimicrobial classes such as fusidic acid and mupirocin.

Indications

- *Clinical indications (FDA):* Treatment of impetigo due to *Staphylococcus aureus* or *Streptococcus pyogenes* in adult and pediatric patients 2 months of age and older.
- *Off-label common uses.*

Formulations

- US: 1% cream [brand: Xepi].
- Canada: 1% cream [brand: Ozanex].
- Europe:

Dosages and Suggested Regimens

- Adults: apply a thin layer of cream to the affected area twice daily for 5 days.
  - The total treatment area should not exceed 100 cm^2 total BSA.
- Infants, children, and adolescents: apply a thin layer of cream to the affected area twice daily for 5 days.
  - The total treatment area should not exceed 2% of the total BSA for patients under 12.
  - The total treatment area should not exceed 100cm^2 total BSA for patients over 12.
- Wash hands after application. The treated area may be covered with a sterile bandage or gauze dressing.
- Missed dose.
- Any sign or symptom of overdose should be treated symptomatically, as no specific antidote is known.

Pharmacokinetics

- Absorption is negligible following topical application.
- Ozenoxacin was not metabolized in the presence of human skin discs and was only minimally metabolized in human hepatocytes.
- Due to negligible systemic absorption, tissue distribution and excretion have not been investigated in humans.

Use in Special Populations

- No dosage change is required for geriatric patients.
- There is no available information to suggest dosing changes would be required in patients with hepatic or renal dysfunction.
- To date, no large studies have been done with the use of topical ozenoxacin. However, due to negligible systemic absorption, exposure of the fetus to the drug is not expected.
- To date, no large studies have been done with the use of topical bacitracin during lactation, and it is not known if ozenoxacin is present in breastmilk. However, due to negligible systemic absorption, exposure of the infant to the drug is not expected.

Contraindications and Cautions

- Contraindicated in those with a hypersensitivity to ozenoxacin or to any component of the formulation of the available product. If signs of allergic reaction occur, discontinue use immediately.
- Prolonged use of ozenoxacin may result in overgrowth of nonsusceptible bacteria and fungi, resulting in a superinfection. Discontinue use and use alternative therapy if superinfection occurs.
- There is no mention of toxicity with the use of topical ozenoxacin.

Important Drug Interactions

- There are no significant drug-drug interactions with ozenoxacin.
- There are no significant drug-food interactions with ozenoxacin.

Adverse Effects and Management

- May cause rosacea or seborrheic dermatitis upon application.

Carcinogenicity

- Long-term animal studies have not been conducted to evaluate the carcinogenicity of ozenoxacin, although ozenoxacin has not been found to induce genotoxicity when evaluated in vitro in the Ames test, mouse lymphoma cell assay, or in a rat micronucleus test with systemic exposure.
- Ozenoxacin has not been found to affect the fertility of male and female rats treated orally with 500 mg/kg/day, which is much greater than the maximum human plasma concentration with topical application of 1% ozenoxacin cream.

Patch Test Concentration

- Patch testing information not available.

Essential Patient Information

- It is recommended to use this medication for the entire duration as prescribed, even if symptoms have improved earlier.
- Ozenoxacin should be stored at room temperature (20–25 °C), though some exposure to temperatures between 15 and 30 °C are permitted.
- If symptoms worsen, ozenoxacin should be discontinued and a healthcare provider consulted.

Polymyxin-B Sulfate

Mahan Maazi

Classification and Mode of Action

- Polymyxin-B sulfate is a cationic, peptide antibiotic mixture of polymyxins B1 and B2 effective against gram-negative bacteria and is obtained from *Bacillus polymyxa.* It acts as a surface detergent and destroys bacterial membranes. It is usually used in combination with other antibiotics such as bacitracin or neomycin.

Indications and Dermatological Uses

- Clinical indications (FDA): Acute infections caused by susceptible strains of *Pseudomonas aeruginosa* (urinary tract, meninges, eyes, bloodstream).
- Serious infections (*H. influenzae*, meningeal; *E.coli*, urinary tract; *Aerobacter aerogenes*, bacteremia; and *Klebsiella pneumoniae*, bacteremia).
- Off-label common uses: inhalation for nebulization (off-label route).

Formulations/Presentation

- US: 10,000 units = 1 mg: 500,000 units (solution injections), 100 million units (powder), 10,000 units per g (ointment), 200,000 units per 1 mL (solution; irrigation).

Dosages and Suggested Regimens

- Topical: apply to affected area one to three times/day.
- Bladder irrigation: 1000 mL/24 h; if urine output exceeds 2000 mL/day increase to 2000 mL/24 h.
- CNS Infections (intrathecal/intraventricular): 50,000 units once daily.
- Ocular infections (ophthalmic): 10,000–25,000 units/mL as one to three drops every hour increasing the interval as response indicates. 100,000 units/day for corneal/conjunctival infections.
- Pulmonary infection (inhalation for nebulization): 500,000 units every 12 h.
- Systemic infections: 20,000–25,000 units/kg loading dose followed by a maintenance dose of 12,500–15,000 units/kg every 12 h.
- Recommended dosage reduction in kidney impairment.
- No dosage adjustments for hepatic impairment.

Pharmacokinetics

- Not absorbed from GI tract. Insignificant absorption from intact skin or mucous membrane.
- Tissue diffusion is poor and does not cross blood brain barrier into CSF or into the eye.
- Protein binding of ~60%.
- Half-life elimination is 10.1–13.6 h.
- Excretion is in the urine with <1% as unchanged drug for first 12 h and up to 60% as therapy continues.

Use in Special Populations

- Use in children approved, however, due to toxicity risks, systemic use should be limited to life-threatening, multidrug-resistant infection when there are no alternatives.

- Listed as FDA pregnancy classification B (former classification system).
- It is unknown whether present in breast milk.
- Kidney insufficiency: manufacturer labelling recommends dosage reduction; however, clinical data shows that clearance is not altered substantially in kidney impairment; dose adjustment is not expected to be needed.
- Hepatic insufficiency: not evaluated; dose adjustment is not expected to be needed.

Monitoring

- Desquamation, skin hyperpigmentation, and urticaria.
- Albuminuria, hypocalcemia, hypochloremia, hypokalemia, hypomagnesemia, and hyponatremia.
- *Clostridioides difficile*-associated diarrhea (CDAD).
- Azotemia.
- Local thrombophlebitis and pain.

Contraindications and Cautions

- Hypersensitivity reaction.
- Nephrotoxicity (mainly IM/IV use)—albuminuria, cellular casts, and azotemia.
- Neurotoxicity (mainly IM/IV use)—respiratory paralysis from neuromuscular blockade.
- Superinfection.

Important Drug Interactions

- Enhance nephrotoxic effects (aminoglycosides, bacitracin (systemic), cefazedone, colistimethate, methoxyflurane, netilmicin (ophthalmic)).
- Enhance neuromuscular-blocking effect (capreomycin, methoxyflurane, neuromuscular-blocking agents).

- Diminish therapeutic effect of typhoid vaccine, sodium picosulfate, lactobacillus and estriol, immune checkpoint inhibitors, cholera vaccine, BCG vaccine, BCG (intravesical), bacillus clausii.
- Overall toxicity with kanamycin.

Adverse Effects and Their Management

- Nephrotoxicity: avoid concurrent or sequential use of other nephrotoxic drugs, if symptoms arise, discontinue therapy with decreasing urinary output and increasing BUN.
- Neurotoxicity (respiratory paralysis): avoid concurrent or sequential use of other neurotoxic drugs.
- Superinfection with prolonged use (CDAD and pseudomembranous colitis. Avoid prolonged use.
- Toxic when given parenteral, avoid parenteral use whenever possible.

Carcinogenicity—If Known

- Long-term studies to assess carcinogenicity in animals have not been conducted.

Patch Test Concentration

- 3% or 5% in petrolatum

Essential Patient Information

- Polymyxin-B sulfate has not been fully studied during pregnancy.
- It may cause kidney problems and/or nerve problems.
- Be aware of signs of an allergic reaction, flushing, dizziness, diarrhea, fever, headache, and stiffness.
- Wash hands before and after use and keep out moth, nose, and eyes if not indicated.

Retapamulin (Altabax)

Parsa Abdi

Classification and Mode of Action

- Primarily acts as a bacteriostatic agent against *Staphylococcus aureus* and *Streptococcus pyogenes* by inhibiting bacterial protein biosynthesis. It achieves this by binding to a unique site, known as protein L3, on the 50S subunit of the ribosome. This blocks peptidyl transfer and P-site interactions at this site, which prevents the formation of active 50S ribosomal subunits.

Indications and Dermatological Uses

- For the treatment of uncomplicated bacterial skin and skin structure infections caused by *Staphylococcus aureus* (methicillin-susceptible isolates only) or *Streptococcus pyogenes*. Primary indications include impetigo and secondarily for infected traumatic lesions (small lacerations, abrasions, and sutured wounds).
- Use in individuals who are 9 months or older, including both adults and pediatric patients. In adults, it can be used on a total area of up to 100 cm^2, while in pediatric patients aged 9 months or older, it can be used on up to 2% of the total body surface area.
- The safety of Retapamulin has not been established in patients younger than 9 months.
- To maintain the effectiveness of Retapamulin and other antibacterial drugs and prevent the development of drug-resistant bacteria, it should only be used to treat or prevent infections that are known or strongly suspected to be caused by susceptible bacteria.

Formulations/Presentation

- The ointment has a concentration of 10 mg of retapamulin per 1 gram and comes in 15 and 30 gram tubes.

Dosages and Suggested Regimens

- To treat the affected area, apply a thin layer of retapamulin twice daily for five days. The area of application should not exceed 100 cm^2 in adults or 2% of the total body surface area in pediatric patients aged 9 months or older. If desired, the treated area may be covered with a sterile bandage or gauze dressing. In the event that a dose of retapamulin is skipped, it is recommended to apply the ointment at earliest recollection and subsequently adhere to the appropriate time interval for the next application. Re-evaluation of patients is advised if they don't exhibit a clinical response after 3–4 days.
- *Missed Dose:* In the event that a dose of retapamulin is skipped, it is recommended to apply the ointment at earliest recollection and subsequently adhere to the appropriate time interval for the next application.
- *Overdosage:* To date, there have been no reported incidents of overdosing on retapamulin. In the event of an overdose, whether resulting from topical application or accidental ingestion, appropriate symptom-based treatment should be administered in accordance with established clinical practices. It is important to note that there is currently no known antidote for retapamulin overdoses.

Pharmacokinetics

- *Absorption:*
  - The absorption of retapamulin through topical application is generally low but increases when applied to abraded skin and is age-dependent, with the highest absorption observed

in younger patients. In infants and children aged 2–24 months receiving twice-daily retapamulin, a measurable serum concentration was observed in 46% of patients, compared to 7% of those aged ≥2 years. Among infants aged 2–9 months, a higher proportion had measurable serum concentrations compared to those aged 9–24 months (69% vs 32%). For children aged ≥2 years, adolescents, and adults, absorption was low but increased when applied to abraded skin.

- *Distribution:*
  - Currently, there is no available information on the tissue distribution of retapamulin in humans. However, it is known that the drug is highly bound to human plasma proteins, with an approximate binding rate of 94%.
- *Metabolism:*
  - Retapamulin is metabolized primarily by the liver through the action of the enzyme CYP 3A4. The drug undergoes extensive metabolic transformation via mono-oxygenation and di-oxygenation, resulting in the formation of multiple metabolites.
- *Excretion:*
  - There is currently no available information on the elimination of retapamulin in humans, as systemic exposure to the drug after topical application is very low. However, in preclinical species, elimination of 14C-labeled retapamulin was found to be rapid, primarily through metabolism and excretion of drug-related materials in the bile.

Use in Special Populations

- *Pediatrics:*
  - Retapamulin has been proven to be both safe and effective for treating impetigo in pediatric patients ranging from 9 months to 17 years of age, exhibiting similar efficacy and safety profiles as those observed in adults. The safety and efficacy of retapamulin have not been established for pediatric patients below 9 months of age, thus the use of retapamulin is contraindicated in this age group.
  - *Geriatrics:* No dosage change is required.

- *Hepatic Insufficiency:*
  - There is no need to adjust the dosage as low systemic exposure to retapamulin is expected following topical application in adults and pediatric patients aged 2 years and older, and hepatic impairment is unlikely to cause systemic exposure of clinical significance; however, caution should be taken for children under 2 years of age due to potential drug interactions.
- *Renal Insufficiency:*
  - There is no need to adjust the dosage as topical application of retapamulin results in low systemic exposure, hence renal impairment is not expected to cause any significant systemic exposure.
- *Pregnancy and Lactation:*
  - There is currently no data available regarding the use of retapamulin in pregnant women, and thus, there is no information about the potential drug-associated risk for fetal harm or miscarriage; however, as retapamulin is only minimally absorbed systemically after topical administration, it is unlikely to result in fetal exposure during maternal use. Additionally, no data is available on the presence of retapamulin in human milk, its impact on the nursing infant, or its effect on milk production, but given the negligible systemic absorption of retapamulin after the topical application of retapamulin, breastfeeding is not anticipated to result in drug exposure to the infant. Caution should be taken when using retapamulin in pregnant or nursing women.

Monitoring

- Retapamulin is indicated for external use only and is intended for the treatment of impetigo that is either proven or suspected to be caused by susceptible bacteria.

Contraindications and Cautions

- The manufacturer's labeling does not specify any contraindications.

Warnings and Precautions

- *General:* Retapamulin should only be applied topically and should not be ingested, and it is not indicated for the management of methicillin-resistant *Staphylococcus aureus* (MRSA) or abscesses.
- *Local Irritation:* If sensitization or severe local irritation occurs with the use of retapamulin, the treatment should be discontinued immediately, the ointment should be removed, and an appropriate alternative therapy should be initiated to treat the infection.
- *Not for Mucosal or Systemic Use:* It is not recommended to use retapamulin through ingestion or oral, intranasal, ophthalmic, or intravaginal routes as it is intended only for topical use, and its efficacy and safety have not been established on mucosal surfaces. The application of retapamulin on nasal mucosa has been linked to incidents of epistaxis.
- *Potential for Microbial Overgrowth:* The utilization of antibiotics can result in the development of non-susceptible organisms. Extended usage of retapamulin may lead to fungal or bacterial superinfection, including *C. difficile*-associated diarrhea (CDAD) and pseudomembranous colitis. It is worth noting that instances of CDAD have been reported to occur over two months after completing a course of antibiotics. Prescribing retapamulin in the absence of confirmed or highly suspected bacterial infection is improbable to provide any advantages to the patient and enhances the probability of the emergence of antibiotic-resistant bacteria.

Important Drug Interactions

- *Drug-Drug Interactions:* There are currently no known clinically significant drug interactions in adults with retapamulin. However, co-administration of oral ketoconazole 200 mg twice daily has been shown to increase retapamulin levels in healthy adult males by 81% after topical application of retapamulin on abraded skin. The effect of co-administration of retapamulin with CYP3A4 inhibitors, such as ketoconazole, has not been studied in children. The systemic exposure of retapamulin was higher in pediatric subjects aged 2–24 months compared to those aged 2 years and older following topical application. Therefore, it is not advised to administer retapamulin concurrently with strong CYP3A4 inhibitors in patients under 24 months of age due to the higher exposure of retapamulin.
- *Drug-Food Interactions:* There is currently no evidence of any interactions between retapamulin and food.

Adverse Effects and Their Management

- According to product labeling (unless otherwise specified), adverse drug reactions and their corresponding incidence rates for the product are reported as follows:
- In the range of 1–10%, adverse reactions include headache (1–2% incidence in the central nervous system), eczema (1% incidence in infants, children, and adolescents in the dermatologic category), diarrhea (1–2% incidence in the gastrointestinal category), nausea (1% incidence in the gastrointestinal category), application site irritation (2% incidence in adults in the local category), and application site pruritus (2% incidence in infants, children, and adolescents in the local category). Nasopharyngitis (1–2% incidence in the respiratory category) is also listed as an adverse drug reaction.
- In addition, there have been reports of several adverse drug reactions with an incidence rate of less than 1%, as well as post-marketing and/or case reports. These include angioedema,

application site burning, application site pain, contact dermatitis, epistaxis, erythema, hypersensitivity reaction, and increased creatine phosphokinase.

Carcinogenicity

- There have been no long-term animal studies conducted to assess the carcinogenic potential of retapamulin. In vitro evaluations of gene mutation and chromosomal effects in the mouse lymphoma cell assay, as well as in cultured human peripheral blood lymphocytes, and in vivo testing in a rat micronucleus test, have revealed no genotoxicity associated with retapamulin. Furthermore, no indications of impaired fertility were observed in male or female rats that received oral doses of retapamulin at 50, 150, or 450 mg/kg/day.

Patch Test Concentration

- 1% in petrolatum. If unavailable, may use 1% retapamulin ointment as is. It is recommended to exclude a contact allergy to butylhydroxytoluene (BHT), when indicated, as some base formulations may contain BHT.

Essential Patient Information

- Patients using retapamulin should follow the instructions given by their healthcare practitioner, using the medication as directed. Hands should be washed after application, except when treating the hands. Retapamulin is for external use only, and should not be swallowed, used in the eyes, mouth, lips, inside the nose, or inside the female genital area. A sterile bandage or gauze dressing may be applied to the treated area, particularly for infants and young children who may accidentally touch or lick the lesion site, to protect the area and prevent accidental transfer of ointment to other areas. The healthcare practitioner should be notified if symptoms do not improve within 3–4 days or if there is worsening of irritation, redness, itching, burning, swelling, blistering, or oozing at the application site.

Silver Sulfadiazine

Rebecca M. Law

Classification and Mode of Action

- Bactericidal activity for many gram-negative and gram-positive bacteria with some activity against yeast.
- Inhibits bacteria resistant to other antibiotics.
- Superior to sulfadiazine.
- Mechanism of action differs from sodium sulfadiazine and from silver nitrate.
- Acts on cell membrane and cell wall to produce its bactericidal effect.

Indications and Dermatological Uses

- *Clinical indications (FDA):* An adjunct for the prevention and treatment of wound sepsis in patients with second- and third-degree burns.

Formulations/Presentation

- US: Each gram of silver sulfadiazine (SILVADENE). Cream 1% contains 10 mg of micronized silver sulfadiazine. The cream vehicle consists of white petrolatum, stearyl alcohol, isopropyl myristate, sorbitan monooleate, polyoxyl 40 stearate, propylene glycol, and water, with methylparaben 0.3% as a preservative.
- Canada:
- Europe:

Dosages and Suggested Regimens

- The cream should be applied once to twice daily to a thickness of approximately 1/16 inch. Whenever necessary, the cream should be reapplied to any areas from which it has been removed by patient activity.
- Reapply immediately after hydrotherapy.
- Treatment should be continued until satisfactory healing has occurred, or until the burn site is ready for grafting. The drug should not be withdrawn from the therapeutic regimen while there remains the possibility of infection except if a significant adverse reaction occurs.

Pharmacokinetics

- Absorption of silver sulfadiazine varies depending upon the percent of body surface area and the extent of the tissue damage.

Use in Special Populations

- Should not be used on pregnant women approaching or at term, on premature infants, or on newborn infants during the first 2 months of life. Sulfonamide therapy is known to increase the possibility of kernicterus.
- It is unknown whether silver sulfadiazine is excreted in human milk.
- Safety and effectiveness in pediatric patients have not been established.
- If hepatic and renal functions become impaired and elimination of drug decreases, accumulation may occur, and drug discontinuation should be weighed against the therapeutic benefit being achieved.

Monitoring

- In the treatment of burn wounds involving extensive areas of the body, the serum sulfa concentrations may approach adult therapeutic levels (8–12 mg%). Therefore, in these patients, it would be advisable to monitor serum sulfa concentrations. Renal function should be carefully monitored, and the urine should be checked for sulfa crystals.
- Absorption of the propylene glycol vehicle has been reported to affect serum osmolality, which may affect the interpretation of laboratory tests.

Contraindications and Cautions

- Although few have been reported, it is possible that any adverse reaction associated with sulfonamides may occur. These include blood dyscrasias including agranulocytosis, aplastic anemia, thrombocytopenia, leukopenia, and hemolytic anemia; dermatologic and allergic reactions, including life-threatening cutaneous reactions [Stevens-Johnson syndrome (SJS), toxic epidermal necrolysis (TEN) and exfoliative dermatitis]; gastrointestinal reactions; hepatitis and hepatocellular necrosis; CNS reactions; and toxic nephrosis.
- There is potential cross-sensitivity between silver sulfadiazine and other sulfonamides. If allergic reactions attributable to treatment with silver sulfadiazine occur, continuation of therapy must be weighed against the potential hazards of the particular allergic reaction.
- Fungal proliferation in and below the eschar may occur. However, the incidence of clinically reported fungal superinfection is low.
- The use of silver sulfadiazine in some cases of glucose-6-phosphate dehydrogenase-deficient individuals may be hazardous, as hemolysis may occur.

Important Drug Interactions

- In considering the use of topical proteolytic enzymes in conjunction with silver sulfadiazine, there is a possibility that silver may inactivate such enzymes.

Adverse Effects and their Management

- Transient leukopenia have been reported, primarily characterized by decreased neutrophil count with maximal WBC depression occurring within 2–4 days of initiation of therapy and normalized within 2–3 days. Recovery is not influenced by the continuation of silver sulfadiazine therapy.
- Other infrequently occurring events include skin necrosis, erythema multiforme, skin discoloration, burning sensation, rashes, and interstitial nephritis.

Carcinogenicity

- Long-term dermal toxicity studies of 24-month duration in rats and 18 months in mice with concentrations of silver sulfadiazine three to ten times the concentration in silver sulfadiazine cream 1% revealed no evidence of carcinogenicity.

Patch Test Concentration

- 5% pet.; test also silver nitrate 1% water and sulfadiazine 5% pet.; test propylene glycol

Essential Patient Information

- The burned areas should be covered by cream at all times. Cream should be reapplied to any areas where it has been removed due to activity or other reasons such as hydrotherapy. Dressings are not required but may be used as needed.

References

Acetic Acid and Hydrocortisone (Acetasol HC)

1. LexiComp drug monograph Acetic Acid and Hydrocortisone (Topical). Available from: LexiComp Online at online.Lexi.com. Copyright 2022 UptoDate, Inc.
2. Falcon Pharmaceuticals. Neomycin and polymyxin B sulfates, and hydrocortisone otic suspension prescribing information. Fort Worth, TX; 2007 Jun.
3. Monarch Pharmaceuticals. Cortisporin® (neomycin and polymyxin B sulfates and hydrocortisone) otic solution prescribing information. Bristol, TN; 2003 Apr.
4. JHP Pharmaceuticals. Coly-Mycin® S (colistin sulfate, neomycin sulfate, thonzonium bromide, and hydrocortisone acetate) otic solution prescribing information. MI: Rochester; 2008 Feb.
5. Taro Pharmaceuticals. Hydrocortisone 1% and acetic acid 2% otic solution prescribing information. NY: Hawthorne; 2004 Jun.

Bacitracin

6. LexiComp drug monograph. Bacitracin (Topical). Available from: LexiComp Online at online.Lexi.com. Copyright 2024 UpToDate Inc.
7. Nguyen, Rosalee, et al. "Bacitracin Topical." *StatPearls*, StatPearls Publishing, 21 November 2022.
8. Bacitracin ointment [prescribing information]. Hawthorne, NY: Taro Pharmacueticals; Revised January 2020.
9. Antibiotic Ointment with Bacitracin Safety Data Sheet. Buffalo, NY: Safetec of America Inc; Revised February 2022.

10. Heal CF, et al. Topical antibiotics for preventing surgical site infection in wounds healing by primary intention. Cochrane Database Syst Rev. 2016;11(11):CD011426. https://doi.org/10.1002/14651858.CD011426.pub2.
11. de Groot AC. Monographs in contact allergy. In: Topical drugs, vol. 3. 1st ed. CRC Press; 2021. https://doi.org/10.1201/9781003159360.

Gentamicin Sulfate

12. LexiComp drug monograph Gentamicin Sulfate (Topical). Available from: LexiComp Online at online.Lexi.com. Copyright 2022 UptoDate, Inc.
13. Tsai CC, Yang PS, Liu CL, Wu CJ, Hsu YC, Cheng SP. Comparison of topical mupirocin and gentamicin in the prevention of peritoneal dialysis-related infections: a systematic review and meta-analysis. Am J Surg. 2018;215(1):179–85. https://doi.org/10.1016/j.amjsurg.2017.03.005.
14. AHFS Drug Information 2007. In: McEvoy GK, editor. Gentamicin sulfate. Bethesda: American Society of Health-System Pharmacists; 2007. p. 3444–5.
15. Fougera. Gentamicin sulfate ointment prescribing information. Melville: From the DailyMed website. Accessed 12 Apr 2023; 1998 Mar.
16. de Groot AC. Monographs in contact allergy. In: Topical drugs, vol. 3. 1st ed. CRC Press; 2021. https://doi.org/10.1201/9781003159360.

Gramicidin

17. FDA Drug Monograph Gramicidin. Available from https://precision.fda.gov/uniisearch/srs/unii/5ie62321p4. Accessed 23 Mar 2023.
18. LexiComp Drug Monograph Gramicidin. Available from: LexiComp Online at online.Lexi.com. Copyright 2022 UptoDate, Inc.
19. Sorochkina AI, Plotnikov EY, Rokitskaya TI, et al. N-terminally glutamate-substituted analogue of gramicidin a as protonophore and selective mitochondrial uncoupler. PLoS One. 2012;7:e41919.
20. David JM, Rajasekaran AK, Gramicidin A. A New Mission for an old antibiotic. Journal of kidney cancer and VHL. 2015;2:15–24.
21. DrugBank Online Monograph Gramicidin D. Available from: DrugBank Online at go.drugbank.com/drugs/DB00027. Accessed 23 Mar 2023.
22. de Groot AC. Monographs in contact allergy. In: Topical drugs, vol. 3. Milton: CRC Press; 2021.

Mupirocin

23. FDA Drug Monograph Mupirocin. Available from https://www.accessdata.fda.gov/drugsatfda_docs/label/2017/050591s034lbl.pdf Accessed 24 Mar 2023.
24. LexiComp Drug Monograph Mupirocin. Available from: LexiComp Online at online.Lexi.com. Copyright 2022 UptoDate, Inc.
25. de Groot AC. Monographs in contact allergy. In: Topical drugs, vol. 3. 1st ed. CRC Press; 2021. https://doi.org/10.1201/9781003159360.
26. Wolverton SE, Wu JJ, ClinicalKey Flex, Elsevier All Access Books, eBook—Specialty Medicine 2020 [EBCSM20]. Comprehensive dermatologic drug therapy. 4th ed. Philadelphia: Elsevier; 2021. p. 2019.
27. de Groot AC. Monographs in contact allergy. In: Topical drugs, vol. 3. Milton: CRC Press; 2021.
28. Katzung BG, Trevor AJ, Access Pharmacy, Access Medicine. Basic and clinical pharmacology 15e. 15th ed. Blacklick: McGraw-Hill Companies; 2021. 2020

Neomycin Sulfate

29. LexiComp drug monograph Neomycin Sulfate (Topical). Available from: LexiComp Online at online.Lexi.com. Copyright 2022 UptoDate, Inc.
30. Johnson & Johnson. Neosporin® original (bacitracin zinc, neomycin sulfate, and polymyxin B sulfate) ointment patient information. Skillman, NJ; Undated. From Dailymed website. Accessed 2023 Apr 18.
31. Johnson & Johnson. Neosporin® Plus (bacitracin zinc, neomycin sulfate, polymyxin B sulfate, and pramoxine hydrochloride) ointment patient information. Skillman, NJ; Undated. From Dailymed website. Accessed 2023 Apr 18.
32. Actavis Pharma. Triple antibiotic (bacitracin zinc, neomycin sulfate, and polymyxin B sulfate) ointment patient information. Parsippany: Undated. From Dailymed website. Accessed; 2023 Apr 18.
33. Cell Novation Technology. Bacitracin zinc, neomycin sulfate, polymyxin B sulfate, and lidocaine hydrochloride cream patient information. Undated. From Dailymed website; 2023. Accessed 2023 Apr 18
34. Hart Health. Tribioticlc LC (bacitracin zinc, neomycin sulfate, polymyxin B sulfate, and lidocaine) ointment patient information. Seattle: Undated. From Dailymed website; 2023. Accessed 2023 Apr 18
35. Pfizer. Neosporin® G.U. Irrigant sterile (neomycin sulfate-polymyxin B sulfate solution for irrigation) prescribing information. New York; 2016 Sep.

36. AHFS Drug Information 2020. In: Snow EK, editor. Neomycin sulfate. Bethesda: American Society of Health-System Pharmacists; 2020.

Ozenoxacin

37. LexiComp Drug Monograph. Ozenoxacin (Topical). Available from: LexiComp Online at online.Lexi.com. Copyright 2024 UpToDate Inc.
38. Xepi (ozenoxacin) [Prescribing information]. Woburn: Biofontera Inc; Revised September 2023.
39. Zhanel GG, et al. In vitro activity and resistance rates of topical antimicrobials fusidic acid, mupirocin and ozenoxacin against skin and soft tissue infection pathogens obtained across Canada (CANWARD 2007-18). J Antimicrob Chemother. 2021;76(7):1808–14. https://doi.org/10.1093/jac/dkab098.

Polymyxin-B Sulfate

40. FDA drug monograph Polymyxin B for Injection USP. Available from https://www.accessdata.fda.gov/drugsatfda_docs/label/2012/060716Orig1s020Lbl.pdf. Accessed 25 Mar 2023.
41. FDA drug monograph Maxitrol. Available from https://www.accessdata.fda.gov/drugsatfda_docs/label/2017/050023s036lbl.pdf Accessed 25 Mar 2023.
42. LexiComp drug monograph Polymyxin B. Available from: LexiComp Online at online.Lexi.com. Copyright 2022 UptoDate, Inc.
43. de Groot AC. Monographs in contact allergy. In: Topical drugs, vol. 3. 1st ed. CRC Press; 2021. https://doi.org/10.1201/9781003159360.
44. Wolverton SE, Wu JJ, ClinicalKey Flex, Elsevier All Access Books, eBook—Specialty Medicine 2020 [EBCSM20]. Comprehensive dermatologic drug therapy. 4th ed. Philadelphia: Elsevier; 2021. p. 2019.
45. de Groot AC. Monographs in contact allergy. In: Topical drugs, vol. 3. Milton: CRC Press; 2021.
46. Katzung BG, Trevor AJ, Access Pharmacy, Access Medicine. Basic and clinical pharmacology 15e. 15th ed. Blacklick: McGraw-Hill Companies; 2021. p. 2020.

Retapamulin (Altabax)

47. FDA drug monograph ALTABAX® (retapamulin ointment), 1%. Available https://www.accessdata.fda.gov/drugsatfda_docs/label/2012/022055s002lbl. Accessed 7 Apr 2023.
48. LexiComp Drug Monograph Retapamulin. Available from: LexiComp Online at online.Lexi.com. Copyright 2022 UptoDate, Inc.
49. de Groot AC. Monographs in contact allergy. In: Topical drugs, vol. 3. 1st ed. CRC Press; 2021. https://doi.org/10.1201/9781003159360.

Silver Sulfadiazine

50. FDA drug monograph (silver sulfadiazine). Available from https://www.accessdata.fda.gov/drugsatfda_docs/label/2013/017381s050lbl.pdf. Accessed 22 June 2024.
51. LexiComp drug monograph (silver sulfadiazine). Available from: LexiComp Online at online.Lexi.com. Copyright 2024 UptoDate, Inc.
52. De Groot AC. Patch testing, vol. 3. 3rd ed. Chapter 3.
53. Caffee F, Bingham H. Leukopenia and silver sulfadiazine. J Trauma. 1982;22:586–7.
54. Jarret F, Ellerbe S, Demling R. Acute leukopenia during topical burn therapy with silver sulfadiazine. Amer J Surg. 1978;135:818–9.
55. Kiker RG, Carvajal HF, Micak RP, Larson DL. A controlled study of the effects of silver sulfadiazine on white blood cell counts in burned children. J Trauma. 1977;17:835–6.

Topical Antifungals 13

Laurie A. Temiz, Austinn C. Miller,
Susuana Adjei, and Stephen K. Tyring

Contents

Introduction

Topical antifungal drugs are used to treat a variety of yeast and dermatophyte infections. Topical formulations are often only effective in treating superficial and localized infections of the

L. A. Temiz
Department of Dermatology and Cutaneous Surgery, University of South Florida, Tampa, FL, USA

Center for Clinical Studies, Webster, TX, USA
e-mail: ltemiz@ccstexas.com

A. C. Miller · S. Adjei
Center for Clinical Studies, Webster, TX, USA
e-mail: fellowwebster@ccstexas.com; fellowtmc@ccstexas.com

S. K. Tyring (✉)
Center for Clinical Studies, Webster, TX, USA

Department of Dermatology, University of Texas Health Science Center, Houston, TX, USA
e-mail: styring@ccstexas.com

R. M. Law, H. I. Maibach (eds.), *Handbook of Topical Drug Treatment in Dermatology*,
https://doi.org/10.1007/978-3-031-93616-6_13

skin, hair, and nails, whereas systemic medications are reserved for more severe disease.

Fungi of medical importance are capable of causing an array of diseases, ranging from asymptomatic superficial skin infections to fatal systemic infections. Fungi are a group of eukaryotic microorganisms often divided into yeasts and molds. Yeasts are single-celled, oval-shaped microorganisms that reproduce primarily through budding. Molds are multicellular microorganisms formed from elongated multinucleate filaments (hyphae) that reproduce by apical extension. While most fungi exist as either a yeast or a mold, dimorphic fungi can switch between each form depending on environmental factors, such as temperature. Regardless of the form, all fungi share common properties: absorptive nutrition (food digestion occurs externally via expulsion of hydrolytic enzymes and absorption of the resulting product), lysine synthesize, chitinous cell wall (rather than peptidoglycan found in mammalian walls), and plasma membranes containing ergosterol (rather than cholesterol found in mammalian membranes).

Many antifungals target steps in the fungal plasma membrane synthesis pathway with high affinity, given that fungi utilize ergosterol, rather than cholesterol as occurs in mammalian sterol synthesis. Most topical antifungals are fungistatic, inhibiting cell growth; however, a few are fungicidal resulting in cell death (amphotericin, echinocandins, and nystatin).

Superficial fungal infections are most likely to be seen in immunocompromised individuals. This includes infants without full immune maturity, elderly with waning immune responses, and those who are immunosuppressed for any other reason. However, anyone can be infected. Other high-risk populations include those who are in frequent contact with people who may be infected (athletes), come in contact with spores in the environment (digging, gardening, contact with animals, and caving), and recent use of antibiotics (vulvovaginal candidiasis).

Like other antimicrobials, resistance to antifungals is increasing, and several factors contribute to this issue. Resistance is defined as persistent fungal infections despite the use of appropriate fungal therapy. These factors range from mutations, biofilm formation, poor medication adherence, and host immunosuppression.

Fungi of medical importance can cause an array of diseases, ranging from asymptomatic superficial skin infections to fatal systemic infections. While immunocompromised individuals are at greatest risk of fungal infections, they may occur in anyone. Topical antifungal drugs are commonly used to treat a superficial yeast and dermatophyte infections. Most antifungals function by taking advantage of cellular processes unique to fungi, allowing for limited cross reactivity with human cells and thus less side effects. However, like other antimicrobials, resistance to antifungals is increasing. When faced with recalcitrant or severe fungal infections, systemic antifungals are typically the treatment of choice.

Allylamines

Naftifine

Classification and Mode of Action

- Synthetic allylamine derivative. Naftifine is a topical, broad-spectrum antifungal agent that works via dose-dependent selective inhibition of squalene-2,3-epoxidase. As this enzyme is crucial to fungal cells' ability to synthesize ergosterol, the result is a buildup of intracellular squalene and the loss of the fungal membrane's primary sterol. Thus, naftifine has both fungicidal and fungistatic activity.

Indications and Dermatological Uses

- *Clinical indications:* Topical treatment of interdigital tinea pedis (athlete's foot), tinea corporis (ringworm), and tinea cruris (jock itch) caused by *Trichophyton rubrum.*
- *Off-label common uses:* Tinea manuum (Level of evidence: C).

Formulations/Presentation

- US: 1% cream, 2% cream, 1% gel, 2% gel.
- Canada: Not on Lexicomp.
- Europe: Not on Lexicomp.

Dosages and Suggested Regimens

- *Cream (1%, 2%):* A thin layer of cream should be applied to clean, dry skin on the affected area(s), plus a ½-inch margin of surrounding tissue once daily until clinical resolution. For tinea pedis and tinea manuum infections, treatment should be continued for 1 week after clinical resolution.
- *Gel (1%, 2%):* A thin layer of gel should be applied to clean, dry skin on the affected area(s), plus a ½-inch margin of surrounding tissue twice daily until clinical resolution. For tinea pedis and tinea manuum, treatment should be continued for 1 week after clinical resolution.
- The selected treatment regimen should be maintained for a minimum of 2 weeks. Clinical effects may take 1–4 weeks to become apparent.
- No suggested dosage adjustment for renal or hepatic impairment due to low systemic absorption.

Baseline Investigations and Considerations

- Culture and KOH exams.

Pharmacokinetics (Percutaneous Absorption, Distribution, Metabolism, Excretion: As Relevant for the Drug)

- When applied topically, naftifine hydrochloride penetrates the stratum corneum but has a low systemic bioavailability. The cream formulation has more systemic penetration, reaching 6% systemic absorption as compared to 4% in the gel form.
- The plasma elimination half-life of naftifine and its metabolites is 2–3 days.
- Unchanged naftifine, as well as its metabolites, is excreted in both the feces and urine.

Use in Special Populations: Pregnancy (FDA Guidance), Lactation, Children, Renal Insufficiency, Hepatic Insufficiency

- The treatment of tinea corporis is approved in children ≥2 years of age and for the treatment of tinea cruris and pedis in children ≥12 years of age. No pediatric dose adjustment is required.

- Naftifine may be present in breast milk. Lactating patients should not apply this product to the nipples or breasts.
- Human studies of naftifine in pregnant or lactating patients have not been performed; however, due to its low systemic bioavailability, application over a limited area is acceptable in these patients.

Monitoring

- Culture and KOH exams *(repeat if no signs of clinical improvement after 4 weeks).*
- Application-site reactions *(exfoliation, erythema, or dermatitis).*

Contraindications and Cautions

- Naftifine is contraindicated in patients with a hypersensitivity to either the drug product or any component of the formulation.
- Naftifine is indicated for topical use only and contact with the eyes, nose, mouth, or mucous membranes should be avoided.
- This medication should not be used with occlusive dressings.

Important Drug Interactions

- This drug has no significant drug interactions.

Adverse Effects and Their Management

- Contact dermatitis is the most commonly reported adverse event seen with the use of naftifine. Other common cutaneous reactions include a burning or stinging sensation of the skin, xeroderma, skin irritation, erythema, and pruritus. Approximately 2% of patients reported local application site reactions. If sensitivity or irritation occurs, naftifine should be discontinued and replaced with an alternative therapy.
- In rare cases, more severe cutaneous and systemic reactions have been reported. Systemic manifestations include agranulocytosis, leukopenia, inflammatory reactions, dizziness, and headache. Rare cutaneous reactions reported were maceration, rash, serous drainage, blistering of the skin, and tenderness and swelling of the skin.

- Despite the structural and mechanistic similarities between naftifine and terbinafine, there is no evidence of cross-reactivity or sensitization to active ingredients across the class of allylamine antifungals.

Patch Test Concentration

- 1% and 5% in alcohol

Essential Patient Information

- This drug is used to treat fungal infections of the skin.
- Hands should be washed before and after use.
- Naftifine should be applied to the affected area and approximately ½ inch of surrounding healthy skin in all directions.
- This drug should only be applied to clean, dry skin. Contact with the eyes, nose, mouth, or intravaginal tissue should be avoided.
- Occlusive dressings should not be used.
- If irritation, redness, peeling, other skin sensitivity, or worsening of condition occurs, a physician should be contacted immediately, and the use of the medication should be discontinued.
- If any signs of an allergic reaction *(rash; hives; itching; red, swollen, blistered, or peeling skin; wheezing; chest or throat tightness; difficulty breathing, swallowing or talking; unusual hoarseness; or swelling of the mouth, face, lips, tongue, or throat) are noticed,* appropriate medical help should be sought immediately. Use of the medication should be discontinued, and any side effects should be reported to the physician.

Terbinafine

Classification and Mode of Action

- Synthetic allylamine derivative. Terbinafine inhibits the enzyme squalene-2,3-epoxidase, limiting fungal cells' ability to synthesize ergosterol, a key component of the fungal cell membrane. Without this sterol, the integrity of the fungal cell membrane is severely compromised, leading to fungal cell death.

Indications and Dermatological Uses

- Clinical indications: Treatment of tinea pedis (athlete's foot), tinea cruris (jock itch), tinea corporis (ringworm), and tinea versicolor *(in Canada only).*
  - **Note: In the United States, the above indications are approved for OTC management**
- *Off-label common uses:* Topical treatment of tinea manuum (Level of evidence: C).

Formulations/Presentation

- US: 1% cream, 1% gel, 1% solution.
- Canada: 1% cream, 1% solution.
- Europe: Not on Lexicomp.

Dosages and Suggested Regimens

- *Tinea corporis:* The cream or gel should be applied to the affected and surrounding area(s) once daily for at least 1 week. Treatment should be continued until clinical resolution.
- *Tinea cruris:* Cream, gel, or spray should be applied to the affected and surrounding area(s) once daily for at least 1 week. Treatment should be continued until clinical resolution.
- *Tinea pedis/manuum:* This drug should be applied to the affected and surrounding area(s) once daily (gel) or twice daily (cream) until 1 week after clinical resolution.
- *Tinea versicolor (Canada only):* This drug should be applied to the affected area once daily (pediatric) or twice daily (adult).
  - The gel formulation should be used for 1 week, while the cream formulation should be used for 2 weeks.
  - Terbinafine spray is approved for pediatric use only.

Baseline Investigations and Considerations

- There is no specific requirement for baseline investigations.

Pharmacokinetics (Percutaneous Absorption, Distribution, Metabolism, Excretion: As Relevant for the Drug)

- When applied topically, less than 5% of a given dose of terbinafine reaches the systemic circulation. The drug is primarily distributed to the sebum and skin with an elimination half-life of 14–35 h.

Use in Special Populations: Pregnancy (FDA Guidance), Lactation, Children, Renal Insufficiency, and Hepatic Insufficiency

- Terbinafine is present in breast milk following oral administration, but systemic absorption is limited following topical application. This drug should be used with caution and should avoid being applied on or near the nipples in lactating patients.
- Infants should not be allowed to come into contact with treated skin.
- Due to low systemic absorption, topical terbinafine may be considered for use in a pregnant population if needed.

Monitoring

- There is no specific requirement for monitoring.

Contraindications and Cautions

- Terbinafine is contraindicated in patients with a hypersensitivity to either the drug product or any component of the formulation.
- If irritation or sensitivity occurs, the medication should be discontinued, and appropriate alternative therapy should be instituted.
- Some dosage forms may be formulated with propylene glycol. Exposure to large amounts of propylene glycol has been associated with potentially fatal neonatal toxicity and may present with metabolic acidosis, renal failure, CNS depression, and seizures. Similar propylene glycol toxicity has also been reported in children and adults and may present with these

findings, in addition to hyperosmolality and respiratory depression.

- Some dosage forms may be formulated with benzyl alcohol; some studies have implicated benzoate in the displacement of bilirubin from protein binding sites. Exposure to benzyl alcohol in doses exceeding 99 mg/kg/day has been associated with a potentially fatal neonatal toxicity known as gasping syndrome. Gasping syndrome presents with metabolic acidosis, hypotension, cardiovascular collapse, seizures, intracranial hemorrhage, other CNS dysfunction, gasping respirations, and respiratory distress. The use of products containing benzyl alcohol should be avoided in this patient population.

Important Drug Interactions

- There are no known significant drug interactions.

Adverse Effects and Their Management

- The most commonly reported adverse reactions are localized skin irritation, contact dermatitis, burning or stinging sensations of the skin, skin dryness, exfoliation, pruritus, and skin rash.
- A wider range of cutaneous reactions have been reported with the use of terbinafine as opposed to naftifine. These reactions are relatively common, occurring in approximately 2.7% of patients. Severity of reactions can vary; however, severe reactions may necessitate the discontinuation of therapy.
- Such reactions may include instances of erythema multiforme, erythroderma, pityriasis rosea, or worsening of the initial skin condition.
- Other reported cutaneous reactions include lichenoid drug eruption, de novo inductions of cutaneous lupus, exacerbations of systemic lupus erythematosus, and symmetrical drug-related intertriginous and flexural exanthema (SDRIFE), acute generalized exanthematous cutaneous pustulosis (AGEP), and drug rash with eosinophilic systemic symptoms (DRESS) syndrome.

Patch Test Concentration

- No data available

Essential Patient Information

- This drug is used to treat fungal infections of the skin.
- For external use only. Contact with the eyes, nose, mouth, or intravaginal tissue should be avoided.
- This drug should not be used on the nails, scalp, or for vaginal yeast infections.
- The affected area should be washed with soap and water and dried completely prior to application. This drug should only be applied to clean, dry skin, in sufficient amounts to cover the affected area. Hands should be washed before and after use.
- If any signs of an allergic reaction *(rash; hives; itching; red, swollen, blistered, or peeling skin; wheezing; chest or throat tightness; difficulty breathing, swallowing, or talking; unusual hoarseness; or swelling of the mouth, face, lips, tongue, or throat)* are noticed, appropriate medical help should be sought immediately. This medication should be discontinued and any side effects should be reported to a physician.

Azoles

Clotrimazole

Classification and Mode of Action

- Imidazole antifungal. By binding to phospholipids within the fungal cell membrane, clotrimazole significantly alters cell wall permeability, resulting in the loss of essential intracellular elements.
- Clotrimazole is not effective in infections caused by *Candida glabrata.*

Indications and Dermatological Uses

- *Clinical indications:* Topical treatment of candidiasis due to *Candida albicans*, tinea versicolor due to *Malassezia furfur*, vulvovaginal candidiasis, and relief of external vulvar itching and irritation.
- *OTC indications:* Topical treatment of tinea cruris, *Candida albicans*, tinea corporis, and tinea pedis.
- *Off-label common uses:* Otomycosis (level of evidence: C) and tinea manuum (level of evidence: C).

Formulations/Presentation

- US: External cream (1%), intravaginal cream (1% and 2%), external ointment (1%), external solution (1%).
- Canada: External cream (1%), intravaginal cream (1% and 2%), 100 mg, 150 mg, 200 mg, 500 mg vaginal tablet/insert.
- Europe: Not on Lexicomp.

Dosages and Suggested Regimens

- *Vulvovaginal candidiasis:* One applicator of vaginal cream should be inserted once daily (preferably at bedtime). Duration of treatment is based on the strength of the product selected with the 1%, 2%, and 10% formulations requiring treatment for 7 days, 3 days, and 1 day, respectively. Cream may also be applied externally twice daily for up to 7 days as needed for itching and irritation.
- *Cutaneous candidiasis:* Cream should be applied to the affected area twice daily for 4 weeks. Alternatively, OTC ointment may be applied twice daily for 2 weeks.
- *Otomycosis:* Four to five drops of topical solution should be instilled into the affected ear(s) twice daily for 10–14 days.
- *Tinea corporis/cruris:* An appropriate amount of cream, ointment, or solution should be applied to the affected and surrounding area(s) twice daily for 4 weeks or until clinical resolution of infection. If treating tinea cruris is in a pediatric patient, the duration of therapy should be limited to 2 weeks.

- *Tinea pedis:* An appropriate amount of cream, ointment, or solution should be applied to the affected and surrounding area(s) twice daily until 1 week after clinical resolution.
- *Tinea versicolor:* An appropriate amount of cream or solution should be applied to the affected area(s) twice daily.

Baseline Investigations and Considerations

- In patients with otomycosis, the provider should perform a thorough cleansing of the ear canal prior to initiating pharmacotherapy.

Pharmacokinetics (Percutaneous Absorption, Distribution, Metabolism, Excretion: As Relevant for the Drug)

- When applied to intact skin, clotrimazole exhibits negligible systemic absorption. When applied intravaginally, 3–10% of the applied dose is absorbed, reaching peak serum concentration in approximately 24 h.

Use in Special Populations: Pregnancy (FDA Guidance), Lactation, Children, Renal Insufficiency, and Hepatic Insufficiency

- It is not known if clotrimazole is excreted in breast milk. Use with caution in lactating patients.
- Approved for the treatment of cutaneous candidiasis in pediatric patients ≥2 years of age and for the treatment of vulvovaginal candidiasis in patients ≥12 years of age.

Monitoring

- This drug should be monitored for both signs of clinical improvement and severe skin irritation.
- In patients with otomycosis, the presence of fungal elements in the ear canal should be assessed following completion of therapy. Several cycles of ear cleansing, pharmacotherapeutic treatment, and reassessment may be necessary to achieve complete resolution. If otomycosis persists after multiple cycles of treatment, the patient should be managed by an otolaryngologist.

- If there is no improvement in clinical signs of cutaneous candidiasis or tinea versicolor after 4 weeks of treatment, the diagnosis should be reassessed.

Contraindications and Cautions

- This drug is contraindicated in patients with a hypersensitivity to either the drug product or any component of the formulation.
- Some cases may require an extended course of therapy for effective management. Up to 14 days or treatment may be indicated for patients with severe or recurrent infections, infections with candida species other than *C. albicans*, or immunocompromised states.
- While rare, there have been reports of severe toxicity and allergic reaction associated with the use of azole antifungals. Allergic reactions have been reported in up to 2% of patients and usually present as a rash or pruritus. More severe dermal reactions, including epidermal necrolysis, serum sickness, and anaphylaxis have been reported with the use of oral formulations. In most cases, allergic reactions may become apparent several days or weeks after starting therapy. In sensitized patients, symptoms may occur within minutes or hours. Allergic reactions to azole antifungals have been found to respond well to corticosteroids and antihistamine.
- Clinical data regarding incidences of cross-reaction is limited; however, there are numerous case reports of significant occurrences. While there is potential for cross-reactivity between all types of azole antifungals, the possibility is greatest in patients who have taken other imidazoles due to the high degree of structural similarity.
- Some dosage forms may be formulated with benzyl alcohol; some studies have implicated benzoate in the displacement of bilirubin from protein binding sites. Exposure to benzyl alcohol in doses exceeding 99 mg/kg/day has been associated with a potentially fatal neonatal toxicity known as gasping syndrome. Gasping syndrome presents with metabolic acidosis, hypotension, cardiovascular collapse, seizures, intracranial hemorrhage, other CNS dysfunction, gasping respirations, and

respiratory distress. The use of products containing benzyl alcohol should be avoided in this patient population.

Important Drug Interactions

- Progesterone *(Risk X)*: Clotrimazole may decrease the efficacy of progesterone. Combinations with these products should be avoided.

Adverse Effects and Their Management

- Vulvovaginal burning associated with the use of vaginal preparations is relatively common and has been reported in up to 10% of patients.
- In addition, burning sensations of the penis (of the sexual partner), polyuria, pruritus vulvae, vaginal discharge, and vulvar pain and swelling have been reported in <1% of patients.
- Hepatotoxicity is a rare adverse event associated with the use of azole antifungals and may represent either direct toxicity or immune system involvement. If cholestatic jaundice or other signs of liver toxicity occur, immediately discontinue medication and initiate appropriate therapy.

Patch Test Concentration

- 1% pet. (SmartPracticeCanada & Europe); generally, alcohol or methyl ethyl ketone (MEK) may be more suitable for patch testing imidazoles.

Essential Patient Information

- This drug is used to treat fungal infections of the skin and vaginal yeast infections.
- Hands should be washed before and after use.
- Medication use should be supervised in children under the age of 12.
- If a patient develops severe skin irritation; sensitivity; burning; or blisters that ooze, drain, or crust over, or if nausea, vomiting, abdominal pain, or foul-smelling vaginal discharge occurs, this medication should immediately be discontinued and a physician should be informed.

- If any signs of an allergic reaction *(rash; hives; itching; red, swollen, blistered, or peeling skin; wheezing; chest or throat tightness; difficulty breathing, swallowing or talking; unusual hoarseness; or swelling of the mouth, face, lips, tongue, or throat)* are noticed, appropriate medical help should be sought immediately. This medication should be discontinued, and any side effects should be reported to a physician.
- Topical formulations are intended for external use only. Contact with the eyes should be avoided.
- Clotrimazole is not effective for the treatment of infections impacting the scalp or nails.
- If a patient has not previously had a vaginal yeast infection diagnosed by a doctor, experienced 3 or more yeast infections within 3 months, or had an exposure to HIV, a physician should be consulted prior to using any formulation of vaginal cream for OTC self-medication.
- If treating vaginal yeast infection, vaginal intercourse and the use of tampons, douches, spermicides, or other vaginal products should be refrained from for the duration of treatment.
- Vaginal preparations may weaken latex condoms and diaphragms, decreasing their efficacy in preventing unwanted pregnancy and sexually transmitted diseases.
- If treating athlete's foot, special attention should be paid to the spaces between the toes and wear well-fitting, ventilated shoes. Patients should change shoes and socks at least once daily.

Econazole

Classification and Mode of Action

- Imidazole antifungal. Econazole inhibits the synthesis of ergosterol, a primary sterol of the fungal cell membrane. By decreasing the availability of ergosterol, this drug fundamentally alters cell wall permeability, causing an accumulation of 14α-methyl sterols and leakage of cellular contents. Econazole may also interfere with lipid metabolism and the synthesis of RNA and proteins.

- In clinical trials, econazole was found to effectively treat interdigital tinea pedis in approximately 48% of cases, achieving mycological cure in 67–68.3% of patients and complete cure in 23.2 = 25.3% of cases. In comparison, luliconazole and sertaconazole were considered to provide effective treatment in 33–48% and 32.3–50.5% of cases, respectively.

Indications and Dermatological Uses

- *Clinical indications:* Topical treatment of cutaneous candidiasis; tinea versicolor; and tinea pedis, tinea cruris, and/or tinea corporis caused by *Trichophyton rubrum, Trichophyton mentagrophytes, Trichophyton tonsurans, Microsporum canis, Microsporum audouinii, Microsporum gypseum,* and/or *Epidermophyton floccosum.*
- *Off-label common uses:* Tinea manuum (level of evidence: C).

Formulations/Presentation

- US: 1% cream, 1% foam.
- Canada: 1% cream, 150 mg vaginal ovule.
- Europe: Not on Lexicomp.

Dosages and Suggested Regimens

- *Cutaneous candidiasis:* Affected area(s) should be applied with treatment twice daily.
- *Tinea versicolor*: The affected and surrounding area(s) should be applied with this drug once daily for 2 weeks (adults) or 4 weeks (pediatric).
- *Other tinea infection*: The affected and surrounding area(s) should be applied with treatment once daily for 4 weeks, or until condition resolves.
- If treating tinea pedis, treatment should be continued for 1 week after clinical resolution.

Baseline Investigations and Considerations

- There is no specific requirement for baseline investigations.

Pharmacokinetics (Percutaneous Absorption, Distribution, Metabolism, Excretion: As Relevant for the Drug)

- Following topical administration, econazole exhibits expansive penetration of the skin, with concentrations exceeding those necessary to achieve minimum inhibitory concentration in the stratum corneum, epidermis, and mid-dermis. Less than 10% of an applied dose reaches the systemic circulation; peak serum concentration is reached in 6.8 ± 5.1 h.
- Econazole undergoes extensive hepatic metabolism, producing more than 20 distinct metabolites. Less than 1% of a given dose is excreted as unchanged drug in the feces and urine.

Use in Special Populations: Pregnancy (FDA Guidance), Lactation, Children, Renal Insufficiency, and Hepatic Insufficiency

- It is not known if econazole is present in breast milk. Use with caution in lactating patients.
- There is little data available regarding the use of econazole in pregnant patients. It is recommended to avoid the use of this drug in this population during the first trimester and use sparingly for the remainder of pregnancy only when necessary.
- Approved for use in pediatric patients ≥12 years of age.

Monitoring

- Signs of clinical improvement should be monitored.
- If there is no improvement after completing the course of therapy, diagnosis should be reassessed.

Contraindications and Cautions

- Econazole cream is contraindicated in patients with a hypersensitivity to either the drug product or any component of the formulation.

- Occlusion, application to the genitals, or use over a large body surface area may increase systemic absorption and subsequent risk for adverse events or drug interaction.
- If sensitivity or irritation occurs, the use of this drug should be discontinued.
- While rare, there have been reports of severe toxicity and allergic reaction associated with the use of azole antifungals. Allergic reactions have been reported in up to 2% of patients and usually present as a rash or pruritus. More severe dermal reactions, including epidermal necrolysis, serum sickness, and anaphylaxis have been reported with the use of oral formulations. In most cases, allergic reactions may become apparent several days or weeks after starting therapy. In sensitized patients, symptoms may occur within minutes or hours. Allergic reactions to azole antifungals have been found to respond well to corticosteroids and antihistamine.
- Clinical data regarding incidences of cross-reaction is limited; however, there are numerous case reports of significant occurrences. While there is potential for cross-reactivity between all types of azole antifungals, the possibility is greatest in patients who have taken other imidazoles due to the high degree of structural similarity.
- Some dosage forms may be formulated with propylene glycol. Exposure to large amounts of propylene glycol has been associated with potentially fatal neonatal toxicity and may present with metabolic acidosis, renal failure, CNS depression, and seizures. Similar propylene glycol toxicity has also been reported in children and adults and may present with these findings, in addition to hyperosmolality and respiratory depression.

Important Drug Interactions

- Vitamin K Antagonists *(Risk: C)*: Econazole may increase the serum concentration of vitamin K antagonist drugs, resulting in an increased anticoagulant effect. Monitor therapy.

Adverse Effects and Their Management

- Adverse events have been noted to occur in approximately 3% of patients and include burning or stinging sensations of the skin, pruritus, and erythema.
- Hepatotoxicity is a rare adverse event associated with the use of azole antifungals and may represent either direct toxicity or immune system involvement. If cholestatic jaundice or other signs of liver toxicity occur, immediately discontinue medication and initiate appropriate therapy.

Patch Test Concentration

- Nitrate, 1.0% alc. (Chemotechnique).

Essential Patient Information

- This drug is used to treat fungal infections of the skin.
- For external use only. Contact with the eyes, nose, mouth, vagina, and other mucous membranes should be avoided.
- The foam canister should be shaken for ~5 s before use.
- Topical foam is flammable. Exposure to heat, flame, and smoking should be avoided during and immediately after foam application.
- Containers should not be punctured, incinerated, or stored at high temperatures (>120 °F/49 °C) or in direct sunlight, even when empty.
- If any signs of an allergic reaction *(rash; hives; itching; red, swollen, blistered, or peeling skin; wheezing; chest or throat tightness; difficulty breathing, swallowing, or talking; unusual hoarseness; or swelling of the mouth, face, lips, tongue, or throat)* are noticed, appropriate medical help should be sought immediately. This medication should be discontinued and any side effects should be reported to a physician.

Ketoconazole

Classification and Mode of Action

- Imidazole antifungal. Ketoconazole inhibits fungal cytochrome P450 and multiple other enzymes, blocking the synthesis of triglycerides and phospholipids, altering the permeability of the cell wall, inhibiting androgen synthesis, and causing accumulation of hydrogen peroxide to detrimental levels in fungi.

Indications and Dermatological Uses

- *Clinical indications:* Topical treatment of tinea (pityriasis) versicolor due to *Pityrosporum orbiculare* also termed *Malassezia furfur*. Topical treatment of tinea corporis (ringworm), tinea cruris (jock itch), and tinea pedis (athlete's foot) due to *Trichophyton rubrum*, *Trichophyton mentagrophytes*, and *Epidermophyton floccosum*. Treatment of cutaneous candidiasis due to *Candida* sp. Treatment of seborrheic dermatitis. Please see Chap. 24: *Seborrheic Dermatitis* for additional discussion.
- *OTC indications:* Control of flaking, scaling, and itching associated with dandruff.
- *Off-label common uses:* Tinea manuum (Level of evidence: C).

Formulations/Presentation

- US: 2% foam, 2% cream, 2% gel, 1% shampoo, 2% shampoo.
- Canada: 2% cream, 2% shampoo.
- Europe: Not on Lexicomp.

Dosages and Suggested Regimens

- *Cutaneous candidiasis:* Topical cream is applied over the entire affected area plus the surrounding area once a day for 2 weeks (2–3 weeks according to Canadian label).

- *Tinea corporis and Tinea cruris:* Topical cream is applied over the entire affected area(s) plus surrounding area once a day for 1–3 weeks or until clinical resolution of the infection.
- *Tinea pedis:* Topical cream is applied over the entire affected area(s) plus surrounding area once a day for 4–6 weeks, or 1 week after clinical resolution.
- *Tinea versicolor:* Topical cream is applied over the entire affected plus the surrounding area for 2 weeks (Canadian label recommends 2–3 weeks).
- *Seborrheic dermatitis:* Topical cream is applied to the entire affected area twice a day for 4 weeks or until clinical resolution.
- *Dandruff:* 5–10 mL of 2% ketoconazole shampoo is applied to the wet scalp. It should be lathered and allowed to sit for 3–5 min before rinsing. This drug is used twice weekly for 2–4 weeks, then once every 1–2 weeks for ongoing control. If self-treating dandruff, 1% ketoconazole shampoo can be used once every 3–4 days for up to 8 weeks, then as needed to control condition.

Baseline Investigations and Considerations

- There is no specific requirement for baseline investigations.

Pharmacokinetics (Percutaneous Absorption, Distribution, Metabolism, and Excretion: As Relevant for the Drug)

- Systemic absorption of ketoconazole following topical application is limited. In patients using ketoconazole shampoo, serum drug levels are undetectable, even after chronic use. Use of the cream, gel, and foam products results in minimal systemic absorption, with observed serum levels 250 times lower than seen with an equivalent oral dose.

Use in Special Populations: Pregnancy (FDA Guidance), Lactation, Children, Renal Insufficiency, and Hepatic Insufficiency

- Topical ketoconazole is approved for use in the treatment of complications secondary to infectious atopic dermatitis in pregnant patients.
- While topically administered ketoconazole demonstrates low systemic absorption, it may be present in breast milk. Use with caution in patients desiring to breastfeed. Do not allow the medication to come into contact with the nipple, surrounding breast, or infant.

Monitoring

- There is no specific requirement for monitoring.

Contraindications and Cautions

- Ketoconazole is contraindicated in patients with a hypersensitivity to either the drug product or any component of the formulation.
- When used for self-medication, do not apply if the scalp is broken or inflamed.
- If sensitivity or irritation occurs, the use of this medication should be discontinued.
- While rare, there have been reports of severe toxicity and allergic reaction associated with the use of azole antifungals. Allergic reactions have been reported in up to 2% of patients and usually present as a rash or pruritus. More severe dermal reactions, including epidermal necrolysis, serum sickness, and anaphylaxis have been reported with the use of oral formulations. In most cases, allergic reactions may become apparent several days or weeks after starting therapy. In sensitized patients, symptoms may occur within minutes or hours. Allergic reactions to azole antifungals have been found to respond well to corticosteroids and antihistamine.
- Some formulations of this product may contain sulfites, posing a risk for severe or life-threatening asthmatic episodes, allergic reactions, and anaphylaxis in patients with a sensitivity.

- Clinical data regarding incidences of cross-reaction is limited; however, there are numerous case reports of significant occurrences. While there is potential for cross-reactivity between all types of azole antifungals, the possibility is greatest in patients who have taken other imidazoles due to the high degree of structural similarity.
- Some dosage forms may be formulated with propylene glycol. Exposure to large amounts of propylene glycol has been associated with potentially fatal neonatal toxicity and may present with metabolic acidosis, renal failure, CNS depression, and seizures. Similar propylene glycol toxicity has also been reported in children and adults and may present with these findings, in addition to hyperosmolality and respiratory depression.

Important Drug Interactions

- There are no known significant drug interactions.

Adverse Effects and Their Management

- Hepatotoxicity is a rare adverse event associated with the use of azole antifungals and may represent either direct toxicity or immune system involvement. If cholestatic jaundice or other signs of liver toxicity occur, immediately discontinue medication and initiate appropriate therapy.
- The shampoo may cause burning, itchy, or dry scalp; changes in hair texture, including straight hair, or discoloration; loss of hair.
- Adverse reactions from dermatologic administration include application-site pruritus from cream in <5% of patients, from shampoo in up to 3% of patients, from foam and gel in <1% of patients; Xeroderma from shampoo in up to 3% of patients, from foam and gel in <1% of patients; stinging from cream in <5% of patients.
- Adverse reactions from local administration include: application-site reactions from cream in <6% of patients, from shampoo in up to 3% of patients, from foam gel in <1% of patients; burning from gel in 4% of patients, from foam and shampoo in

<1% of patients; local irritation from cream in <5% of patients, from foam and shampoo in less than 1% of patients.

- Other reported adverse events include: urticaria, anaphylaxis, angioedema, application-site dermatitis and/or discharge, erythema, pain, contact dermatitis, skin irritation, skin rash; cheilitis; dizziness; eye irritation, swelling of the eye, dry eye syndrome, eye irritation; swelling of the face; headache; hypersensitivity reaction; impetigo; nail discoloration; localized warm feeling; paresthesia; pustules; pyogenic granuloma; acne vulgaris.

Patch Test Concentration

- 1% alcohol

Essential Patient Information

- For external use only. Contact with the eyes, nose, mouth, vagina, and other mucous membranes should be avoided.
- Topical gel and foam preparations are flammable. Exposure to heat, flame, and smoking should be avoided during and immediately after application.
- Foam canister contains alcohol and propane/butane. Containers should not be punctured or incinerated.
- If any signs of an allergic reaction *(rash; hives; itching; red, swollen, blistered, or peeling skin; wheezing; chest or throat tightness; difficulty breathing, swallowing, or talking; unusual hoarseness; or swelling of the mouth, face, lips, tongue, or throat)* are noticed, appropriate medical help should be sought immediately. This medication should be discontinued, and any side effects should be reported to a physician.
- Foam application is best performed when the foam is kept in cool temperatures. Warm surfaces, including hands and fingers, will cause the foam to melt prematurely. Utilizing the cap or hands previously rinsed in cool water prior to application is preferable. After obtaining a small amount in the fingers, application of the foam to the affected area will cause it to disappear. It should be ensured that hair is parted away from the application site in order to apply to skin in hair-bearing areas.

- For gel application, the entire affected area should be treated. Application of products such as sunscreen or makeup should be delayed for 20 min. Washing of the affected area after gel application should be delayed for 3 h.

Luliconazole

Classification and Mode of Action

- Imidazole antifungal: By inhibiting the CYP450-dependent enzyme 14α-lanosterol demethylase, luliconazole interferes with the conversion of lanosterol to ergosterol, the primary sterol of the fungal cell wall. This results in decreased availability of ergosterol and a subsequent buildup of the precursor component.
- In clinical trials, luliconazole was found to effectively treat interdigital tinea pedis in between 33% and 48% of cases, achieving mycological cure in 56–62% of patients and complete cure in 14–26% of cases. In comparison, econazole and sertaconazole were considered to provide effective treatment in 48.4–48.8% and 32.3–50.5% of cases, respectively.

Indications and Dermatological Uses

- *Clinical indications:* Topical treatment of interdigital tinea pedis, tinea cruris, and/or tinea corporis secondary to infection with *Trichophyton rubrum* or *Epidermophyton floccosum.*
- *Off-label common uses:* Tinea manuum (level of evidence: C).

Formulations/Presentation

- US: 1% cream.
- Canada: Not in Health Canada Drug Product Database.
- Europe: Not on Lexicomp.

Dosages and Suggested Regimens

- Luliconazole should be applied to affected area(s) and 1 inch of surrounding healthy tissue once daily until condition resolves.
- For the treatment of tinea pedis or tinea manuum, treatment should be continued for 1 week following clinical resolution.
- Clinical efficacy may take up to 3 weeks to become evident.

Baseline Investigations and Considerations

- There is no specific requirement for baseline investigations.

Pharmacokinetics (Percutaneous Absorption, Distribution, Metabolism, and Excretion: As Relevant for the Drug)

- Luliconazole demonstrates limited systemic absorption following topical application.
- Within the serum, luliconazole exhibits >99% binding to plasma proteins.
- This drug is a weak-to-moderate inhibitor of CYP2C19. It also inhibits the activity of CYP2B6, CYP2C8, CYP2C19, and CYP3A4.

Use in Special Populations: Pregnancy (FDA Guidance), Lactation, Children,Renal Insufficiency, and Hepatic Insufficiency

- It is not known if luliconazole is present in the breast milk; however, small amounts of drug can be found in the serum following topical administration. Use with caution in lactating patients.
- There are no studies evaluating the use of luliconazole in pregnant or lactating patients; however, animal reproduction studies have demonstrated an increased risk for adverse outcomes. Extrapolated risks of birth defect and miscarriage within the United States population reach up to 4% and 20%, respectively.
- This product is approved for use in pediatric patients ≥2 years of age.

Monitoring

- Luliconazole should be monitored for localized dermatitis, cellulitis, application site reactions, and irritation during use.

Contraindications and Cautions

- There are no known contraindications.
- While rare, there have been reports of severe toxicity and allergic reaction associated with the use of azole antifungals. Allergic reactions have been reported in up to 2% of patients and usually present as a rash or pruritus. More severe dermal reactions, including epidermal necrolysis, serum sickness, and anaphylaxis have been reported with the use of oral formulations. In most cases, allergic reactions may become apparent several days or weeks after starting therapy. In sensitized patients, symptoms may occur within minutes or hours. Allergic reactions to azole antifungals have been found to respond well to corticosteroids and antihistamine.
- Clinical data regarding incidences of cross-reaction is limited; however, there are numerous case reports of significant occurrences. While there is potential for cross-reactivity between all types of azole antifungals, the possibility is greatest in patients who have taken other imidazoles due to the high degree of structural similarity.

Important Drug Interactions

- Clobazam; Fosphenytoin; Phenytoin *(Risk C)*: Luliconazole is a weak inhibitor of CYP2C19, though some studies have reported moderate enzyme inhibition. Concurrent use may result in increased serum concentrations of fosphenytoin, phenytoin, or clobazam and its active metabolites. Therapy should be monitored.
- CYP Interactions: May inhibit the breakdown of drugs metabolized by CYP2B6, 2C8, 2C19, and 3A4.

Adverse Effects and Their Management

- Reports of adverse events with the use of luliconazole are rare. Post-marketing reports of adverse drug effects include application site reactions, contact dermatitis, and cellulitis; however, these occurred in <1% of patients.
- Hepatotoxicity is a rare adverse event associated with the use of azole antifungals and may represent either direct toxicity or immune system involvement. If cholestatic jaundice or other signs of liver toxicity occur, medication should be discontinued immediately, and appropriate therapy should be initiated.

Patch Test Concentration

- 2% pet.

Essential Patient Information

- This drug is used to treat fungal infections of the skin.
- Hands should be washed after use.

Miconazole Nitrate

Classification and Mode of Action

- Imidazole Antifungal: The exact mechanism by which miconazole exerts its fungicidal action is not fully understood; however, azole antifungals as a group are known to inhibit the synthesis of ergosterol, a key component of the fungal cell membrane, resulting in a toxic accumulation of methylated sterols.
- Clinical studies of miconazole have demonstrated interference with triglyceride and fatty acid synthesis, damage to actin cables, and inhibition of fungal oxidative and peroxidase enzymes. It has been postulated that the cumulative result of these actions is increased accumulation of reactive oxygen species (ROS), mitochondrial dysregulation, and, ultimately, the induction of cellular apoptosis.

Indications and Dermatological Uses

- *Clinical indications:* Topical treatment of cutaneous and mucocutaneous fungal infections, vulvovaginal candidiasis, and adjunctive treatment of diaper dermatitis complicated by documented evidence of comorbid candidiasis in immunocompetent patient ≥4 weeks of age.
- *Off-label common uses:* Tinea manuum.

Formulations/Presentation

- US: Aerosol powder (2%), non-aerosol powder (2%), cream (2%), fungoid tincture/solution (2%), ointment (2%).
- Canada: Spray (2%), cream (2%), vaginal cream (2%).
- Europe: Not on Lexicomp.

Dosages and Suggested Regimens

- *Diaper dermatitis:* A thin layer of ointment should be applied to clean, dry skin of the affected area using the tips of the fingers at each diaper change for 7 days. The ointment should not be rubbed in.
- *Other dermatologic infection:* This drug should be applied to the affected area twice daily for up to 4 weeks or clinical resolution. If treating tinea pedis or tinea manuum, treatment should be continued for 1 week following clinical resolution.

Baseline Investigations and Considerations

- Prior to initiating treatment for diaper dermatitis, confirmation of candidal infection should be obtained with microscopic evidence of pseudohyphae and/or budding yeast.
- KOH Prep.

Pharmacokinetics (Percutaneous Absorption, Distribution, Metabolism, Excretion: As Relevant for the Drug)

- Although topical miconazole is negligibly absorbed into the systemic circulation, it is widely distributed and highly protein bound (91–93%) with detectable concentrations in the body tissues, joint spaces, and fluid spaces. There is very little evidence of penetration into the saliva, urine, sputum, and CSF. Absorption is slightly increased when applied vaginally but is still low. Miconazole is primarily metabolized in the liver and exhibits multiphasic degradation; its alpha, beta, and terminal half-lives are 40 min, 126 min, and 24 h, respectively. Excretion occurs mostly via the feces; 50% of absorbed miconazole is excreted unchanged in the feces, as opposed to <1%, which appears in the urine.

Use in Special Populations: Pregnancy (FDA Guidance), Lactation, Children, Renal Insufficiency, and Hepatic Insufficiency

- Miconazole has not been evaluated for use in pregnant, lactating, or geriatric patients.
- In animal studies, miconazole given at high doses was found to be associated with prolonged gestation and a decreased rate of live births.
- It is not known if miconazole is expressed in breast milk. Only the cream formulation is approved for treatment of candidiasis affecting the breasts or nipples. Miconazole gel should not be applied to these areas and prolonged administration of any dosage form should be avoided.
- This drug is not approved for OTC use in children <2 years of age.
- Clinical efficacy has not been demonstrated in infants <4 weeks of age. Safety and efficacy have not been evaluated in very-low-birthweight or premature infants.
- Some dosage forms may be formulated with propylene glycol. Exposure to large amounts of propylene glycol has been associated with potentially fatal neonatal toxicity and may present with metabolic acidosis, renal failure, CNS depression, and seizures. Similar propylene glycol toxicity has also been reported in children and adults and may present with these findings, in addition to hyperosmolality and respiratory depression.
- Some dosage forms may be formulated with benzyl alcohol; some studies have implicated benzoate in the displacement of

bilirubin from protein binding sites. Exposure to benzyl alcohol in doses exceeding 99 mg/kg/day has been associated with a potentially fatal neonatal toxicity known as gasping syndrome. Gasping syndrome presents with metabolic acidosis, hypotension, cardiovascular collapse, seizures, intracranial hemorrhage, other CNS dysfunction, gasping respirations, and respiratory distress. The use of products containing benzyl alcohol should be avoided in this patient population.

Monitoring

- There is no specific requirement for monitoring.

Contraindications and Cautions

- Miconazole is contraindicated in patients with a hypersensitivity to either the drug product or any component of the formulation.
- If skin sensitivity, irritation, or worsening of condition occurs, use of this medication should be discontinued, and a healthcare provider should be contacted.
- While rare, there have been reports of severe toxicity and allergic reaction associated with the use of azole antifungals. Allergic reactions have been reported in up to 2% of patients and usually present as a rash or pruritus. More severe dermal reactions, including epidermal necrolysis, serum sickness, and anaphylaxis have been reported with the use of oral formulations. In most cases, allergic reactions may become apparent several days or weeks after starting therapy. In sensitized patients, symptoms may occur within minutes or hours. Allergic reactions to azole antifungals have been found to respond well to corticosteroids and antihistamine.
- Clinical data regarding incidences of cross-reaction is limited; however, there are numerous case reports of significant occurrences. While there is potential for cross-reactivity between all types of azole antifungals, the possibility is greatest in patients who have taken other imidazoles due to the high degree of structural similarity.

- May inhibit the metabolism of oral sulfonylureas. Caution should be used in diabetic patients and counseling should be provided on appropriate blood glucose testing procedures.

Important Drug Interactions

- Progesterone *(Risk X)*: Miconazole may decrease the efficacy of progesterone. Combinations should be avoided with these products.
- Vitamin K Antagonists *(Risk: D)*: Miconazole may increase the serum concentration of vitamin K antagonist drugs, resulting in an increased anticoagulant effect. Coadministration with warfarin may lead to elevations in INR, prothrombin time, and bleeding risk. The use of miconazole-containing drug products should be avoided in patients treated with warfarin. If use of both agents is unavoidable, therapy modification should be strongly considered. The anticoagulant dose can be decreased by 10–20%; close monitoring for signs of excessive anticoagulant activity should be performed for the duration of therapy.
- Miconazole may inhibit the metabolism of orally administered sulfonylureas. Patients should monitor blood glucose regularly.

Adverse Effects and Their Management

- The primary adverse event for this drug is allergic contact dermatitis, a burning sensation of the skin, and skin maceration. Notably, clinical trials have evidenced similar incidences of adverse events in patients treated with either miconazole preparations or the inactive vehicle alone.
- The following adverse events have been reported in <1% of patients: blistering and exfoliation of the skin, skin dryness, diaper dermatitis, pruritus, erythema, vomiting, pain, and inflammation.
- Hepatotoxicity is a rare adverse event associated with the use of azole antifungals and may represent either direct toxicity or immune system involvement. If cholestatic jaundice or other signs of liver toxicity occur, medication should be immediately discontinued, and appropriate therapy should be initiated.

- If any signs of an allergic reaction *(rash; hives; itching; red, swollen, blistered, or peeling skin; wheezing; chest or throat tightness; difficulty breathing, swallowing or talking; hoarseness; or swelling of the mouth, face, lips, tongue, or throat)* are noticed, appropriate medical help should be sought immediately. This medication should be discontinued, and any side effects should be reported to a physician.

Patch Test Concentration

- 1% alc. (Chemotechnique)

Essential Patient Information

- This product is indicated for topical use only. Contact with the eyes and mouth should be avoided.
- Miconazole preparations (e.g., *ointment, cream,* and *powder)* should not be used for intravaginal treatment unless specifically directed by either the package labeling or a physician.
- Prior to application, skin should be washed with lukewarm water and patted dry with a towel.
- The safety of long-term treatment with miconazole ointment has not been evaluated. Miconazole should not be used for longer than 7 days.
- Diapers should be changed frequently to minimize the occurrence of diaper dermatitis. This medication is not a substitute for routine diaper changes, and it should not be used as prophylactic therapy. Diaper dermatitis should be treated for the full recommended 7 days, even if symptoms resolve.
- Inappropriate, preventive, or extended use of this medication may lead to the development of drug resistance.

Oxiconazole Nitrate

Classification and Mode of Action

- Imidazole antifungal: Oxiconazole inhibits the synthesis of ergosterol, a key component of the fungal cell membrane, resulting in the loss of cytoplasmic membrane integrity.

- Oxiconazole has fungicidal activity and is known to be active against *Trichophyton rubrum, Trichophyton mentagrophytes, Epidermophyton floccosum,* and *Malassezia furfur*.
- Clinical studies have found that oxiconazole reaches a minimum inhibitory concentration (MIC) sufficient to inhibit growth for several other fungal species, however its safety and efficacy in the treatment of these infections has not been established. These include most strains of *Candida albicans, Trichophyton violaceum, Trichophyton tonsurans, Microsporum canis, Microsporum audouinii*, and *Microsporum gypseum*.

Indications and Dermatological Uses

- *Clinical indications:* Topical treatment of tinea (pityriasis) versicolor due to *Malassezia furfur*. Topical treatment of tinea pedis (athlete's foot), tinea cruris (jock itch), and/or tinea corporis (ringworm) due to *Trichophyton rubrum*, *Trichophyton mentagrophytes*, or *Epidermophyton floccosum*.
- *Off-label common uses:* Tinea manuum (level of evidence: C).

Formulations/Presentation

- US: 1% cream, 1% lotion.
- Canada: Cancelled Post Market (Health Canada).
- Europe: Not on Lexicomp.

Dosages and Suggested Regimens

- Oxiconazole should be applied to clean, dry skin on the affected area(s), plus a ½-inch margin of surrounding tissue one to two times daily for 2 weeks or until clinical resolution.
- For tinea pedis and tinea manuum infections, treatment should be for a minimum of 4 weeks and continued until 1 week after clinical resolution.

Baseline Investigations and Considerations

- Culture and KOH preparation.
- Clinical signs of infection.

Pharmacokinetics (Percutaneous Absorption, Distribution, Metabolism, and Excretion: As Relevant for the Drug)

- A topical dose can penetrate the epidermis, upper corium, and deeper corium within 5 h of application.
- Oxiconazole exhibits low systemic absorption with <0.3% of an administered dose reaching the urine 5 days after application.

Use in Special Populations: Pregnancy (FDA Guidance), Lactation, Children, Renal Insufficiency, and Hepatic Insufficiency

- Although systemic absorption of oxiconazole is very limited, it has been found to be excreted in breast milk. Caution should be used in patients desiring to breastfeed.
- There are insufficient human trials of oxiconazole in geriatric patients to effectively establish safety and efficacy.
- Animal studies and Phase IV marketing have not evidenced any notable teratogenic effects; however, due to the lack of human trial data, this drug should only be used in pregnant patients if clearly needed.
- This product is approved for use in children ≥12 years of age.

Monitoring

- Signs of clinical resolution should be monitored.
- Culture and KOH preparation can be used to evaluate for mycological cure (no evidence of baseline pathogen) 2 weeks after completion of treatment.
- Treatment is considered successful if both mycological cure and a 90% improvement in clinical signs are achieved.
- If there is no improvement within 3 weeks of initiation, the diagnosis should be reassessed.

Contraindications and Cautions

- Hypersensitivity to oxiconazole or any component of the formulation.
- If sensitivity or irritation occurs, this medication should be discontinued.
- While there are no reports of topical oxiconazole overdose in humans, clinical trials have evidenced dermal reactions due to drug toxicity in animal models.
- While rare, there have been reports of severe toxicity and allergic reaction associated with the use of azole antifungals. Allergic reactions have been reported in up to 2% of patients and usually present as a rash or pruritus. More severe dermal reactions, including epidermal necrolysis, serum sickness, and anaphylaxis have been reported with the use of oral formulations. In most cases, allergic reactions may become apparent several days or weeks after starting therapy. In sensitized patients, symptoms may occur within minutes or hours. Allergic reactions to azole antifungals have been found to respond well to corticosteroids and antihistamine.
- Clinical data regarding incidences of cross-reaction is limited; however, there are numerous case reports of significant occurrences. While there is potential for cross-reactivity between all types of azole antifungals, the possibility is greatest in patients who have taken other imidazoles due to the high degree of structural similarity.

Important Drug Interactions

- There are no known significant drug interactions.

Adverse Effects and Their Management

- The most commonly reported adverse events for this medication are pruritus and localized burning; however, these have been reported in <2% of patients.
- Other reported adverse events include allergic contact dermatitis; dyshidrotic eczema; erythema; pain; stinging or tingling sensations of the skin; maceration, folliculitis, or exfoliation of

the skin; development of skin fissures, papules, and nodules; erythema; pain; and rashes and irritation.
- If sensitivity, irritation, or worsening of condition occurs, the drug should be discontinued.
- Hepatotoxicity is a rare adverse event associated with the use of azole antifungals and may represent either direct toxicity or immune system involvement. If cholestatic jaundice or other signs of liver toxicity occur, the medication should be immediately discontinued, and appropriate therapy should be initiated.

Patch Test Concentration
- 1% alcohol or MEK (methyl ethyl ketone)

Essential Patient Information
- This medication is not intended for ophthalmic or intravaginal use. For external use only on clean, dry, intact skin as directed by a physician.
- Contact with the eyes, nose, mouth, vagina, and other mucous membranes should be avoided.
- The use of occlusive dressings should be avoided, unless otherwise directed.
- Hands should be washed before and after use. This drug should be shaken well before using.
- If there is no improvement after 2–4 weeks of therapy, or if the condition gets worse, a physician should be contacted.
- Tinea (pityriasis) versicolor may present with patches of skin discoloration on the trunk, neck, arms, and upper thighs. The timing for pigment normalization is highly variable and depends on such factors as individual skin type and incidental sun exposure. Restoration of normal or consistent skin tone may not occur for several months following successful treatment. Further, although tinea versicolor is not contagious, the causative organism is part of the normal skin flora. Therefore, it is possible for this condition to recur even after successful treatment.

- The use of this medication should be continued for the full duration of the prescribed treatment, even if symptoms have improved.
- If a patient experiences a severe skin reaction at the application site such as blistering, swelling, burning, oozing, or bleeding, immediate medical help should be sought.

Sertaconazole Nitrate

Classification and Mode of Action

- Imidazole antifungal: By inhibiting the CYP450-dependent enzyme 14α-lanosterol demethylase, sertaconazole interferes with the conversion of lanosterol to ergosterol, the primary sterol of the fungal cell wall. This results in increased permeability of the fungal cell membrane and cellular injury secondary to leakage of cytoplasmic contents from the cell.
- Sertaconazole is active against most strains of *Trichophyton rubrum, Trichophyton mentagrophytes,* and *Epidermophyton floccosum*.

Indications and Dermatological Uses

- *Clinical indications:* Topical treatment of interdigital tinea pedis caused by *Trichophyton rubrum, Trichophyton mentagrophytes*, and *Epidermophyton floccosum.*
- *Off-label common uses:* Cutaneous candidiasis (level of evidence: B), seborrheic dermatitis (level of evidence: B), tinea corporis/cruris (level of evidence: B), tinea manuum (level of evidence: C), tinea versicolor (level of evidence: C).

Formulations/Presentation

- US: 2% cream.
- Canada: Not on Health Canada Drug Product Database.
- Europe: Not on Lexicomp.

Dosages and Suggested Regimens

- Sertaconazole should be applied to clean, dry skin on the affected area(s), plus a ½-inch margin of surrounding tissue twice daily for 4 weeks. If treating tinea pedis or tinea manuum, regimen should be continued for 1 week after clinical resolution of infection.
- For the treatment of tinea corporis or tinea cruris, this drug should be applied one to ttwo times daily until clinical resolution of infection. It may take 1–3 weeks for clinical effect to become apparent.

Baseline Investigations and Considerations

- There is no specific requirement for baseline investigations.

Pharmacokinetics (Percutaneous Absorption, Distribution, Metabolism, Excretion: As Relevant for the Drug)

- The systemic bioavailability of sertaconazole is negligible. Following the application of a topical dose, serum drug concentrations are undetectable.

Use in Special Populations: Pregnancy (FDA Guidance), Lactation, Children, Renal Insufficiency, and Hepatic Insufficiency

- This drug is only approved for use in immunocompetent patients ≥12 years of age.
- Animal studies and Phase IV marketing have not evidenced any notable teratogenic effects. It is not known if sertaconazole is present in breast milk, however, systemic absorption is very low. Use with caution in lactating women.
- Due to the low systemic bioavailability of this product, no dosage adjustments are required for patients with hepatic or renal dysfunction.

Monitoring

- Clinical improvement should be monitored. If there is no improvement after 2 weeks of treatment, diagnosis and therapy should be reevaluated.

Contraindications and Cautions

- There are no known contraindications to the use of this medication.
- While rare, there have been reports of severe toxicity and allergic reaction associated with the use of azole antifungals. Allergic reactions have been reported in up to 2% of patients and usually present as a rash or pruritus. More severe dermal reactions, including epidermal necrolysis, serum sickness, and anaphylaxis have been reported with the use of oral formulations. In most cases, allergic reactions may become apparent several days or weeks after starting therapy. In sensitized patients, symptoms may occur within minutes or hours. Allergic reactions to azole antifungals have been found to respond well to corticosteroids and antihistamine.
- Clinical data regarding incidences of cross-reaction is limited; however, there are numerous case reports of significant occurrences. While there is potential for cross-reactivity between all types of azole antifungals, the possibility is greatest in patients who have taken other imidazoles due to the high degree of structural similarity.

Important Drug Interactions

- Progesterone *(Risk X)*: Sulconazole may decrease the efficacy of progesterone. Combinations with these products should be avoided.

Adverse Effects and Their Management

- The most commonly reported adverse events are skin dryness, contact dermatitis, skin tenderness, and a burning sensation of the skin.

- Phase IV reports have noted desquamation, erythema, hyperpigmentation, pruritus, and vesicular eruptions in <1% of patients.
- Hepatotoxicity is a rare adverse event associated with the use of azole antifungals and may represent either direct toxicity or immune system involvement. If cholestatic jaundice or other signs of liver toxicity occur, immediately discontinue medication and initiate appropriate therapy.

Patch Test Concentration

- 1% and 5% pet.; imidazoles are usually tested 1% alcohol or MEK (methyl ethyl ketone)

Essential Patient Information

- This drug is used to treat fungal infections of the skin.
- This product is for external use only and contact with the eyes, nose, mouth, or mucous membranes should be avoided.
- Sertaconazole should be applied only to skin which has been thoroughly cleansed and dried. Hands should be washed before and after application. Contact with the eyes, nose, mouth, vagina, and other mucous membranes should be avoided.
- This medication should be used for the entire duration of treatment recommended by a physician, even if symptoms improve.
- This medication should not be used with occlusive dressings.
- If irritation, redness, peeling, change in skin color, other skin sensitivity, or worsening of condition occurs, a physician should be contacted immediately, and the use of this medication should be discontinued.
- If any signs of an allergic reaction *(rash; hives; itching; red, swollen, blistered, or peeling skin; wheezing; chest or throat tightness; difficulty breathing, swallowing, or talking; unusual hoarseness; or swelling of the mouth, face, lips, tongue, or throat)* are noticed, appropriate medical help should be sought immediately. This medication should be discontinued, and any side effects should be reported to a physician.

Sulconazole

Classification and Mode of Action

- Imidazole antifungal. Sulconazole inhibits the synthesis of ergosterol, a key component of the fungal cell membrane, resulting in decreased growth of dermatophytes and other fungal organisms. In most cases, the drug effect is primarily fungistatic; however, in the treatment of some *Candida albicans* and *Candida parapsilosis* infections, its activity is actually fungicidal.

Indications and Dermatological Uses

- *Clinical indications:* Topical treatment of tinea pedis (athlete's foot), tinea corporis (ringworm), and tinea cruris (jock itch) caused by *Trichophyton rubrum, Trichophyton mentagrophytes, Epidermophyton floccosum*, and *Microsporum canis*. Topical treatment of tinea versicolor.
- *Off-label common uses:* Topical treatment of tinea manuum (level of evidence: C).

Formulations/Presentation

- US: 1% cream, 1% solution.
- Canada: Not on Health Canada Drug Product Database.
- Europe: Not on Lexicomp.

Dosages and Suggested Regimens

- A small amount of sulconazole should be applied to the affected and surrounding area(s) and gently rubbed in one to two times daily for at least 3 weeks, or until clinical resolution.
- For tinea pedis infections, this medication should be used twice daily and continue treatment for 1 week after clinical resolution.

Baseline Investigations and Considerations

- There are no known significant drug interactions.

Pharmacokinetics (Percutaneous Absorption, Distribution, Metabolism, Excretion: As Relevant for the Drug)

- Following topical administration, sulconazole exhibits between 8.7% and11% percutaneous absorption. The drug is primarily excreted in the urine.

Use in Special Populations: Pregnancy (FDA Guidance), Lactation, Children, Renal Insufficiency, and Hepatic Insufficiency

- There are insufficient human studies concerning the use of this drug in pediatric, geriatric, pregnant, or lactating patients. In animal studies, sulconazole given at high doses was found to be embryotoxic, but not teratogenic. High-dose sulconazole was also found to cause prolonged gestation and dystocia, resulting in maternal death in several animal models.
- It is not known if sulconazole is present in breast milk. This drug should be used with caution and should not be applied on or near the nipples in lactating patients.

Monitoring

- Signs of clinical improvement should be monitored. If the condition does not improve following 4–6 weeks of appropriate therapy, the diagnosis should be reevaluated.

Contraindications and Cautions

- This drug is contraindicated in patients with a hypersensitivity to either the drug product or any component of the formulation.
- Effectiveness has not been proven in the treatment of tinea pedis; tinea pedis infections should be treated for a minimum of 4 weeks.
- If sensitivity or irritation occurs, this medication should be discontinued,

- While rare, there have been reports of severe toxicity and allergic reaction associated with the use of azole antifungals. Allergic reactions have been reported in up to 2% of patients and usually present as a rash or pruritus. More severe dermal reactions, including epidermal necrolysis, serum sickness, and anaphylaxis have been reported with the use of oral formulations. In most cases, allergic reactions may become apparent several days or weeks after starting therapy. In sensitized patients, symptoms may occur within minutes or hours. Allergic reactions to azole antifungals have been found to respond well to corticosteroids and antihistamine.
- Clinical data regarding incidences of cross-reaction is limited; however, there are numerous case reports of significant occurrences. While there is potential for cross-reactivity between all types of azole antifungals, the possibility is greatest in patients who have taken other imidazoles due to the high degree of structural similarity.

Important Drug Interactions

- There are no known significant drug interactions.

Adverse Effects and Their Management

- The most commonly reported adverse events are localized burning, erythema, pruritus, and stinging of the skin.
- Hepatotoxicity is a rare adverse event associated with the use of azole antifungals and may represent either direct toxicity or immune system involvement. If cholestatic jaundice or other signs of liver toxicity occur, immediately discontinue medication and initiate appropriate therapy.

Patch Test Concentration

- 1% alcohol or MEK (methyl ethyl ketone)

Essential Patient Information

- This drug is used to treat fungal infections of the skin.
- Symptomatic relief typically occurs within the first few days of treatment; however, it may take a full week for signs of clinical improvement to become apparent.

- This product is intended for external use only. Contact with the eyes and mucous membranes should be avoided.
- Exposing solution to light or excessive heat (> 104 °F/40 °C) should be avoided.
- If any signs of an allergic reaction *(rash; hives; itching; red, swollen, blistered, or peeling skin; wheezing; chest or throat tightness; difficulty breathing, swallowing, or talking; unusual hoarseness; or swelling of the mouth, face, lips, tongue, or throat)* are noticed, appropriate medical help should be sought immediately. This medication should be discontinued, and any side effects should be reported to a physician.

Butenafine HCl

Classification and Mode of Action

- Benzylamine antifungal. Butenafine inhibits the enzyme squalene-2,3-epoxidase, limiting fungal cells' ability to synthesize ergosterol, a key component of the fungal cell membrane.

Indications and Dermatological Uses

- *Clinical indications:* Topical treatment of tinea (pityriasis) versicolor due to *Malassezia furfur.*
- *OTC indications:* Topical treatment of interdigital tinea pedis (athlete's foot), tinea corporis (ringworm), and tinea cruris (jock itch) and relief of burning, itching, scaling, or cracking associated with these infections.
- *Off-label common uses:* Topical treatment of tinea manuum.

Formulations/Presentation

- US: 1% cream.
- Canada: 1% cream.
- Europe: Not on Lexicomp.

Dosages and Suggested Regimens

- *Tinea versicolor:* A thin layer should be applied to clean, dry skin on the affected area(s), plus a ½-inch margin of surrounding tissue once daily for 2 weeks.

- *Tinea corporis and cruris:* A thin layer should be applied to clean, dry skin on the affected area(s), plus a ½-inch margin of surrounding tissue once daily for 2 weeks. Treatment should be continued until clinical resolution of infection.
- *Tinea pedis and manuum:* A thin layer should be applied to clean, dry skin on the affected area(s), plus a ½-inch margin of surrounding tissue twice daily for 2 weeks or once daily for 4 weeks. Treatment should be continued until 1 week after clinical resolution of infection.
- Clinical effects may take 1–3 weeks to become apparent.

Baseline Investigations and Considerations

- There are no known significant drug interactions.

Pharmacokinetics (Percutaneous Absorption, Distribution, Metabolism, Excretion: As Relevant for the Drug)

- Following topical application, butenafine demonstrates minimal systemic bioavailability. Absorbed drug undergoes hepatic metabolism via hydroxylation, reaching its peak serum concentration in 6–15 h. Butenafine undergoes biphasic elimination with the alpha phase having a $t_{1/2}$ of 35 h, and the beta phase having a $t_{1/2}$ of over 150 h.

Use in Special Populations: Pregnancy (FDA Guidance), Lactation, Children, Renal Insufficiency, and Hepatic Insufficiency

- This product is approved for use in children ≥12 years of age.
- Human studies of naftifine in pregnant or lactating patients have not been performed; however, animal studies have not evidenced any notable adverse events. Butenafine should be used with caution in patients desiring to breastfeed.

Monitoring

- Patients should be monitored for signs of clinical efficacy using fungal cultures and a KOH exam. Tinea pedis can also be monitored by its clinical signs.

Contraindications and Cautions

- Butenafine is contraindicated in patients with a hypersensitivity to either the drug product or any component of the formulation.
- When used for OTC self-medication, butenafine should not be used for any treatment of the nails, scalp, or mucous membranes, or for intravaginal yeast infections. This drug should not be used in or near the mouth and/or eyes.
- Butenafine should not be used with occlusive dressings.
- This drug should be used with caution in patients with sensitivities to allylamine antifungals. Cross sensitivity may occur due to the structural similarity between benzylamines and allylamines.

Important Drug Interactions

- This drug has no known significant drug interactions.

Adverse Effects and Their Management

- Primary adverse events are contact dermatitis, application site irritation, and burning and stinging of the skin. This medication should be discontinued if sensitivity or irritation occurs.

Patch Test Concentration

- No data available

Essential Patient Information

- The area of skin to be treated can be washed with soap and water and dried completely before application.
- If treating athlete's foot, well-fitting, ventilated shoes should be worn, and shoes and socks should be changed at least once per day.
- Hands should be washed after each use.
- If skin irritation occurs or worsens, this medication should be discontinued, and a physician should be notified.
- In case of contact with the eye(s), a patient should rinse thoroughly with water. If swallowed, a patient should seek immediate medical help or contact a Poison Control Center.

Ciclopirox Olamine

Classification and Mode of Action

- Hydroxypyridinone derivative. Ciclopirox is a hydroxypyridone that chelates trivalent cations, thereby inhibiting metal dependent enzymes. Its broad mechanism of action targets fungi in a variety of ways: inhibition of cytochromes, oxidative damage, affects nutrient uptake, synthesis of proteins, and nucleic acids.
- Less effective than Efinaconazole and Tavaborole solutions in complete clearance of onychomycosis.

Indications and Dermatological Uses

- *Clinical indications:* Tinea (pedis, cruris, corporis, versicolor), onychomycosis, candidiasis, and seborrheic dermatitis.
- *Off-label common uses:* Tinea manuum (level of evidence: D).

Formulations/Presentation

- US: 0.77% gel, 0.77% cream, 0.77% solution, 1% shampoo, 8% nail lacquer.
- Canada: 1% cream, 1% lotion, 1.5% shampoo, 8% nail lacquer.
- Europe: Not on LexiComp.

Dosages and Suggested Regimens

- Tinea: Application is once to twice daily, reassess after 4 weeks.
- Onychomycosis: Application is once daily for 24 weeks (fingernails) to 48 weeks (toenails).
- Candidiasis: Application is twice daily, reassess after 4 weeks.
- Seborrheic dermatitis: Application is twice daily (gel) or twice weekly (shampoo).
- No suggested dosage adjustment for renal or hepatic impairment due to low systemic absorption.

Baseline Investigations and Considerations

- There are no known significant drug interactions.

Pharmacokinetics (Percutaneous Absorption, Distribution, Metabolism, Excretion: As Relevant for the Drug)

- Minimal topical absorption. Elimination half-life is between 1.7 h (cream), 5.5 h (gel). Excreted in urine, feces.
- Onset of effect: < 4 weeks (gel, cream).

Use in Special Populations: Pregnancy (FDA Guidance), Lactation, Children, Renal Insufficiency, and Hepatic Insufficiency

- Approved for use in children. Internal use should be avoided.
- Listed as FDA pregnancy classification B (former classification system).
- Unknown whether ciclopirox is present in breast milk.
- Renal insufficiency: not evaluated; dose adjustment is not expected to be needed.
- Hepatic insufficiency: not evaluated; dose adjustment is not expected to be needed.

Monitoring

- Skin irritation (dryness, itching, erythema, pain/burning, blistering, swelling, oozing) at the application site.
- Allergy (angioedema, lip swelling, facial edema, tachycardia—reported with shampoo).

Contraindications and Cautions

- Contraindication: Hypersensitivity to ciclopirox or any component of the formulation.
- Ophthalmic, oral, and intravaginal use should be avoided.
- Occlusive dressings should not be placed over treated areas.

Important Drug Interactions

- There are no known significant drug interactions.

Adverse Effects and Their Management

- Skin irritation can occur. Erythema, stinging/burning, dryness, or pruritus may occur especially during the initial 2–4 weeks of use. These may lessen with continued use.
- May cause headaches.
- Hypersensitivity reactions including facial edema and tachycardia have been reported with shampoo. Use must be discontinued immediately as anaphylactoid/anaphylactic reactions may occur.

Patch Test Concentration

- 1% pet.

Essential Patient Information

- Contact with broken, sunburned, eczematous or abraded skin should be avoided.
- Contact with eyes, lips, or other mucous membranes (e.g., inside nose) should be avoided.
- For external use only. This drug should not be ingested.
- Occlusive dressings should be avoided.
- Nail polish should not be used during the treatment of onychomycosis.

Nystatin

Classification and Mode of Action

- Polyene antifungal derived from *Streptomyces noursei*. Nystatin binds to sterols in fungal cell membranes, fundamentally altering permeability across the cell wall and allowing for leakage of cellular contents.
- Active against a wide variety of yeasts and yeast-like fungi, including *Candida albicans, C. parapsilosis, C. tropicalis, C. guilliermondii*, *C. pseudotropicalis*, *C. krusei*, *Torulopsis glabrata, Trichophyton rubrum*, and *T. mentagrophytes*.

- *Candida albicans* does not develop resistance to nystatin. Other *Candida* species (*C. tropicalis, C. guilliermondii, C. krusei*, and *C. stellatoidea*) develop significant resistance to nystatin and can simultaneously become cross-resistant to amphotericin. Resistance is lost following removal of the antibiotic.

Indications and Dermatological Uses

- *Clinical indications:* Treatment of cutaneous and mucocutaneous fungal infections caused by *Candida albicans* or other susceptible *Candida* species.

Formulations/Presentation

- US: 100,000 units/g cream, 100,000 units/g ointment, 100,000 units/g powder.
- Canada: 100,000 units/g cream, 100,000 units/g ointment.
- Europe: Not on Lexicomp.

Dosages and Suggested Regimens

- When using cream or ointment, this drug can be applied liberally and gently massaged into the affected area(s) of skin twice daily until condition resolves. For treatment of candidal diaper dermatitis, medication can be applied up to four times daily.
- When using powder, the affected area(s) should be applied two to three times daily until condition resolves.
- For application to particularly moist areas, nystatin powder is the preferred dosage form. The cream formulation is preferred over ointment for intertriginous areas.

Baseline Investigations and Considerations

- Confirm fungal origin of infection and diagnosis of cutaneous or mucocutaneous candidiasis via KOH smears, cultures, or other appropriate diagnostic methods.

Pharmacokinetics (Percutaneous Absorption, Distribution, Metabolism, Excretion: As Relevant for the Drug)

- Nystatin is not absorbed systemically from the skin or mucous membranes.
- Symptomatic relief from candidiasis is typically achieved within 24–72 h after initiation of therapy.

Use in Special Populations: Pregnancy (FDA Guidance), Lactation, Children, Renal Insufficiency, and Hepatic Insufficiency

- This drug has not been evaluated in human or animal models for use in pregnant or lactating patients; however, due to the lack of systemic absorption, nystatin may be used with caution in such patients.
- It is not known whether nystatin is excreted in human milk.
- Safe for use in pediatric patients of all ages.

Monitoring

- Clinical response should be monitored.
- If condition does not improve with treatment, a repeat assessment of KOH smears, cultures, or other diagnostic methodology may be used to confirm diagnosis.

Contraindications and Cautions

- Nystatin is contraindicated in patients with a hypersensitivity to either the drug product or any component of the formulation.
- Hypersensitivity or skin irritation may occur. This medication should be discontinued if a hypersensitivity reaction occurs.
- This product is approved for external use only. Contact with the eyes, nose, mouth, or intravaginal tissue should be avoided.
- Some dosage forms may be formulated with propylene glycol. Exposure to large amounts of propylene glycol has been associated with potentially fatal neonatal toxicity and may present with metabolic acidosis, renal failure, CNS depression, and seizures. Similar propylene glycol toxicity has also been

reported in children and adults and may present with these findings, in addition to hyperosmolality and respiratory depression.

Important Drug Interactions

- Progesterone *(Risk X)*: Nystatin may decrease the efficacy of progesterone. Combinations with these products should be avoided.

Adverse Effects and Their Management

- Contact dermatitis, Stevens-Johnson Syndrome, and hypersensitivity reactions are the most commonly reported adverse events seen with the use of nystatin; however, the overall incidence of adverse events in patients treated with Nystatin is <0.1%.

Patch Test Concentration

- 2% pet. (SmartPractice Canada, Smart Practice Europe); testing in polyethylene glycol 400 (100,000 IU nystatin/gr) may be preferable over petrolatum

Essential Patient Information

- This drug is used to treat fungal infections of the skin.
- For external use only. Contact with the eyes, nose, mouth, vagina, and other mucous membranes should be avoided.
- Nystatin powder should be stored at room temperature. Exposures to excessive heat *(≥ 104 °F/40 °C)* should be avoided.
- This medication should be used for the full duration of treatment as prescribed by a physician, even if a patient's condition appears to have resolved.
- If severe skin irritation occurs or condition worsens, this medication should be discontinued, and a physician should be notified.

- If using the powder formulation for the treatment of tinea pedis, the powder can be dusted in all footwear in addition to being applied to the feet as directed by a physician.
- If any signs of an allergic reaction *(rash; hives; itching; red, swollen, blistered, or peeling skin; wheezing; chest or throat tightness; difficulty breathing, swallowing, or talking; unusual hoarseness; or swelling of the mouth, face, lips, tongue, or throat)* are noticed, appropriate medical help should be sought immediately. This medication should be discontinued and any side effects should be reported to a physician.

Tavaborole

Classification and Mode of Action

- Benzoxaborole derivative. Tavaborole is a benzoxaborole that prevents fungal synthesis through inhibition of fungal aminoacyl-transfer RNA (tRNA) synthetase. It has broad-spectrum antifungal activity against dermatophytes, non-dermatophyte molds, and yeasts.
- More effective than Ciclopirox but less effective than Efinaconazole in complete clearance of onychomycosis.

Indications and Dermatological Uses

- *Clinical indications:* Onychomycosis (toenails).
- *Off-label common uses:* None.

Formulations/Presentation

- US: 5% solution.
- Canada: Not on Health Canada Drug Product Database.
- Europe: Not on Lexicomp.

Dosages and Suggested Regimens

- Onychomycosis: Application is once daily for 48 weeks (toenails).
- No suggested dosage adjustment for renal or hepatic impairment due to low systemic absorption.

Baseline Investigations and Considerations

- There are no known significant drug interactions.

Pharmacokinetics (Percutaneous Absorption, Distribution, Metabolism, Excretion: As Relevant for the Drug)

- Minimal topical absorption. Elimination half-life 28.5 h. Excreted in urine.
- Onset of effect: 2–3 months.

Use in Special Populations: Pregnancy (FDA Guidance), Lactation, Children, Renal Insufficiency, and Hepatic Insufficiency

- Safety and efficacy have not been determined in children. Internal use should be avoided.
- Listed as FDA pregnancy classification C (former classification system).
- Unknown whether tavaborole is present in breast milk.
- Renal insufficiency: not evaluated; dose adjustment is not expected to be needed.
- Hepatic insufficiency: not evaluated; dose adjustment is not expected to be needed.

Monitoring

- Skin irritation (erythema, exfoliation, and dermatitis) at the application site.

Contraindications and Cautions

- There are no contraindications listed in the manufacturer's labeling.
- Ophthalmic and mucous membrane use should be avoided.

Important Drug Interactions

- There are no known significant drug interactions.

Adverse Effects and Their Management

- Skin irritation can occur at the application site. Exfoliation, erythema, and dermatitis are most common.
- Ingrown nails may occur.
- Hypersensitivity reactions such as allergic contact dermatitis may occur.

Patch Test Concentration

- No data available

Essential Patient Information

- This drug should be applied to the entire toenail surface including underside near the hyponychium.
- Nail polish should not be used during the treatment of onychomycosis.
- Contact with skin should be avoided. Excess solution from surrounding skin can be wiped.
- Tavaborole is flammable. Heat and flame should be avoided when applied.
- Contact with eyes, lips, or other mucous membranes should be avoided (e.g. inside nose).
- For external use only. This drug should not be ingested.

Tolnaftate

Classification and Mode of Action

Synthetic thiocarbamate. Tolnaftate works by distorting susceptible fungi hyphae and thereby stunting mycelial growth.

Indications and Dermatological Uses

- *Clinical indications:* Tinea corporis, tinea cruris, tinea pedis treatment and prevention.
- *Off-label common uses:* Tinea manuum (level of evidence: D).

Formulations/Presentation

- US: 1% aerosol, 1% aerosol powder, 1% cream, 1% powder, 1% solution.
- Canada: 1% w/w spray, 1% cream, 1% tincture, 1% powder.

Dosages and Suggested Regimens

- This drug should be applied to the affected and surrounding area(s) twice a day until resolution in tinea corporis and tinea cruris but until 1 week after resolution for tinea pedis and tinea manuum.
- There is no suggested dosage adjustment for renal or hepatic impairment due to low systemic absorption.

Baseline Investigations and Considerations

- There are no known significant drug interactions.

Pharmacokinetics (Percutaneous Absorption, Distribution, Metabolism, Excretion: As Relevant for the Drug)

- Data on pharmacokinetics is unknown.
- Onset of effect: 24–72 h.

Use in Special Populations: Pregnancy (FDA Guidance), Lactation, Children, Renal Insufficiency, Hepatic Insufficiency

- Approved for use in children but not for self-medication for children under 2 years of age.
- There are no known effects of tolnaftate use in pregnancy or during lactation.
- There are no dosage adjustments recommended for use in hepatic or renal insufficiency.

Monitoring

- Skin irritation.
- Contact dermatitis.
- Pruritus.

Contraindications and Cautions

- Some dosage forms may be formulated with propylene glycol. Exposure to large amounts of propylene glycol has been associated with potentially fatal neonatal toxicity and may present with metabolic acidosis, renal failure, CNS depression, and seizures. Similar propylene glycol toxicity has also been reported in children and adults and may present with these findings, in addition to hyperosmolality and respiratory depression.

Important Drug Interactions

- There are no known significant drug interactions.

Adverse Effects and Their Management

- Skin irritation, stinging, and pruritus may occur and will improve when use is reduced.
- Contact dermatitis. Will improve when use is reduced. Topical steroids can improve symptoms.

Patch Test Concentration

- 1% pet.

Essential Patient Information

- Does not work for nail or scalp infections.
- May cause skin irritation.
- Affected area should be cleaned before use.
- The treated area should be dried well and should not be covered unless specified by healthcare provider.
- Hands should be washed before and after use.
- Contact with eyes should be avoided.
- This drug should not be used for diaper rash.

Summary

Fungi of medical importance are capable of causing an array of diseases, ranging from asymptomatic superficial skin infections to fatal systemic infections. While immunocompromised individuals are at greatest risk of fungal infections, they may occur in anyone. Topical antifungal drugs are commonly used to treat a superficial yeast and dermatophyte infections. Most antifungals function by taking advantage of cellular processes unique to fungi, allowing for limited cross reactivity with human cells and thus less side effects. However, like other antimicrobials, resistance to antifungals is increasing. When faced with recalcitrant or severe fungal infections, systemic antifungals are typically the treatment of choice.

References

Allylamines

1. FDA drug monograph. https://www.accessdata.fda.gov/drugsatfda_docs/label/2018/019356s008,019599s014,204286s003lbl.pdf. Accessed: 15 Dec 2021.
2. Naftifine monograph from LexiComp Online at online.lexi.com. Copyright 2021 UpToDate, Inc.

Terbinafine

3. FDA drug monograph. https://www.accessdata.fda.gov/drugsatfda_docs/label/1999/20846s001lbl.pdf. Accessed: December 16, 2021.
4. Terbinafine monograph from LexiComp Online at online.lexi.com. Copyright 2021 UpToDate, Inc.

Azoles: Clotrimazole

5. FDA drug monograph. https://www.accessdata.fda.gov/drugsatfda_docs/label/2009/020010s021lbl.pdf. Accessed: 17 Dec 2021.
6. https://nctr-crs.fda.gov/fdalabel/services/spl/set-ids/78d792a0-15d5-4c71-a63b-91c24e469df1/spl-doc?hl=Clotrimazole. Accessed 17 Dec 2021.
7. Clotrimazole monograph from LexiComp Online at online.lexi.com. Copyright 2024 UpToDate, Inc.
8. Health Canada Drug & Health Products Register—Clotrimazole: https://hpr-rps.hres.ca/query.php?drugquery=clotrimazole. Accessed 28 Feb 2024.

Econazole

9. FDA drug monograph. https://www.accessdata.fda.gov/drugsatfda_docs/label/2013/205175s000lbl.pdf. Accessed 18 Dec 2021.
10. https://www.accessdata.fda.gov/drugsatfda_docs/label/2017/018751s024lbl.pdf. Accessed 18 Dec 2021.
11. https://fda.report/DailyMed/3ACC5E03-0339-4B23-945D-641746E81923.pdf. Accessed 18 Dec 2021.
12. Econazole monograph from LexiComp Online at online.lexi.com. Copyright 2021 UpToDate, Inc.

Ketoconazole

13. FDA drug monograph. https://www.accessdata.fda.gov/drugsatfda_docs/label/2013/019927s032lbl.pdf. Accessed 20 Dec 2021.
14. https://www.accessdata.fda.gov/drugsatfda_docs/label/2019/021946s007lbl.pdf. Accessed 20 Dec 2021.
15. https://www.accessdata.fda.gov/drugsatfda_docs/label/2007/021738lbl.pdf. Accessed 20 Dec 2021.
16. Ketoconazole monograph from LexiComp Online at online.lexi.com. Copyright 2021 UpToDate, Inc.
17. Health Canada Drug & Health Products Register—Ketoconazole: https://hpr-rps.hres.ca/query.php?drugquery=ketoconazole. Accessed 28 Feb 2024.

Luliconazole

18. FDA drug monograph. https://www.accessdata.fda.gov/drugsatfda_docs/label/2013/204153s000lbl.pdf. Accessed 22 Dec 2021.
19. https://fda.report/DailyMed/7CCDA3BA-9C98-468D-83C6-7F0CC7C88C33.pdf. Accessed 22 Dec 2021.
20. Luliconazole monograph from LexiComp Online at online.lexi.com. Copyright 2021 UpToDate, Inc.

Miconazole Nitrate

21. FDA drug monograph. https://www.accessdata.fda.gov/drugsatfda_docs/label/2018/021026s013lbl.pdf. Accessed 27 Dec 2021.
22. https://www.accessdata.fda.gov/drugsatfda_docs/label/2006/021026s000lbl.pdf. Accessed 27 Dec 2021.
23. Miconazole Nitrate monograph from LexiComp Online at online.lexi.com. Copyright 2021 UpToDate, Inc.

24. Health Canada Drug & Health Products Register—Miconazole: https://hpr-rps.hres.ca/query.php?drugquery=miconazole. Accessed 28 Feb 2024.
25. Barasch A, Griffin AV. Miconazole revisited: new evidence of antifungal efficacy from laboratory and clinical trials. Future Microbiol. 2008;3(3):265–9. https://doi.org/10.2217/17460913.3.3.265.

Oxiconazole Nitrate

26. FDA drug monograph. https://www.accessdata.fda.gov/drugsatfda_docs/label/2004/19828slr009,20209slr005_oxistat_lbl.pdf. Accessed 29 Dec 2021.
27. https://nctr-crs.fda.gov/fdalabel/services/spl/set-ids/b87a89d2-6e45-4eb8-be2c-7f55f34d61e5/spl-doc?hl=oxiconazole%20nitrate. Accessed 29 Dec 2021.
28. Oxiconazole Nitrate monograph from LexiComp Online at online.lexi.com. Copyright 2021 UpToDate, Inc.
29. Health Canada Drug & Health Products Register—Oxiconazole: https://hpr-rps.hres.ca/query.php?drugquery=oxiconazole. Accessed 19 Apr 2024.

Sertaconazole Nitrate

30. FDA drug monograph. https://www.accessdata.fda.gov/drugsatfda_docs/label/2020/021385s006lbl.pdf. Accessed 1 Jan 2021.
31. Sertaconazole Nitrate monograph from LexiComp Online at online.lexi.com. Copyright 2021 UpToDate, Inc.

Sulconazole

32. FDA drug monograph. https://www.accessdata.fda.gov/drugsatfda_docs/label/2003/18737slr003_exelderm_lbl.pdf. Accessed 3 Jan 2021.
33. https://www.accessdata.fda.gov/drugsatfda_docs/label/2009/018738s009lbl.pdf. Accessed 3 Jan 2021.
34. https://dailymed.nlm.nih.gov/dailymed/fda/fdaDrugXsl.cfm?setid=cf6f4340-940c-4a61-b675-456e3297d810&type=display. Accessed 3 Jan 2021.
35. https://nctr-crs.fda.gov/fdalabel/services/spl/set-ids/cf6f4340-940c-4a61-b675-456e3297d810/spl-doc?hl=sulconazole%20nitrate. Accessed 3 Jan 2021.

36. https://nctr-crs.fda.gov/fdalabel/services/spl/set-ids/5b731aa0-fb3f-4a96-9034-636138cbca03/spl-doc?hl=sulconazole%20nitrate. Accessed 3 Jan 2021.
37. Sulconazole monograph from LexiComp Online at online.lexi.com. Copyright 2021 UpToDate, Inc.

Butenafine HCl

38. FDA drug monograph. https://www.accessdata.fda.gov/drugsatfda_docs/label/2002/21408lbl.pdf. Accessed 4 Jan 2021.
39. Butenafine HCl monograph from LexiComp Online at online.lexi.com. Copyright 2021 UpToDate, Inc.
40. Health Canada Drug & Health Products Register—Butenafine: https://hpr-rps.hres.ca/query.php?drugquery=butenafine. Accessed 19 Apr 2024.

Ciclopirox Olamine

41. FDA drug monographs. https://www.accessdata.fda.gov/drugsatfda_docs/label/2013/018748s024,019824s023,020519s016lbl.pdf. Accessed 11 Nov 2021.
42. https://www.accessdata.fda.gov/drugsatfda_docs/label/2004/21022s004lbl.pdf. Accessed 11 Nov 2021.
43. Ciclopirox olamine monograph from LexiComp Online at online.lexi.com. Copyright 2021 UpToDate, Inc.
44. Lipner SR, Scher RK. Onychomycosis: treatment and prevention of recurrence. J Am Acad Dermatol. 2019;80(4):853–67.

Nystatin

45. FDA drug monograph. https://nctr-crs.fda.gov/fdalabel/services/spl/set-ids/629d2b7e-a5b8-4b6d-ba59-46e1c51da5bf/spl-doc?hl=nystatin. Accessed: 5 Jan 2021.
46. https://nctr-crs.fda.gov/fdalabel/services/spl/set-ids/e1b4622c-0f9f-4c00-b42c-2aa85a5e3d4f/spl-doc?hl=nystatin. Accessed 5 Jan 2021.
47. https://nctr-crs.fda.gov/fdalabel/services/spl/set-ids/6a3bb3da-adf9-46d2-a5ff-f796e7aae7a1/spl-doc?hl=nystatin. Accessed 5 Jan 2021.
48. Nystatin monograph from LexiComp Online at online.lexi.com. Copyright 2021 UpToDate, Inc.
49. Health Canada Drug & Health Products Register—Nystatin: https://hpr-rps.hres.ca/query.php?drugquery=nystatin. Accessed 28 Feb 2024.

Tavaborole

50. FDA drug monograph. https://www.accessdata.fda.gov/drugsatfda_docs/label/2014/204427s000lbl.pdf. Accessed 11 Nov 2021.
51. Tavaborole monograph from LexiComp Online at online.lexi.com. Copyright 2021 UpToDate, Inc.
52. Elewski BE, Aly R, Baldwin SL, Soto RF, Rich P, Weisfeld M, Wiltz H, Zane LT, Pollak R. Efficacy and safety of tavaborole topical solution, 5%, a novel boron-based antifungal agent, for the treatment of toenail onychomycosis: results from 2 randomized phase-III studies. J Am Acad Dermatol. 2015;73(1):62–9.

Tolnaftate

53. FDA drug monograph. https://www.accessdata.fda.gov/scripts/cdrh/cfdocs/cfcfr/CFRSearch.cfm?fr=333.210. Accessed 3 Jan 2021.
54. Tolnaftate monograph from LexiComp Online at online.lexi.com. Copyright 2021 UpToDate, Inc.
55. Health Canada Drug & Health Products Register—Tolnaftate: https://hpr-rps.hres.ca/query.php?drugquery=tolnaftate. Accessed 19 Apr 2024.

Topical Antineoplastics in Dermatology

14

Christina Huang, Paola A. Baker, Chavy Chiang, Anuk Burli, Enzo Berardesca, Bradley D. Kwinta, Larisa J. Geskin, and Jack L. Arbiser

Contents

C. Huang
Sidney Kimmel Medical College, Thomas Jefferson University, Philadelphia, PA, USA
e-mail: christina.huang@students.jefferson.edu

P. A. Baker
Department of Dermatology, Emory University School of Medicine, Atlanta, GA, USA
e-mail: pao-olaya@hotmail.com

C. Chiang
Department of Dermatology, University of Rochester Medical Center, Rochester, NY, USA
e-mail: chavyz@gmail.com

R. M. Law, H. I. Maibach (eds.), *Handbook of Topical Drug Treatment in Dermatology*,
https://doi.org/10.1007/978-3-031-93616-6_14

Introduction

Topical antineoplastic agents have been effective against various cutaneous lesions for multiple decades and serve as useful therapeutic tools in clinical dermatology [1]. Of note, efficacy of topical antineoplastics against basal cell carcinoma and actinic keratosis has been well acknowledged [2, 3]. Beyond these applications, certain antineoplastic agents have shown utility in treating multiple skin conditions outside of their FDA-approved indications. For instance, imiquimod has been used to treat various cutaneous conditions such as mycosis fungoides and Kaposi's sarcoma, despite it being only FDA approved for perianal warts, basal cell carcinoma, and actinic keratosis [4]. Topical antineoplastics also have various mechanisms of action, from 5-fluorouracil, which inhibits metabolism, to imiquimod, which modulates the immune system [1, 5, 6]. With diversity in clinical applications and mechanism of action, topical antineoplastics have significant potential for future research regarding clinical efficacy or new compounds under development [7].

The use of topical antineoplastics is clinically beneficial in multiple ways. Topical antineoplastics serve as a valuable alternative

A. Burli
Department of Dermatology, Stanford University School of Medicine, Redwood City, CA, USA
e-mail: anukb@stanford.edu

E. Berardesca
Dr. Phillip Frost Department of Dermatology and Cutaneous Surgery, Miller School of Medicine, University of Miami, Miami, FL, USA
e-mail: Berardesca@berardesca.it

B. D. Kwinta · K. L. Geskin
Department of Dermatology at Columbia University Irving Medical Center, New York, NY, USA
e-mail: bdk2123@cumc.columbia.edu; ljg2145@cumc.columbia.edu

J. L. Arbiser (✉)
Department of Dermatology, Emory University School of Medicine, Winship Cancer Institute, Atlanta Veterans Administration Health Center, Atlanta, GA, USA
e-mail: jarbise@emory.edu

to surgical treatment in conditions such as basal cell carcinoma, especially if the presentation or preferences of the individual patient disfavor surgery [8]. One study found that patients with low-risk nodular and superficial basal cell carcinoma valued 5% imiquimod cream more highly than excisional surgery, with patients considering cosmetic outcome and potential adverse effects [9]. Another study found that although surgical outcomes were superior to topical imiquimod in low-risk nodular or superficial basal cell carcinoma, there is still sustained treatment benefit for lesions that respond to topical antineoplastics [10]. When compared to systemic therapies, topical antineoplastic agents have less systemic absorption, limiting potential adverse effects [11, 12]. Topical administration also increases the local concentration of a drug, resulting in higher efficacy in the area of administration, which is particularly useful for localized cutaneous tumors [7]. Overall, topical antineoplastics serve as an important option in the individualized clinical treatment of cutaneous tumors.

Antineoplastic Retinoids

Enzo Beradesca

There are two retinoids which are used topically as antineoplastic agents.

Alitretinoin is a retinoic acid derivative used as an antineoplastic (topical) and anti-inflammatory (oral) agent. It is a naturally occurring endogenous retinoid that binds to and activates intracellular retinoid receptors (RAR and RXR subtypes); this results in altered expression of the genes controlling cellular differentiation and proliferation in normal and neoplastic cells, inhibiting the growth of Kaposi sarcoma.

Bexarotene binds to and activates retinoid X receptor subtypes. Once activated, these receptors function as transcription factors that regulate the expression of genes which control cellular differentiation and proliferation, resulting in decreased cell proliferation, apoptosis of some cancer cell types, and tumor regression. It is indicated for treatment of cutaneous T-cell lymphoma.

See Chap. 23: Retinoids for the alitretinoin and bexarotene drug monographs.

Fluorouracil (5-FU)

Chavy Chiang and Anuk Burli

Fluorouracil prevents methylation of deoxyuridylic acid to thymidylic acid to block DNA and, to a lesser extent, RNA synthesis, particularly so in rapidly growing cells.

It is indicated for the treatment of actinic keratosis and basal cell carcinoma (superficial). There are off-label uses for other neoplasms as well.

See Chap.10: Drug Treatment for Actinic Keratosis for the Drug Monograph.

Mechlorethamine Gel

B. Kwinta and L. Geskin

Classification and Mode of Action

- Mechlorethamine, known as nitrogen mustard, is an alkylating agent. When used systemically, it forms DNA cross-links and inhibits DNA synthesis in rapidly dividing cells. Topically, the mechanism of action is not fully understood but may be immune mediated [22, 23].
- Mechlorethamine HCl 0.016% gel (equivalent to 0.02% chlormethine/mechlorethamine ointment) was shown to be noninferior to Aquaphor®-based mechlorethamine HCl 0.02% ointment in a pivotal 2013, phase 2, randomized controlled trial in patients with persistent or recurrent stage IA, IB, and IIA mycosis fungoides who had received at least one skin directed therapy [24].

Indications and Dermatological Uses

- *Clinical indications (FDA):* Topical treatment of stage IA and IB mycosis fungoides in adult patients who have received prior skin-directed therapy.
- *Off-label common uses:* Not applicable.

Formulations/Presentation

- USA: Brand name Valchlor. 60 g tube of Valchlor 0.016% gel (equivalent to 0.02% mechlorethamine HCl). No generic.
- Canada: Brand name Legada. 60 g tube of Legada 0.016% gel (equivalent to 0.02% mechlorethamine HCl).
- Europe: Brand name Legada. 60 g tube of Legada 0.016% gel (equivalent to 0.02% mechlorethamine HCl).

Dosages and Suggested Regimens

- Mechlorethamine gel should be stored in a refrigerator, at a temperature between 36 °F and 46 °F (2 °C–8 °C).
- Apply within 30 min of removal from the refrigerator.
- Apply to dry skin at least 4 h before or 30 min after showering or washing.
- Using disposable nitrile gloves, apply a thin film once daily to affected areas of the skin. Safely dispose of gloves after application.
- Wash hands after application, and let skin dry for 5–10 min before covering area with clothing.
- Avoid open flames as the gel is alcohol-based and flammable.
- Moisturizer can be applied within 2 h of application.
- Do not apply water or air-tight dressings to the area.
- The pivotal randomized trial prohibited topical corticosteroid use. Some studies suggest that dose frequency modifications and concomitant therapy use (primarily corticosteroids, phototherapy, systemic retinoids) are generally well tolerated [25, 26].

- Experts generally recommend concurrent intermittent use of topical corticosteroids to minimize skin irritation and avoid dose modifications [26].

Baseline Investigations and Considerations

Pharmacokinetics

- No systemic absorption was detected in the pivotal trial.

Use in Special Populations: Pregnancy

- Women should avoid becoming pregnant while using this medication.
- It is unknown whether mechlorethamine passes into breastmilk. Nursing mothers should discontinue drug or nursing.
- Not approved for use in children.
- No special considerations are needed for renal or hepatic insufficiency.

Monitoring

- Dermatitis.
- Non-melanoma skin cancers.

Contraindications and Cautions

- Patients with known severe hypersensitivity reactions to this medication, including anaphylaxis, should avoid using it. Patients who experience a severe hypersensitivity reaction should seek immediate medical help.

Important Drug Interactions

- Drug interaction studies have not been conducted, though are unlikely due to lack of systemic absorption.

Adverse Effects and Their Management

- May cause dermatitis. Patients should be monitored and report any redness, swelling, inflammation, itchiness, blisters, ulceration, or secondary skin infections. Treatment should be stopped or dose frequency reduced.
- May increase risk of developing non-melanoma skin cancers. Patients should undergo full body skin examinations during and after treatment. Patients should report new skin lesions to their healthcare provider.

Carcinogenicity

- Painting studies in mice at a dose of 4 mg/kg weekly for up to 33 weeks resulted in squamous cell tumors in 9 of 33 mice—however, at maximum, over the total body surface, patients use 0.034 mg/kg daily, 100 times less. More recent studies show no increased risk of secondary malignancies [27].

Patch Test Concentration

- 0.02% water; perform an open test first.

Essential Patient Information

- For use on the skin only.
- Avoid contact with the eyes, lips, or other mucous membranes (e.g., inside the nose). Exposure can cause permanent damage or blindness. If exposure occurs, irrigate the area for 15 min with water and then seek immediate medical help.

Caregivers and individuals other than the patient should avoid direct skin contact. Risks of exposure are the same as in the patient including dermatitis, non-melanoma skin cancers, and eye/mucosa injury. If contact occurs, wash the area with soap and water for at least 15 min and remove contacted clothing.

Romidepsin

C. Huang, P. Baker, and J. Arbiser

Classification and Mode of Action

- Romidepsin is a histone deacetylase (HDAC) inhibitor. By inhibiting histone deacetylation, romidepsin causes accumulation of acetylated histones. This leads to a wide profile of epigenetic modifications and gene expression. This is thought to result in arrest cell cycle at G1 and G2/M phase and induce apoptosis [30].
- Romidepsin may also have other effects that target survival of malignant T cells, including activation of stress signal pathways and DNA hypomethylation [31].
- A Phase II clinical trial showed romidepsin had a relatively high response rate in the treatment of cutaneous T-cell lymphoma (CTCL), leading to its approval as a monotherapy for CTCL patients who had failed at least one prior systemic therapy [32].
- A Phase III clinical trial showed the addition of romidepsin to cyclophosphamide, doxorubicin, vincristine, and prednisone (CHOP) therapy did not significantly improve outcomes as a first-line treatment for peripheral T-cell lymphoma (PTCL) [33].

Indications and Dermatological Uses

- *Clinical indications (FDA):* Romidepsin is indicated for the treatment of CTCL in patients who had received at least one prior systemic therapy.
- *Off-label common uses:* Evidence previously supported romidepsin use to treat PTCL that has either relapsed or been refractory to treatment. However, after Phase III clinical trial results of romidepsin and CHOP, the indication for romidepsin in PTCL has been withdrawn [34].

Formulations/Presentation

- USA: Brand name Istodax. 10 mg of romidepsin in lyophilized powder and 20 mg of povidone with a 20-mL dilutant (80% propylene glycol, USP, and 20% dehydrated alcohol, USP). Generic: 27.5 mg/5.5 mL IV solution or 10 mg powder.
- Canada: Brand name Istodax. 10 mg of romidepsin in lyophilized powder and 20 mg of povidone with a 20-mL dilutant (80% propylene glycol, USP, and 20% dehydrated alcohol, USP).
- Europe: Not approved for use in Europe.

Dosages and Suggested Regimens

- Romidepsin should be administered intravenously (IV) at a dose of 14 mg/m^2 over a 4-hour period on days 1, 8, and 15 of a 28-day cycle.
- Repeat this treatment cycle every 28 days as long as the patient benefits from and tolerates romidepsin.
- Romidepsin powder, romidepsin solution, and provided dilutant should be stored at 20 °C to 25 °C.
- Once romidepsin powder is reconstituted, the solution is stable for 8 h at room temperature.

- If romidepsin powder or romidepsin solution is diluted for infusion in normal saline, the solution can be stable for up to 24 h at room temperature. However, manufacturer instructions recommend infusing as soon as possible.

Baseline Investigations and Considerations

- Antiemetics are recommended as romidepsin has a moderate emetic potential.
- Electrolyte imbalances either before or during treatment should be corrected.
- Antiviral prophylaxis should be considered in patients with a history of hepatitis B infection.
- Romidepsin binds to estrogen receptors and may reduce effectiveness of estrogen-containing contraceptives.

Pharmacokinetics

- Romidepsin has linear pharmacokinetics at the recommended dose.
- Distribution: Romidepsin is 92–94% bound to plasma protein (mostly α1-acid-glycoprotein).
- Metabolism: Romidepsin is primarily metabolized hepatically by CYP3A4, with minor CYP3A5, CYP1A1, CYP2B6, and CYP2C19 activity.
- Excretion: The terminal half-life of romidepsin is approximately 3 h.

Use in Special Populations

- Pregnancy: FDA former Category D. Not to be used in pregnancy.
- Lactation: No information.
- Children: No information about safety and efficacy of romidepsin in children.

- Renal insufficiency: Renal function is not expected to affect safety of romidepsin; however, patients with end-stage renal disease should be treated with caution.
- Hepatic insufficiency: Mild hepatic impairment does not impair romidepsin metabolism; patients with moderate to severe hepatic impairment should be treated with caution.

Monitoring

- Monitor potassium and magnesium levels to avoid QT prolongation.
- Monitor hematological parameters to avoid thrombocytopenia, leukopenia, and/or anemia.
- Monitor for prolonged prothrombin time (PT) and International Normalized Ratio. (INR) in patients receiving romidepsin and coumadin derivatives.
- Monitor for tumor lysis syndrome.
- Monitor for toxicity in patients with moderate or severe hepatic impairment.

Contraindications

- Hypersensitivity reaction to romidepsin.

Cautions

- QT interval prolongation, especially in patients with congenital long QT syndrome, patients taking medications that may increase QT length, or patients with current or previous cardiac disease.
- Thrombocytopenia, leukopenia, anemia—note that serious infections may occur because of leukopenia.
- Tumor lysis syndrome, especially in patients with advanced disease/high tumor burden.

Important Drug Interactions

- CYP3A4 inhibitors/inducers might increase/decrease concentrations of romidepsin, respectively.
- Coumadin with romidepsin may excessively increase PT/INR.
- Drugs that inhibit P-glycoprotein, an efflux transporter, may increase concentrations of romidepsin.

Adverse Effects and Their Management

- Nausea/vomiting—antiemetics are recommended as romidepsin is associated with moderate emetic potential.
- Fatigue—patients can seek medical help if fatigue is persistent or bothersome.
- Infections—patients should seek medical advice for more severe adverse effects such as infections.
- Anorexia—patients can seek medical help if fatigue is persistent or bothersome.
- Anemia—patients should have hematologic parameters monitored.
- Thrombocytopenia—patients should have hematologic parameters monitored.
- ECG T-wave changes—patient electrolyte levels (especially sodium and potassium) should be monitored and corrected as needed to prevent cardiologic adverse effects.
- Neutropenia—patients should have hematologic parameters monitored.
- Lymphopenia—patients should have hematologic parameters monitored.

Carcinogenicity

- No studies done.

Patch Test Concentration

- Not available.

Essential Patient Information

- Patients should be cautioned that romidepsin could prolong the QT interval, potentially leading to torsades de pointes if given with other medications that prolong the QT interval.

Vorinostat

P. Baker, C. Huang, and J. L. Arbiser

Classification and Mode of Action

- Vorinostat, known as suberoylanilide hydroxamic acid or SAHA, is a histone deacetylase (HDAC) class I and II inhibitor. Vorinostat induces cell cycle arrest, differentiation, or apoptosis of transformed cells. Vorinostat inhibits HDAC activity by binding to the active site and inducing accumulation of acetylated proteins. The antiproliferative effects of vorinostat are believed to be due to a drug-induced accumulation of acetylated proteins, including the core nucleosomal histones and other proteins such as BCL6, p53, and Hsp90. These effects include an alteration in the transcription of genes via acetylation of histones and transcription factors, and non-transcriptional effects such as inhibition of mitosis. Vorinostat has shown to impact the expression of several genes, some of which are induced such as $p21^{WAF1}$, histone H2B, metallothionein 1 L, TBP-2, and gelsolin, while others are repressed including cyclin D1, thymidylate synthase, ErbB2, and importin b [37, 38].

- Vorinostat has shown to be active against hematologic malignancies and solid tumors as oral and intravenous preparations in Phase I development trial. In two Phase II clinical trials, vorinostat shown to be safe and effective at an oral dose of 400 mg/day with an overall response rate of 24–30% in refractory advanced patients with cutaneous T-cell lymphoma (CTCL) including large cell transformation and Sezary syndrome [39]. One of these trials led vorinostat's approval as treatment of cutaneous manifestation of CTCL in refractory patients [40, 41].

Indications and Dermatological Uses

- *Clinical indications (FDA):* Oral systemic therapy of cutaneous manifestation of CTCL in patients with progressive, persistent, or recurrent disease on or following two systemic therapies.
- *Off-label common uses:* No data available.

Formulations/Presentation

- USA: Brand name Zolinza. Capsules 100 mg. No generic.
- Canada: Brand name Zolinza. Capsules 100 mg.
- Europe: Not approved for use in the EU.

Dosages and Suggested Regimens

- Zolinza capsules should be stored at 68 °F to 77 °F (20 °C to 25 °C); excursions are permitted to 59 °F to 86 °F (15 °C to 30 °C).
- The recommended dose is 400 mg orally once daily with food. It's important to maintain adequate hydration (≥2 L/day fluids) during treatment. The treatment may be continued until disease progression or unacceptable toxicity.
- The capsules shouldn't be opened, broken, or chewed.

Baseline Investigations and Considerations

- If patient is intolerant to therapy, the dose may be reduced to 300 mg orally once daily with food. The dose may be further reduced to 300 mg orally once daily with food for 5 consecutives days each week.

Pharmacokinetics

- Time to peak plasma with high-fat meal is 4 h (range 2–10 h).
- Distribution: Vorinostat is approximately 71% bound to human plasma proteins.
- Metabolism: Vorinostat is glucuronidated and hydrolyzed followed by beta-oxidation to inactive metabolites. Vorinostat has negligible biotransformation by cytochromes P450.
- Excretion: Vorinostat is eliminated predominantly through metabolism. Renal excretion is ~52 as inactive metabolites and <1% as unchanged drug in urine.
- Vorinostat half-life elimination is ~2 h.

Use in Special Populations

- Pregnancy: FDA former category D. Not to be used in pregnancy.
- Lactation: It is not known whether vorinostat is excreted in human milk. Due to the potential for serious adverse reactions, breastfeeding is not recommended during therapy and for at least 7 days after the last dose.
- Children: Safety and effectiveness in pediatric patients have not been stablished.
- Renal insufficiency: Vorinostat was not evaluated in patients with renal impairment. However, renal excretion does not play a role in the elimination of vorinostat, patients with preexisting renal impairment should be treated with caution.
- Hepatic insufficiency: Vorinostat is contraindicated in patients with severe hepatic impairment and should be used with caution in patients with mild and moderate hepatic impairment.

Mild to moderate hepatic impairment (total bilirubin one to three times ULN or AST > ULN): Initial dose 300 mg once daily.

Monitoring

- Monitor CBC Classification and (with differential) and serum chemistry including potassium, calcium, magnesium, glucose, and creatinine at baseline, then every 2 weeks during the first 2 months of therapy, and monthly thereafter, or as clinically necessary.
- Monitor hepatic function to avoid hepatic toxicity.
- Monitor INR if on concomitant warfarin therapy.
- Monitor fluid status.
- Monitor for signs/symptoms of thromboembolism.

Contraindications and Cautions

- Patients with severe hepatic impairment (total bilirubin ≥3 times ULN) should avoid use.
- Patients with known hypersensitivity to vorinostat should avoid use.
- Patients with mild and moderate hepatic impairment should be treated with caution.
- Screening for hepatitis B virus should be performed prior to starting therapy.

- Correct electrolyte abnormalities prior to starting therapy.
- Use vorinostat with caution in patients with a history of QT prolongation or with medications known to prolong the QT interval.

Important Drug Interactions

- Coumarin-derivate anticoagulants might increase PT/INR.
- Other HDAC inhibitors might increase risk of thrombocytopenia and gastrointestinal bleeding.
- 5-Aminosalicylic acid derivates might enhance myelosuppressive effect.

Adverse Effects and Their Management

- Gastrointestinal symptoms: diarrhea/constipation, nausea, dry mouth, and dysgeusia. Vorinostat is associated with low emetic potential (<30%): Patients can seek medical help if symptoms are persistent or bothersome. Patient fluid status and electrolyte levels should be monitored and corrected as needed.
- Constitutional symptoms: fatigue, anorexia, and weight decrease: Patients can seek medical help if fatigue/anorexia is persistent or bothersome.
- Hematologic abnormalities: thrombocytopenia and anemia: Patients should have hematologic parameters monitored. If toxicity, consider dose reduction.
- Cardiopulmonary: pulmonary embolism: Monitor for sings/symptoms especially in patients with a history of thrombotic events. Patients should seek immediate medical help if symptoms of thromboembolism occur. Prolonged QT interval on ECG: Monitor and correct potassium, calcium, and magnesium levels during therapy.
- Signs of an allergic reaction/anaphylaxis: Patients should seek immediate medical help if symptoms of allergy occur.
- Laboratory abnormalities: hyperglycemia and increased serum creatinine: Patients should have metabolic parameters monitored.

Carcinogenicity

- Carcinogenicity studies have not been performed with vorinostat.

Patch Test Concentration

- Not available.

Essential Patient Information

- Avoid pregnancy: pregnancy testing should be conducted within 7 days prior to treatment in females of reproductive potential, and use an effective contraceptive during therapy and for at least 6 months after the last vorinostat dose.

References

1. Ceilley RI. Mechanisms of action of topical 5-fluorouracil: review and implications for the treatment of dermatological disorders. J Dermatolog Treat. 2012;23:83–9. https://doi.org/10.3109/09546634.2010.507704.
2. Micali G, Lacarrubba F, Nasca MR, Schwartz RA. Topical pharmacotherapy for skin cancer: part I. pharmacology. J Am Acad Dermatol. 2014;70(965):e961–965.e912. https://doi.org/10.1016/j.jaad.2013.12.045.
3. Micali G, Lacarrubba F, Nasca MR, Ferraro S, Schwartz RA. Topical pharmacotherapy for skin cancer: part II. Clinical applications. J Am Acad Dermatol. 2014;70(979):e971–979.e912. https://doi.org/10.1016/j.jaad.2013.12.037.
4. Hanna E, Abadi R, Abbas O. Imiquimod in dermatology: an overview. Int J Dermatol. 2016;55:831–44. https://doi.org/10.1111/ijd.13235.
5. Rhodes J. Discovery of immunopotentiatory drugs: current and future strategies. Clin Exp Immunol. 2002;130:363–9. https://doi.org/10.1046/j.1365-2249.2002.02016.x.
6. Grossberg AL, Gaspari AA. Topical antineoplastic agents in the treatment of mucocutaneous diseases. Curr Probl Dermatol. 2011;40:71–82.
7. Cullen JK, Simmons JL, Parsons PG, Boyle GM. Topical treatments for skin cancer. Adv Drug Deliv Rev. 2020;153:54–64. https://doi.org/10.1016/j.addr.2019.11.002.

8. Kash N, Silapunt S. A review of emerging and non-US FDA-approved topical agents for the treatment of basal cell carcinoma. Future Oncol. 2021;17:3111–32. https://doi.org/10.2217/fon-2020-1147.
9. Tinelli M, Ozolins M, Bath-Hextall F, Williams HC. What determines patient preferences for treating low risk basal cell carcinoma when comparing surgery vs imiquimod? A discrete choice experiment survey from the SINS trial. BMC Dermatol. 2012;12:19. https://doi.org/10.1186/1471-5945-12-19.
10. Williams HC, et al. Surgery versus 5% imiquimod for nodular and superficial basal cell carcinoma: 5-year results of the SINS randomized controlled trial. J Invest Dermatol. 2017;137:614–9. https://doi.org/10.1016/j.jid.2016.10.019.
11. Dillaha CJ, Jansen GT, Honeycutt WM, Holt GA. Further studies with topical 5-fluorouracil. Arch Dermatol. 1965;92:410–7. https://doi.org/10.1001/archderm.1965.01600160066015.
12. Bubna AK. Imiquimod—its role in the treatment of cutaneous malignancies. Ind J Pharmacol. 2015;47:354–9. https://doi.org/10.4103/0253-7613.161249.

Antineoplastic Retinoids: Alitretinoin

13. Panretin (alitretinoin) [prescribing information]. Concordia Pharmaceuticals; May 2020.
14. Walmsley S, Northfelt DW, Melosky B, Conant M, Friedman-Kien AE, Wagner B. Treatment of AIDS-related cutaneous Kaposi's sarcoma with topical alitretinoin (9-cis-retinoic acid) gel. Panretin Gel North American Study Group. J Acquir Immune Defic Syndr. 1999;22(3):235–46. [PubMed 10770343]

Antineoplastic Retinoids: Bexarotene

15. Breneman D, Duvic M, Kuzel T, Yocum R, Truglia J, Stevens VJ. Phase 1 and 2 trial of bexarotene gel for skin-directed treatment of patients with cutaneous T-cell lymphoma [published correction appears in Arch Dermatol. 2002;138(10):1386]. Arch Dermatol. 2002;138(3):325–32. https://doi.org/10.1001/archderm.138.3.325. [PubMed 11902983]
16. Heald P, Mehlmauer M, Martin AG, Crowley CA, Yocum RC, Reich SD, Worldwide Bexarotene Study Group. Topical bexarotene therapy for patients with refractory or persistent early-stage cutaneous T-cell lymphoma: results of the phase III clinical trial. J Am Acad Dermatol. 2003;49(5):801–15. https://doi.org/10.1016/s0190-9622(03)01475-0. [PubMed 14576658]
17. Targretin (bexarotene) [prescribing information]. Bridgewater, NJ: Valeant; October 2016.

Fluorouracil (5-FU)

18. https://www.accessdata.fda.gov/drugsatfda_docs/label/2016/012209s040lbl.pdf
19. LexiComp drug monograph Fluorouracil. Available from: LexiComp Online at online.Lexi.com. Copyright 2024 UptoDate, Inc.

Mechlorethamine Gel

20. FDA drug monograph VALCHLOR (mechlorethamine) gel, for topical use. Available from: https://www.accessdata.fda.gov/drugsatfda_docs/label/2013/202317lbl.pdf. Accessed 5 Jan 2022.
21. LexiComp drug monograph Mechlorethamine (nitrogen mustard) topical gel. Available from: LexiComp Online at online.lexi.com Copyright 2021 UpToDate, Inc.
22. Kim YH, Martinez G, Varghese A, Hoppe RT. Topical nitrogen mustard in the management of mycosis fungoides: update of the Stanford experience. Arch Dermatol. 2003;139:165–73.
23. Tang L, Cao L, Bernardo O, Chen Y, Sundberg JP, Lui H, et al. Topical mechlorethamine restores autoimmune-arrested follicular activity in mice with an alopecia areata-like disease by targeting infiltrated lymphocytes. J Invest Dermatol. 2003;120:400–6.
24. Lessin SR, Duvic M, Guitart J, Pandya AG, Strober BE, Olsen EA, et al. Topical chemotherapy in cutaneous T-cell lymphoma: positive results of a randomized, controlled, multi-center trial testing the efficacy and safety of a novel mechlorethamine, 0.02%, gel in mycosis fungoides. JAMA Dermatol. 2013;149:25–32.
25. Kim EJ, Guitart J, Querfeld C, Girardi M, Musiek A, Akilov OE, Angello JT, Bailey WL, Geskin LJ. The PROVe study: US real-world experience with chlormethine/mechlorethamine gel in combination with other therapies for patients with mycosis Fungoides cutaneous T-cell lymphoma. Am J Clin Dermatol. 2021 May;22(3):407–14. https://doi.org/10.1007/s40257-021-00591-x. Epub 2021 Mar 3. PMID: 33656660; PMCID: PMC8068681
26. Garcia-Saleem TJ, Stonesifer CJ, Khaleel AE, Geskin LJ. Management of mycosis fungoides with topical Chlormethine/Mechlorethamine Gel: a Columbia University cutaneous lymphoma center experience. Acta Derm Venereol. 2021;101(9):adv00544. https://doi.org/10.2340/00015555-3911. PMID: 34436621
27. Lindahl LM, Fenger-Grøn M, Iversen L. Secondary cancers, comorbidities and mortality associated with nitrogen mustard therapy in patients with mycosis fungoides: a 30-year population-based cohort study. Br J Dermatol. 2014 Mar;170(3):699–704. https://doi.org/10.1111/bjd.12620. PMID: 24024659

Romidepsin

28. FDA drug monograph ISTODAX (romidepsin) for injection. Available from: https://www.accessdata.fda.gov/drugsatfda_docs/label/2009/022393lbl.pdf. Accessed 17 Dec 2022.
29. LexiComp drug monograph RomiDEPsin. Available from: LexiComp Online at online.Lexi.com. Copyright 2022 UptoDate, Inc.
30. Jain S, Zain J. Romidepsin in the treatment of cutaneous T-cell lymphoma. J Blood Med. 2:37–47. https://doi.org/10.2147/jbm.S9649.
31. Valdez BC, et al. Romidepsin targets multiple survival signaling pathways in malignant T cells. Blood Cancer J. 5:e357–7. https://doi.org/10.1038/bcj.2015.83.
32. Whittaker SJ, et al. Final results from a multicenter, international, pivotal study of romidepsin in refractory cutaneous T-cell lymphoma. J Clin Oncol. 28:4485–91. https://doi.org/10.1200/jco.2010.28.9066.
33. Bachy E, et al. Romidepsin plus CHOP versus CHOP in patients with previously untreated peripheral T-Cell lymphoma: results of the Ro-CHOP Phase III study (conducted by LYSA). J Clin Oncol. 40:242–51. https://doi.org/10.1200/jco.21.01815.
34. Bristol Myers Squibb Statement on Istodax® (romidepsin) Relapsed/Refractory Peripheral T-cell Lymphoma U.S. Indication. Available from: https://news.bms.com/news/details/2021/Bristol-Myers-Squibb-Statement-on-Istodax-romidepsin-Relapsed-Refractory-Peripheral-T-cell-Lymphoma-U.S.-Indication/default.aspx. Accessed 17 Dec 2022.

Vorinostat

35. FDA drug monograph (name of monograph). Available from (FDA weblink). Accessed (date).
36. LexiComp drug monograph (name of monograph). Available from: LexiComp Online at online.Lexi.com. Copyright 2022 UptoDate, Inc.
37. Eckschlager T, Plch J, Stiborova M, Hrabeta J. Histone deacetylase inhibitors as anticancer drugs. Int J Mol Sci. 2017;18(7)
38. Richon VM. Cancer biology: mechanism of antitumour action of vorinostat (suberoylanilide hydroxamic acid), a novel histone deacetylase inhibitor. Br J Cancer. 2006;95(1):S2–6.
39. Duvic M, Vu J. Update on the treatment of cutaneous T-cell lymphoma (CTCL): focus on vorinostat. Biologics. 2007;1(4):377–92.
40. Mann BS, Johnson JR, Cohen MH, Justice R, Pazdur R. FDA approval summary: Vorinostat for treatment of advanced primary cutaneous T-cell lymphoma. Oncologist. 2007;12(10):1247–52.
41. Olsen EA, Kim YH, Kuzel TM, Pacheco TR, Foss FM, Parker S, et al. Phase IIb multicenter trial of vorinostat in patients with persistent, progressive, or treatment refractory cutaneous T-cell lymphoma. J Clin Oncol. 2007;25(21):3109–15.

Antipruritic Agents

15

Nadia Kashetsky and Aileen Feschuk

Contents

Note

Other topical agents with antipruritic properties are discussed elsewhere. See Chap. 17 *for Calcineurin Inhibitors. See* Chap. 18 *for topical corticosteroids.*

Other topical anesthetics, e.g., lidocaine benzocaine creams, etc., are not included in this textbook as they are sensitizing and should not be used.

N. Kashetsky (✉)
Department of Dermatology and Skin Science, Faculty of Medicine, University of British Columbia, Vancouver, BC, Canada
e-mail: nkashetsky@mun.ca

A. Feschuk
Faculty of Medicine, Memorial University of Newfoundland, St. John's, NL, Canada
e-mail: afeschuk@mun.ca

R. M. Law, H. I. Maibach (eds.), *Handbook of Topical Drug Treatment in Dermatology*,
https://doi.org/10.1007/978-3-031-93616-6_15

Doxepin 5% Cream (Zonalon)

Classification and Mode of Action

- Zonalon (doxepin hydrochloride) cream, 5%, is a topical drug approved by the FDA in 1994 [1, 2]. Each gram contains that active ingredient: 50 mg of doxepin hydrochloride (equivalent to 44.3 mg of doxepin) [1]. Zonalon cream also contains the following ingredients: sorbitol, cetyl alcohol, isopropyl myristate, glyceryl stearate, PEG-100 stearate, petrolatum, benzyl alcohol, titanium dioxide, and purified water [1].
- Doxepin hydrochloride is part of the classification of agents called dibenzoxepin tricyclic antidepressant compounds [1].
- The exact mechanism of action of the active ingredient doxepin is unknown [1]. Doxepin HCl does have H1 and H2 histamine receptor blocking actions; however, it is suggested that the drowsiness produced by Zonalon cream may reduce awareness of pruritis [1].

Indications and Dermatological Uses

- Clinical indications recommended by the FDA include short-term management (up to 8 days) of moderate pruritus in atopic dermatitis or lichen simplex chronicus in adult patients [1].
- Off-label common uses include neuropathic pain [2].

Formulations/Presentation

- *United States*: Available in the United States as Zonalon cream in 30-g (NDC 62436-523-30) and 45-g (NDC 62436-523-45) tubes [1]. Store at or below 27 °C (80 °F) [2].
- *Canada*: Available in Canada as Zonalon cream, doxepin HCL cream 5%, in 30-g aluminum tubes [3].

Dosages and Suggested Regimens

- Application and dosing: Apply a thin film of Zonalon Cream, four times daily, with at least a 3-to-4-hour interval between applications, for up to 8 days [1]. Data does not exist establishing safety and efficacy for more than 8 days [1]. Use beyond 8 days may result in increased systemic levels and risk of contact sensitization [1].

- Greater body surface area application (>10%) may increase the risk of sedation and drowsiness [1]. Patients treating more than 10% of their body surface area should therefore be cautious to monitor for drowsiness and other systemic adverse effects of doxepin [1]. If sedation occurs, it is suggested that patients decrease the body surface area treated, number of applications per day, amount of cream applied, or discontinue Zonalon cream [1].
- Absorption of topical drugs are increased by occlusive dressings and thus should not be used with Zonalon cream [1].

Baseline Investigations and Considerations

- No baseline investigations are recommended. Review contraindications, warnings, precautions, and drug interactions and special populations before commencing the drug.

Pharmacokinetics

- Plasma concentrations of doxepin from topical application of Zonalon cream ranges from undetectable 47 ng/mL from percutaneous absorption, which may affect the central nervous system and result in other systemic side effects [1]. After systemic absorption, hepatic metabolism converts digoxin to pharmacologically active desmethyldoxepin [1].

- Urinary excretion of the drug and its metabolites follows subsequent glucuronidation [1].
- The half-life of desmethyldoxepin is not affected by multiple dosing and ranges from 28 to 52 hours [1].

- Doxepin and desmethyldoxepin plasma levels are variable and poorly correlated with dosing [1].
- Distribution occurs widely across the body including the liver, brain, lungs, and heart [1].
- Metabolism and elimination of doxepin are impacted by the following variables: renal disease, genetic factors, age, and other medications [1].

Use in Special Populations

- *Pregnancy (FDA Guidance)*
  - Studies evaluating doxepin hydrochloride carcinogenesis, mutagenesis, and impairment of fertility have not been completed [1].
  - In vivo animal studies with rats and rabbits exposed to oral doxepin have revealed no evidence of harm to rat or rabbit fetuses due to doxepin [1]. However, as in vivo animal studies are not always predictive of human clinical response, Zonalon should be used only if necessary and with caution in pregnant women [1].

- *Lactation*
  - Following oral administration, doxepin is excreted in human milk, and thus following topical application, it is possible that doxepin may also be excreted in human milk [1]. Clinically, one case of apnea and drowsiness in a nursing infant has been reported where the mother was taking oral doxepin HCl [1]. Thus, a decision should be made to discontinue nursing versus discontinuing the drug based on the importance of Zonalon cream to the mother [1].

- *Children*
  - Zonalon cream is not recommended in pediatrics, as safe use has not been established [1]. Additionally, a 2.5-year-old pediatric patient receiving treatment with Zonalon cream, 27 grams had been applied over 3 days for eczema, was reported to developed somnolence, grand mal seizure, respiratory depression, ECG abnormalities, and coma [1]. He had complete resolution with supportive care, activated charcoal, and systemic alkalization [1].

- *Geriatrics*
  - Studies do not have large enough sample sizes of geriatric patients to determine whether they respond differently from younger adults [1]. However, reported clinical data has not identified differences in responses between these two groups [1].
  - As discussed above, monitoring for confusion and oversedation in the geriatric population is advised [1]. Caution should be used when determining dosing, starting at lower levels of the dosing range due to greater frequency in the geriatric population of decreased hepatic, renal or cardiac function, and of concomitant drug treatment or disease [1]. Of note, clinically a geriatric patient has been reported to develop probable systemic anticholinergic toxicity (urinary retention and delirium) after the application of Zonalon cream to their arms, legs, and back three times daily over 2 days [1].

- *Renal Insufficiency*
  - Renal excretion of doxepin extent has not been determined [1], and thus there are no dosage adjustments provided [2].

- *Hepatic Insufficiency*
  - Be cautious in dose selection for hepatic insufficiency, because once absorbed into the systemic circulation, doxepin undergoes hepatic metabolism [1]; however there are no dosage adjustments provided [2].

Monitoring

- Monitor for drowsiness, other systemic effects, and anticholinergic effects [2]. Monitor sites of application for pruritus, redness, and irritation [2]. Monitor for efficacy [2].

Contraindications and Warnings and Precautions

- *Contraindications*: Patients with previous sensitivity to any of *Zonalon's* components or untreated narrow angle glaucoma or a tendency to urinary retention, due to the anticholinergic effects of doxepin HCl [1].

- *Warnings*
  - Deaths may occur with overdosage of this drug (see Management of Overdose section) [1].
  - Drowsiness and sedation occur in over one fifth of patients, especially in patients receiving Zonalon on greater than 10% of their body surface area. Patients should be cautioned regarding driving or operating hazardous machinery while receiving Zonalon treatment [1].
  - Excessive drowsiness may warrant reduced frequency of applications, amount of dose applied, or amount of body surface area treated or discontinuation of Zonalon [1].
  - Potentiating of alcohol, antihistamine, and other central nervous system depressant sedating effects while being treated with Zonalon [1].
  - Keep Zonalon away from the eyes [1].

- *Precautions*
  - Drowsiness: As described under warnings, patients should be cautioned regarding driving or operating hazardous machinery while receiving Zonalon treatment due to potential drowsiness. Similarly, as described above, patients should also be cautioned that alcohol, antihistamine, and other central nervous system depressant sedating effects

may be potentiated. Additionally, geriatric patients should be monitored closely as Zonalon may cause confusion or oversedation in this population [1].

- Occlusive dressings should not be used with Zonalon as this may increase absorption [1].
- Contact sensitization, or a type IV hypersensitivity reaction, may be caused by doxepin [1].

Important Drug Interactions

There are many significant potential drug interactions, even for the topical use of doxepin (c.f. LexiComp drug monograph). Please check for drug interactions with the patient's list of medications using drug interaction checkers or other methods of verification prior to using doxepin.

The following table (Table 15.1) provides potential drug interactions with the topical use of doxepin.

For more details about each of the listed drugs, please visit Lexicomp drug monograph [2].

Although most drug interactions with Zonalon cream have not been investigated by studies [1], topical application of Zonalon leads to plasma levels of doxepin that can reach levels obtained with oral doxepin HCl therapy [1]. Thus, the following interactions are possible with topical Zonalon cream [1].

Drugs Metabolized by P450 2D6

Poor metabolizers or people with reduced biochemical activity of the drug-metabolizing isozyme cytochrome P450 2D6 have increased plasma concentrations of tricyclic antidepressants (TCAs). Approximately 7–10% of Caucasians are poor metabolizers. Unfortunately, prevalence estimates of reduced P450 2D6 isozyme activity among Asian, African, and other populations are not yet available.

Table 15.1 Topical doxepin drug interactions and associated action to be taken

Drugs that should concomitantly be avoided	Drugs that should be considered for modification	Drugs that should be monitored	Drugs that require no action
Aclidinium	Alpha–/beta-agonists	Acetylcholinesterase Inhibitors	Hydrocortisone (ophthalmic)
Azelastine (nasal)	Alpha2-agonists	Alcohol (ethyl)	Levodropropizine
Bromopride	Barbiturates	Alizapride	Procarbazine
Bromperidol	Blonanserin	Almotriptan	QT-prolonging agents (indeterminate risk: avoid)
Cimetropium	Buprenorphine	Alosetron	QT-prolonging agents (indeterminate risk: caution)
Dapoxetine	Chlormethiazole	Alpha1-agonists	Hydrocortisone (ophthalmic)
Dronedarone	Clozapine	Alpha2-agonists (ophthalmic)	Levodropropizine
Eluxadoline	Domperidone	Altretamine	Procarbazine
Glycopyrrolate (oral inhalation)	Droperidol	Amantadine	

Glycopyrronium (topical)	Flunitrazepam	Amifampridine	
Iobenguane radiopharmaceutical products	Fluoxetine	Amisulpride (oral)	
Ipratropium (oral inhalation)	Iohexol *depends on route*	Amphetamines	
Kratom	Iomeprol *depends on route*	Anticholinergic agents	
Levosulpiride	Iopamidol *depends on route*	Antiemetics (5HT3 antagonists)	
Linezolid	Lemborexant	Antipsychotic agents	
Methylene blue	Lofexidine	Aspirin	
Monoamine oxidase inhibitors (antidepressant)	Methadone	Baclofen	
Orphenadrine	Methotrimeprazine	Beta2-agonists	
Oxatomide	Opioid agonists	Botulinum toxin-containing products	
Oxomemazine	Oxybate salt products	Brexanolone	

(continued)

Table 15.1 (continued)

Drugs that should concomitantly be avoided	Drugs that should be considered for modification	Drugs that should be monitored	Drugs that require no action
Paraldehyde	Oxcodone	Brimonidine (topical)	
Pimozide	Paroxetine	Bupropion	
Pitolisant *depends on international labeling*	QT-prolonging agents (highest risk: consider alternatives. Patients with other risk factors: (older age, female, bradycardia, hypokalemia, hypomagnesemia, and heart disease are at increased risk))	Buspirone	
Potassium chloride *depends on dosage form*	Ropeginterferon Alfa-2b	Cannabinoid-containing products	
Potassium citrate	Secretin	Carbamazepine	
Pramlintide	Serotonergic opioids (high risk)	Chloral betaine	
Rasagiline	Suvorexant	Chlorphenesin carbamate	
Revefenacin	Zolpidem *depends on brand name*	Cimetidine	
Safinamide		Citalopram	
Selegiline		CNS depressants	
Thalidomide		Cocaine (topical)	
Tiotropium		Cyclobenzaprine	
Umeclidinium		CYP2D6 inhibitors (moderate)	

		CYP2D6 inhibitors (strong)	
		Desmopressin	
		Dexmethylphenidate-methylphenidate	
		Dextromethorphan	
		Difelikefalin	
		Dimethindene (topical) *depends on route*	
		Doxylamine *depends on brand name*	
		Duloxetine	
		Eletriptan	
		CNS depressants	
		Ergot derivatives	
		Escitalopram	
		Esketamine	
		Fenfluramine	
		Fexinidazole	

(continued)

Table 15.1 (continued)

Drugs that should concomitantly be avoided	Drugs that should be considered for modification	Drugs that should be monitored	Drugs that require no action
		Fluvoxamine	
		Gastrointestinal agents (prokinetic)	
		Gilteritinib	
		Glucagon *depends on indication*	
		Guanethidine	
		Haloperidol *depends on route*	
		Hydroxyzine	
		Itopride	
		Kava kava	
		Lasmiditan	
		Levodopa-containing products	
		Lisuride	
		Lorcaserin (withdrawn from the US market)	

		Magnesium sulfate *depends on dose*	
		Metaxalone	
		Metoclopramide	
		Metyrosine	
		Mianserin	
		Minocycline (systemic) *depends on route*	
		Mirabegron	
		Nefazodone	
		Nicorandil	
		Nitroglycerin *depends on dosage form*	
		Nonsteroidal anti-inflammatory agents (COX-2 selective)	
		Nonsteroidal anti-inflammatory agents (nonselective)	
		Ondansetron *depends on route*	

(continued)

Table 15.1 (continued)

Drugs that should concomitantly be avoided	Drugs that should be considered for modification	Drugs that should be monitored	Drugs that require no action
		Oxitriptan	
		Ozanimod	
		Pentamidine (systemic) *depends on route*	
		Perampanel	
		Piribedil	
		Pramipexole	
		QT-prolonging antipsychotics (moderate risk)	
		QT-prolonging class IC antiarrhythmics (moderate risk)	
		QT-prolonging kinase inhibitors (moderate risk)	
		QT-prolonging miscellaneous agents (moderate risk)	

		QT-prolonging moderate CYP3A4 inhibitors (moderate risk)	
		QT-prolonging quinolone antibiotics (moderate risk)	
		QT-prolonging strong CYP3A4 inhibitors (moderate risk)	
		Ramosetron	
		Ropinirole	
		Rotigotine	
		Rufinamide	
		Serotonergic agents (high risk, miscellaneous)	
		Serotonergic non-opioid CNS depressants	
		Serotonin 5-HT1D receptor agonists (triptans)	

(continued)

Table 15.1 (continued)

Drugs that should concomitantly be avoided	Drugs that should be considered for modification	Drugs that should be monitored	Drugs that require no action
		Serotonin/norepinephrine reuptake inhibitors	
		Sertraline	
		Sodium phosphates *depends on dose*	
		St. John's wort	
		Sulfonylureas	
		Syrian rue	
		Thiazide and thiazide-like diuretics	
		Thyroid products	
		Topiramate	
		Tricyclic antidepressants	
		Trimeprazine	
		Valerian	
		Valproate products	
		Vasopressin	
		Vilazodone	
		Vortioxetine	

Normal metabolizers can act as poor metabolizers with the addition of drugs that inhibit isozyme cytochrome P450 2D6 activity. These drugs include medications not metabolized by the enzyme (quinidine; cimetidine) and substrates (many other antidepressants, phenothiazines, and the type 1C antiarrhythmics propafenone and flecainide).

Selective serotonin reuptake inhibitors (SSRIs) also inhibit P450 2D6, but vary in their extent of inhibition. Thus, caution is advised for concomitant TCAs with any SSRIs, and sufficient time must elapse before initiating a TCA in a patient previously on an SSRI (at least 5 weeks may be necessary).

For these reasons, TCAs used concomitantly with drugs that can inhibit cytochrome P450 2D6 activity may require lower doses for either drug. Additionally, monitoring plasma levels of TCA whenever it will be co-administered with a P450 2D6 inhibitor is advised.

MAO Inhibitors

MAO inhibitors should be discontinued at least 2 weeks prior to initiation of Zonalon cream as serious adverse events, and death have been reported with concomitant use of certain drugs with MAO inhibitors.

Cimetidine

Concomitant use of TCA and cimetidine have produced serious anticholinergic symptoms including severe dry mouth, urinary retention, and blurred vision. Additionally, higher TCA plasma levels have been observed in patients already taking cimetidine.

Alcohol

As discussed above, alcohol ingestion may exacerbate the potential sedative effects of Zonalon cream.

Tolazamide

Severe hypoglycemia has been reported in a type two diabetic patient on tolazamide (1 gm/day) 11 days after the addition of oral doxepin (75 mg/day).

Adverse Effects and Overdose

Adverse Reactions

Adverse events from clinical trials are reported in Table 15.2 [1]. The most common systematic side effect was drowsiness occurring in 22% (*n* = 71/330) patients with Zonalon cream versus 2% (*n* = 7/334) patients with vehicle cream [1]. In these controlled trials, drowsiness lead to discontinuation of Zonalon cream prematurely in approximately 5% of patients [1]. The most common local site adverse reaction was stinging and/or burning in 23% (76/330) of patients with Zonalon cream versus 16% (54/334) using vehicle cream [1]. Approximately 1% of patients treated

Table 15.2 Adverse events during clinical trials at incidence ≥1% while using vehicle cream versus Zonalon cream[a]

Adverse reaction	Vehicle cream, % (n/N)	Zonalon cream, % (n/N)
Burning/stinging	16% (54/334)	23% (76/330)
Drowsiness	2% (7/334)	22% (71/330)
Dry mouth	1% 4/334)	10% (32/330)
Pruritus	6% (20/334)	4% (13/330)
Fatigue	2% (5/334)	3% (10/330)
Eczema exacerbation	2% (8/334)	3% (10/330)
Other reaction at application site	5% (16/334)	3% (10/330)
Dizziness	1% (3/334)	2% (7/330)
Emotional changes	0.5% (1/334)	2% (6/330)
Taste changes	0.5% (1/334)	2% (5/330)
Edema	0.5% (1/334)	1% (4/330)
Headache	4% (14/334)	1% (3/330)

[a]Table is adapted from FDA Zonalon Drug Label [1]

with Zonalon cream finished the study prematurely second to stinging and/or burning [1].

Additionally, nervousness/anxiety, tongue numbness, fever, and nausea occurred in less than 1% of participants [1].

Overdosage and Management

As previously stated, overdosage with this class of drugs may cause death [1]. Physicians should recognize signs and symptoms of overdosage and contact their local poison control center for current information on treatment [1].

Signs and symptoms of tricyclic antidepressant toxicity develop rapidly and include the following:

- Cardiac dysrhythmias
- Severe hypotension
- Convulsions
- CNS depression (including coma)
- Electrocardiogram changes (QRS axis or width)
- Confusion
- Disturbed concentration
- Transient visual hallucinations
- Dilated pupils
- Agitation
- Hyperactive reflexes
- Stupor
- Drowsiness
- Muscle rigidity
- Vomiting
- Hypothermia
- Hyperpyrexia
- Any of the symptoms listed under section "Adverse Reactions" [1]

A general guide to the management of overdosage is outlined as follows. Hospital monitoring is required immediately [1]. Patient's airway should be protected, electrocardiogram obtained, and cardiac monitoring should be commenced immediately [1]. Intravenous access should be established, and then gastric decontamination should be initiated [1]. The time of observation for the central nervous system of respiration depression should be a minimum of 6 hours [1]. During these 6 hours, patients should also be closely monitored for hypotension, cardiac dysrhythmias and/or conduction blocks, and seizures [1]. Any signs of toxicity within the 6-hour time period suggest an extended period of monitoring [1]. Management should not be guided by plasma levels of drug [1]. Early intubation is recommendation for patients with central nervous system depression second to the potential for abrupt deterioration [1]. Seizures should be controlled with benzodiazepines which are recommended as first line to control seizures, with other anticonvulsants including phenobarbital or phenytoin if benzodiazepines are ineffective [1]. Physostigmine is reserved for life-threatening symptoms that are unresponsive to other therapies, and only after consultation with a poison control center [1]. The best indication of overdose severity may be a maximal limb-lead QRS duration of ≥0.10 seconds [1]. Serum pH should be maintained with intravenous sodium bicarbonate, with hyperventilation being used if response is inadequate [1]. Their concomitant use should be done with extreme caution and monitoring [1]. Lidocaine, bretylium, or phenytoin are third line if response is inadequate [1]. Hemoperfusion may be beneficial in rare cases of acute toxicity leading acute refractory cardiovascular instability [1].

Patch Test Concentration

- One percent and 5% pet.
- There have been at least 20 cases documented that have had a positive patch test to doxepin 5% cream [1, 4].

Essential Patient Information

- Patients should be provided the following information:
  - This drug is used for itching [2]. It may also be given for other reasons, and if this is the case for you, please talk to your doctor [2]. Speak with your physician if you have dry mouth, burning, stinting, and increased thirst that bothers you or does not go away [2]. Although very rare, it is possible that some people have severe or deadly side effects; when taking this drug, tell your doctor or seek medical care if you have severe fatigue; confusion; severe skin irritation; signs of an allergic reaction, including rash, hives, itching, red, swollen, blistered, or peeling skin with or without fever; wheezing; tightness in the chest or throat, trouble breathing, swallowing, or talking; unusual hoarseness; or swelling of the mouth, face, lips, tongue, or throat [2].

Pramoxine

Classification and Mechanism of Action

- Pramoxine is classified as a local anesthetic agent [4].
- The mechanism of action is identical to other anesthetics: decreasing neurons' membrane permeability to sodium ions, leading to blockage of both initiation and conduction nerve impulses, and inhibition of neuron depolirization [4].

Indications and Dermatological Uses

- Clinical indications (FDA) include the following:
  - Perianal pruritus, hemorrhoidal irritations, and anorectal cleaning;
  - Minor skin irritations (pain and pruritus) including rashes, sunburns, hives, minor burns, minor cuts and scrapes, insect bites, poison ivy, oak, and sumac

- Mouth irritations (pain and pruritus) including fever blisters and cold sores
- Vaginal irritations (pruritus and burning) including minor vaginal skin irritations

Off-Label Common Uses

- No off-label common uses are reported [4].

Formulations/Presentation

- Pramoxine can be administered alone or in combination with hydrocortisone or other ingredients in several forms including gel, lotion, solution, aerosol foam, cream, ointment, or pledget [4].
- Typical formulation for pramoxine is 1% concentration [4].

Formulations in the United States are as follows:
As hydrochloride

Foams
- Proctofoam: 1% (15 g) (steroid free; contains cetyl alcohol, methylparaben, propylene glycol, propylparaben, trolamine (triethanolamine))
- Generic: 1% (15 g)

Gels
- Itch-X: 1% (35.4 g)
- PrameGel: 1% (118 mL)
- Pramox: 1% (113 g) (contains methylparaben, propylene glycol, propylparaben)

Lotions

- Calaclear: Pramoxine hydrochloride 1% and zinc acetate 0.1% (177 mL) (contains alcohol, usp, methylparaben, polysorbate 80, propylene glycol, propylparaben)
- Caladryl Clear: Pramoxine hydrochloride 1% and zinc acetate 0.1% (177 mL) (contains methylparaben, propylene glycol, propylparaben, sd alcohol)
- Caldyphen Clear: Pramoxine hydrochloride 1% and zinc acetate 0.1% (177 mL) (contains alcohol, usp, methylparaben, polysorbate 80, propylene glycol, propylparaben)
- Callergy Clear: Pramoxine hydrochloride 1% and zinc acetate 0.1% (177 mL) (contains alcohol, usp, methylparaben, propylene glycol, propylparaben)
- DerMend Moisturizing Anti-Itch: 1% (237 mL) (fragrance free, paraben free, steroid free; contains cetyl alcohol, coconut oil (copra/cocos nucifera oil), trolamine (triethanolamine))
- GoodSense Clear Anti-Itch: Pramoxine hydrochloride 1% and zinc acetate 0.1% (177 mL) (contains alcohol, usp, methylparaben, propylene glycol, propylparaben)
- Ivy Wash Poison Ivy Cleanser: 1% (177 mL) (contains disodium edta, methylparaben, propylene glycol, propylparaben)
- Prax: 1% (118 mL, 237 mL) (contains cetyl alcohol, trolamine (triethanolamine))
- Sarna Sensitive: 1% (222 mL) (fragrance free, steroid free; contains benzyl alcohol, cetyl alcohol)

Approved drugs in Canada containing pramoxine include the following [5]:

Foams

- Proctofoam-HC (hydrocortisone acetate 1%, pramoxine hydrochloride 1%): Each application delivers approximately 375 mg of foam containing approximately 1% hydrocortisone acetate (3.75 mg/dose) and 1% pramoxine hydrochloride (3.75 mg/dose).

Ointment

- Anusol Plus (pramoxine HCl-zinc sulfate monohydrate): Each tube of smooth, colorless, translucent ointment contains pramoxine HCl 1% w/w and zinc sulfate monohydrate 0.5% w/w. Nonmedicinal ingredients: calcium phosphate, mineral oil, oleth-2, parabens, and petrolatum. Tubes of 30 g with applicator. Store between 15 and 30 °C.
- Proctodan-HC (pramoxine HCl-hydrocortisone acetate-zinc sulfate monohydrate): Each g of ointment contains pramoxine HCl 1%, hydrocortisone acetate 0.5%, and zinc sulfate monohydrate 0.5%. Nonmedicinal ingredients: methylparaben, propylparaben, and petrolatum. Tubes of 15 and 30 g with rectal applicator.

Suppositories

- Anusol Plus (pramoxine HCl-zinc sulfate monohydrate): Each white, opaque suppository contains pramoxine HCl 20 mg and zinc sulfate monohydrate 10 mg. Nonmedicinal ingredients: calcium phosphate, magnesium stearate, parabens, and vegetable oil. Boxes of 12 and 24. Store between 15 and 30 °C.
- Proctodan-HC (pramoxine HCl-hydrocortisone acetate-zinc sulfate monohydrate): Each suppository contains pramoxine HCl 20 mg, zinc sulfate monohydrate 10 mg, and hydrocortisone acetate 10 mg in a triglyceride base. Nonmedicinal ingredients: dibasic calcium phosphate, magnesium stearate, methylparaben, propylparaben, and triglyceride. Boxes of 12. Store between 15 and 30 °C. Avoid freezing.

Europe: Not listed in LexiComp monograph

Dosages and Suggested Regimens

As described above pramoxine can be administered topically alone or in combination with other ingredients in several forms summarized below [4].

- Anorectal cleaning wipes: use topically up to five times daily.
- For hemorrhoidal irritations and/or perianal itching: gel can be applied topically to the affected local area three to four times daily, or foam, wipes, or lotion can be applied topically to the affected area up to five times daily [4].
- For minor skin irritations: cream, gel, lotion, or spray can be applied to the affected local area up to three to four times daily [4].
- For mouth irritations: liquid can be topically applied up to three to four times daily, beginning at the first sign of a fever blister or cold sore [4].
- For vaginal irritation: wipes should be applied topically—applied externally to vaginal area as needed (Luvena) or applied to affected area up to three to four times daily (Vagisil) [4].

Baseline Investigations and Considerations

No baseline investigations are recommended. Review contraindications, warnings, precautions, and drug interactions and special populations before commencing the drug.

Pharmacokinetics

A study by Lewis and Wingold in 1985 concluded that pramoxine was not systemically absorbed [6].

Use in Special Populations

- *Pregnancy*
  - Pramoxine has been suggested to be compatible and safe with pregnancy. A study by Lewis and Wingold in 1985 concluded that pramoxine was not systemically absorbed [6]. Accordingly, insignificant systemic absorption results in negligible risk to the embryo or fetus [4]. Although, theoretically the low molecular weight of the drug would allow it to cross the placenta and reach the fetus, the amount, if any of the mother's plasma concentration, is negligible [4].
  - A second study by Ebrahimi et al. in 2011 studied the effects of using pramoxine during the third trimester of pregnancy in 204 women and found no adverse effects on fetal gestational age, birth weight, prematurity rates, or pericomplications. Insignificant systemic absorption results in negligible risk to the embryo or fetus [7].

- *Lactation*
  - There are no human studies that describe the use of pramoxine during lactation [4]. Theoretically, it is suggested that the risk to a nursing infant is negligible [4]. Although the molecular weight of the drug's free base is low enough that excretion into the breast milk is possible, the drug is thought not to be systemically absorbed [4].

- *Children*
  - Pramoxine should not be used in patients younger than 2 for minor skin irritations [4].
  - Pramoxine should not be used in patients younger than 12 years for hemorrhoidal/anorectal itching [4].

- *Geriatrics*
  - There are no dosage adjustments provided for the geriatric population [4].

- *Renal Insufficiency*
  - There are no dosage adjustments provided.

- *Hepatic Insufficiency*
  - There are no dosage adjustments provided.

Monitoring

- None recommended

Contraindications and Cautions

- *Contraindications*
  - Use is contraindicated in patients with known hypersensitivity to pramoxine or any ingredient in the formulation [4].

- *Warnings/Cautions*
  - This drug is for external use only; do not ingest this drug [4]. Keep away from the eyes and nose [4]. If condition does not improve within a week, worsens, resolves, and then reoccurs again within a few days, or additional symptoms arise including edema, rash, and irritation, contact a health care provider [4]. This drug is not to be used over open wounds or large body surface areas [4]. When using the foam or gel anorectal products, do not put the foam or gel into the rectum [4].

Important Drug Interactions

- Pramoxine has two important drug interactions.
  - The first is bupivacaine as pramoxine may enhance adverse effects and toxicity of this drug [4]. Thus, pramoxine should be avoided within 96 hours of a bupivacaine implant insertion or bupivacaine and meloxicam periarticular solution, and pramoxine should be avoided within 168 hours after subacromial infiltration [4].

  - The second drug interaction is methemoglobinemia-associated agents, as these drugs may enhance the adverse effects and toxicity of pramoxine, specifically they may increase the risk of methemoglobinemia [4].

Adverse Effects and Their Management

- Local effects after topical application of the drug, including burning or stinging [4].
- Pramoxine has a low index of sensitization and a low index of cross-sensitization with other local anesthetics [4].

Patch Test Concentration

- Hydrochloride 2% pet. (Chemotechnique)

Essential Patient Information

- This drug is used for several conditions including hemorrhoids or rectal irritation, itching, and pain from insect bites, skin irritation, poison oak, ivy, and sumac rashes [4].
- Although very rare, it is possible that some people have severe or deadly side effects when taking this drug; tell your doctor or seek medical care if you have irritation; swelling, warmth, or redness of the skin; signs of an allergic reaction, like rash; hives; itching; red, swollen, blistered, or peeling skin with or without fever; wheezing; tightness in the chest or throat; trouble breathing, swallowing, or talking; unusual hoarseness; or swelling of the mouth, face, lips, tongue, or throat; or bleeding from the rectum or rectal pain [4].

Topical Anesthetics

Topical Anesthetics such as benzocaine and lidocaine are numbing; thus, they have antipruritic properties. However, they are not recommended due to the risk of sensitization. (Intradermal lidocaine is often used prior to skin biopsies which is an appropriate use of the injectable lidocaine formulation.)

References

Topical Antipruritic Agents

1. ZONALON® (doxepin hydrochloride) CREAM, 5%.
2. Lexicomp. http://online.lexi.com.qe2a-proxy.mun.ca/lco/action/doc/retrieve/docid/patch_f/1827022?cesid=9NQ6ESUDebI&searchUrl=%2Flco%2Faction%2Fsearch%3Fq%3Dzonalon%26t%3Dname%26va%3Dzonalon. Accessed 7 Jan 2022.
3. Unknown. Zonalon (doxepin hydrochloride) 5% cream [product monograph]. 2013.
4. Lexicomp. http://online.lexi.com.qe2a-proxy.mun.ca/lco/action/doc/retrieve/docid/patch_f/7540?cesid=5sAl3gVckA5&searchUrl=%2Flco%2Faction%2Fsearch%3Fq%3Dpramoxine%26t%3Dname%26va%3Dpramoxine#thclist. Accessed 7 Jan 2022.
5. Woodby R. Compendium of Pharmaceuticals and Specialties (CPS) Database: Canadian Standard for Drug Monographs. https://library.rrc.ca/RxTx/drug. Accessed 8 Jan 2022.
6. Lewis JH, Weingold AB. The use of gastrointestinal drugs during pregnancy and lactation. Am J Gastroenterol. 1985;80(11):912–23.
7. Ebrahimi N, Vohra S, Gedeon C, et al. The fetal safety of hydrocortisone-pramoxine (Proctofoam-HC) for the treatment of hemorrhoids in late pregnancy. J Obstet Gynaecol Can. 2011;33:153. https://doi.org/10.1016/S1701-2163(16)34802-2.

Antiviral Agents 16

Rebecca M. Law, Drake Carter, Sean Mangion, and Howard I. Maibach

Contents

R. M. Law (✉)
School of Pharmacy and Faculty of Medicine (Discipline of Family Medicine), Memorial University of Newfoundland, St. John's, NL, Canada
e-mail: rlaw@mun.ca; rlawUCSF@gmail.com

D. Carter
Chicago Medical School, Rosalind Franklin University of Medicine & Science, North Chicago, IL, USA
e-mail: drake.carter@my.rfums.org

R. M. Law, H. I. Maibach (eds.), *Handbook of Topical Drug Treatment in Dermatology*,
https://doi.org/10.1007/978-3-031-93616-6_16

Introduction

Rebecca M. Law

Antiviral agents discussed in this chapter are those non-HIV antiviral agents which have topical formulations. Some of the agents are precursors/prodrugs for others, and both agents have been included as separate mographs. The clinical uses discussed in the monographs include herpes simplex virus (HSV) infections such as recurrent herpes labialis (HSV-1) and genital infections (HSV-2), varicella-zoster virus (VZV) infections such as shingles, and molluscum contagiosum.

The drug monographs included are the following:

Acyclovir
Berdazimer
Famciclovir
Penciclovir
Valaciclovir

S. Mangion
UniSA: Clinical and Health Sciences, University of South Australia, Adelaide, SA, Australia

Therapeutics Research Centre, Basil Hetzel Institute of Translational Health Research, The Queen Elizabeth Hospital, Woodville, SA, Australia

Sydney Medical School, The University of Sydney, Camperdown, NSA, Australia
e-mail: sean.mangion@hotmail.com

H. I. Maibach
Department of Dermatology, University of California San Francisco (UCSF), San Francisco, CA, USA
e-mail: howard.maibach@ucsf.edu

Acyclovir (Zovirax)

Rebecca M. Law

Classification and Mode of Action

- Acyclovir is a synthetic purine nucleoside analogue with cell culture and in vivo inhibitory activity against herpes simplex virus (HSV) types 1 (HSV-1) and 2 (HSV-2).
- The inhibitory activity of acyclovir is highly selective due to its affinity for the enzyme thymidine kinase (TK) encoded by HSV. This viral enzyme converts acyclovir into acyclovir monophosphate, a nucleotide analogue. The monophosphate is further converted into diphosphate by cellular guanylate kinase and into triphosphate by a number of cellular enzymes.
- In cell culture, acyclovir triphosphate stops the replication of herpes viral DNA. This inhibition is accomplished in three ways: (1) competitive inhibition of viral DNA polymerase, (2) incorporation into and termination of the growing viral DNA chain, and (3) inactivation of the viral DNA polymerase.

Indications and Dermatological Uses

- *Clinical indications (FDA)*: Indicated for the treatment of recurrent herpes labialis (cold sores) in immunocompetent adults and adolescents 12 years of age and older

Formulations/Presentation

- USA: Acyclovir 5% cream
- Canada: Acyclovir 5% cream

Dosages and Suggested Regimens

- Apply five times per day for 4 days.
- Initiate therapy as soon as possible after onset of signs or symptoms.

Pharmacokinetics

- Absorption: In one study, the average daily urinary excretion of acyclovir was approximately 0.04% of the daily applied topical dose. Plasma acyclovir concentrations were below the limit of detection (0.01 μM) in five subjects and barely detectable (0.014 μM) in one subject. Systemic absorption of acyclovir from 5% cream is minimal in adults.

Use in Special Populations

- Pregnancy: No adequate and well-controlled studies of acyclovir cream in pregnant women. Acyclovir cream should be used during pregnancy only if the potential benefit justifies the potential risk to the fetus (formerly FDA pregnancy category B).
- Lactation: Unknown whether topically applied acyclovir is excreted in breast milk. However, after oral administration, acyclovir concentrations have been seen in breast milk (0.6–4.1 times the corresponding plasma levels). Thus nursing mothers with active herpetic lesions near or on the breast should avoid breastfeeding.
- Pediatrics: Safety profile in children 12–17 years was similar to that observed in adults. Safety in children under 12 years is not established.
- Geriatrics: Systemic absorption after topical administration is minimal. Clinical experience have shown no differences in responses between the elderly and younger adults.

Monitoring

- Monitor for adverse effects including irritant skin reactions (cumulative) and hypersensitivity reactions.

Contraindications and Cautions

- Contraindicated in patients with known hypersensitivity to acyclovir, valacyclovir.
- Cream should only be applied on the affected external aspects of the lips and face in patients with herpes labialis. Because no data are available, application to human mucous membranes is not recommended. Zovirax cream is intended for cutaneous use only and should not be used in the eye or inside the mouth or nose.

Important Drug Interactions

- None known

Adverse Effects and Their Management

- There is a potential for irritation and contact sensitization. In particular, there is a high and cumulative irritation potential.
- The most common adverse reactions at the site of topical application were dry lips, desquamation, dryness of the skin, cracked lips, burning skin, pruritus, flakiness of the skin, and stinging on the skin (each adverse reaction occurred in less than 1% of patients receiving Zovirax cream).
- Postmarking adverse events included angioedema, anaphylaxis, contact dermatitis, and eczema.

Carcinogenicity

- Unknown

Patch Test Concentration

- Ten percent pet (Chemotechnique); scratch-patch tests may be performed in the case of a? + reaction or a negative reaction to acyclovir with highly suspected history for allergy.

Essential Patient Information

- Should be used for cold sores on the lips and around the mouth only. It should not be used in the eyes, mouth, nose, or on the genitals.
- Acyclovir cream is not a cure for cold sores.
- Acyclovir cream should be used as soon as the first symptoms of a cold sore occur, such as itching, redness, burning or tingling, or when the cold sore appears.
- Apply to the affected area five times daily for 4 days, including the outer edge.
- Do not apply other skin products to the affected area during treatment with acyclovir cream.
- Do not rub the cold sore, since this may cause spread to other areas around the mouth or make the cold sore worse.

Berdazimer

Sean Mangion

Classification and Mode of Action

- First-in-class nitric oxide (NO)-releasing topical agent for molluscum contagiosum.
- NO has antimicrobial activity related to protein nitrosylation that influences immunomodulation, apoptosis, cytokine production, and inflammation. It may also affect viral replication through cytotoxic reactive oxygen and nitrogen species.

- In a 12-week pivotal Phase 3 trial (B-SIMPLE4), 891 patients with a mean age of 6.6 years (range, 0.9–47.5 years) were randomly assigned to treatment with berdazimer gel 10.3% or a vehicle gel applied in a thin layer to all lesions once daily. At 12 weeks, 32.4% of patients in the berdazimer group achieved complete clearance of lesions compared with 19.7% in the vehicle group ($P < 0.001$).
- It is also being explored for use in acne (phase 3 trial currently underway for a 3.4% containing gel).

Indications and Dermatological Uses

- *Clinical indications (FDA)*: Molluscum contagiosum: adults and pediatric patients ≥1 year of age
- *Off-label common uses*: None

Formulations/Presentation

- USA: Berdazimer sodium (Zelsuvmi®), 10.3% gel

Dosages and Suggested Regimens

- Apply to lesions once daily.
- The product comes with two tubes of gel that must be mixed according to the dosing guide before application. The drug should be applied immediately after mixing, by thin layer on the affected lesion/s. The drug should dry for at least 10 minutes before occlusion with clothes or gloves.
- Bathing, showering, or swimming should not occur for 1 hour after application.

Baseline Investigations and Considerations

- None

Pharmacokinetics

- Measurement of NO metabolite hMAP3 during the Phase I study showed that once-daily application of berdazimer resulted in minimal systemic absorption in children aged 2–12 years old. Efficacy and safety data for use in molluscum contagiosum is so far limited to a maximum of 12 weeks of use.

Use in Special Populations

Pediatrics

- Approved for use in children aged over 1 year.

Pregnancy and Lactation

- Not currently classified as limited human data available.

Renal insufficiency

- Not evaluated; dose adjustment is not expected to be needed.

Hepatic insufficiency

- Not evaluated; dose adjustment is not expected to be needed.

Monitoring

- Signs of an allergic reaction, like rash; hives; itching; red, swollen, blistered, or peeling skin with or without fever; wheezing; tightness in the chest or throat; trouble breathing, swallowing, or talking; unusual hoarseness; or swelling of the mouth, face, lips, tongue, or throat.

Contraindications and Cautions

- None reported.

Important Drug Interactions

- None reported.

Adverse Effects and their Management

- Signs of skin infection like oozing, heat, swelling, redness, or pain.
- Skin breakdown where this drug is used.
- Dry skin, blisters, peeling, flaking, or change in the color of the skin.
- Pain, burning, stinging, itching, swelling, or redness.
- Product should be discontinued, and medical advice should be sought on management.

Carcinogenicity (if Known, Including Mouse Painting Studies)

- The carcinogenic potential of berdazimer gel was assessed in a 2-year dermal mouse carcinogenicity study. There were no drug-related tumor findings associated with daily topical administration of berdazimer gel to mice at doses up to 4% berdazimer gel. Berdazimer was mutagenic in a bacterial mutagenicity assay (Ames assay) but was not clastogenic in an in vitro chromosomal aberration assay in human peripheral blood lymphocytes or in an in vivo micronucleus assay in rats.

Patch Test Concentration

- Not available

Essential Patient Information

- Not to be taken orally, ophthalmologically, or intravaginally.
- Not to be mixed until ready for use.
- Not to be applied on healthy skin or on open wounds.
- Wash hands after application unless the hand is the affected site.

Famciclovir

Drake Carter

Classification and Mode of Action

- Famciclovir is a prodrug that undergoes biotransformation into its active metabolite, penciclovir. This metabolite is phosphorylated by HSV-1, HSV-2, and VZV thymidine kinase into penciclovir monophosphate. Cellular enzymes then convert this into penciclovir triphosphate, which competes with deoxyguanosine triphosphate to inhibit viral DNA polymerase by chain termination.
- Famciclovir was found to be less effective than valacyclovir for suppression of genital HSV infections and the resolution and pain management of acute herpes zoster (VZV).

Indications and Dermatological Uses

- *Clinical indications (FDA)*: HSV (orolabial and genital infections), varicella-zoster (shingles)
- *Off-label common uses*: Varicella (chickenpox) infection in patients with uncomplicated HIV (level of evidence: G); HSV prevention in solid organ transplant recipients (level of evidence: G)

Formulations/Presentation

- USA: 125-mg, 250-mg, and 500-mg tablets
- Canada: 125-mg, 250-mg, and 500-mg tablets

Dosages and Suggested Regimens

- Genital HSV infections (immunocompetent patients)
  - Initial episode: 250 mg three times daily for 7–10 days
  - Recurrent episodes: 1 g twice daily for 1 day; 500 mg as single dose followed by 250 mg twice a day for 5 days
- Orolabial HSV infections (immunocompetent patients)
  - Initial episode (gingivostomatitis): 250 mg three times daily for 1 day; 500 mg twice daily for 7–10 days
  - Recurrent episodes: 1.5 g as a single dose
- HSV infections (immunocompromised patients, including those with HIV)
  - 500 mg twice daily for 5–10 days
- Herpes zoster (shingles)
  - Dermatomal lesions: 500 mg three times daily for 7–10 days

Baseline Investigations and Considerations

Pharmacokinetics

- Famciclovir undergoes deacetylation and oxidation by the liver to turn into penciclovir.
- Oral bioavailability is 77 ± 8%.
- Half-life is 2.8 ± 1.0 hour following a 500-mg dose in patients with herpes zoster.
- Time to maximum plasma concentration is 0.9 hour.
- Excreted primarily in urine. Active tubular secretion contributes to renal clearance.

Use in Special Populations

- Listed as FDA pregnancy classification B (former classification scheme).
- Unknown whether famciclovir is excreted in breast milk.
- The efficacy and safety of famciclovir has not been determined in children due to limited data available.
- Dosage adjustments due to renal impairment should be made based on the patient's measured creatinine clearance (CrCl).

- For recurrent HSV infections (genital-immunocompetent)
  When CrCl is 40–59 mL/minute: 500 mg every 12 hours for 1 day
  When CrCl is 20–39 mL/minute: 500 mg as single dose
  When CrCl is <20 mL/minute: 250 mg as single dose
- For recurrent HSV infections (oral-immunocompetent)
  When CrCl is 40–59 mL/minute: 750 mg as single dose
  When CrCl is 20–39 mL/minute: 500 mg as single dose
  When CrCl is <20 mL/minute: 250 mg as single dose
- For HSV infections in immunocompromised (including those with HIV)
  When CrCl is 20–39 mL/minute: 500 mg every 24 hours
  When CrCl is <20 mL/minute: 250 mg every 24 hours
- For herpes zoster dermatomal lesions
  When CrCl is 40–59 mL/minute: 500 mg every 12 hours
  When CrCl is 20–39 mL/minute: 500 mg every 24 hours
  When CrCl is <20 mL/minute: 250 mg every 24 hours

• No suggested dose adjustment for hepatic impairment as it has not been studied.

Monitoring

• Renal impairment. Change dosing as indicated above, as needed

Contraindications and Cautions

• Contraindicated in patients with known allergy to famciclovir or its active metabolite, penciclovir.
• Tablets contain lactose; use with caution in cases of lactase deficiency, galactose intolerance, or glucose-galactose malabsorption syndromes.

Important Drug Interactions

- Concurrent use of other drugs eliminated by active renal tubular secretion may increase the plasma concentrations of famciclovir (e.g., probenecid).
- Famciclovir may decrease the efficacy of other drugs that undergo intracellular phosphorylation (e.g., cladribine).
- Famciclovir may diminish the efficacy of other antiherpetic antivirals (e.g., talimogene laherparepvec).
- Famciclovir may reduce the efficacy of both varicella virus and zoster vaccinations.

Adverse Effects and Their Management

- The most commonly reported adverse effects are headache and nausea (>10%).
- Other adverse reactions include fatigue (5%), migraine (3%), paresthesia (3%), pruritus (2–4%), rash (3%), diarrhea (2–8%), flatulence (5%), vomiting (5%), dysmenorrhea (8%), neutropenia (3%), leukopenia (1%), increased serum ALT (3%), increased serum AST (2%), and increased serum bilirubin (2%).
- Cases of acute renal failure have occurred in patients with underlying renal impairment; dose adjustment is needed in patients with renal impairment to avoid giving an inappropriately high dose.

Carcinogenicity (if Known, Including Mouse Painting Studies)

- A 2-year carcinogenicity study found a higher incidence of mammary adenocarcinoma in female rats receiving famciclovir in high doses of 600 mg/kg/day (1.1 to 4.5x the human systemic exposure at the recommended dose range of 500–2000 mg daily).

- No increases in tumor incidence were found in male rats receiving doses up to 240 mg/kg/day.
- No increases in tumor incidence were seen in male and female mice receiving high doses of 600 mg/kg/day.

Patch Test Concentration

- Not available

Essential Patient Information

- Famciclovir can be taken with or without food.
- Alert medical provider if there is a known history of renal impairment.
- Use with caution if there is a known history of lactose intolerance.

Penciclovir (Denavir)

Drake Carter

Classification and Mode of Action

- Penciclovir is phosphorylated by viral thymidine kinases in HSV-1 and HSV-2 infected cells into a monophosphate form. This form is then converted to penciclovir triphosphate by cellular kinases, which then competitively inhibits HSV DNA polymerase via competing with deoxyguanosine triphosphate.

Indications and Dermatological Uses

- *Clinical indications (FDA)*: herpes labialis (cold sores)
- *Off-label common uses:*

Formulations/Presentation

- USA: 1% cream
- Canada:
- Europe:

Dosages and Suggested Regimens

- Apply (topically) at the first indication of cold sore (during prodrome or when symptoms appear). During waking hours, apply every 2 hours for 4 days.

Baseline Investigations and Considerations

Pharmacokinetics

- No systemic percutaneous absorption has been reported.
- Concentrations of penciclovir were not detected in urine or plasma of healthy male volunteers (n = 12) following single or repeat topical application of 1% penciclovir cream in doses of 180 g daily (about 67 times the usual dose).

Use in Special Populations

- Listed as FDA pregnancy classification B. No well-controlled studies have been conducted in pregnant women.
- There is no data on whether topically applied penciclovir is excreted in breast milk. However, penciclovir has been shown to be excreted in breast milk following oral administration of famciclovir, a prodrug that is converted into penciclovir.

- The frequency of adverse effects in children aged 12–17 was similar to adult patients. However, safety and efficacy in patients <12 has not been established.
- No dosage adjustment required in patients with impaired renal function.
- No dosage adjustment required in patients with impaired hepatic function.

Monitoring

- Skin irritation following application
- Taste distortion
- Local anesthesia
- Erythematous rash

Contraindications and Cautions

- Penciclovir is contraindicated in patients with known hypersensitivity to the product or any of its components.

Important Drug Interactions

- No drug interaction studies have been performed. Since penciclovir is minimally absorbed percutaneously, systemic drug interactions are unlikely.

Adverse Effects and Their Management

- Application site reaction
- Hypesthesia/local anesthesia
- Taste perversion
- Erythematous rash

Carcinogenicity (if Known, Including Mouse Painting Studies)

- Two-year carcinogenicity studies were conducted with the prodrug of penciclovir, famciclovir. After oral doses of 600 mg/kg/day (395 times the maximum theoretical human exposure following topical penciclovir application), an increase in the incidence of mammary adenocarcinoma was seen in female rats. No increases in tumor incidence were seen in male rats treated with 240 mg/kg/day (190 times the maximum theoretical exposure to penciclovir) or in male and female mice receiving doses of 600 mg/kg/day (100 times the maximum theoretical exposure to penciclovir).
- Testicular toxicity was observed in rats and dogs following repeated intravenous administration of penciclovir following doses of 160 mg/kg/day (1155x the maximum theoretical human AUC) in rats and 100 mg/kg/day (3255x the maximum theoretical human AUC) in dogs. Adverse reactions reported include atrophy of the seminiferous tubules, reduced sperm count, and increased incidence of sperm with altered morphology that affected motility.

Patch Test Concentration

- Not available

Essential Patient Information

- Wash your hands before applying to a clean, dry skin.
- Only apply over affected areas. Rub in the cream until it disappears.
- Do not ingest. For topical use only.

Valacyclovir (Valtrex)

Drake Carter

Classification and Mode of Action

- Valacyclovir is a nucleoside analog viral DNA polymerase inhibitor. It is converted to its active metabolite, acyclovir, via intestinal and hepatic metabolism. Acyclovir is then converted to acyclovir monophosphate by viral thymidine kinase and then further converted to acyclovir triphosphate by cellular enzymes. Acyclovir triphosphate competes with deoxyguanosine triphosphate in order to be incorporated into viral DNA and act as a terminator of the growing DNA chain.
- Valacyclovir was found to be better than famciclovir for suppression of genital herpes in a comparative study.
- Valacyclovir showed to accelerate the resolution of herpes zoster-associated pain compared to acyclovir, while maintaining a simpler dosing and favorable safety profile.

Indications and Dermatological Uses

- *Clinical Indications (FDA)*
  - Cold sores (herpes labialis) in both pediatric and adult patients
  - Genital herpes in adults
  - Herpes zoster (shingles) in adults
  - Chickenpox (varicella) in pediatric patients
- *Off-Label Common Uses*
  - VZV prevention in immunocompromised patients (level of evidence: G)

Formulations/Presentation

- USA: 500-mg tablet, 1-g tablet
- Canada: 500-mg tablet, 1-g tablet

Dosages and Suggested Regimens

- *Genital Herpes: Adult*
  - Initial episode (immunocompetent): Take 1 g twice daily for 7–10 days; extend duration of treatment if lesion is not healed after 10 days.
  - Initial episode (immunocompromised): Take 1 g twice daily for 5–10 days; extend duration of treatment if lesion is not healed after 10 days.
  - Initial episode (pregnant): Take 1 g daily for 7–10 days; extend duration of treatment if lesion is not healed after 10 days.
  - Recurrent episode (immunocompetent): Take 500 mg twice daily for 3 days *or* 1 g once daily for 5 days; most effective when initiated either during prodrome phase or within 1 day of onset of lesion.
  - Recurrent episode (pregnant): Take 500 mg twice daily for 3 days *or* 1 g once daily for 5 days.
  - Suppressive therapy (immunocompetent): Take 500 mg *or* 1 g once daily. Reassess the need for continued treatment annually.
  - Suppressive therapy (immunocompromised): Take 500 mg twice daily. Reassess the need for continued treatment annually.
  - Suppressive therapy (pregnant): Take 500 mg twice daily beginning at 36 weeks of gestation until delivery; for patients with primary infection during the third trimester, suppressive therapy may be considered before 36 weeks of gestation.

- *Genital Herpes: Pediatric*
  - First episode: Take 20 mg/kg/dose orally every 12 hours, with a maximum dose of 1 g/dose. Treat for 7–10 days. Some patients may need extension of treatment duration if lesion has not healed by 10 days.
  - Recurrent episode: Take 20 mg/kg/dose orally every 12 hours, with a maximum dose of 1 g/dose. Treat for 5–10 days. Adolescents without HIV may receive 500 mg every 12 hours for 3 days alternatively.
  - Suppressive therapy (patients without HIV): Take 20 mg/kg/dose orally once daily, with a maximum dose of 500 mg/dose. Doses of 1 g/day may be more effective in patients with ≥10 occurrences per year. Reassess the need for continued treatment annually.
  - Suppressive therapy (patients with HIV: take 500 mg orally every 12 hours). Reassess the need for continued treatment annually.
- *Orolabial HSV (Gingivostomatitis, Cold Sores): Adult*
  - Initial infection (immunocompetent): Take 1 gram twice daily for 7–10 days.
  - Initial infection (immunocompromised): Take 1 g twice daily for 5–10 days until complete resolution of lesion.
  - Recurrent infection (immunocompetent): Take 2 g twice daily for 1 day.
  - Recurrent infection (immunocompromised): Take 1 g twice daily for 5–10 days until complete resolution of lesion.
  - Suppressive therapy (immunocompetent): Take 500 mg once daily *or* 1 g once daily.
  - Suppressive therapy (immunocompromised): Take 500 mg twice daily.
- *Orolabial HSV (Gingivostomatitis, Cold Sores): Pediatric*
  - Patients without HIV treatment

    Infants ≥3 months, children, and adolescents: Dose is 20 mg/kg/dose orally every 12 hours. Maximum dose of 1000 mg/dose. Treat immunocompromised patients for 5–7 days and immunocompromised patients 10–14 days.

Patients ≥12 years old: Take 2 g orally every 12 hours for 1 day.

- Patients with HIV

  Treatment (adolescents): Take 1 g orally every 12 hours for 5–10 days

  Suppressive therapy (adolescents): Take 500 mg orally every 12 hours

- *Herpes Zoster (Shingles): Adults*
  - Acute localized dermatomal lesions: Take 1 g three times a day for 7–10 days. Initiate at the earliest sign of lesion. Treatment is most effective within 72 hours of rash onset.
  - Disseminated zoster: Take 1 g three times daily for 10–14 days after receiving initial therapy with IV acyclovir and the formation of new lesions has ceased.
- *Chickenpox (Varicella): Pediatric*
  - Infants ≥3 months, children, adolescents: Take 20 mg/kg/dose orally every 8 hours for 5 days with a maximum dose of 1 g/dose. Initiate treatment within 24 hours of rash onset for best results. Immunocompromised patients should be treated for 7–14 days depending upon clinical response. Patients with HIV may require 4–6 weeks of treatment.
- *VZV Prevention in Hematopoietic Cell Transplant (HCT) Recipients (off-label): Adult*
  - *Post-exposure prophylaxis*: Take 1 g orally three times daily within 96 hours of exposure. Continue for 22 days after exposure.
  - *Prevention of VZV reactivation in seropositive patients*: Take 500 mg orally twice daily for 1 year following transplantation.
- *VZV Prevention in Hematopoietic Cell Transplant (HCT) Recipients (Off-Label): Pediatric*
  - *Post-exposure prophylaxis*: Take 500 mg (if <40 kg) or 1 g (if ≥40 kg) orally three times daily within 48 hours of exposure. Continue for 22 days after exposure.
  - *Prevention of VZV reactivation in seropositive patients*: Take 250 (if <40 kg) or 500 mg (if ≥40 kg) orally twice daily.

- *VZV Prevention in Solid Organ Transplant Recipients (Off-Label): Adult*
  - *Solid organ transplant recipients* (VZV-seropositive patients not requiring CMV prophylaxis): Take 500 mg orally twice daily for 3–6 months after transplantation and during periods of lymphodepletion.

Baseline Investigations and Considerations

Pharmacokinetics

- Valacyclovir is converted to acyclovir and *L*-valine by first-pass metabolism.
- Bioavailability is 54.5% ± 9.1% and is not altered by administration with food.
- Half-life ranges from 2.5 to 3.3 hours.
- Excretion is primarily excreted through urine.

Use in Special Populations

- Approved for use in children. Dosing adjustments based on weight may need to be done.
- Listed as FDA pregnancy category B (former FDA classification).
- Caution should be exercised when prescribing to lactating women. A 500-mg dose of valacyclovir to a lactating mother provides a nursing infant with less than 2% of the exposure obtained after a standard neonatal dose of 30 mg/kg/day. The decision to continue or discontinue breastfeeding while a mother is on valacyclovir should consider the risk of infant virus exposure, the benefits of breastfeeding to the infant, and the benefits of valacyclovir to the mother. Valacyclovir is considered compatible with breastfeeding.
- Dosage adjustments are required in patients with renal impairment, with lower doses indicated as the patient's creatinine clearance decreases

- Dosage modification is not necessary for those with hepatic impairment. Data shows that the rate but not the extent of conversion to active acyclovir is decreased in patients with hepatic impairment.

Monitoring

- Kidney function (especially in elderly patients)
- CNS function (altered mental status, mood changes, seizures, hallucinations)
- CBC (risk of thrombotic thrombocytopenic purpura and hemolytic uremic syndrome)

Contraindications and Cautions

- Valacyclovir is contraindicated in patients with known hypersensitivity to valacyclovir, acyclovir, or other components in the formulation.

Important Drug Interactions

- *No significant drug or food interactions with valacyclovir are known.*

Adverse Effects and Their Management

- Acute kidney injury, including obstructive nephropathy
- Neurotoxicity: including confusion, agitation, lethargy, hallucination, impaired consciousness, aphasia, ataxia, myoclonus, tremor, and seizures
- Thrombotic thrombocytopenic purpura (TTP)
- Hemolytic uremic syndrome (HUS)
- Gastrointestinal: abdominal pain and nausea
- Headache

- Nasopharyngitis
- Skin rash
- Dysmenorrhea

Carcinogenicity (if Known, Including Mouse Painting Studies)

- No studies have shown that valacyclovir was carcinogenic.

Patch Test Concentration

- Not available

Essential Patient Information

- Take medications as directed at the first sign of lesion onset.
- Alert your provider if your lesions are not healed after finishing the medication.
- Monitor for signs of altered CNS function (confusion, headaches, hallucinations, seizures).
- Monitor for signs of kidney injury (pain with urination, blood in urine, back pain).
- Monitor for excess bruising, rash, or yellowing of the skin.

References

Acyclovir (Zovirax)

1. FDA drug monograph (acyclovir). Available from (https://www.accessdata.fda.gov/drugsatfda_docs/label/2014/021478s007lbl.pdf). Accessed 27 June 2024.
2. De Groot AC. Patch testing. 3rd ed. Volume 3 Chapter 3.

Berdazimer

3. FDA drug monograph (Berdazimer). Available from (https://www.accessdata.fda.gov/drugsatfda_docs/label/2024/217424s000lbl.pdf). Accessed 9 Feb 2024.
4. LexiComp drug monograph (Berdazimer). Available from: LexiComp Online at online.Lexi.com. Copyright 2024 UptoDate, Inc.
5. Browning JC, Cartwright M, Thorla I, et al. A patient-centered perspective of molluscum contagiosum as reported by B-SIMPLE4 clinical trial patients and caregivers: global impression of change and exit interview substudy results. Am J Clin Dermatol. 2023;24:119–33. https://doi.org/10.1007/s40257-022-00733-9.
6. Browning JC, Enloe C, Cartwright M, et al. Efficacy and safety of topical nitric oxide–releasing berdazimer gel in patients with molluscum contagiosum. JAMA Dermatol. 2022;158(8):871–8. https://doi.org/10.1001/jamadermatol.2022.2721.
7. Cartwright M, Enloe C, Stripling S, Maeda-Chubachi T. Pharmacokinetic profile, safety, and tolerability of topical Berdazimer gel, 10.3% in patients with molluscum contagiosum. J Drugs Dermatol. 2022;21(10):1104–10. https://doi.org/10.36849/jdd.6938.
8. Hebert AA, Siegfried EC, Durham T, et al. Efficacy and tolerability of an investigational nitric oxide–releasing topical gel in patients with molluscum contagiosum: a randomized clinical trial. J Am Acad Dermatol. 2020;82(4):887–94. https://doi.org/10.1016/j.jaad.2019.09.064.

Famciclovir

9. FDA drug monograph (FAMVIR). Available from https://www.accessdata.fda.gov/drugsatfda_docs/label/2011/020363s037lbl.pdf. Accessed 04/12/2023.
10. LexiComp drug monograph (Famciclovir). Available from: LexiComp Online at online.Lexi.com. Copyright 2022 UptoDate, Inc.
11. Wald A, Selke S, Warren T, Aoki FY, Sacks S, Diaz-Mitoma F, Corey L. Comparative efficacy of famciclovir and valacyclovir for suppression of recurrent genital herpes and viral shedding. Sex Transm Dis. 2006;33(9):529–33. https://doi.org/10.1097/01.olq.0000204723.15765.91. PMID: 16540883.
12. Bist A, Savitha A, Gumma KM. Efficacy of valacyclovir and famciclovir in herpes zoster: a comparative study. Indian J Pharmacol.

2020;52(6):472–5. https://doi.org/10.4103/ijp.IJP_555_18. PMID: 33666187; PMCID: PMC8092181.

Penciclovir (Denavir)

13. FDA drug monograph (DENAVIR). Available from https://www.accessdata.fda.gov/drugsatfda_docs/label/2013/020629s016lbl.pdf. Accessed 04/14/2023.
14. LexiComp drug monograph (Penciclovir). Available from: LexiComp Online at online.Lexi.com. Copyright 2022 UptoDate, Inc.

Valacyclovir (Valtrex)

15. FDA drug monograph (VALTREX – valacyclovir hydrochloride). Available from https://www.accessdata.fda.gov/drugsatfda_docs/label/2008/020487s014lbl.pdf. Accessed 04/17/2023.
16. LexiComp drug monograph (Valacyclovir). Available from: LexiComp Online at online.Lexi.com. Copyright 2022 UptoDate, Inc.
17. Wald A, Selke S, Warren T, Aoki FY, Sacks S, Diaz-Mitoma F, Corey L. Comparative efficacy of famciclovir and valacyclovir for suppression of recurrent genital herpes and viral shedding. Sex Transm Dis. 2006;33(9):529–33. https://doi.org/10.1097/01.olq.0000204723.15765.91. PMID: 16540883.
18. Lin WR, Lin HH, Lee SS, Tsai HC, Huang CK, Wann SR, Chen YS, Chiang SC, Yen MY, Liu YC. Comparative study of the efficacy and safety of valaciclovir versus acyclovir in the treatment of herpes zoster. J Microbiol Immunol Infect. 2001;34(2):138–42. PMID: 11456360.

Atopic Dermatitis: Topical Therapy

17

Rebecca M. Law

Contents

Introduction

Atopic dermatitis is primarily a disease seen in infants and young children. Treatment with topical therapies is the standard of care, although for severe cases systemic therapies such as biologic agents are effective. Topical pharmacologic therapies include the use of topical corticosteroids (TCS), topical calcineurin inhibitors (TCI), and phosphodiesterase (PDE)-4 inhibitors. Topical non-pharmacologic treatment modalities include the copious use of moisturizers, wet wrap therapy, etc. which are not discussed in this chapter.

R. M. Law (✉)
School of Pharmacy and Faculty of Medicine (Discipline of Family Medicine), Memorial University of Newfoundland, St. John's, NL, Canada
e-mail: rlaw@mun.ca; rlawUCSF@gmail.com

R. M. Law, H. I. Maibach (eds.), *Handbook of Topical Drug Treatment in Dermatology*,
https://doi.org/10.1007/978-3-031-93616-6_17

Topical Corticosteroids (TCS)

Topical corticosteroids (TCS) are first-line treatments for atopic dermatitis. They remain the standard of care. See Chap. 18: Topical Corticosteroids for a discussion of TCS and the monographs for individual TCS. Not all TCS have been FDA approved for use in infants and children.

Topical Calcineurin Inhibitors (TCI)

Topical calcineurin inhibitors (TCI) are usually considered second-line treatments for atopic dermatitis. They are efficacious but have potential side effects including a carcinogenicity concern. They are not FDA approved for use in children <2 years of age. There are two calcineurin inhibitors used topically for atopic dermatitis: tacrolimus (Protopic) and pimecrolimus (Elidel). Tacrolimus 0.03% ointment is approved for children 2–15 years and adults, whereas the 0.1% ointment is approved only for adults. Pimecrolimus 1% cream is not FDA approved for use in children <2 years of age. The drug monographs for tacrolimus and pimecrolimus are provided below.

Phosphodiesterase (PDE)-4 Inhibitors

Crisaborole and apremilast are small-molecule phosphodiesterase (PDE)-4 inhibitors. Cyclic nucleotide PDEs break down cAMP and cGMP into inactive metabolites, and there is increased PDE activity in AD, creating a proinflammatory state that may result in the stimulation of Th_2 cells to release inflammatory mediators. PDE-4 inhibitors inhibit the increased PDE activity; and crisaborole ointment is FDA approved for the treatment of mild-to-moderate AD in adults and children 2 years of age or older [1]. Crisaborole is applied topically, whereas apremilast is an oral medication. Thus, only the drug monograph for crisaborole is provided below.

Janus Kinase (JAK) Inhibitors

Janus kinase (JAK) inhibitors target JAK/STAT and signal transducers and activators of transcription. JAK inhibitors inhibit this signal pathway, thus blocking the transcription of proinflammatory cytokines that play a central role in the pathogenesis of many inflammatory and autoimmune diseases, including atopic dermatitis, psoriasis, and vitiligo [2]. There are topical and systemic JAK inhibitors—systemic JAK inhibitors are also useful as treatment of steroid refractory graft-versus-host disease, myelofibrosis, and polycythemia vera [3]. Ruxolitinib (topical) is a JAK inhibitor approved for atopic dermatitis and vitiligo and investigated for psoriasis. See Chap. 21: Psoriasis for the ruxolitinib (topical) drug monograph.

Drug Monographs

Topical Corticosteroids (TCS)

See Chap. 18: Topical Corticosteroids

Ruxolitinib

See Chap. 21: Psoriasis

Tacrolimus (Topical) [4, 5, 6]

Classification and Mode of Action

- Tacrolimus is a topical calcineurin inhibitor (TCI). Tacrolimus inhibits T-cell activation by first binding to an intracellular protein, FKBP-12. A complex of tacrolimus-FKBP-12, calcium, calmodulin, and calcineurin is then formed, and the calcineurin phosphatase activity is inhibited.

Indications and Dermatological Uses

- *Clinical indications (FDA)*: Atopic dermatitis (moderate to severe) in immunocompetent patients not responsive to conventional therapy or when conventional therapy (i.e., corticosteroids) is not appropriate.
- *Off-label common uses*: Oral lichen planus, psoriasis (intertriginous and facial), pyoderma gangrenosum, vitiligo.
- Not approved for <2 years of age. 0.03% ointment is approved for 2–15 years old.

Formulations/Presentation

- USA: 0.03% and 0.1% ointment
- Canada: 0.03% and 0.1% ointment

Dosages and Suggested Regimens

- For atopic dermatitis: Apply a thin layer twice daily. Duration of use: Either discontinue use when symptoms have cleared or (off-label use) go to maintenance therapy using 0.03% or 0.1% ointment twice daily twice a week.
- For oral lichen planus (off-label use): Apply 0.1% ointment up to four times daily. Treatment period in clinical trials ranged from 4 to 6 weeks.
- For psoriasis (intertriginous and facial) (off-label use): 0.1% ointment twice daily for 6–8 weeks.
- For pyoderma gangrenosum (off-label use): 0.1% ointment once daily and may taper to 0.03% once daily after improvement is seen.
- For vitiligo (off-label use): 0.1% ointment twice daily and reassess every 3–6 months for adequate response.

Pharmacokinetics

- Minimally absorbed. Serum concentration is about 2 ng/mL in the majority of adult patients studied (range: undetectable to 20 ng/mL) using the 0.1% ointment.
- Bioavailability about 0.5%.

Use in Special Populations

- Children 2–15 years should use 0.03% ointment only (FDA approved).
- Not for use in children <2 years of age.
- Tacrolimus is transferred across the placenta. The use of systemically administered tacrolimus during pregnancy has been associated with neonatal hyperkalemia and renal dysfunction. Tacrolimus should be used during pregnancy only if the potential benefit to the mother justifies a potential risk to the fetus.
- Although systemic absorption of tacrolimus following topical applications of tacrolimus is minimal relative to systemic administration, it is known that tacrolimus is excreted in human milk. Because of the potential for serious adverse reactions in nursing infants from tacrolimus, a decision should be made whether to discontinue nursing or to discontinue the drug, taking into account the importance of the drug to the mother.
- No manufacturer recommendations for dosage adjustments in renal or hepatic failure.
- Adverse profile in the elderly (>65) was consistent with other adult patients. No manufacturer recommendations for dosage adjustments in the elderly.

Contraindications and Cautions

- Should not be used in patients with Netherton's syndrome or skin diseases with a potential for increased systemic absorption.
- Avoid treatment on malignant or premalignant skin conditions, as these can present as dermatitis.

Important Drug Interactions

- Formal topical drug interaction studies with Protopic ointment have not been conducted. Based on its minimal extent of absorption, interactions of Protopic ointment with systemically administered drugs are unlikely to occur but cannot be ruled out.

- The concomitant administration of known CYP3A4 inhibitors in patients with widespread and/or erythrodermic disease should be done with caution.

Adverse Effects and Their Management

- Local symptoms such as skin burning (burning sensation, stinging, soreness) or pruritus, most commonly during the first few days of use and typically improve as the lesions of atopic dermatitis heal.
- Use in patients with Netherton's syndrome is not recommended due to the potential for increased systemic absorption of tacrolimus.
- Safety has not been established in patients with generalized erythroderma.
- No phototoxicity and no photoallergenicity was detected in clinical studies of 12 and 216 normal volunteers, respectively.
- One out of 198 normal volunteers showed evidence of sensitization in a contact sensitization study.

Carcinogenicity

- Although a causal relationship has not been established, rare cases of malignancy (e.g., skin and lymphoma) have been reported in patients treated with TCIs.
- The enhancement of ultraviolet carcinogenicity is not necessarily dependent on phototoxic mechanisms. Despite the absence of observed phototoxicity in humans, Protopic ointment shortened the time to skin tumor formation in an animal photocarcinogenicity study. Therefore, it is prudent for patients to minimize or avoid natural or artificial sunlight exposure.
- No evidence of genotoxicity was seen in bacterial (*Salmonella* and *E. coli*) or mammalian (Chinese hamster lung-derived cells) in vitro assays of mutagenicity, the in vitro CHO/HGPRT assay of mutagenicity, or in vivo clastogenicity assays performed in mice. Tacrolimus did not cause unscheduled DNA synthesis in rodent hepatocytes.
- In a 52-week photocarcinogenicity study, the median time to the onset of skin tumor formation was decreased in hairless

mice following chronic topical dosing with concurrent exposure to UV radiation (40 weeks of treatment followed by 12 weeks of observation) with tacrolimus ointment at ≥0.1% tacrolimus.

Patch Test Concentration

- 5% alcohol

Essential Patient Information

- Use sun protection. Limit sun exposure even when the medication is not on the skin.
- Minimize or avoid exposure to natural or artificial sunlight (tanning beds or UVA/B treatment).
- Do not use sun lamps, tanning beds, or get treatment with ultraviolet light therapy during treatment with tacrolimus.
- Tacrolimus ointment is not for oral use. Oral ingestion may lead to adverse effects associated with systemic administration of tacrolimus. If oral ingestion occurs, seek medical advice.

Pimecrolimus [6, 7, 8]

Classification and Mode of Action

- Pimecrolimus is a topical calcineurin inhibitor indicated as second-line therapy for the short-term and noncontinuous chronic treatment of mild to moderate atopic dermatitis in non-immunocompromised adults and children 2 years of age and older, who have failed to respond adequately to other topical prescription treatments, or when those treatments are not advisable
- See tacrolimus for the mode of action.

Indications and Dermatological Uses

- *Clinical indications (FDA)*: Atopic dermatitis.
- *Off-label common uses*: Oral lichen planus, psoriasis (intertriginous and facial), rosacea, and vitiligo.
- Not FDA approved for children <2 years of age.

- FDA black box warning: Although a causal relationship has not been established, rare cases of malignancy (e.g., skin and lymphoma) have been reported in patients treated with topical calcineurin inhibitors, including Elidel cream, 1%.
  - Therefore: Continuous long-term use of topical calcineurin inhibitors, including Elidel cream, 1%, in any age group should be avoided, and application limited to areas of involvement with atopic dermatitis.

Formulations/Presentation

- USA: 1% cream (Elidel)
- Canada: 1% cream (Elidel)

Dosages and Suggested Regimens

- Atopic dermatitis: Apply a thin layer twice daily. Limit application to affected area. Discontinue use when symptoms resolve, and re-evaluate if symptoms persist >6 weeks.
- Oral lichen planus (off-label use): Apply twice daily for 1 month.
- Psoriasis (intertriginous and facial) (off-label use): Apply twice daily.
- Vitiligo (off-label use): Apply twice daily for 6 months. Treatment beyond 12 months may be useful.
- Rosacea (off-label use): Apply twice daily.

Pharmacokinetics

- Low systemic concentrations after topical use. Usually <2 ng/mL
- Protein binding 99.5% primarily to various lipoproteins
- Metabolized in the liver via CYP 3A4. Elimination half-life 30–40 hours. Excreted by fecal route (78% as metabolites, < 1% as unchanged drug)

Use in Special Populations

- Not recommended for use in children <2 years of age.
- Pregnancy: No adverse effects seen in animal reproduction studies after topical application.

- Breastfeeding: Unknown whether pimecrolimus is excreted in breast milk. Manufacturer recommends deciding whether to discontinue the drug or discontinue nursing, taking into account the importance of treatment to the mother.
- No manufacturer recommendations for dosage adjustments in renal or hepatic failure, or in the elderly.

Contraindications and Cautions

- Continuous long-term use should be avoided. Safety of intermittent use for >1 year has not been established.
- Avoid treatment on malignant or premalignant skin conditions, as these can present as dermatitis.
- Should not be used in patients with Netherton's syndrome or skin diseases with a potential for increased systemic absorption.
- Should not be used in immunocompromised adults and children, including patients on systemic immunosuppressive medications.
- Safety has not been established in patients with generalized erythroderma.
- Before commencing treatment, bacterial or viral infections at treatment sites should be resolved. Trials have not evaluated the safety and efficacy of Elidel cream 1% in the treatment of clinically infected atopic dermatitis.

Important Drug Interactions

- Avoid combination with systemic corticosteroids or other immunosuppressive agents, as pimecrolimus may enhance the immunosuppressive effect.
- Due to low blood levels of pimecrolimus detected in some patients after topical application, systemic drug interactions are not expected, but cannot be ruled out. Since pimecrolimus is metabolized by CYP 3A4, CYP 3A4 inhibitors may reduce its metabolism. Monitoring is recommended.
- Alcohol may enhance the dermatologic adverse effects of pimecrolimus. Monitoring is recommended.

Adverse Effects and Their Management

- The most commonly reported adverse reactions (≥1%) were application site burning, headache, nasopharyngitis, cough, influenza, pyrexia, and viral infection.
- While patients with atopic dermatitis are predisposed to superficial skin infections including eczema herpeticum (Kaposi's varicelliform eruption), treatment with Elidel cream 1% may be independently associated with an increased risk of varicella zoster virus infection (chicken pox or shingles), herpes simplex virus infection, or eczema herpeticum.
- In clinical trials, 15/1544 (1%) cases of skin papilloma (warts) were observed in subjects using Elidel cream 1%. The youngest subject was age 2 and the oldest was age 12. In cases where there is worsening of skin papillomas or they do not respond to conventional therapy, discontinuation of pimecrolimus should be considered until complete resolution of the warts is achieved.
- From clinical trial experience, no phototoxicity or photoallergenicity were detected. Also, there was no contact sensitization or cumulative irritation.
- From post-marketing experience (causal relationship to pimecrolimus use not established), the following have been reported: anaphylactic reactions, ocular irritation after application of the cream to the eye lids or near the eyes, angioneurotic edema, facial edema, skin flushing associated with alcohol use, skin discoloration, lymphomas, basal cell carcinoma, malignant melanoma, and squamous cell carcinoma.

Carcinogenicity

- Although a causal relationship has not been established, rare cases of malignancy (e.g., skin and lymphoma) have been reported in patients treated with topical calcineurin inhibitors

Patch Test Concentration

- 1% pet. If not available, test 1% pimecrolimus cream and its base.

Essential Patient Information

- Use sun protection. Limit sun exposure even when the medication is not on the skin. Do not use sun lamps, tanning beds, or get treatment with ultraviolet light therapy during treatment with pimecrolimus.
- Not for prolonged continuous use.

Crisaborole [9, 10]

Classification and Mode of Action

- Crisaborole is a phosphodiesterase 4 (PDE-4) inhibitor. PDE-4 inhibition results in increased intracellular cyclic adenosine monophosphate (cAMP) levels.

Indications and Dermatological Uses

- *Clinical indications (FDA)*: Treatment of mild to moderate atopic dermatitis in adults and pediatric patients >3 months of age

Formulations/Presentation

- USA: 2% ointment
- Canada: 2% ointment

Dosages and Suggested Regimens

- Apply thin film to affected area(s) twice daily. Consider reducing to once daily once clinical response is achieved.

Pharmacokinetics

- Crisaborole is absorbed systemically after topical application.
- Crisaborole is 97% protein bound.
- Crisaborole is metabolized by the liver.

Use in Special Populations

- Pregnancy: adverse effects not seen in animal reproduction studies, except with high oral doses that also produced maternal toxicity.
- Breastfeeding: Unknown whether excreted in breast milk.
- There are no dosage adjustments provided in the manufacturer's labeling for patients with altered kidney or liver function.
- There are no dosage adjustments provided in the manufacturer's labeling for use in pediatrics.

Contraindications and Cautions

- Riociguat (see below)

Important Drug Interactions

- Riociguat: Crisaborole may enhance the hypotensive effect of riociguat. This is a contraindication.

Adverse Effects and Their Management

- Pain at application site, including burning and stinging of the skin (1–10%), urticaria (<1%). Post marketing: allergic contact dermatitis and other hypersensitivity reactions have been reported.

Carcinogenicity

- No information yet available

Patch Test Concentration

- Not available

Essential Patient Information

- If there is severe application site irritation or if signs of an allergic reaction are seen (rash, hives), contact a medical professional.

References

1. Law RM, Gulliver W. Chapter 119: atopic dermatitis. In: Dipiro's pharmacotherapy: a pathophysiologic approach. 12th ed. NY: McGraw-Hill Medical; 2023. p. 1661–72.
2. Sluczanowska-Glabowska S, Ziegler-Krawczyk A, Szumilas K, Pawlik A. Role of Janus kinase inhibitors in therapy of psoriasis. J Clin Med. 2021;10(19):4307.
3. LexiComp drug monograph (Ruxolitinib). Available from: LexiComp Online at online.Lexi.com. Copyright 2024 UptoDate Inc.
4. FDA drug monograph (tacrolimus). Available from https://www.accessdata.fdau.gov/drugsatfda_docs/label/2000/50777lbl.pdf. Accessed 1 Aug 2024.
5. LexiComp drug monograph (Tacrolimus). Available from: LexiComp Online at online.Lexi.com. Copyright 2024 UptoDate, Inc.
6. De Groot AC. Patch testing. 3rd ed. Volume 3 Chapter 3.
7. FDA drug monograph (pimecrolimus). Available from https://www.accessdata.fda.gov/drugsatfda_docs/label/2014/021302s018lbl.pdf. Accessed 3 Aug 2024.
8. LexiComp drug monograph (pimecrolimus). Available from: LexiComp Online at online.Lexi.com. Copyright 2024 UptoDate, Inc.
9. FDA drug monograph (crisaborole). Available from https://www.accessdata.fda.gov/drugsatfda_docs/label/2020/207695s007s009s010lbl.pdf. Accessed 3 Aug 2024.
10. LexiComp drug monograph (crisaborole). Available from: LexiComp Online at online.Lexi.com. Copyright 2024 UptoDate, Inc.

18 Topical Corticosteroids

Kiha Kim, Taylor Skinner,
and Rebecca M. Law

Contents

K. Kim
Faculty of Medicine, Memorial University of Newfoundland,
St. John's, NL, Canada
e-mail: kihak@mun.ca

T. Skinner (✉)
Faculty of Medicine, Memorial University of Newfoundland,
St. John's, NL, Canada
e-mail: tcskinner@mun.ca

R. M. Law
School of Pharmacy and Faculty of Medicine (Discipline of Family
Medicine), Memorial University of Newfoundland, St. John's, NL, Canada
e-mail: rlaw@mun.ca; rlawUCSF@gmail.com

R. M. Law, H. I. Maibach (eds.), *Handbook of Topical Drug Treatment in Dermatology*,
https://doi.org/10.1007/978-3-031-93616-6_18

Introduction

Indications for Use

Topical corticosteroids (TCS) are a classification of anti-inflammatory drugs applied directly on the skin to treat various skin-related inflammatory diseases. They are effective in providing relief for ailments such as psoriasis, atopic dermatitis (eczema), rash, and multiple other miscellaneous skin conditions. TCS are first-line therapies for atopic dermatitis and psoriasis. Some TCS are also indicated for vitiligo (e.g., some of the fluorinated/higher potency TCS have this indication).

Although systemic corticosteroids can be an alternative effective method of combating severe or urgent/life-threatening inflammatory disease, they are not routinely used for atopic dermatitis or psoriasis—the TCS are. TCS provide more localized/focused areas of treatment with fewer adverse systemic effects.

Mechanisms of Action

TCS have anti-inflammatory, immunosuppressive, and vasoconstrictive properties. TCS induce phospholipase A2 inhibitory proteins which suppress the production of arachidonic acid and interleukin-1 that are responsible for inducing inflammation, thus reducing endogenous inflammation mediators. TCS have anti-inflammatory properties that aim to suppress the immune response at the site of application.

During the inflammatory process, blood vessels become dilated around the site of inflammation. TCS also work to reduce skin inflammation by constricting the blood vessels around the site of inflammation and reducing capillary wall permeability for leukocytes to enter.

These drugs also decrease the complement components and histamine activity, while inhibiting macrophage recruitment into the site of inflammation.

Formulations

TCS can be delivered in various dosage forms such as creams, ointments, gels, lotions, sprays, and foams. The mode of delivery varies based on the site of application and the severity of disease. For example, lotions and gels are commonly used in hairy areas (e.g. scalp), while ointments are used for dry scaly lesions or more severe cases (e.g. psoriasis on the palms), as ointments provide better occlusion and hence increased potency. Formulation bases in decreasing occlusion order are ointment > creams > lotions. Specific formulations available for each TCS are discussed in the drug monographs.

Suggested Regimens and Usage Guidance

Apply TCS sparingly. For hydrocortisone (the lowest potency corticosteroid), the frequency of use is up to three times daily for atopic dermatitis or 2–4 times daily for other corticosteroid-responsive dermatoses. Hair should be moved to allow direct application of the topical agent to the skin for a hairy skin. For betamethasone valerate (a medium potency corticosteroid), the frequency of use is once to twice daily depending on the formulation. Augmented ointment formulations of betamethasone dipropionate (a high potency corticosteroid) are often used once daily. for conditions such as plaque psoriasis, and can be used twice daily if needed. Reassessment at two weeks for efficacy is essential, and duration of use should be limited to minimize the risk of adverse effects, including systemic side effects. If continuing TCS use is needed, step down to a lower potency TCS as soon as possible.

TCS is for external use only, not for oral, ophthalmic, or intravaginal use; wash hands after use unless hands are part of the treatment area. Avoid contact with eyes; wash eyes thoroughly with water if contact occurs.

Do not use occlusive dressing unless otherwise stated, including the diaper area for pediatric populations, as they can significantly increase percutaneous absorption; occlusive dressings may be used for some TCS in some situations (e.g., for managing psoriasis or recalcitrant conditions) if their use is deemed necessary.

Therapy should usually be stopped once control has been met unless otherwise directed by a healthcare professional. If no improvements is seen, reassessment of diagnosis should be done.

Anti-inflammatory Potency Classifications

As mentioned above, the potency of TCS can vary greatly based on the innate anti-inflammatory potency of the drug, the vehicle/formulation, and whether the drug has been augmented or not. A drug in a tape, due to its occlusive properties, may be very potent (e.g., flurandrenolide tape). An ointment base provides more occlusion than a cream or lotion, and the same TCS in an ointment base may be more potent than in a cream or lotion. Augmented betamethasone dipropionate 0.05% ointment is one of the most potent TCS. Furthermore, the salt form of the drug may affect potency—for example, betamethasone dipropionate is more potent than betamethasone valerate. In addition, the site of application, the individual patient, and whether an occlusive dressing used may affect potency.

TCS have been classified from Groups 1 to 7, with Group 1 being the most potent and Group 7 being the least potent. The Topical Corticosteroid Potency Table in this chapter (Appendix A) is an updated table from a reference textbook chapter (Law and Gulliver 2023) using a seven-group classification [1]. This was collated from several classification systems and is currently a classification system used in the USA. There are other classification systems from different countries where TCS potencies are sorted into three, four, or five groups. We recently published an updated seven-group topical corticosteroid potency classification system [2].

Pharmacokinetic Considerations

Topical corticosteroids need to have sufficient percutaneous absorption on the skin for topical efficacy. Topical corticosteroids have low bioavailability in systemic circulation, as most is retained in the epidermal and dermal layers of the skin. There is a general consensus that most TCS are not significantly absorbed into the systemic circulation; however, this varies based on the innate characteristics of the particular TCS. Fluorinated TCS are more potent than non-fluorinated TCS, for example. See monographs for specific pharmacokinetics relating to a particular TCS.

Sites and Methods of Application Affecting Potency

When topical corticosteroids are applied onto the skin, only a small amount of the drug is percutaneously absorbed into the inner layer of the dermis and into the systemic circulation. This percutaneous absorption of the drug can be increased by using occlusive dressings, by using different vehicles, by increasing the dose concentration, or when a layer of the skin has been damaged due to skin conditions such as psoriasis and eczema. Hence, these drugs have higher rates of absorption when applied to the face, scalp, eyelid, axilla, or scrotum, compared to thicker surfaces of the skin with a stratum corneum layer such as the elbow, palm, or sole.

Adverse Effects

Common side effects include mild sensations of burning and stinging that occur within the first few application cycles of TCS, which is transient. However, prolonged uses of TCS at high doses can cause skin thinning or reddening (erythema) which in turn makes the skin more susceptible to bruises and stretching. Therefore, people with sensitive skin, including young infants and elders, are more likely to experience these side effects. Other dermatologic adverse effects of TCS include acne vulgaris, alopecia, pruritus, xeroderma, dermatitis, folliculitis, skin discoloration, skin rashes, and telangiectasia.

Non-dermatologic adverse effects of TCS include the following:

Ophthalmic: conjunctivitis
Endocrine: hyperglycemia
Gastrointestinal: dysgeusia

Nervous system: paresthesia.

Adverse systemic effects can occur especially from prolonged use of TCS and especially if used on large areas of the skin, and in particular with the high potency TCS groups (classified in Groups 1 and 2 of the TCS Potency Table included as Appendix A). Transient manifestations of Cushing's syndrome, hyperglycemia, and reversible hypothalamic-pituitary-adrenal axis suppression have occurred for certain patients.

Although rare, some patients have had very negative side effects that require drug discontinuation. The possible side effects that should be monitored are Cushing syndrome-like symptoms, adrenal gland problems, vision changes, high blood pressure, excessive skin changes including stretching, irritation, and thinning.

Adverse Effects in Special Populations, Pregnancy, and Lactation Concerns

- Although the use of TCS is not associated with a significant risk of adverse pregnancy outcomes, however, newborn infants have an increased risk of being low weight and birth, though the risk is shown to be low.
- Pregnant populations should avoid application of the drug to high absorptive areas such as the arm pit, skin folds, and vulva; extra precaution should be taken for application to abdomen, breast, and thighs, as they are more prone to developing striae. In general, medium potency TCS should be used with avoidance of very-high-potency agents.
- Pregnant women should use low- to medium-potency TCS and avoid using very-high-potency agents; rectal corticosteroids may be used for flares in pregnant patients with inflammatory bowel disease, but maintenance therapy should be avoided.
- Regular doses of rectal corticosteroids are not expected to suppress lactation.
- For many TCS, no specific human data can be found for breastfeeding populations, although it is speculative to be probably

compatible; however, for some TCS traces of drug can be detected in breastmilk. The decision to breastfeed during TCS use should be considered based on the benefits provided to the mother versus the potential drug exposure to the infant. If the decision is to breastfeed, avoid application of TCS to the nipple and areola when breastfeeding.

- Topical corticosteroids can be used for parents who are planning a pregnancy; although the use of rectal corticosteroid for ulcerative colitis does not decrease fertility, patients with inflammatory bowel disease may have decreased fertility and should plan pregnancy after a 3–6-month remission.
- Children are more prone to systemic effects and may absorb proportionally higher amounts of TCS (due to larger body surface area to body mass ratio in comparison to adults). When used in children, HPA suppression, intracranial hypertension, and Cushing syndrome have been reported; growth of the child should be monitored routinely as prolonged use may stunt growth velocity. Use with caution in pediatric patients; generally, TCS should not be used in neonates and infants under 1 year of age. Use of augmented formulations in children <13 years of age is generally not recommended. (Refer to Chaps. 4 and 5 for further discussion.)
- Topical corticosteroids should be used cautiously for older populations in the smallest possible effective dose for the shortest duration possible.

Contraindications

TCS should not be used in combination with calcipotriene or with clotrimazole. Do not use if the patient is hypersensitive to corticosteroids.

Monitoring Considerations

Ocular Effects

TCS may increase the risk of cataracts and glaucoma. Monitor for ocular symptoms and avoid contact with eyes.

Skin Reactions

Discontinue if skin rashes, contact dermatitis, or other dermatologic reactions occur (as described above). As noted, mild stinging or burning may be transient and do not require drug discontinuation. Prolonged use of TCS may lead to steroid atrophy, and striae may be seen.

Systemic Effects

TCS may be absorbed percutaneously. Absorption of TCS may cause manifestations of Cushing syndrome, hyperglycemia, or glycosuria. Absorption can be increased by using occlusive dressings, application to denuded skin, application to large surface areas, or prolonged use.

HPA axis suppression and adrenal insufficiency can occur, especially in children or with augmented formulation use: foam, gel, lotion (augmented), and ointment (augmented):

- ACTH stimulation test, morning plasma cortisol test, and urinary free-cortisol test can be obtained when signs of adrenal suppression have been detected; reassess again after 2 weeks.

Monitor and assess for hyperglycemia (showing confusion, fatigue, increased thirst, hunger, polyuria).

Some TCS formulations may contain benzyl alcohol and other derivatives; large amounts of benzyl alcohol (e.g. ≥99 mg/kg/day) have been associated with a potentially fatal toxicity; avoid benzyl alcohol-containing formulations for newborn patients; monitor for signs and symptoms of hypotension, respiratory distress, gasping respirations, CNS dysfunction, and cardiovascular collapse. Some TCS formulations may contain propylene glycol; in neonates large amounts of propylene glycol even topically may be associated with metabolic acidosis, seizures, renal failure, and CNS depressions potentially resulting in fatalities. Toxicities of propylene glycol reported in children and adults have included lactic acidosis, seizures and respiratory depression.

Patch Test Concentration

In general, TCS may be tested at 0.1% and 1% in alcohol; late readings (6–10 days) are strongly recommended [3]. Other patch test formulations for specific TCS listed in deGroots have been included with each monograph, as available.

Drug Interactions

- General contraindications within TCS applies. TCS may suppress the wheal and flare reactions to skin test antigens.
- Aldesleukin: Corticosteroids may diminish the antineoplastic effect of aldesleukin; combination should be avoided.
- CYP3A4 inhibitors may increase the serum concentration of betamethasone (topical).
- Nirmatrelvir and ritonavir may increase the serum concentration of topical corticosteroids.

Use in Special Populations

- See Under Adverse Effects Above
- Pregnancy and Breastfeeding
  - The systemic bioavailability of topical corticosteroids may be variable (see Chap. 1). In general, the use of topical corticosteroids is not associated with a significant risk of adverse pregnancy outcomes. However, there may be an increased risk of low birth weight infants following maternal use of very potent topical products especially in high doses. In general, the use of the least potent product in limited amounts for the shortest time period is recommended during pregnancy.
  - Not adequate data – may be teratogenic in certain animal populations.
  - Use only if necessary; do not used in large amounts for prolonged time periods.
  - Extra caution for nursing women, as TCS (and systemic corticosteroids) can be distributed in milk.

  - Avoid application of TCS to the nipple and areola when breastfeeding. If needed, apply TCS immediately after breastfeeding, then clean nipples prior to the next feeding.
- Pediatrics
  - Extra precaution should be used for young children, as adrenal suppression may be increased with decreasing age. Other adverse effects as described above under Systemic Effects.
  - Example: Seventy-three percent of children 6–12 years old and 32% of children 3 months–12 years for betamethasone dipropionate-augmented ointment or cream experienced adrenal suppression. Thus this product is not recommended for patients younger than 13 years old for augmented ointment or cream.
- Renal or Hepatic Insufficiency
  - In general, there are no dosage adjustments needed for patients with altered renal or hepatic insufficiency. Any specific concerns will be discussed in the individual monographs.

Essential Patient Information

- Apply TCS sparingly to a clean, dry skin. Clean the hands before and after application.
- Do not use occlusive dressing unless otherwise stated, including in the diaper area.
- Do not apply very-high-potency agents to the face, groin, axillae, or diaper area—not for oral, ophthalmic, or intravaginal use.
- TCS are not generally subject to restriction in sporting activities, but competitors should check with the appropriate sports authorities; furthermore, care may be advisable with TCS if conditions liable to promote systemic absorption are present.

Individual drug monographs follow. These are arranged in order of potency, as per Appendix A. Where potency changes based on drug augmentation, formulation, or concentration, the drug monograph is placed at the first occurrence of the drug, i.e., the highest drug potency.

If part of a monograph is similar to what has been discussed in the Introduction to TCS (e.g., mechanisms of action or adverse effects), that section will be omitted.

High to Super High Potency

Betamethasone Dipropionate (Augmented and Nonaugmented)

(not augmented is included in this monograph)

Classification and Mode of Action

- Class of betamethasone dipropionate augmented to become more potent.
  - Betamethasone dipropionate not augmented (classic) is also available.
- A synthetic fluorinated corticosteroid.
- *Potency varies with the formulation as follows:*
  - Betamethasone dipropionate (augmented) ointment 0.05% and gel 0.05% are Class 1: super potent.
  - Betamethasone dipropionate (not augmented) ointment 0.05% and gel 0.05% are Class 2: highly potent.
  - Betamethasone dipropionate (augmented) cream 0.05% and lotion 0.05% are Class 2: highly potent.
  - Betamethasone dipropionate (not augmented) cream 0.05% is Class 3: mid-high potent.
  - Betamethasone dipropionate (not augmented) lotion 0.05%, emulsion 0.05% (Sernivo), and spray 0.05% (Sernivo) are Class 4 or 5: mid- to mid-low potent.
- See under Introduction for other details.

Formulations/Presentation

- USA: 0.05% ointment, gel, lotion.
- Canada: Ointment, as dipropionate augmented: diprolene: 0.05% (50 g), generic: 0.05% (15 g, 50 g)

Dosages and Suggested Regimens

Cream 0.05% and ointment 0.05%: adolescents (topical): Apply a thin film to affected area once or twice daily; maximum dose: 50 g/week; evaluate continuation of therapy if no improvement within 2 weeks of treatment.

Gel 0.05%: children ≥12 years and adolescents (topical): Apply a thin layer to the affected area once or twice daily; rub in gently; maximum dose: 50 g/week; not recommended for use longer than 2 weeks.

Lotion 0.05%: adolescents (topical): Apply a few drops to the affected area once or twice daily; rub in gently; maximum dose: 50 mL/week; not recommended for use for longer than 2 weeks.

Pharmacokinetics

- Percutaneous absorption.
  - Can be increased by increasing concentration and using occlusive dressings.
  - Percutaneous absorption using occlusive dressings increased notably for up to 96 hours, but no real differences for the first 24 hours vs regular topical application.
  - Up to 30–90% absorption when administered rectally.
- Metabolized by liver.
- Excreted by the kidneys or sometimes in the bile.
- Half-life is 8.5 days, while the drug was completely eliminated 48 days after withdrawal.

Use in Special Populations

- See under Introduction.

  - Studies: Seventy-three percent of children 6–12 years old and 32% of children 3 months–12 years using augmented ointment or cream experienced adrenal suppression.
  - Thus, augmented ointment or creams are not recommended for patients younger than 13 years old.

Contraindications

- Contraindications associated when used in combination with calcipotriene or with clotrimazole
- Not to use if hypersensitive to corticosteroids

Drug Interaction

- General contraindications within the topical corticosteroids applies.
- Aldesleukin: Corticosteroids may diminish the antineoplastic effect of aldesleukin; combination should be avoided.
- CYP3A4 inhibitors May increase the serum concentration of betamethasone (topical).
- Nirmatrelvir and ritonavir may increase the serum concentration of topical corticosteroids.

Patch Test Concentration

- 1.0% pet. (Chemotechnique); 0.5% pet., 0.1% pet. (SmartPracticeCanada)

Essential Patient Information

- Apply topical sparingly to affected areas.
- Do not use if atrophy is present at the treatment site.
- Do not cover with occlusive dressing unless directed otherwise by a healthcare provider.
- Do not apply very-high-potency agents to the face, groin, axillae, or diaper area—not for oral, ophthalmic, or intravaginal use.
- Wash the hands after use.
- Product use should be stopped if irritation or allergic reactions occur; consult your doctor immediately.

Clobetasol Propionate

Classification and Mode of Action

- Clobetasol is a synthetic fluorinated corticosteroid.
- Indicated for the relief of the inflammatory and pruritic manifestations of corticosteroid-responsive dermatoses in patients 12 years of age and older.
- See Introduction.

Formulation/Presentation

- US: 0.05% as cream, ointment, shampoo, lotion, solution, foam, and gel
- Canada: 0.05% as cream, ointment, shampoo, solution, foam, and liquid

Dosages and Suggested Regimens

- Clobetasol propionate cream, foam gel, lotion, and ointment use should not exceed 14 days, while the shampoo formulas should not exceed 4 consecutive weeks—due to a possibility of HPA-axis suppression.
- The total dosage should not exceed 50 grams per week.
- Topical clobetasol propionate should be applied sparingly in thin films and applied gently onto the skin twice daily; shampoo and solutions are applied to the scalp once and twice daily, respectively.
- Do not use occlusion.

Pharmacokinetics

- Follows pharmacokinetic elimination of general topical corticosteroids.
- However, systemic metabolism not fully characterized.
- Excreted in the bile and in urine.

- Percutaneous absorption varies among individuals; absorption with gel is greater than cream; absorption increased with occlusive dressings and with an inflamed skin.
- Peak plasma concentration occurred after 3 hours of a single application.
- Mean peak plasma of 0.63 ng/mL of clobetasol propionate concentrations occurred 8 hours after a second 30-g dose (applied 13 hours after first dose) of 0.05% ointment for healthy individuals with normal skin; mean peak plasma was slightly higher when using the 0.05% cream; another study showed mean peak plasma concentration of 2.3 or 4.6 ng/mL which occurred 3 hours after a single application of a 25-g dose of 0.05% ointment for subjects with psoriasis or eczema, respectively.

Use in Special Populations

- Not recommended for children under the age of 12
  - Can lead to HPA axis suppression, intracranial hypertension, and Cushing syndrome for children who received the topical
- Clobex and Clodan shampoo not recommended for patients under the age of 17
- Adverse effects reported in geriatric patients over 65 years of age similar to pediatric patients, although clinical studies are insufficient
- Pregnancy
  - Teratogenic properties for pregnant women are not known; however, clinical studies in mice and rabbits have shown harm to the fetus (cleft palate, skeletal abnormalities, cranioschisis).
  - Clinical studies in rats demonstrated decrease in viable fetuses from increased fetal resorptions when the dose was higher than 50 mcg/kg daily.
- No human data for breastfeeding patients

Contraindications and Cautions

- See Introduction.
- This is also contraindicated for individuals with primary infections of the scalp.
- Canadian labelling: The product should not be used children under 2 years of age (for shampoo and spray formulas) and under 1 year of age (for cream, ointment, scalp formulas); avoid application to eyes and eyelids; should be careful for treatment of rosacea, acne vulgaris, perioral dermatitis, or perianal and genital pruritus, viral (herpes or varicella) lesions of the skin, bacterial or fungal skin infections, parasitic infections, skin manifestations relating to tuberculosis or syphilis, and eruptions following vaccinations.

Carcinogenicity

- No evidence of clobetasol-induced mutagenesis for in vitro studies

Patch Test Concentration

- 1% pet. (Chemotechnique, SmartPracticeCanada, SmartPracticeEurope), 0.25% pet. (SmartPracticeCanada, SmartPracticeEurope), 0.1% alc. (SmartPracticeCanada)

Essential Patient Information

- Applied sparingly in thin films and applied gently to the skin. Do not use for longer than 2 weeks (4 weeks for shampoos).
- Cream, ointment, gel, lotion, foam, and shampoo for vehicles should not be applied to the face and intertriginous areas (axilla and groin).
- Dosage of the drug should not exceed 50 g/week in a 0.05% cream, ointment, foam, or shampoo.
- Clobetasol propionate cream, foam, gel, lotion, ointment, solution, or shampoo should *not* be used with occlusive dressings or be covered with bandages.

Desoximetasone

Classification, Mechanism of Action, and Clinical Uses

- Desoximetasone is a synthetic fluorinated corticosteroid.
- *Potency varies with formulation.* See Appendix A.
  - Has intermediate potency to high potency, dependent on the dosage form and concentration

    0.25% spray. *Class 1: super potent*

    0.25% ointment, 0.25% cream. *Class 2: highly potent*

    0.05% gel, 0.05% ointment. *Class 3: mid-high potent*

    0.05% cream. *Class 4: mid potent*
- See Introduction for other information.

Indications and Dermatological Uses

- Clinical Indications (FDA)
  - See Introduction.
- Off-Label Common Uses
  - Used for short-term relief of inflammation and cortical-responsive dermatosis for dental purposes

Formulations/Presentation

- USA: Desoximetasone cream, ointment, spray (0.25%), desoximetasone gel (0.05%, Topicort and Topicort LP (0.05%))
- Canada: Desoxi cream and gel (0.05%), desoximetasone, Topicort gel and ointment

Use in Special Populations

- No dosing adjustments for patients with altered renal or hepatic impairments,
- Pediatric populations are more prone to develop systemic side effects (e.g. HPA suppression) due to a larger skin surface area to body mass ratio; use with caution in pediatric patients.

Contraindications and Cautions

- In Canadian labelling, contraindications for untreated bacterial, tubercular, fungal, and most viral lesions of the skin (including herpes simplex, vaccinia, and varicella); not for ophthalmic use.
- Not recommended for use in infants and neonates less than 1 year of age due to a possibility of adrenal suppression.
- See Introduction for other information.

Adverse Effects and Their Management

- Greater than 10% of patients experienced HPA-axis suppression (especially with the 0.25% formulations).
- If skin infections occur, use appropriate antibacterial or antifungal agents to treat the skin; discontinue use of the desoximetasone topical if the infection persists.
- The use of the topical may increase the risk of posterior subcapsular cataracts and glaucoma; consult an ophthalmologist if visual abnormalities persist with the use of the drug.

Carcinogenicity

- No mention on the drug's carcinogenicity

Patch Test Concentration

- 1.0% pet. (Chemotechnique, SmartPracticeCanada)

Essential Patient Information

- Not to use with occlusive dressing unless otherwise stated.
- Spray: Avoid contact with eyes; avoid using on the face, axilla, groin, or in the presence of atrophy at the treatment site; avoid heat, flame, or smoking when applying topical.
- Cream, gel, and ointment: Avoid contact with eyes.
- Desoximetasone preparations should be stored in well-closed containers at 15–30 °C.

Diflucortolone Valerate

Formulations/Presentation

- Cream and ointment: 0.1% and 0.3%

Dosages and Suggested Regimens

- Cream and ointment: 0.1% and 0.3%
  - Apply a thin layer using only enough to cover affected area one to two times daily. The drug can be used for a maximum of 4 weeks, where a lack of improvement or worsening of condition after 2 weeks of application should be assessed for further evaluation.

Contraindications and Cautions

- Do not use for infants under 1 year of age.
- Do not use for viral lesions of the skin; discontinue use if bacterial, fungal, or parasitic skin infections; eruptions following vaccinations; or skin manifestations relating to tuberculosis or syphilis occur.
- This should not be used with occlusive dressings.
- Application to chronic leg ulcers induce increased chance of hypersensitivity.
- See under Introduction.

Adverse Effects and Their Management

- See under Introduction. Since this is a high-potency TCS, adverse reactions have included adrenal suppression, immunosuppression, Cushing syndrome, and hyperglycemia.
- Special caution should be used for patients with psoriasis as systemic toxicity due to impaired skin have been previously observed.
- Other side effects have included folliculitis, contact dermatitis, and hypersensitivity.
- Skin infections (fungal, bacterial) have been observed after prolonged or repeated use.

Carcinogenicity

- Kaposi sarcoma has been reported as being associated.

Patch Test Concentration

- In general, TCS may be tested at 0.1% and 1% in alcohol; late readings (6–10 days) are strongly recommended.

Essential Patient Information

- For topical use only; apply a thin layer of the topical to cover the affected area.
- Clean hands and affected skin area before use.
- Do not use occlusive dressings or apply nearby eye or mucous membranes.
- Diflucortolone valerate is restricted for certain sports as a prohibited agent; patients should check with the sporting officials to see if the drug is suitable for use in competition.

Fluocinonide

Classification and Mechanism of Action and Clinical Uses

- Fluocinonide is a fluorinated TCS considered to be of high potency.
- See under Introduction.
- *Please note that this is a different TCS than fluocinolone acetonide, in structure and in potency.* (See fluocinolone acetonide for its drug monograph.)

Formulations/Presentation

- Cream, gel, ointment, and solution (0.05%)
- Cream (0.1%)

Dosages and Suggested Regimens

- Cream, gel, ointment, and solution (0.05%): Apply a thin layer to affected area two to four times daily.
- Cream (0.1%): Apply a thin layer to affected areas once daily. Seek consultation with a physician if no improvement is seen within 2 weeks; not recommended for use of over 2 weeks or a dose higher than 60 g per week.
- Lower strength 0.05% formulations may be used carefully on the face and areas of the skin folds around the groin, axilla, and breasts; higher strength 0.1% formulas should not be used on these surfaces.

Pharmacokinetics

- No specified differences in pharmacokinetics compared to other TCS

Use in Special Populations

- Fluocinonide can be used for atopic dermatitis for patients planning pregnancy. A milder version of the drug should be used and refrained from using in highly absorptive areas (armpit, skin folds, vulva) during pregnancy.
- Avoid 0.1% fluocinonide concentration for patients who are breastfeeding.
- Due to skin changes related to old age, older adults should limit the use of TCS.
- See under Introduction for other considerations.

Monitoring

- HPA axis suppression test (ACTH stimulation test, AM plasma cortisol test, urinary free cortisol test) should be administered, especially for children.
- Signs of fungal and bacterial infections should be monitored for.

Contraindications, Cautions, and Important Drug Interactions

- See Introduction.

Adverse Effects and Their Management

- See under Introduction.
- Higher strength formulas (0.1%) should not be used on the face, groin, and axilla.
- When using lower strength formulas (0.05%), special care should be taken so the opposing skin surfaces do not rub or touch.
- Children are more prone to systemic effects and may absorb proportionally higher amounts; growth signs of adrenal suppression should be regularly monitored for.

Patch Test Concentration

- In general, TCS may be tested at 0.1% and 1% in alcohol; late readings (6–10 days) are strongly recommended.

Carcinogenicity

- No data available

Essential Patient Information

- See under Introduction.
- Do not use occlusive dressing unless otherwise stated, including the diaper area for pediatric populations, as they significantly increase percutaneous absorption; occlusive dressings may be used with 0.05% fluocinonide for managing psoriasis or recalcitrant conditions if they are deemed necessary by a healthcare professional.
- Store cream, gel, ointment, solution, and shampoo between 15 and 30 °C, and discard shampoo after 3 months of use; do not freeze or heat above 40 °C.

Flurandrenolide: Tape, Cream, and Lotion

Classification, Mechanism of Action, and Clinical Use

- Flurandrenolide is a synthetic fluorinated corticosteroid.
- *Potency varies with the formulation as follows*:
  - *Ultra-high to high:* Flurandrenolide tape 4 ug/cm^2 (Cordran)
  - *Mid to mid-low:* Flurandrenolide 0.025%, 0.05% cream, and 0.05% lotion
  - See TCS Potency Table (Appendix A)
- See Introduction for other details.

Formulations/Presentation

USA

- Cream: 0.025%, 0.05%
- Lotion: 0.05%
- Ointment: 0.05%
- Tape: 4 mcg/cm^2

Dosages and Suggested Regimens

- See Introduction for cream, lotion, and ointment.
- For tape (4 mcg/cm^2): Apply every 12 hours. Measure the appropriate amount of tape to be used. If used on the face, apply carefully and avoid contact with eyes. Do not use in intertriginous areas. Tape application is most effective for dry, scaling, localized lesions.

Contraindications and Cautions

- Do not use in intertriginous areas for drug administered via tape.

Patch Test Concentration

- In general, TCS may be tested at 0.1% and 1% in alcohol; late readings (6–10 days) are strongly recommended.

Carcinogenicity

- No animal studies for carcinogenicity, mutagenicity, or fertility are reported. See introduction for TCS.

Essential Patient Information

- Flurandrenolide cream, lotion, and ointment should be protected from light and stored in tight containers at a temperature less than 40 °C, preferably between 15 and 30 °C; freezing should be avoided. Flurandrenolide tape should be stored at 15–30 °C.

Halobetasol Propionate

Indications and Dermatological Uses

- Clinical Indications (FDA)
  - For treating plaque psoriasis in patients older than 18 years of age with the generic foam and 0.01% lotion, or with patients greater than 12 years of age with the 0.05% foam (Lexette).
  - See Introduction.

Formulations/Presentation

- USA: Cream (0.05%), foam (0.05%), lotion (0.01%, 0.05%), and ointment (0.05%)
- Canada: cream (0.05%), lotion (0.01%), and ointment (0.05%)

Dosages and Suggested Regimens

- See Introduction.
- Apply a thin layer to the affected skin once daily for up to 8 weeks (lotion 0.01%) or 2 weeks (foam, lotion 0.05%). Total dosage should not exceed 50 g/week.

Pharmacokinetics

- See Introduction.
- Study: Less than 6% of the topical dose enters the systemic circulation within 96 hours of application.

Use in Special Populations

- No human data on pregnant populations suing the drug; animal data suggests moderate risk due to the high potency of the drug.
- In animal data, rats which were exposed with 13–33 times the human topical dose resulted in cleft lip and omphalocele.
- See Introduction.

Contraindications and Cautions

- Contraindications for Canadian labelling includes untreated bacterial, tubercular, and fungal skin infections and viral diseases (such as herpes simplex, chicken pox, vaccinia).
- See Introduction.

Patch Test Concentration

- No data available

Carcinogenicity

- No data available

Amcinonide

Classification, Mechanism of Action, and Clinical Uses

- Amcinonide is a synthetic fluorinated corticosteroid.
- *Potency varies with the formulation as follows:*

  - *Ointment:* 0.1% (Class 2 high potency)
  - *Cream & lotion:* 0.1% (Class 3 mid-high potency)
- See Introduction.

Formulations/Presentation

- USA: Cream (0.1%), ointment (0.1%), and lotion (0.1%)
- Canada: Cream (0.1%)

Patch Test Concentration

- 0.1% pet. (SmartPracticeCanada; SmartPraxticeEurope)

Carcinogenicity

- No indications of its carcinogenicity

Essential Patient Information

- Store in well-closed containers at a temperature less than 40 °C, preferably between 15 and 30 °C; freezing should be avoided. Amcinonide lotion and ointment should be stored at 15–30 °C; freezing of the lotion should be avoided.
- Should not be used in neonates and infants under 1 year of age due to higher risk of adrenal suppression.
- See Introduction.

Diflorasone Diacetate

Classification, Mechanism of Action, and Clinical Use

- Diflorasone diacetate is a synthetic fluorinated corticosteroid.
- See Introduction.

Formulations/Presentation

- USA: Cream (0.05%) and ointment (0.05%)
- Appears white or a buff-colored powder and is insoluble in water.

Use in Special Populations

- Follows similar precautions for special populations compared to other topical corticosteroids. See Introduction.
- Pediatric populations are prone to develop HPA suppression due to larger skin surface to body mass ratio; use with caution in pediatric patients; should not be used in neonates and infants under 1 year of age.

Important Drug Interactions

- Does fall under the category of corticosteroids, which may diminish antineoplastic effect of aldesleukin.
- Concurrent use of diflorasone may result in false-negative results for the nitroblue tetrazolium test for bacterial infection.

Adverse Effects and Their Management

- See Introduction.
- Very few (less than 1%) of cases reported the following adverse effects: Acne rosacea, aggravation reaction (cutaneous candidiasis, herpes, demodex, cataract, dermal ulcer, glaucoma, hirsutism, hyperpigmentation, Kaposi's sarcoma, nonthrombocytopenic purpura, ocular hypertension, psoriasis flare, purpura, skin photosensitivity, spontaneous star-shaped scar-like lesions, telangiectasia, and tinea).

Carcinogenicity

- No mention on the drug's carcinogenicity

Patch Test Concentration

- In general, corticosteroids may be tested at 0.1% and 1% in alcohol; late readings (6–10 days) are strongly recommended.

Halcinonide

Classification, Mechanism of Action, and Clinical Use

- Halcinonide is a synthetic fluorinated corticosteroid.
- Halcinonide's potency varies with formulation: 0.1% ointment is Class 1: super potent, and 0.1% cream and solution are Class 2: highly potent.
- See Introduction.

Formulations/Presentation

- USA
  - Cream: Halog, generic at 0.1%
  - Ointment: Halog 0.1% (60 g)
  - Solution: Halog 0.1%

Use in Special Populations

- Follows similar precautions for special populations compared to other topical corticosteroids
- No dosing adjustments for patients with altered renal or hepatic impairments

Adverse Effects and Their Management

- Some formulations may contain propylene glycol, where large amounts can be toxic and be associated with hyperosmolarity, lactic acidosis, seizures, and respiratory depression.
- See Introduction for other adverse effects.

Patch Test Concentration

- In general, corticosteroids may be tested at 0.1% and 1% in alcohol; late readings (6–10 days) are strongly recommended.

Carcinogenicity

- No mention on the drug's carcinogenicity

Essential Patient Information

- Topical cream, ointment, and solution should be stored in closed containers at room temperature; freezing or refrigeration should be avoided; excess heat should be avoided.
- Apply to affected area externally two to three times daily; administration of drug should be discontinued when control is achieved.
- If no improvement is seen, reassessment of diagnosis may be necessary.
- For pediatric populations, experts suggest once or twice daily application.
- Occlusive dressings may be used for managing and treating psoriasis; apply a small amount of topical onto the affected area, and cover with nonporous film to seal the edges; a damp cloth may be applied before occlusive dressing is used; topical should be reapplied for each dressing change; discontinue occlusive dressings if infections arise.

Mid-High to Mid-Low Potency (Class 3 to 5)

Betamethasone Valerate

- See betamethasone dipropionate monograph for further information; mechanism of action and clinical indications; etc. are similar as both are classified as betamethasone topicals. However, there are structural differences: betamethasone dipropionate contains two esters—this makes it more fat soluble and increases its ability to penetrate skin. This makes betamethasone dipropionate more potent than betamethasone valerate, which only contains one ester. This is a clinically significant potency difference: betamethasone dipropionate formulations, especially when augmented, are TCS potency Class 1 and Class 2, in comparison to *betamethasone valerate formulations being TCS potency Class 3 to Class 5*. Thus, betamethasone dipropionate has greater efficacy and greater risk for adverse effects *than betamethasone* valerate. *For details of potency classification differences for the various formulations, see Appendix A.*

Formulations/Presentation

- USA: Foam 0.12%, lotion 0.1%, cream 0.1%, and ointment 0.1%
- Canada: Lotion 0.1%, cream 0.1%, ointment 0.1%, and patch 2.25 mg (Beteflam)

Patch Test Concentration

- 1.0% pet. (Chemotechnique, SmartPracticeCanada); 0.12% pet. (SmartPracticeCanada, SmartPracticeEurope); 0.1% alc. (SmartPracticeCanada)

Fluticasone Propionate

Classification and Mechanism of Action

- Fluticasone propionate is a mid-range potency TCS with the ointment more potent than the cream, even at 1/10th the concentration. Fluticasone propionate 0.005% ointment is considered Class 3: mid-high potent, whereas fluticasone propionate 0.05% cream is Class 4: mid-potent. See Appendix A.

Indications and Dermatological Uses

- Clinical Indications (FDA)
  - Used for the relief of various skin rashes, irritation, and steroid-responsive dermatosis
  - Used for the treatment and management of psoriasis and vitiligo
  - Used for the treatment of atopic dermatitis for infants

Formulations/Presentation

- US: Ointment (0.005%) and cream (0.05%)
- Canada: Ointment (0.005%)

Patch Test Concentration

- In general, corticosteroids may be tested at 0.1% and 1% in alcohol; late readings (6–10 days) are strongly recommended.

Carcinogenicity

- No mention of the drug's carcinogenicity

Essential Patient Information

- For pediatric patients, do not apply topical to diaper area; safety and efficacy in cream have not been established for use in children beyond 4 weeks; children may absorb proportionally higher amounts of topical and may be prone to more systemic side effects.
- Cream and ointment should be stored between 2 and 30 °C (36 and 86 °F).
- Cream may be used for corticosteroid-responsive dermatoses in patients 3 months of age or older. Ointment is for adult use only.
- Avoid contact with eyes; not recommended for routine use around the face, underarms, and groin.

Mometasone Furoate

Classification, Mechanism of Action, and Clinical Use

- See Introduction.

Formulations/Presentation

- USA: Cream (0.1%), ointment (0.1%), and solution (0.1%)
- Canada: Cream (0.1%), ointment (0.1%), and lotion (0.1%)

Pharmacokinetics

- Percutaneous absorption of cream is 0.4%; lotion, ointment, and solution have an absorption rate of 0.7%; both absorptions can be increased with skin inflammation.
- No mention on the drug's metabolism or excretion.

Adverse Effects and Their Management

- Do not use with occlusive dressing or on weeping/exudative lesions.
- 1–10% of the population may experience the following adverse reactions:
  - Central nervous system: paresthesia (1–3%)
  - Dermatologic: dyschromia (loss of normal skin markings: ≤6%), taut and shiny skin (≤6%), folliculitis (lotion: 3%; cream, children: <1%), telangiectasia (≤3%), dermatologic disorders (2%), bacterial skin infection (infants and children: ≤2%), and epidermal thinning (≤2%)
  - Endocrine and metabolic: decreased cortisol (infants and children: lotion: ≤6%, cream and ointment: ≤2%), and endocrine disease (lotion: 2%)
  - Gastrointestinal: xerostomia (infants and children: 2%)
  - Hematologic and oncologic: bruise (1%)
  - Local: application site burning (2%) and application site pruritus (≤2%)

- Less than 1% or an undefined frequency of the population may experience the following adverse reactions:
  - Tingling of the skin, furunculosis, skin atrophy, stinging of the skin at site of application, acneiform eruption, cataract, cutaneous candidiasis, glaucoma, skin and depigmentation
- Not for treatment of diaper dermatitis for pediatric populations; discontinue therapy when control is met for pediatric patients and reassess from a physician if no improvements is seen in 2 weeks.

Patch Test Concentration

- 0.1% alc. (SmartPracticeCanada); late readings (6–10 days) are strongly recommended.

Carcinogenicity

- No mention of the carcinogenicity of the drug

Essential Patient Information

- Store at 25 °C.
- Reassess diagnosis if no improvements is seen after 2 weeks of use for pediatric populations.

Triamcinolone Acetonide

Classification and Mechanism of Action

- Triamcinolone has intermediate to mid-high-range potency dependent on dosage, concentration, and what type of vehicles are used (Class 3 to 5); more information listed on the table below and in Appendix A.

Indications and Dermatological Uses

- Clinical Indications (FDA)
  - Used for relief of inflammatory and pruritic manifestations of corticosteroid-responsive dermatoses, such as atopic dermatitis, contact/vulvar/seborrheic dermatitis, and psoriasis)
  - Can provide temporary relief of symptoms associated with oral inflammation and oral ulcers resulting from trauma in a form of oral paste, such as Aphthous stomatitis
- Off-Label Common Uses
  - Used for stasis dermatitis, where the use of topical triamcinolone showed evidence of management; the evidence is derived from observational studies, unsystematic clinical experience, or potentially controlled and flawed randomized trials; the estimate of effect is uncertain.

Formulations/Presentation

- USA
  - Aerosol (0.147 mg/g)
  - Cream (0.1%, 0.025%)
  - Lotion (0.025%)
  - Ointment (0.05%, 0.025%)
  - Oral paste (0.1%)
  - Therapy pack (0.1%)
- Canada
  - Cream (0.5%, 0.1%, 0.025%)
  - Ointment (0.1%)
  - Oral paste (0.1%)

Potencies Related to Formulation Differences

- Potency of topical triamcinolone varies depending on the dosage, concentration, and vehicle used; it is best to start with the lowest potency agent.
- The various potency of topical triamcinolone is listed on the table below.

Vehicle	Strength	Potency (according to the US classification system)
Ointment	0.5%	High (Class 3)
Cream	0.5%	Medium (Class 4)
Aerosol spray	(delivering ~0.2 mg per 2-second spray)	Medium-low (Class 5)
Ointment	0.1%	Medium (Class 4)
Cream, oral/ dental paste	0.1%	Medium-low (Class 5)
Ointment	0.05%	Medium-low (Class 5)
Lotion	0.1%	Medium-low (Class 5)
Ointment	0.025%	Medium-low (Class 5)
Cream, lotion	0.025%	Low (Class 6)

Goldstein 2019; Tadicherla 2009, DiPiro 12th ed

Pharmacokinetics

- Triamcinolone acetonide is percutaneously absorbed; epidermal integrity, formulation used, and use of occlusive dressings may affect absorption rates.
- The drug is metabolized in the liver.
- The drug is excreted mostly by feces (60%) and urine (40%).
- The drug has a biologic half-life of 18–36 hours.

Use in Special Populations

- See Introduction.

Contraindications and Cautions

- Fungal, viral, or bacterial infections within the oral cavity and throat when using oral topical formulations.

Important Drug Interactions

- Triamcinolone is a class of corticosteroid that may diminish the antineoplastic effects of Aldesleukin; recommended to avoid the combination of both drugs.

- CYP3A4 inhibitors may strongly increase the serum concentration of mometasone, and therapy should be monitored when used in conjunction.
- Nirmatrelvir and ritonavir may increase the serum concentration of corticosteroids, and therapy should be monitored when used in conjunction.

Adverse Effects and Their Management

- The following adverse reactions may occur when using triamcinolone:
  - Dermatologic: acneiform eruption, allergic contact dermatitis, atrophic striae, desquamation, folliculitis, hypertrichosis, hypopigmentation, local dryness, maceration of the skin, miliaria, perioral dermatitis, skin atrophy, and skin blister
  - Endocrine and metabolic: Cushing syndrome, glycosuria, HPA-axis suppression, and hyperglycemia
  - Gastrointestinal: Oral mucosa changes (paste; atrophy or maceration)
  - Local: application site burning, application site irritation, and application site pruritus
- Minor side effects such as burning, itching, or dry skin may occur.
- See Introduction for other adverse effects and cautions.

Patch Test Concentration

- 1% pet. (Chemotechnique, SmartPracticeCanada, SmartPracticeEurope); 0.1% pet. (SmartPracticeCanada); the lower concentration may be preferable; late readings (6–10 days) are strongly recommended

Carcinogenicity

- No mention on drug's carcinogenicity

Essential Patient Information

- See Introduction.
- When using oral paste, do not apply the same paste onto skin or eyes; if noticeable improvement around oral cavity is not seen after a week of use, reassessment of the etiology of oral lesion is recommended.
- Store cream, ointment, lotion, and oral paste at 20–25 °C; do not freeze oral paste.
- Store aerosol spray at room temperature; avoid excessive heat and puncturing the spray.

Clocortolone Pivalate

Classification, Mechanism of Action, and Clinical Use

- Clocortolone is a mid-potent TCS (Class 4).
- See under Introduction for sections not listed below.

Formulations/Presentation

- USA: Cream (0.1%) (Cloderm and generic)

Carcinogenicity

- No mention on the drug's carcinogenicity

Essential Patient Information

- Store drug between 15 and 30 °C and do not freeze.
- See Introduction.

Fluocinolone Acetonide

Classification, Mechanism of Action, and Clinical Use

- Fluocinolone acetonide is a fluorinated corticosteroid. Fluocinolone acetonide and fluocinonide are both synthetic fluorinated corticosteroids that share the action of other TCS *but differ significantly in potency*. Fluocinolone acetonide is low-mid potency depending on the dosage formulation and concentration. Fluocinolone acetonide 0.025% ointment is considered mid-potency; 0.025% cream is considered mid-low potency; 0.01% cream, shampoo, solution and oil are considered low potency (weakly potent).
- *Please note that this is a different TCS than fluocinonide, in structure and in potency.* Refer to fluocinonide monograph for info relating to fluocinonide.
- Fluocinolone acetonide is generally most effective in acute or chronic dermatoses such as seborrheic or atopic dermatitis, localized neurodermatitis, anogenital pruritus, psoriasis, late phase of allergic contact dermatitis, and inflammatory phase of xerosis.

Formulations/Presentation

- USA
  - Cream (0.025%, 0.01%)
  - Ointment (0.025%)
  - Oil (0.01%)
  - Shampoo (0.01%)
  - Solution (0.01%)
- Canada
  - Cream (0.025%, 0.01%) (discontinued)
  - Ointment (0.025%, 0.01%)
  - Oil (0.01%)
  - Solution (0.01%) (discontinued)

Formulations, Packaging, and Manufacturer (Included for Clarification)

- Cream as acetonide
  - Synalar: 0.025% (120 g) (contains cetyl alcohol, edetate (edta) disodium, methylparaben, propylene glycol, propylparaben)
  - Generic: 0.01% (15 g, 60 g); 0.025% (15 g, 60 g)
- Kit as acetonide
  - Synalar (cream): 0.025% (contains cetyl alcohol, edetate (edta) disodium, methylparaben, propylene glycol, propylparaben)
  - Synalar (ointment): 0.025%
  - Synalar TS: 0.01% (contains propylene glycol)
  - Xilapak: 0.01% (discontinued) (contains butylparaben, cetyl alcohol, methylparaben, propylene glycol, propylparaben)
- Oil as acetonide
  - Derma-Smoothe/FS Body: 0.01% (118.28 mL) (contains isopropyl alcohol, peanut oil)
  - Derma-Smoothe/FS Scalp: 0.01% (118.28 mL) (contains isopropyl alcohol, peanut oil)
  - Generic: 0.01% (118.28 mL)
- Ointment as acetonide
  - Synalar: 0.025% (120 g)
  - Generic: 0.025% (15 g, 60 g)
- Shampoo, external, as acetonide
  - Capex: 0.01% (120 mL)
- Solution, external, as acetonide
  - Synalar: 0.01% (60 mL) (contains propylene glycol)
  - Generic: 0.01% (60 mL)

For further clarification, below are two tables outlining the various forms of fluocinolone acetonide and fluocinonide that are available:

Fluocinolone acetonide				
Routes	Dosage forms	Strengths	Brand names	Manufacturer
Topical	Cream	0.01%*		
		0.025%*		
			Synalar®	Medicis
			Synemol® emollient cream	Medicis
	For shampoo	0.01%	*Capex® shampoo*	Galderma
	Oil	0.01%	*Derma-Smoothe/FS®*	Hill
	Ointment	0.025%*	*Fluocinolone acetonide ointment*	
			Synalar®	Medicis
	Solution	0.01%*		
			Synalar®	Medicis

Fluocinonide				
Routes	Dosage forms	Strengths	Brand names	Manufacturer
Topical	Cream	0.05%*	*Fluocinonide E emollient cream*	
			Lidex®	Medicis
			Lidex®-E emollient cream	Medicis
	Gel	0.05%*	*Fluocinonide gel*	
			Lidex® gel	Medicis
	Ointment	0.05%*		
			Lidex®	Medicis
	Solution	0.05%*		
			Lidex®	Medicis

Pharmacokinetics

- Metabolized in the liver
- Excreted primarily by urine, and the rest by bile

Contraindications and Cautions

- See Introduction.
- For Canadian labelling, additional contraindications state as following:
  - Viral lesions of the skin
  - Bacterial/fungal/parasitic infections
  - Skin manifestations relating to tuberculosis or syphilis
  - Eruptions after vaccinations
  - Application to the eye or surrounding areas
- Certain fluocinolone acetonide 0.01% topical is made with 48% refined peanut oil; as peanut protein is undetected at 2.5 ppm, this formulation should be used with caution for patients with hypersensitivity to peanuts; discontinue use if wheal and flare-type hypersensitivity reactions occur.

Patch Test Concentration

- In general, TCS may be tested at 0.1% and 1% in alcohol; late readings (6–10 days) are strongly recommended.

Carcinogenicity

- Although some corticosteroids have exhibited mutagenic activity in some in vivo and in vitro microbial/mammalian tests, no studies have been performed to evaluate the carcinogenicity of fluocinolone acetonide (or the similar fluocinonide formula).

Essential Patient Information

- For scalp psoriasis, apply a thin layer of oil or topical onto scalp and massage thoroughly on wet hair; leave overnight or for at least 4 hours before washing hair with shampoo.
- For seborrheic dermatitis of the scalp, apply no more than 1 ounce of shampoo onto the scalp once daily; leave for at least 5 minutes before washing hair with shampoo.

- If no improvements is seen, reassessment of diagnosis should be met.
- May use occlusive dressings for the management of psoriasis or recalcitrant conditions; if skin infection occurs, discontinue use and seek appropriate antimicrobial therapy.
- Store oil and shampoo between 20 and 25 °C, and discard shampoo after 2 months of use; store cream, ointment, and topical solution between 15 and 25 °C, and avoid freezing or exposing it to excessive heat above 40 °C.
- Only use shampoo solution for seborrheic dermatitis of the scalp, as this formulation has not been proven to be effective in other corticosteroid responsive dermatoses.
- See Introduction.

Flurandrenolide

- Cordran 0.05% Ointment is mid-potency.
- See flurandrenolide above for further details.

Hydrocortisone Salts (Valerate, Butyrate, Acetate, Probutate, Etc.)

Classification, Mechanism of Action, and Clinical Uses

- *Hydrocortisone salts differs from hydrocortisone* (*base*) and has low to intermediate range potency depending on the salt form, dosage form and formulation, and concentration. In general, salt forms are more potent than hydrocortisone base (Class 7: lowest potency). See table below for comparisons, and Appendix A Potency table.

Hydrocortisone	Vehicle	Strength	Potency (according to the US classification system)
Valerate	Ointment	0.2%	Medium (Class 4)
Butyrate	Ointment	0.1%	Medium (Class 4)
Butyrate	Cream, lotion, and solution	0.1%	Lower-mid (Class 5)
Probutate	Cream	0.1%	Lower-mid (Class 5)
Valerate	Cream	0.2%	Lower-mid (Class 5)
Acetate	Ointment	1%	Weakly potent (Class 6)
Acetate	Cream, lotion	1%, 2%, and 2.5%	Least potent (Class 7)
Base	Cream, gel, lotion, ointment, solution, spray	0.5%, 1%, 2%, and 2.5%	Least potent (Class 7)

Goldstein (2021), Tadicherla (2009)

- See Introduction for Clinical Uses
  - For OTC hydrocortisone products, the drug can be used for temporary relief of itching associated with minor skin irritations, inflammation, and rashes (such as eczema, psoriasis, poison ivy or insect bites, seborrheic dermatitis) and temporary relief of external anal and genital itching.
- Off-Label Common Uses
  - For the management of stasis dermatitis.
  - The 10% hydrocortisone (base) cream, but not the valerate derivative, has been used for desquamative inflammatory vaginitis.

Use in Special Populations

- See Introduction.
- Pregnant woman have been prescribed hydrocortisone products and gave birth to infants with congenital malformations, but the relationship between the drug and the outcome could not be determined for human data.

- Although hydrocortisone may cross the placenta to the fetus for pregnant populations, there is a low transfer to the fetus as the placenta is rich with enzymes called 11β-ol-dehydrogenase that metabolize the hydrocortisone into an inactive 11-ketosteroid compound.
- Some formulations of the drug may contain propylene glycol, which can cause fatal toxicities in neonates when delivered orally, topically, or intravenously (over 3000 mg/day); symptoms include metabolic acidosis, seizures, renal failure, and CNS depression; symptoms such as hyperosmolality, lactic acidosis, respiratory depression, and seizures have been observed in adults and children when exposed to high amounts of this substance.

Contraindications and Cautions

- Do not use for the treatment of diaper dermatitis when treating it as an OTC self-medication.
- See Introduction.

Important Drug Interactions

- Topical hydrocortisone may diminish the therapeutic effects of calcipotriene; combined use should be monitored by detecting if there is a reduced efficacy of calcipotriene when used with hydrocortisone; separating the administration of both drugs by 10–12 hours may minimize the risk of this interaction.
- See Introduction.

Adverse Effects and Their Management

- See Introduction.

Patch Test Concentration

- Hydrocortisone (base): 1.0% pet. (SmartPracticeCanada, SmartPracticeEurope): late readings (6–10 days) are strongly recommended. Testing with this preparation probably results in many false-negative reactions. In general, corticosteroids can be tested 0.1% and 1% alcohol.

- Hydrocortisone acetate: 1.0% pet. (Chemotechnique; SmartPracticeCanada); late readings (6–10 days) are strongly recommended. Hydrocortisone acetate 1% in alc./DMSO is irritant.
- Hydrocortisone butyrate: 1.0% pet. (Chemotechnique, SmartPracticeCanada); 1% alc. (Chemotechnique, SmartPracticeCanada); 0.1% pet. (SmartPracticeCanada, SmartPracticeEurope); alcohol may be a better vehicle for testing hydrocortisone butyrate than petrolatum. Late readings (6–10 days) are strongly recommended.
- Hydrocortisone hemisuccinate/hydrocortisone probutate/hydrocortisone valerate: In general, corticosteroids may be tested at 0.1% and 1% in alcohol; late readings (6–10 days) are strongly recommended.

Carcinogenicity

- No available information

Essential Patient Information

- Store at 20–25 °C; do not freeze or heat the medication.
- For topical products, apply topical corticosteroids to moist skin immediately after bathing for optimal absorption.
- Clean and dry the skin at the site of topical application, removing offending agents surrounding the skin; do not use on scars or damaged skin.
- Occlusive dressings may be used when instructed by healthcare professional; the use of occlusive dressings may increase absorption of the drug by a factor of 10.
- Shake lotion well before use.
- Hydrocortisone is a larger class of corticosteroids with different derivatives. Instructions for hydrocortisone valerate use for certain corticosteroid-responsive dermatoses are listed below, but may not be a comprehensive list.

- Atopic dermatitis: Apply hydrocortisone valerate cream once or twice daily to affected areas for 2 to 4 weeks; apply valerate ointment for moderate to severe cases once or twice daily to affected areas for 2 to 4 weeks, with intermittent application once daily for 2 consecutive days per week for patients seeing improvement; lower-potency preparations are recommended for areas affecting the groin, face, and areas of skin folds.
- Contact dermatitis: Apply valerate cream or ointment once or twice daily for 1–2 weeks for allergic dermatitis; apply valerate cream once or twice daily for 1–2 weeks for irritant dermatitis.
- Genital pruritus: Apply valerate ointment once daily for 2–4 weeks; therapy can be continued indefinitely at minimum frequency until pruritus is effectively controlled.
- Seborrheic dermatitis: Apply valerate cream once or twice daily until symptoms subside for chest and upper back symptoms, usually lasting 1–2 weeks
- Stasis dermatitis: Apply valerate ointment once or twice daily for 1–2 weeks; avoid prolonged use due to a risk of ulceration and skin atrophy at site of application.

Hydrocortisone (Topical) (Geriatric Lexi-Drugs)

Hydrocortisone valerate (Martindale: The Complete Drug Reference)

Hydrocortisone, hydrocortisone acetate, hydrocortisone butyrate, hydrocortisone butyrate, hydrocortisone valerate (topical) (AHFS Essentials (adult and pediatric))

Hydrocortisone, hydrocortisone acetate, hydrocortisone butyrate, hydrocortisone butyrate, hydrocortisone valerate (topical) (AHFS DI (adult and pediatric))

Hydrocortisone (topical) (Pediatric and Neonatal Lexi-Drugs)

Hydrocortisone (Briggs Drugs in Pregnancy and Lactation)

Alclometasone Dipropionate

Classification, Mechanism of Action, and Clinical Use

- Alclometasone dipropionate is a synthetic corticosteroid.
- Unlike other topical corticosteroids, alclometasone dipropionate should not be used for the treatment of acne, rosacea, or perioral dermatitis.
- *Potency varies with formulation.* Alclometasone dipropionate 0.05% ointment is Class 5: mid-low potency, and other formulations (0.05% cream) are Class 6: weakly potent.
- Cream as alclometasone dipropionate is as follows:
  - Generic: 0.05% (15 g, 45 g, 60 g)
  - Aclovate: 0.05%
- Ointment as alclometasone dipropionate is as follows:
  - Generic: 0.05% (15 g, 45 g, 60 g)
  - Aclovate: 0.05% (with propylene glycol)
- Indicated for patients more than 1 year of age.

Pharmacokinetics

- About 3% of the drug is reportedly absorbed into the systemic circulation during an 8-hour period of a single application of a 0.05% ointment; systemic absorption may be increased with skin disease and inflammation.
- Onset of initial response occurs after 5.3 days of drug use for eczema and 6.7 days after for psoriasis.
- There is a peak response of the drug 13.9 days after for eczema and 14.8 days after for psoriasis.
- Metabolism of drug is not fully characterized; in animal testing, topical drug did not accumulate in tissues and is thought to be completely metabolized to unidentifiable metabolites.
- Drug and its metabolites are excreted in feces by biliary elimination and by urine.

Use in Special Populations

- Although teratogenic properties of alclometasone dipropionate is unknown, some potent corticosteroid have shown to be teratogenic in animals after topical application; reproduction studies in rabbit with dosages of 1.2 g/kg oral or 0.75 mg/kg topical application has shown maternal toxicity, inability to maintain pregnancy, increased resorption, inhibition of weight gain, decreased litter size, and death; evidence of fetal harm (such as cleft palate, developmental problems, increased malformations) as a secondary effect from the mother's toxicity was been shown in this animal study.
- See Introduction.

Contraindications and Cautions

- Unlike other topical corticosteroids, alclometasone dipropionate should not be used for the treatment of acne, rosacea, or perioral dermatitis.
- Alclometasone shares toxic properties with other topical corticosteroids and precautions should be taken; no evidence of local irritation, anesthetic effect, phototoxicity/photosensitization, or local antigenic/immunogenic effects when 0.1% of alclometasone dipropionate ointment was applied in animal studies.
- Alclometasone dipropionate does not appear to suppress the HPA axis with usual doses; no effect on plasma cortisol levels in patients with psoriasis or atopic dermatitis after 15 g of 0.05% ointment applied to 30% of body twice daily for 7 days with 12/24-hour occlusive dressings on certain patients; essentially unchanged levels of plasma cortisol concentrations before and after the drug use for children 3 months to 12 years old using drug therapy for various dermatosis such as atopic eczema, seborrheic eczema, diaper dermatitis or psoriasis; slightly decreased cortisol, urinary-free cortisol, and 17-hydroxysteroid concentration for healthy individuals using

30 g of 0.05% cream covering 80% of body twice daily for 21 days with daily 12 hour occlusive dressing use—however, the treatment values were within normal ranges, and the application was higher than usual dosages.

- Efficacy and safety of drug has not been established for pediatric use over 3 weeks of duration or for children under 1 year of age.

Patch Test Concentration

- 1.0% pet. (Chemotechnique)

Carcinogenicity

- No evidence of alclometasone-induced mutagenesis in the Ames microbial mutagen test and in in vitro mammalian cell systems; studies have also shown certain other topical corticosteroids such as hydrocortisone or prednisolone to be mutagenic.
- Long-term studies determining carcinogenicity has not be performed to date.

Essential Patient Information

- Generally not for use on the face, underarms, or groin area unless specifically directed to do so.
- Store cream and ointment between 2 and 30 °C.

Desonide

Classification, Mechanism of Action, and Clinical Use

- Desonide is Class 5: mid-low potent and Class 6: weakly potent. *Potency is formulation dependent.* See Appendix A.
- Can be used for atopic dermatitis in infants greater than 3 months old.

Formulations/Presentation

- USA
  - Cream (0.05%)
  - Foam (0.05%)
  - Gel (0.05%)
  - Lotion (0.05%)
  - Ointment (0.05%)
- Canada
  - Cream (0.05%)
  - Ointment (0.05%)

Contraindications and Cautions

- Some dosages of the drug may contain propylene glycol, which can cause fatal toxicities in neonates when delivered orally, topically, or intravenously (over 3000 mg/day); symptoms include metabolic acidosis, seizures, renal failure, and CNS depression; symptoms such as hyperosmolality, lactic acidosis, respiratory depression, and seizures have been observed in adults and children when exposed to high amounts of this substance.

Adverse Effects and Their Management

- 1–10% of patients using this drug may experience the following adverse reactions:
  - Cardiovascular: increased blood pressure (2%)
  - Central nervous system: headache (2%) and irritability (1%)
  - Dermatologic: stinging of the skin (≤3%), atopic dermatitis (<2%; exacerbation), contact dermatitis (<2%), exfoliation of skin (<2%), pruritus (<2%), skin irritation (<2%), xeroderma (<2%), and skin rash (≤1%)
  - Endocrine and metabolic: hyperglycemia (2%) and HPA-axis suppression (more common in pediatric patients)

- Hepatic: abnormal liver function (1%)
- Infection: viral infection (2%)
- Local: application site reaction (1% to 6%), application site burning (≤3%), and application site atrophy (1%)
- Respiratory: Upper respiratory tract infection (10%), cough (4%), asthma (1%), and pharyngitis (1%)

Patch Test Concentration

- In general, corticosteroids may be tested at 0.1% and 1% in alcohol; late readings (6–10 days) are strongly recommended.

Carcinogenicity

- No mention on the drug's carcinogenicity

Essential Patient Information

- When applying onto the face, apply desonide first into hands, and gently massage into affected areas of the face.
- Desonide may be directly applied onto the affected area if not applied onto the face.
- Wash hands after use unless hands are part of the treatment area .
- Do not use on open wounds, cuts, or damaged skin.
- Not recommended for use with occlusive dressings unless told otherwise.
- Do not use for diaper dermatitis for pediatric populations.
- When using foam or lotion solution, shake well before use.
- Foam solution is flammable; patients should not smoke during or immediately following application.
- Store cream, lotion, and ointment between 2 and 30 °C (tridesilon cream at 20–25 °C); store foam between 20 and 25 °C, and keep away from excessive heat and refrain from puncturing container; store gel at 15–30 °C but 25 °C is optimal.

Prednicarbate

Classification, Mechanism of Action, and Clinical Use

- Prednicarbate is a synthetic corticosteroid
- Prednicarbate is Class 5: mid-low potent

Formulations/Presentation

- USA: Cream (0.1%) and ointment (0.1%).
- Canada: Cream (0.1%) and ointment (0.1%).
- In Canada, similar formulas can be found as the name "Dermatop" Canadian Labelling:
  - Cream, external

    Dermatop: 0.1% (20 g, 60 g) (contains benzyl alcohol, edetate, sodium (tetrasodium))
  - Ointment, external

    Dermatop: 0.1% (60 g) (contains propylene glycol)

Contraindications and Cautions

- See Introduction.
- Do not use for diaper dermatitis for pediatric populations.
- For Canadian labelling, additional contraindications are as follows:
  - Hypersensitivity to wool or lanolin
  - Treatment of bacterial/fungal/viral skin infections
  - Diseases such as tuberculosis, syphilis, and chicken pox
  - Eruptions after vaccination

Patch Test Concentration

- 1.0% alc. (SmartPracticeCanada); late readings (6–10 days) are strongly recommended.

Carcinogenicity

- No mention on the carcinogenic properties of prednicarbate

Essential Patient Information

- Store cream at 5–25 °C and ointment at 20–25 °C.

Least Potent Class 7

Hydrocortisone (Base ≥2%)

- *Refer back to "hydrocortisone salts" monograph for further details.*

Indications and Dermatological Uses

- Clinical Indications (FDA)
  - Hydrocortisone topical is used for relief and treatment of inflammatory and pruritic manifestations of corticosteroid-responsive dermatoses such as atopic dermatitis, contact dermatitis, vulvar dermatitis, psoriasis, and seborrheic dermatitis.
  - Can be used for the treatment and relief of psoriasis and vitiligo.
  - Can be used for anal and genital pruritus for genital and anal itching.
  - Hydrocortisone is often used in combination with another agent such as a hemorrhoidal agent (e.g., Anusol-HC). Some of these combination products are listed here.
- Off-Label Common Uses
  - Topical hydrocortisone can be used for the management of stasis dermatitis and desquamative inflammatory vaginitis when administered intravaginally.
  - Both treatments for off-label uses have a "Level of Evidence C" which shows evidence from observational studies, unsystematic clinical experience, or potentially flawed randomized, or controlled trials, where the estimate of effect is uncertain.

Formulations/Presentation

- USA
  - Ointment (2.5%), cream (2.5%), lotion (2%, 2.5%), and solution (2.5%)
- Canada
- Europe

The following hydrocortisone products have a base equal to or greater than 2%:

- Cream as hydrocortisone base
  - Ala-Cort: 2.5% (30 g) (contains cetyl alcohol, propylene glycol)
  - Anusol-HC: 2.5% (30 g)
  - Procto-Med HC: 2.5% (28 g, 30 g) (contains cetearyl alcohol, methylparaben, propylene glycol, propylparaben)
  - Proctosol HC: 2.5% (28.35 g)
  - Proctozone-HC: 2.5% (30 g)
  - Proctozone-HC: 2.5% (30 g) (contains cetearyl alcohol, methylparaben, propylene glycol, propylparaben)
  - Hytone (with propylene glycol): 2.5% (volume not available)
  - Generic: 2.5% (20 g, 28 g, 28.35 g, 30 g, 453.6 g, 454 g)
- Kit as hydrocortisone base
  - Advanced allergy collection: 2.5% (contains cetyl alcohol, methylparaben, propylene glycol, propylparaben)
  - Dermasorb HC: 2% (discontinued) (contains menthol, methylparaben, propylene glycol, propylparaben)
  - Scalacort DK: hydrocortisone lotion 2% and salicylic acid 2% and sulfur 2% (contains benzalkonium chloride, isopropyl alcohol, methylparaben, propylene glycol, propylparaben, soybean lecithin)
- Lotion as hydrocortisone base
  - Ala Scalp: 2% (29.6 mL, 59.2 mL) (contains benzalkonium chloride, isopropyl alcohol, propylene glycol)
  - Hytone (with propylene glycol): 2.5% (volume not available)
- Ointment as hydrocortisone base

- Hytone (with propylene glycol): 2.5% (volume not available)
- Generic: 0.5% (28 g (discontinued), 30 g); 2.5% (20 g, 28.35 g, 453.6 g, 454 g)

- Solution, external, as base
  - Texacort: 2.5% (30 mL) (lipid free, paraben free; contains alcohol, usp)

Use in Special Populations

- Pregnant women prescribed hydrocortisone produced infants with congenital malformations, but the relationship between the drug and the outcome could not be determined for human data.
- Although hydrocortisone may cross the placenta to the fetus for pregnant populations, there is a low transfer to the fetus as the placenta is rich with enzymes called 11β-ol-dehydrogenase that metabolize the hydrocortisone into an inactive 11-ketosteroid compound.
- Some dosages of the drug may contain propylene glycol, which can cause fatal toxicities in neonates when delivered orally, topically, or intravenously (over 3000 mg/day); symptoms include metabolic acidosis, seizures, renal failure, and CNS depression; symptoms such as hyperosmolality, lactic acidosis, respiratory depression, and seizures have been observed in adults and children when exposed to high amounts of this substance.
- See Introduction.

Monitoring

- Signs of HPA axis suppression should be monitored via ACTH stimulation test, morning plasma cortisol test, or urinary free cortisol test.
- Skins of skin atrophy should be noted and monitored.
- As topical absorption may be minimal due to the low potency of this product, there is no additional monitoring for healthcare professionals.

Contraindications and Cautions

- Hypersensitivity to hydrocortisone or other components of the drug.
- Systemic fungal infections and ileocolostomy during the immediate or early postoperative period.
- Cases such as obstruction, abscess, perforation, peritonitis, fresh intestinal anastomoses, and extensive fistulas.
- Possibility of allergenic cross-sensitivity cannot be ruled out for certainty, as documentation of allergenic cross-reactivity is limited.
- Do not use for the treatment of diaper dermatitis when treating it as an OTC self-medication.

Important Drug Interactions

- Hydrocortisone is a class of corticosteroid that may diminish the antineoplastic effects of aldesleukin; recommended to avoid the combination of both drugs.
- Topical hydrocortisone may diminish the therapeutic effects of calcipotriene; combined use should be monitored by detecting if there is a reduced efficacy of calcipotriene when used with hydrocortisone; separating the administration of both drugs by 10–12 hours may minimize the risk of this interaction.

Patch Test Concentration

- Hydrocortisone (base): 1.0% pet. (SmartPracticeCanada, SmartPracticeEurope): late readings (6–10 days) are strongly recommended. Testing with this preparation probably results in many false-negative reactions. In general, corticosteroids can be tested 0.1% and 1% alcohol.

Carcinogenicity

- No available information

Essential Patient Information

- Store at 20–25 °C; do not freeze or heat the medication.
- For topical products, apply topical corticosteroids to moist skin immediately after bathing for optimal absorption.
- Clean and dry the skin at the site of topical application, removing offending agents surrounding the skin; do not use on scars or damaged skin.
- Occlusive dressings may be used when instructed by healthcare professional; the use of occlusive dressings may increase absorption of the drug by a factor of 10.
- Shake lotion well before use.
- Hydrocortisone is a larger class of corticosteroids with different derivatives. Instructions for hydrocortisone use for certain corticosteroid-responsive dermatoses are listed below, but may not be a comprehensive list; also, some of the conditions not listed here may have directions to treat with other hydrocortisone derivatives, for example, contact dermatitis treated with hydrocortisone butyrate or probutate.
  - Atopic dermatitis: Apply 2.5% hydrocortisone base cream or ointment once or twice daily to affected areas for 2 to 4 weeks for mild cases; lower-potency preparations are recommended for areas affecting groin, face, and areas of skin folds.
  - Genital pruritus: Apply 0.5–2.5% hydrocortisone base ointment once daily for 2–4 weeks for vulvar dermatitis; therapy can be continued indefinitely at minimum frequency until pruritus is effectively controlled.
  - Hemorrhoids: Apply 1% or 2.5% hydrocortisone base cream up to twice daily
  - Psoriasis: Apply 1–2.5% hydrocortisone base ointment or cream twice daily until lesions resolve, typically for 2 weeks.
  - Seborrheic dermatitis: Apply 0.5–2.5% hydrocortisone base (cream, ointment, lotion) once or twice daily until signs subside for symptoms on the face or intertriginous areas.

- Vaginitis (off-label): Apply 3–5 g of 10% hydrocortisone cream intravaginally once daily at bedtime for 4–6 weeks; as this is nor commercially available, it must be prepared at a compounding facility or substituted for a 0.5% base hydrocortisone cream.
- For pediatric populations: Hydrocortisone base can be used for dermatologic irritation for up to 3–4 times daily for children over 2 years of age; children over 12 years of age can use hydrocortisone base for anal and genital itching; hydrocortisone base can be used for corticosteroid-responsive dermatosis including psoriasis up to 2–4 times daily.

Hydrocortisone (Base <2%)

See above hydrocortisone base ≥2%, and the hydrocortisone salts monograph for further details.

Dosages and Suggested Regimens

The following hydrocortisone products have a base less than 2%:

- Cream as base
  - Ala-Cort: 1% (28.4 g) (contains cetyl alcohol, propylene glycol)
  - Cortaid Maximum Strength: 1% (28 g (discontinued)) (contains cetyl alcohol, disodium edta, ethylparaben, methylparaben, propylparaben)
  - Cortizone-10 (with parabens and propylene glycol): 1%
  - Curad hydrocortisone: 1% (1.5 g (DSC), 28.4 g (discontinued)) (latex free; contains methylparaben, polysorbate 80, propylene glycol, propylparaben)
  - Hydrocortisone anti-itch: 1% (28 g) (contains cetyl alcohol, chlorocresol (chloro-m-cresol), propylene glycol)
  - Hydrocortisone Max St: 1% (28.4 g)
  - Hydrocortisone Max St/12 Moist: 1% (28.4 g) (contains cetearyl alcohol, methylparaben, propylene glycol, propylparaben)

  - Hydrocortisone/Aloe Max Str: 1% (28 g) (contains cetyl alcohol, edetate (edta) trisodium, isopropyl alcohol, methylparaben, propylparaben, trolamine (triethanolamine))
  - Hytone (with propylene glycol): 1%
  - Instacort 5: 0.5% (28.4 g)
  - Medpura hydrocortisone: 1% (28 g) (contains benzyl alcohol, cetyl alcohol)
  - Preparation H: 1% (26 g) (contains cetyl alcohol, edetate (edta) disodium, methylparaben, propylene glycol, propylparaben, sodium benzoate)
  - Procto-Pak: 1% (28.4 g)
  - Proctocort: 1% (28.4 g) (contains cetyl alcohol, propylene glycol)
  - Recort Plus: 1% (30 g)
  - Generic: 0.5% (15 g, 28.35 g (discontinued), 28.4 g); 1% (1 g, 1.5 g (discontinued), 14.2 g, 20 g, 28 g, 28.35 g, 28.4 g, 30 g, 453.6 g, 454 g)
- Lotion as base
  - Aquanil HC: 1% (120 mL)
  - Beta HC: 1% (60 mL)
  - Nutracort (with parabens): 1%
  - Sarnol-HC: 1% (59 mL)
  - Generic: 1% (114 g, 120 mL)
- Ointment as base
  - Hydrocortisone in Absorbase: 1% (110 g (discontinued))
  - Hydrocortisone Max St: 1% (28 g (discontinued))
  - Generic: 0.5% (28 g (discontinued), 30 g); 2.5% (20 g, 28.35 g, 453.6 g, 454 g); 1% (28 g, 28.35 g, 28.4 g, 30 g, 453.6 g)
- Ointment as base (preservative free)
  - Hydrocortisone in Absorbase: 1% (110 g (discontinued))
- Solution as base:
  - Scalpicin Maximum Strength: 1% (44 mL (discontinued)) (contains disodium edta, menthol, propylene glycol)
  - Cortaid® FastStick® Maximum Strength (with alcohol and methylparaben): 1%

 - Cortaid® Spray Maximum Strength (with alcohol and methylparaben): 1%
 - Cortizone-10® Scalp Itch Formula Liquid (with alcohol SD 40–2 60% v/v, benzyl alcohol, and propylene glycol): 1%
 - Penecort® (with alcohol SD 40–2 57%, benzyl alcohol, and propylene glycol): 1%
 - Texacort® (with SD alcohol 33% and propylene glycol): 1%

Essential Patient Information

- Store at 20–25 °C; do not freeze or heat the medication.
- For topical products, apply topical corticosteroids to the moist skin immediately after bathing for optimal absorption.
- Clean and dry the skin at the site of topical application, removing offending agents surrounding the skin; do not use on scars or damaged skin.
- Occlusive dressings may be used when instructed by healthcare professional; the use of occlusive dressings may increase absorption of the drug by a factor of 10.
- Shake lotion or cream well before use.
- Hydrocortisone is a larger class of corticosteroids with different derivatives. Instructions for hydrocortisone use for certain corticosteroid-responsive dermatoses are listed below, but may not be a comprehensive list; also, some of the symptoms not listed here may have directions to treat for other hydrocortisone derivatives, for example, contact dermatitis treated with hydrocortisone butyrate or probutate.
  - Genital pruritus: Apply 0.5–2.5% hydrocortisone base ointment once daily for 2–4 weeks for vulvar dermatitis; therapy can be continued indefinitely at minimum frequency until pruritus is effectively controlled; apply 1% hydrocortisone base cream or ointment for balanitis twice daily for 1–2 weeks.
  - Hemorrhoids: Apply 1% or 2.5% hydrocortisone base cream up to twice daily.

- Psoriasis: Apply 1–2.5% hydrocortisone base ointment or cream twice daily until lesions resolve, typically for 2 weeks.
- Seborrheic dermatitis: Apply 0.5–2.5% hydrocortisone base (cream, ointment, lotion) once or twice daily until signs subside for symptoms on the face or intertriginous areas.
- Vaginitis (off-label): Apply 3–5 g of 10% hydrocortisone cream intravaginally once daily at bedtime for 4–6 weeks; as this is nor commercially available, it must be prepared at a compounding facility or substituted for a 0.5% base hydrocortisone cream.
- For pediatric populations: Hydrocortisone base can be used for dermatologic irritation for up to 3–4 times daily for children over 2 years of age; children over 12 years of age can use hydrocortisone base for anal and genital itching; Hydrocortisone base can be used for corticosteroid-responsive dermatosis including psoriasis up to 2–4 times daily.

Appendix A: Topical Corticosteroid Potency Table [2]

Potency rating	Topical corticosteroid
Class 1: super potent	Betamethasone dipropionate (augmented) 0.05% Ointment (Diprolene) Gel (generic only) Clobetasol propionate 0.05% Cream, ointment (Dermovate [cr, ung]) Lotion, spray, shampoo (Clobex [ltn, sp., shmp], Clodan [shmp]) Foam (Olux-E, Tovet) Gel (generic only) Desoximetasone 0.25% Spray (Topicort, generic) Diflucortolone valerate 0.3% Ointment, oily cream (Nerisone Forte, Temetex Forte) Fluocinonide 0.1% Cream (Vanos) Flurandrenolide tape 4ug/cm^2 Tape roll (Cordran) Halcinonide 0.1% Ointment (Halog) Halobetasol propionate 0.05% Cream, lotion, ointment (Ultravate) Foam (Lexette)
Class 2: highly potent	Amcinonide 0.1% Ointment (generic only) Betamethasone dipropionate augmented 0.05% Cream (generic only) Betamethasone dipropionate 0.05% Ointment (Diprosone) Gel (generic only) Clobetasol propionate 0.025% Cream (Impoyz) Diflorasone diacetate 0.05% Ointment (generic only) Emollient cream (ApexiCon-E) Desoximetasone 0.25% Cream, ointment (Topicort [cr, ung]) Spray (Topicort spray) Fluocinonide 0.05% Gel, ointment (Lidemol [ung, g], Lidex [ung, g]) Solution (generic only) Halcinonide 0.1% Cream, solution (Halog) Halobetasol propionate 0.01% Lotion (Bryhali)

(continued)

Potency rating	Topical corticosteroid

Class 3: mid-high potent	Amcinonide 0.1%
	  Cream, lotion (generic only)
	Betamethasone dipropionate 0.05%
	  Cream (Diprosone, TARO-sone)
	Betamethasone valerate 0.1%
	  Ointment (Betaderm)
	  Patch (Betaflam) 2.25 mg
	Desoximetasone 0.05%
	  Gel, ointment (Topicort)
	Diflorasone diacetate 0.05%
	  Cream (generic only)
	Diflucortolone valerate 0.1%
	  Ointment, oily cream (Nerisone, Temetex)
	Fluocinonide 0.05%
	  Cream (Lidemol, Lidex, Lyderm, Tiamol)
	Fluticasone propionate 0.005%
	  Ointment (Cutivate)
	Mometasone furoate 0.1%
	  Ointment (Elocom)
	Triamcinolone acetonide 0.5%
	  Ointment (generic only)

Class 4: mid-potent	Betamethasone dipropionate 0.05%
	  Spray (Sernivo)
	Betamethasone valerate 0.12%
	  Foam (generic only)
	Clocortolone pivalate 0.1%
	  Cream (Cloderm)
	Desoximetasone 0.05%
	  Cream (Topicort)
	Fluocinolone acetonide 0.025%
	  Ointment (Synalar)
	Fluticasone propionate 0.05%
	  Cream, lotion (generic only)
	Hydrocortisone butyrate 0.1%
	  Ointment (generic only)
	Hydrocortisone valerate 0.2%
	  Ointment (Hydroval)
	Mometasone furoate 0.1%
	  Cream, lotion (Elocom [cr, ltn])
	  Solution (generic only)
	Prednicarbate 0.1%
	  Ointment (Dermatop)
	Triamcinolone acetonide 0.1%
	  Ointment (Aristocort R)
	Triamcinolone acetonide 0.5%
	  Cream (generic only)

(continued)

Potency rating	Topical corticosteroid
Class 5: mid-low potent	Alclometasone dipropionate 0.05%
	Ointment (generic only)
	Betamethasone dipropionate 0.05%
	Lotion (Diprosone)
	Betamethasone valerate 0.1%
	Cream, lotion (Betaderm [cr, ltn])
	Desonide 0.05%
	Ointment (generic only)
	Gel (generic only)
	Flurandrenolide 0.05%
	Cream, lotion (Cordran [cr. ltn])
	Fluocinolone acetonide 0.025%
	Cream (Synalar)
	Hydrocortisone butyrate 0.1%
	Cream (Locoid Lipocream))
	Lotion (Locoid)
	Solution (generic only)
	Hydrocortisone probutate 0.1%
	Cream (Pandel)
	Hydrocortisone valerate 0.2%
	Cream (Hydroval)
	Prednicarbate 0.1%
	Cream (Dermatop)
	Triamcinolone acetonide 0.05%
	Ointment (generic only)
	Triamcinolone acetonide 0.1%
	Cream (Aristocort R)
	Lotion (generic only)
	Oral paste (Oracort, Kourzeq, Oralone)
	Triamcinolone acetonide 0.147 mg/g
	Aerosol solution (Kenalog)
Class 6: weakly potent	Alclometasone dipropionate 0.05%
	Cream (generic only)
	Desonide 0.05%
	Cream (DesOwen)
	Lotion (generic only)
	Foam (Verddeso)
	Fluocinolone acetonide 0.01%
	Cream (generic only)
	Solution (Synalar)
	Shampoo (Capex)
	Oil (Derma-Smoothe, FS Body, FS Scalp)
	Hydrocortisone acetate 1%
	Ointment (generic only)

(continued)

Potency rating	Topical corticosteroid
Class 7: lowest potency	Hydrocortisone acetate Cream (Vanicream HC) 1% Lotion (NuCort) 2% Foam (Cortifoam) 10% Suppository (Anucort-HC, Anusol-HC, Hemmorex-HC (25 mg), Proctocort (30 mg)) Hydrocortisone base Cream (Instacort 0.5%, Ala-cort 1%, Preparation H 1%, Proctocort 1%, Barriere-HC 1%, Hyderm 1%, Anusol-HC 2.5%, Proctomed-HC 2.5%, Proctosol-HC 2.5%, Proctozone-HC 2.5%, generics 0.5%, 1%, and 2.5%) Enema (Cortenema 100 mg/60 mL) Gel (Hydroxym 2%) Lotion (Aquanil HC 1%, Beta HC 1%, Sarnol-HC 1%, Sarna-HC 1%, Ala Scalp 2%, generics 1% and 2.5%) Ointment (Hydrocortisone Max Strength 1%, Cortoderm 1%, generics 0.5%, 1%, and 2%) Solution (Texacort 2.5%)

References

Introduction

1. Law RM, Gulliver W. Chapter 118: psoriasis. In: Dipiro's pharmacotherapy: a pathophysiologic approach. 12th ed. NY: McGraw-Hill Medical; 2023. p. 1639–60.
2. Skinner TC, Law RM, Maibach HI. Topical corticosteroid potencies: reimagining a new universal classification system. J Drugs Dermatol. 2025;24(5):458–64. https://doi.org/10.36849/JDD.8426
3. De Groot AC. Patch testing. 3rd ed. Volume 3 Chapter 3 & De Groot AC. Patch testing, 4th edition: Update 2018–2022. Wapserveen, The Netherlands: acdegroot publishing, 2022 (37 pages). ISBN/EAN 978-90-813233-7-6.
4. http://online.lexi.com.qe2a-proxy.mun.ca/lco/action/doc/retrieve/docid/disandproc/6577603?cesid=aI9TMWNASqF&searchUrl=%2Flco%2Faction%2Fsearch%3Fq%3Dcorticosteroid%26t%3Dname%26acs%3Dtrue%26acq%3Dcorticosteo#monograph-tab-content
5. https://pubmed.ncbi.nlm.nih.gov/2533778/#:~:text=Corticosteroids%20modify%20the%20functions%20of,form%20a%20steroid%2Dreceptor%20complex
6. https://www.verywellhealth.com/how-topical-steroids-work-1068833

7. https://www.rxlist.com/how_do_topical_corticosteroids_work/drug-class.htm
8. https://www.ncbi.nlm.nih.gov/pmc/articles/PMC3508578/

High to Super High Potency: Betamethasone Dipropionate

9. LexiComp drug monograph (betamethasone dipropionate). Available from: LexiComp Online at online.Lexi.com. Copyright 2024 UptoDate, Inc.
10. FDA drug monograph available at: https://pubmed.ncbi.nlm.nih.gov/29128828/#:~:text=The%20half%2Dlife%20of%20betamethasone,was%20estimated%20up%20to%2048days
11. De Groot AC. Patch testing. 3rd ed. Volume 3 Chapter 3.

High to Super High Potency: Clobetasol Propionate

12. FDA drug monographs (Clobetasol propionate). Available from (https://www.accessdata.fda.gov/drugsatfda_docs/label/2020/213691s000lbl.pdf for the lotion and https://www.accessdata.fda.gov/drugsatfda_docs/label/2012/021835s006lbl.pdf for the spray and https://www.drugs.com/pro/clobetasol-cream.html for the cream). Accessed 7 July 2024.
13. LexiComp drug monograph (clobetasol propionate). Available from: LexiComp Online at online.Lexi.com. Copyright 2024 UptoDate, Inc.
14. De Groot AC. Patch testing. 3rd ed. Volume 3 Chapter 3.

High to Super High Potency: Desoximetasone

15. US FDA PMR Final Study Report for 0.25% desoximetasone spray https://www.fda.gov/media/154879/download (Accessed 17 July 2024).
16. LexiComp drug monograph (Desoximetasone). Available from: LexiComp Online at online.Lexi.com. Copyright 2024 UptoDate, Inc.
17. De Groot AC. Patch testing. 3rd ed. Volume 3 Chapter 3.

High to Super High Potency: Diflucortolone Valerate

18. Health Canada HRES (diflucortolone valerate). Available from: https://pdf.hres.ca/dpd_pm/00037898.PDF Accessed 7 July 2024.
19. LexiComp drug monograph (diflucortolone valerate). Available from: LexiComp Online at online.Lexi.com. Copyright 2024 UptoDate, Inc.
20. De Groot AC. Patch testing. 3rd ed. Volume 3 Chapter 3.

High to Super High Potency: Fluocinonide

21. FDA Drug Monograph (fluocinonide cream—Vanos) Available at: https://www.accessdata.fda.gov/drugsatfda_docs/label/2006/021758s00lbl.pdf
22. LexiComp drug monograph (fluocinonide). Available from: LexiComp Online at online.Lexi.com. Copyright 2024 UptoDate, Inc.
23. De Groot AC. Patch testing. 3rd ed. Volume 3 Chapter 3.

High to Super High Potency: Flurandrenolide: Tape, Cream, and Lotion

24. FDA Drug Monographs for flurandrenolide ointment, cream, lotion (Cordran cream & ointment available at: https://www.accessdata.fda.gov/drugsatfda_docs/label/2013/012806s037lbl.pdf Cream available at https://www.accessdata.fda.gov/drugsatfda_docs/label/2016/205342Orig1s000lbl.pdf).
25. LexiComp drug monograph (flurandrenolide). Available from: LexiComp Online at online.Lexi.com. Copyright 2024 UptoDate, Inc.
26. De Groot AC. Patch testing. 3rd ed. Volume 3 Chapter 3.

High to Super High Potency: Halobetasol Propionate

27. FDA Drug Monograph (Halobetasol propionate). Available at: https://www.accessdata.fda.gov/drugsatfda_docs/label/2012/019968s011lbl.pdf Accessed 9 July 2024.
28. LexiComp drug monograph (halobetasol propionate). Available from: LexiComp Online at online.Lexi.com. Copyright 2024 UptoDate, Inc.

High to Super High Potency: Amcinonide

29. NIH monograph Amcinonide. Available at: https://dailymed.nlm.nih.gov/dailymed/fda/fdaDrugXsl.cfm?setid=ac5c3e79-52f7-434e-92ae-24bd32b45edc&type=display Accessed 8 July 2024.
30. LexiComp drug monograph (amcinonide). Available from: LexiComp Online at online.Lexi.com. Copyright 2024 UptoDate, Inc.
31. De Groot AC. Patch testing. 3rd ed. Volume 3 Chapter 3.

High to Super High Potency: Diflorasone Diacetate

32. FDA drug monograph (diflorasone diacetate 0.05% ointment). Available at: https://www.accessdata.fda.gov/drugsatfda_docs/label/2017/019260s009lbl.pdf Accessed 17 July 2024.
33. LexiComp drug monograph (diflorasone diacetate). Available from: LexiComp Online at online.Lexi.com. Copyright 2024 UptoDate, Inc.
34. De Groot AC. Patch testing. 3rd ed. Volume 3 Chapter 3.

High to Super High Potency: Halcinonide

35. FDA drug monograph (halcinonide 0.1% cream). https://www.accessdata.fda.gov/drugsatfda_docs/label/2009/017556s038lbl.pdf Accessed 18 July 2024.
36. http://online.lexi.com.qe2a-proxy.mun.ca/lco/action/doc/retrieve/docid/complete_ashp/413472?cesid=0z1zhOU0oEu&searchUrl=%2Flco%2Faction%2Fsearch%3Fq%3DHalcinonide%26t%3Dname%26acs%3Dfalse%26acq%3DHalcinonide
37. LexiComp drug monograph (halcinonide). Available from: LexiComp Online at online.Lexi.com. Copyright 2024 UptoDate, Inc.
38. De Groot AC. Patch testing. 3rd ed. Volume 3 Chapter 3.

Mid-High to Mid-Low Potency (Class 3 to 5): Betamethasone Valerate

39. Drugs.com. https://www.drugs.com/betamethasone-topical.html#:~:text=Betamethasone%20dipropionate%20contains%20two%20esters,which%20only%20contains%20one%20ester. Accessed 19 July 2024.
40. http://online.lexi.com/lco/action/doc/retrieve/docid/patch_f/5004842?cesid=6xmrwv6Xokb&searchUrl=%2Flco%2Faction%2Fsearch%3Fq%3DBetamethasone%2Bvalerate%26t%3Dname%26acs%3Dfalse%26acq%3DBetamethasone%2Bvalerate
41. LexiComp drug monograph (Betamethasone valerate). Available from: LexiComp Online at online.Lexi.com. Copyright 2024 UptoDate, Inc.
42. De Groot AC. Patch testing. 3rd ed. Volume 3 Chapter 3.

Mid-High to Mid-Low Potency (Class 3 to 5): Fluticasone Propionate

43. http://online.lexi.com/lco/action/doc/retrieve/docid/patch_f/341?cesid=9U5dGrCLvPk&searchUrl=%2Flco%2Faction%2Fsearch%3Fq%3DFluticasone%2Bpropionate%26t%3Dname%26acs%3Dfalse%26acq%3DFluticasone%2Bpropionate#adr

44. http://online.lexi.com/lco/action/doc/retrieve/docid/3/3674
45. LexiComp drug monograph (Fluticasone propionate). Available from: LexiComp Online at online.Lexi.com. Copyright 2024 UptoDate, Inc.
46. De Groot AC. Patch testing. 3rd ed. Volume 3 Chapter 3.

Mid-High to Mid-Low Potency (Class 3 to 5): Mometasone Furoate

47. http://online.lexi.com/lco/action/doc/retrieve/docid/patch_f/1799125?cesid=3B3LcXIiZK6&searchUrl=%2Flco%2Faction%2Fsearch%3Fq%3Dmometasone%2Bfuroate%26t%3Dname%26acs%3Dtrue%26acq%3DMometasone%2Bfuroate#adr
48. http://online.lexi.com/lco/action/doc/retrieve/docid/pdh_f/2850861?cesid=3B3LcXIiZK6&searchUrl=%2Flco%2Faction%2Fsearch%3Fq%3Dmometasone%2Bfuroate%26t%3Dname%26acs%3Dtrue%26acq%3DMometasone%2Bfuroate
49. LexiComp drug monograph (Mometasone furoate). Available from: LexiComp Online at online.Lexi.com. Copyright 2024 UptoDate, Inc.
50. De Groot AC. Patch testing. 3rd ed. Volume 3 Chapter.

Mid-High to Mid-Low Potency (Class 3 to 5): Triamcinolone Acetonide

51. http://online.lexi.com/lco/action/doc/retrieve/docid/patch_f/1802822?cesid=9uAZSL1oLGH&searchUrl=%2Flco%2Faction%2Fsearch%3Fq%3DTriamcinolone%2Bacetonide%26t%3Dname%26acs%3Dfalse%26acq%3DTriamcinolone%2Bacetonide#
52. http://online.lexi.com/lco/action/doc/retrieve/docid/pdh_f/2860023?cesid=9uAZSL1oLGH&searchUrl=%2Flco%2Faction%2Fsearch%3Fq%3DTriamcinolone%2Bacetonide%26t%3Dname%26acs%3Dfalse%26acq%3DTriamcinolone%2Bacetonide#coi
53. http://online.lexi.com/lco/action/doc/retrieve/docid/essential_ashp/410301?cesid=9uAZSL1oLGH&searchUrl=%2Flco%2Faction%2Fsearch%3Fq%3DTriamcinolone%2Bacetonide%26t%3Dname%26acs%3Dfalse%26acq%3DTriamcinolone%2Bacetonide
54. http://online.lexi.com/lco/action/doc/retrieve/docid/complete_ashp/413424?cesid=9uAZSL1oLGH&searchUrl=%2Flco%2Faction%2Fsearch%3Fq%3DTriamcinolone%2Bacetonide%26t%3Dname%26acs%3Dfalse%26acq%3DTriamcinolone%2Bacetonide
55. Goldstein BG, Goldstein AO. Comparison of representative topical corticosteroid preparations (classified according to the United States system). Waltham, MA: UpToDate. Available at: https://www.uptodate.com/contents/topical-corticosteroidsuse-and-adverse-effects
56. Tadicherla S, Ross K, Shenefelt PD, Fenske NA. Topical corticosteroids in dermatology. J Drugs Dermatol. 2009;8(12):1093–1105.

57. LexiComp drug monograph (Triamcinolone acetonide). Available from: LexiComp Online at online.Lexi.com. Copyright 2024 UptoDate, Inc.
58. De Groot AC. Patch testing. 3rd ed. Volume 3 Chapter.

Mid-High to Mid-Low Potency (Class 3 to 5): Clocortolone Pivalate

59. LexiComp drug monograph (clocortolone pivalate). Available from: LexiComp Online at online.Lexi.com. Copyright 2024 UptoDate, Inc.
60. De Groot AC. Patch testing. 3rd ed. Volume 3 Chapter 3.

Mid-High to Mid-Low Potency (Class 3 to 5): Fluocinolone Acetonide

61. http://online.lexi.com/lco/action/doc/retrieve/docid/patch_f/1796619?cesid=73uymJBy3vC&searchUrl=%2Flco%2Faction%2Fsearch%3Fq%3DFluocinolone%2Bacetonide%26t%3Dname%26acs%3Dfalse%26acq%3DFluocinolone%2Bacetonide#coi
62. http://online.lexi.com/lco/action/doc/retrieve/docid/pdh_f/2850762?cesid=73uymJBy3vC&searchUrl=%2Flco%2Faction%2Fsearch%3Fq%3DFluocinolone%2Bacetonide%26t%3Dname%26acs%3Dfalse%26acq%3DFluocinolone%2Bacetonide
63. http://online.lexi.com/lco/action/doc/retrieve/docid/patch_f/6925?cesid=73uymJBy3vC&searchUrl=%2Flco%2Faction%2Fsearch%3Fq%3DFluocinolone%2Bacetonide%26t%3Dname%26acs%3Dfalse%26acq%3DFluocinolone%2Bacetonide
64. http://online.lexi.com/lco/action/doc/retrieve/docid/complete_ashp/413471?cesid=73uymJBy3vC&searchUrl=%2Flco%2Faction%2Fsearch%3Fq%3DFluocinolone%2Bacetonide%26t%3Dname%26acs%3Dfalse%26acq%3DFluocinolone%2Bacetonide#cauts-nested-1
65. LexiComp drug monograph (clocortolone pivalate). Available from: LexiComp Online at online.Lexi.com. Copyright 2024 UptoDate, Inc.
66. De Groot AC. Patch testing. 3rd ed. Volume 3 Chapter 3.

Mid-High to Mid-Low Potency (Class 3 to 5): Hydrocortisone Salts (Valerate, Butyrate, Acetate, Probutate, Etc.)

67. De Groot AC. Patch testing. 3rd ed. Volume 3 Chapter 3.
68. http://online.lexi.com/lco/action/search?q=Hydrocortisone&t=name&acs=false&acq=Hydrocortisone
69. http://online.lexi.com/lco/action/doc/retrieve/docid/pdh_f/2848040?cesid=7j2fFT9cLDV&searchUrl=%2Flco%2Faction%2Fsearch%3Fq%3DHydrocortisone%2Bvalerate%26t%3Dname%26acs

%3Dfalse%26acq%3DHydrocortisone%2Bvalerate#peds-pated-tab-content
70. http://online.lexi.com/lco/action/doc/retrieve/docid/complete_ashp/413425?cesid=7j2fFT9cLDV&searchUrl=%2Flco%2Faction%2Fsearch%3Fq%3DHydrocortisone%2Bvalerate%26t%3Dname%26acs%3Dfalse%26acq%3DHydrocortisone%2Bvalerate
71. http://online.lexi.com/lco/action/doc/retrieve/docid/essential_ashp/410302?cesid=7j2fFT9cLDV&searchUrl=%2Flco%2Faction%2Fsearch%3Fq%3DHydrocortisone%2Bvalerate%26t%3Dname%26acs%3Dfalse%26acq%3DHydrocortisone%2Bvalerate
72. http://online.lexi.com/lco/action/doc/retrieve/docid/martindale_f/1353657?cesid=7j2fFT9cLDV&searchUrl=%2Flco%2Faction%2Fsearch%3Fq%3DHydrocortisone%2Bvalerate%26t%3Dname%26acs%3Dfalse%26acq%3DHydrocortisone%2Bvalerate
73. http://online.lexi.com/lco/action/doc/retrieve/docid/gdh_f/2151227?cesid=7j2fFT9cLDV&searchUrl=%2Flco%2Faction%2Fsearch%3Fq%3DHydrocortisone%2Bvalerate%26t%3Dname%26acs%3Dfalse%26acq%3DHydrocortisone%2Bvalerate

Mid-High to Mid-Low Potency (Class 3 to 5): Alclometasone Dipropionate

74. http://online.lexi.com/lco/action/doc/retrieve/docid/complete_ashp/413970?cesid=7xU0f4TrK0M&searchUrl=%2Flco%2Faction%2Fsearch%3Fq%3DAlclometasone%2Bdipropionate%26t%3Dname%26acs%3Dfalse%26acq%3DAlclometasone%2Bdipropionate#cauts-nested-1
75. http://online.lexi.com/lco/action/doc/retrieve/docid/patch_f/6293?cesid=7xU0f4TrK0M&searchUrl=%2Flco%2Faction%2Fsearch%3Fq%3DAlclometasone%2Bdipropionate%26t%3Dname%26acs%3Dfalse%26acq%3DAlclometasone%2Bdipropionate#
76. http://online.lexi.com/lco/action/doc/retrieve/docid/essential_ashp/988197#uses-nested (Alclometasone Dipropionate (AHFS Essentials (Adult and Pediatric)).
77. http://online.lexi.com/lco/action/doc/retrieve/docid/martindale_f/1353588?cesid=7xU0f4TrK0M&searchUrl=%2Flco%2Faction%2Fsearch%3Fq%3DAlclometasone%2Bdipropionate%26t%3Dname%26acs%3Dfalse%26acq%3DAlclometasone%2Bdipropionate
78. De Groot AC. Patch testing. 3rd ed. Volume 3 Chapter 3.

Mid-High to Mid-Low Potency (Class 3 to 5): Desonide

79. (http://online.lexi.com/lco/action/doc/retrieve/docid/complete_ashp/413426?cesid=8MJLM9VlShJ&searchUrl=%2Flco%2Faction%2Fsearch%3Fq%3Ddesowen%26t%3Dname%26acs%3Dfalse%26acq%3Ddesowen - Desonide (Topical) (AHFS DI (Adult and Pediatric))
80. http://online.lexi.com/lco/action/doc/retrieve/docid/pdh_f/128606?cesid=98lgc24liE9&searchUrl=%2Flco%2Faction%2Fsearch%3Fq%3Ddesonide%26t%3Dname%26acs%3Dfalse%26acq%3Ddesonide
81. http://online.lexi.com/lco/action/doc/retrieve/docid/complete_ashp/413426?cesid=98lgc24liE9&searchUrl=%2Flco%2Faction%2Fsearch%3Fq%3Ddesonide%26t%3Dname%26acs%3Dfalse%26acq%3Ddesonide
82. http://online.lexi.com/lco/action/doc/retrieve/docid/patch_f/6708?cesid=98lgc24liE9&searchUrl=%2Flco%2Faction%2Fsearch%3Fq%3Ddesonide%26t%3Dname%26acs%3Dfalse%26acq%3Ddesonide#monograph-tab-content
83. De Groot AC. Patch testing. 3rd ed. Volume 3 Chapter 3.

Mid-High to Mid-Low Potency (Class 3 to 5): Prednicarbate

84. http://online.lexi.com/lco/action/doc/retrieve/docid/patch_f/7545?cesid=6g1fi79RDiT&searchUrl=%2Flco%2Faction%2Fsearch%3Fq%3Dprednicarbate%26t%3Dname%26acs%3Dtrue%26acq%3DPrednicarbate#spg
85. http://online.lexi.com/lco/action/doc/retrieve/docid/pdh_f/129094?cesid=6g1fi79RDiT&searchUrl=%2Flco%2Faction%2Fsearch%3Fq%3Dprednicarbate%26t%3Dname%26acs%3Dtrue%26acq%3DPrednicarbate
86. http://online.lexi.com/lco/action/doc/retrieve/docid/complete_ashp/4-14086?cesid=6g1fi79RDiT&searchUrl=%2Flco%2Faction%2Fsearch%3Fq%3Dprednicarbate%26t%3Dname%26acs%3Dtrue%26acq%3DPrednicarbate
87. De Groot AC. Patch testing. 3rd ed. Volume 3 Chapter 3.

Least Potent Class 7: Hydrocortisone (Base ≥2%)

88. http://online.lexi.com/lco/action/doc/retrieve/docid/patch_f/1797823?cesid=3ACyDCSl90w&searchUrl=%2Flco%2Faction%2Fsearch%3Fq%3Dscalacort%26t%3Dname%26acs%3Dfalse%26acq%3Dscalacort#
89. (Hydrocortisone (Topical) (Lexi-Drugs)).
90. http://online.lexi.com/lco/action/doc/retrieve/docid/essential_ashp/410302?cesid=9NCqUUuKIvZ&searchUrl=%2Flco%2Faction%2Fsearch%3Fq%3Dhytone%26t%3Dname%26acs%3Dfalse%26acq%3Dhytone
91. Hydrocortisone, Hydrocortisone Acetate, Hydrocortisone Buteprate, Hydrocortisone Butyrate, Hydrocortisone Valerate (Topical) (AHFS Essentials (Adult and Pediatric)).
92. http://online.lexi.com/lco/action/doc/retrieve/docid/pdh_f/2848040?cesid=6ThRPQaITq3&searchUrl=%2Flco%2Faction%2Fsearch%3Fq%3Dhydrocortisone%26t%3Dname%26acs%3Dfalse%26acq%3Dhydrocortisone
93. De Groot AC. Patch testing. 3rd ed. Volume 3 Chapter 3.

Least Potent Class 7: Hydrocortisone (Base <2%)

94. http://online.lexi.com/lco/action/doc/retrieve/docid/patch_f/1797823?cesid=3ACyDCSl90w&searchUrl=%2Flco%2Faction%2Fsearch%3Fq%3Dscalacort%26t%3Dname%26acs%3Dfalse%26acq%3Dscalacort#
95. (Hydrocortisone (Topical) (Lexi-Drugs)).
96. http://online.lexi.com/lco/action/doc/retrieve/docid/essential_ashp/410302?cesid=9NCqUUuKIvZ&searchUrl=%2Flco%2Faction%2Fsearch%3Fq%3Dhytone%26t%3Dname%26acs%3Dfalse%26acq%3Dhytone
97. Hydrocortisone, Hydrocortisone Acetate, Hydrocortisone Buteprate, Hydrocortisone Butyrate, Hydrocortisone Valerate (Topical) (AHFS Essentials (Adult and Pediatric)).
98. http://online.lexi.com/lco/action/doc/retrieve/docid/pdh_f/2848040?cesid=6ThRPQaITq3&searchUrl=%2Flco%2Faction%2Fsearch%3Fq%3Dhydrocortisone%26t%3Dname%26acs%3Dfalse%26acq%3Dhydrocortisone

Ectoparasiticides 19

Dirk B. Robertson

Contents

Ivermectin

Note that ivermectin also has anti-inflammatory properties and is used for treatment of rosacea. Please refer to Chap. 9 for discussion of its use in rosacea.

Classification and Mode of Action

- Antiparasitic agent, topical; pediculicide
- Ivermectin 0.5% lotion (Sklice) is a topical antiparasitic agent approved for the treatment of pediculosis capitis (head lice).

D. B. Robertson (✉)
Department of Dermatology, Emory University School of Medicine, Atlanta, GA, USA
e-mail: robertsons@prodigy.net

R. M. Law, H. I. Maibach (eds.), *Handbook of Topical Drug Treatment in Dermatology*,
https://doi.org/10.1007/978-3-031-93616-6_19

The FDA initially approved ivermectin lotion, 0.5% for the treatment of head lice infestation in patients 6 months of age and older as a prescription drug in February 2012. Recently the FDA approved its use as an over-the-counter (OTC) nonprescription drug.

- Mechanism of action.
  - Ivermectin is a semisynthetic anthelminthic agent.
  - It binds selectively and with strong affinity to glutamate-gated chloride ion channels which occur in invertebrate nerve and muscle cells. This leads to increased permeability of cell membranes to chloride ions, then hyperpolarization of the nerve or muscle cell, and death of the parasite.

Indications and Dermatologic Uses

- Topical treatment of head lice in patients 6 months and older

Formulations

- Topical 0.5% lotion brand name Sklice. It is available as a generic.

Dosages and Administration

- Topical lotion.
- Apply sufficient amount (up to 1 tube) to dry scalp and hair closest to the scalp first, and then apply outward toward ends of the hair, completely covering the scalp and hair. Leave on for 10 minutes (start timing treatment after the scalp and hair have been completely covered). The hair should then be rinsed thoroughly with warm water. Avoid contact with the eyes.
- Nit combing is not required, although a fine-tooth comb may be used to remove treated lice and nits.

Pharmacokinetics

- Ivermectin is greater than 99% protein bound. It is metabolized hepatically by CYP3A4. Half-life elimination is approximately 6–7 days.

Use in Special Populations

- Breastfeeding considerations
  - Following oral administration, ivermectin is measurable in low concentrations in breast milk. Breastfeeding is not recommended by the manufacturer.
- Use in Pregnancy
  - Although risk with use in pregnancy is likely low risk, other agents are currently recommended for the treatment of pediculosis pubis or scabies in breastfeeding women.
- Pediatric considerations
  - In infants <6 months, systemic absorption may be increased due to higher skin surface area to body mass ratio and immature skin barrier; risk for ivermectin toxicity is potentially increased. Avoid use in these patients.
- Renal insufficiency: No alterations in dosing recommended in renal insufficiency
- Hepatic insufficiency: No alterations in dosing recommended in hepatic insufficiency

Contraindications and Cautions

- There are no contraindications listed in the US manufacturer's labeling.

Adverse Effects

- Localized burning sensation and skin irritation has been noted in less than 1% of patients.

Patch Test Concentration

- Not available

Essential Patient Information

- For external use only. Avoid contact with the eyes while using on the scalp.
- Not for use in the eye, mouth, or vagina.
- Lotion is for one-time use; discard any unused portion.

Lindane

Classification and Mode of Action

- Antiparasitic agent, topical; pediculicide
- Lindane is an ectoparasiticide and ovicide agent used for the topical treatment of scabies and pediculosis capitis and pubis. It is directly absorbed by parasites and ova and overstimulates the neural system resulting in the death of the parasite.

Indications and Dermatologic Uses

- Lindane is clinically indicated for the topical treatment of scabies (*Sarcoptes scabiei*) and pediculosis capitis or pubis. It is not recommended as a first line of treatment and should be reserved for patients who cannot tolerate other approved therapies or have failed first line treatments.

Formulations

- 1% shampoo, 1% lotion

Dosages and Administration

- Pediculosis: Apply lindane shampoo to clean dry hair and massage into the hair for 4 minutes. Add small amounts of water to form a lather, and then rinse thoroughly. Comb with a fine-tooth comb to remove nits. An average patient will need 30 ml. Do not exceed 60 ml. Do not retreat.
- Scabies: Apply a thin layer of lindane lotion over all the skin from the neck down. One ounce is sufficient for an average adult. Do not prescribe more than 2 ounces for larger adults. Apply only once. Wash off in 8 to 12 hours. Do not retreat.

Pharmacokinetics

- Approximately 10% is absorbed percutaneously. Elimination half-life is approximately 20 hours with secretion in urine and feces.

Use in Special Populations

- Pregnancy: Lindane should be given to pregnant women only if clearly needed and alternatives cannot be used.
- Lactation: Lindane is lipophilic and is present in human breast milk, but exact quantities are not known. Nursing mothers who require treatment with lindane lotion should be advised of the potential risks and be counseled to avoid large areas of skin-to-skin contact with the infant following lindane application. They should also interrupt breastfeeding, with expression and discarding of milk, for at least 24 hours following use.
- Pediatrics.
  – Lindane is contraindicated for premature infants because their skin may be more permeable than that of full-term infants, and their liver enzymes may not be sufficiently developed to metabolize lindane.

  - Lindane is on the KIDs (Key Potentially Inappropriate Drugs in Pediatrics) list for pediatric patients less than 10 years of age or weighing less than 50 Kg and should be avoided due to the risk of seizure or spasm.
- Renal insufficiency: No dosage adjustments provided in the manufacturer's labeling.
- Hepatic insufficiency: No dosage adjustments provided in the manufacturer's labeling.

Contraindications and Cautions

- Lindane lotion is contraindicated for patients with crusted (Norwegian) scabies and other skin conditions (e.g., atopic dermatitis and psoriasis) that may increase systemic absorption of the drug.
- Lindane lotion is contraindicated for patients with known uncontrolled seizure disorders
- Lindane lotion is contraindicated for individuals with a known sensitivity to the product or any of its components.

US Boxed Warnings

- **Lindane should only be used in patients who cannot tolerate or have failed first-line treatment with safer medications for the treatment of lice/scabies.**
- **Neurologic toxicity including seizures and deaths have been reported following lindane use with repeat or prolonged application but also in rare cases following a single application according to directions. Lindane should be used with caution in infants, children, the elderly, individuals with other skin conditions, and those who weigh < 110 lbs (50 kg) as they may be at risk of serious neurotoxicity.**
- **Lindane is contraindicated in premature infants and individuals with known uncontrolled seizure disorders.**

- **Instruct patients on the proper use of Lindane, the amount to apply, how long to leave it on, and avoiding re-treatment.**

Essential Patient Information

- Inform patients that itching occurs after the successful killing of lice and is not necessarily an indication for retreatment with lindane.
- **A Lindane Medication Guide must be given to the patient each time lindane is dispensed, as required by law.**

Adverse Effects

- Lindane has been reported to cause central nervous system stimulation ranging from dizziness to seizures. Although seizures were almost always associated with ingestion or misuse of the product, including repeat treatment, seizures and deaths have been reported when lindane lotion was used according to directions.
- Irritant dermatitis from contact with this product has been reported.

Patch Test Concentration

- Not available

Permethrin

Classification and Mode of Action

- Antiparasitic agent, topical; pediculicide
- Permethrin (synthetic pyrethroid cyclopropanecarboxylate ester); an ectoparasiticide and ovicide agent

- Inhibits sodium ion influx through nerve cell membrane channels in parasites, resulting in delayed repolarization and thus paralysis and death

Indications and Dermatologic Uses

- Labeled indications for permethrin include the topical treatment of scabies (*Sarcoptes scabiei*) and head lice (pediculosis capitis).
- Off-label use in adults include pubic lice (*Pediculosis pubis*) and crusted scabies (Norwegian scabies).

Formulations

- 5% cream brand name Elimite (generic available)
- 1% cream rinse/lotion OTC brand name Nix. (generic available)

Dosages and Administration

Dosing: Adult

- Head lice: Topical cream rinse/lotion 1%: Prior to application, wash hair with conditioner-free shampoo; rinse with water and towel dry. Apply a sufficient amount of lotion, or cream rinse to saturate the hair and scalp (especially behind the ears and nape of neck). Leave on hair for 10 minutes (but no longer), and then rinse off with warm water. Remove remaining nits with nit comb. A single application is generally sufficient. However, may repeat 7 days after first treatment if lice or nits are still present.
- Pubic lice (off-label use): Topical cream rinse/lotion 1%: Apply to affected areas and wash off after 10 minutes.
- Scabies: Topical cream 5%: Thoroughly massage cream (30 g for average adult) from the head to the soles of the feet. Leave on for 8 to 14 hours before removing (shower or bath). For

elderly patients, also apply onto the hairline, neck, scalp, temple, and forehead. May repeat if living mites are observed 14 days after the first treatment. One application is generally curative.

- Scabies, crusted (Norwegian scabies) (off-label use): Topical cream 5%: Apply to the entire body; leave on for 8 to 14 hours before washing off with water. Repeat this regimen daily for 7 days, and then twice weekly until symptoms have resolved.

Dosing: Pediatric

- Head lice: Note first-line treatment if community resistance is not an issue.
- Infants ≥2 months, children, and adolescents: Topical: cream rinse, lotion 1%: After hair has been washed with conditioner-free shampoo, rinse with water, and towel dry. Apply a sufficient volume of permethrin cream/rinse lotion to saturate the hair and scalp. Also apply behind the ears and at the base of the neck. Leave on hair for 10 minutes before rinsing off with water; remove remaining nits. May repeat in 7 to 10 days if live lice or nits observed.
- Scabies: Infants ≥2 months, children, and adolescents: Topical: cream 5%: Apply and massage in cream from the head to toe (average adult requires 30 g). Leave on for 8 to 14 hours before washing off with water. For infants, also apply on the hairline, neck, scalp, temple, and forehead. May reapply in 14 days if live mites appear.

Pharmacokinetics

- Permethrin is rapidly metabolized by ester hydrolysis to inactive metabolites which are excreted primarily in the urine.
- Although the amount of permethrin absorbed after a single application of the 5% cream has not been determined precisely, data from studies with 14C-labeled permethrin and absorption studies of the cream applied to patients with moderate to severe scabies indicate it is 2% or less of the amount applied.

Use in Special Populations

- Pregnancy Considerations
  - The amount of permethrin absorbed systemically following topical application is ≤2%. The CDC considers the use of permethrin or pyrethrins with piperonyl butoxide the drugs of choice for the treatment of pubic lice during pregnancy. Permethrin is the preferred treatment for scabies during pregnancy.
- Breastfeeding Considerations
  - It is not known if permethrin is present in breast milk following topical administration for the treatment of scabies or lice. Permethrin exhibits minimal systemic absorption following topical administration (≤2% of applied amount), and any absorbed drug is rapidly metabolized to inactive metabolites. Therefore, breastfeeding is not expected to result in significant exposure to a breastfed child.
- Pediatrics
  - When used for self-medication, do not use on infants <2 months of age.

Carcinogenicity

- No data on the carcinogenicity of permethrin in humans.
- Evidence of permethrin's possible carcinogenicity in humans is derived from bioassays in rodents. Based on the weight of evidence from animal studies, EPA has classified permethrin as "likely to be carcinogenic to humans" by ingestion. This rating is based on benign lung and liver tumors found in mice and similar, though inconclusive, evidence in rats, as well as corroborative Structure-Activity Relationships (SAR) information.

Contraindications and Cautions

- Contraindications: Hypersensitivity to permethrin, pyrethroid, pyrethrin, or any component of the formulation.
- OTC labeling (cream rinse/lotion): When used for self-medication, do not use on infants <2 months of age.
- Do not use near the eyes or inside the nose, ear, mouth, or vagina. Consult health care provider for use on eyebrows or eyelashes.

Adverse Effects

- Central nervous system: Local discomfort (scalp), localized burning, localized numbness, and tingling of the skin
- Dermatologic: Pruritus, erythema, skin rash (scalp), and stinging of the skin

Patch Test Concentration

- Not available

Spinosad

Classification and Mode of Action

- Antiparasitic agent, topical; pediculicide
- Spinosad (a mixture of two glycosylated macrolactones spinosyn A and spinosyn D) is pediculicidal and ovicidal used for the topical treatment of scabies and pediculosis capitis and pubis. Insect paralysis and death is caused by central nervous system excitation and involuntary muscle contractions.

Comparative Efficacy

- Spinosad, which does not require nit combing, is significantly more effective than permethrin in the comparative efficacy studies reflecting actual-use conditions. Most spinosad-treated participants required only one application. Spinosad is a more convenient and effective treatment for pediculosis capitis than permethrin.

Indications and Dermatologic Uses

- Clinically indicated for the topical treatment of scabies (*Sarcoptes scabiei*) in adults and pediatric patients greater than 4 years of age and pediculosis capitis in adults and pediatric patients greater than 6 months of age

Formulations

- Natroba 0.9% topical suspension (brand name), generic formulations are available.

Dosages and Administration

Dosing: Adult

- Head lice, topical: Apply sufficient amount to cover dry scalp and completely cover dry hair. One hundred twenty mL may be necessary depending on hair length. If live lice are seen 7 days after the first treatment, repeat with second application.
- Scabies, topical: Apply sufficient amount to completely cover body from the neck to the toes (including soles of the feet). Apply to the forehead, hairline, scalp, and temples in patients who are balding. Leave on the skin for ≥6 hours prior to bathing or showering.

Dosing: Pediatric

- Head lice: Infants ≥6 months, children, and adolescents: Topical suspension: Apply sufficient amount to cover dry scalp and completely cover dry hair (maximum single application dose: 120 mL). Leave on for 10 minutes and then rinse out with warm water. If live lice are seen 7 days after the first treatment, repeat with second application.
- Scabies: Children ≥4 years and adolescents: Topical suspension: Apply sufficient amount to cover the body from the neck to the toes (including the soles of feet). If patient is bald, apply to the forehead, hairline, scalp, and temples. Allow to absorb into the skin for 10 minutes before putting on clothes. Leave on the skin for ≥6 hours prior to bathing or showering.

Pharmacokinetics

Absorption: Spinosad is not absorbed topically (<3 ng/mL in a pediatric patient plasma sampling study). Absorption of the benzyl alcohol was not analyzed in this study.

Use in Special Populations

- Pregnancy considerations
  - The amount of spinosad absorbed systemically following topical administration is below the limit of quantification (<3 ng/mL). Human studies did not assess the absorption of benzyl alcohol, an ingredient in the product. However, maternal use is not likely to result in fetal exposure.
- Breastfeeding considerations
  - It is not known if spinosad is present in breast milk following topical application.

- The amount of spinosad absorbed systemically following topical administration is below the limit of quantification (<3 ng/mL). Maternal use is not likely to result in infant exposure to spinosad or benzyl alcohol via breast milk. According to the manufacturer, the decision to breastfeed during therapy should take into consideration the risk of infant exposure, the benefits of breastfeeding to the infant, and the benefits of treatment to the mother.
- Spinosad should be removed from the breast area with soap and water prior to breastfeeding to minimize direct infant exposure.

- Pediatric considerations
  - Some dosage forms may contain benzyl alcohol. Large amounts of benzyl alcohol (≥99 mg/kg/day) have been associated with a potentially fatal toxicity ("gasping syndrome") in neonates. The "gasping syndrome" consists of metabolic acidosis, respiratory distress, gasping respirations, CNS dysfunction (including convulsions, intracranial hemorrhage), hypotension, and cardiovascular collapse.
  - Avoid or use dosage forms containing benzyl alcohol with caution in neonates. See manufacturer's labeling.

Carcinogenicity

- In multiple studies, animals were fed low to moderate amounts of spinosad in their diet for 1.5 to 2 years. No increased incidence of cancer was observed. Moreover, spinosad has not been found to be mutagenic. As a result of these experiments, the EPA has classified spinosad as not likely to cause cancer.

Contraindications and Cautions

- There are no contraindications listed in the US manufacturer's labeling.

- Appropriate use: For topical use only; not for oral, ophthalmic, or intravaginal use. Avoid contact with eyes. Wash hands after application.
- See cautions discussed under Use in Special Populations above.

Monitoring Parameters

Patients should be monitored for persistence of scabies or lice.

Adverse Effects

- Dermatologic: Erythema of eyelid (2%), xeroderma (2%)
- Local: Application site burning (≤3%), application site erythema (3%), application site irritation (≤3%), and application site pain (≤3%)

References

Ivermectin

1. FDA drug monograph (Ivermectin) FDA drug monograph SKLICE lotion. Available from https://www.accessdata.fda.gov/drugsatfda_docs/label/2017/202736s003lbl.pdf.
2. LexiComp drug monograph (name of monograph). Available from: LexiComp Online at online.Lexi.com. Copyright 2024 UptoDate, Inc.
3. Frankowski BL, Bocchini JA Jr. Head lice. Pediatrics. 2010;126(2):392–403. [PubMed 20660553].

Lindane

4. FDA drug monograph (Lindane).
5. LexiComp drug monograph (Lindane).
6. Feldmann RJ, Maibach HI. Toxicol Appl Pharmacol. 1974;28:126.
7. Leone PA. Scabies and pediculosis pubis. An update of treatment regimens and general review. Clin Infect Dis. 2007;44(Suppl 3):S153.

Permethrin

8. FDA drug monograph (Permethrin).
9. LexiComp drug monograph (Permethrin).
10. Devore CD, Schutze GE, Council on School Health and Committee on Infectious Diseases, American Academy of Pediatrics. Head lice. Pediatrics. 2015;135(5):e1355–65. [PubMed 25917986].

Spinosad

11. FDA drug monograph (Spinosad).
12. LexiComp drug monograph (Spinosad).
13. Stough D, Shellabarger S, Quiring J, Gabrielsen AA Jr. Efficacy and safety of spinosad and permethrin creme rinses for pediculosis capitis (head lice). Pediatrics. 2009;124(3):e389–95. [PubMed 19706558].
14. Centers for Disease Control (CDC). Neonatal deaths associated with use of benzyl alcohol—United States. MMWR Morb Mortal Wkly Rep. 1982;31(22):290–1. http://www.cdc.gov/mmwr/preview/mmwrhtml/00001109.htm [PubMed 6810084].
15. Shehab N, Lewis CL, Streetman DD, Donn SM. Exposure to the pharmaceutical excipients benzyl alcohol and propylene glycol among critically ill neonates. Pediatr Crit Care Med. 2009;10(2):256–9. [PubMed 19188870].

Depigmenting and Pigmenting Agents

20

Anuk Burli and Chavy Chiang

Contents

Hyper−/hypopigmentation in dermatology patients remains a challenge for many physicians. Treatment options for hyperpigmentation in conditions such as melasma include hydroquinone/triluma. Mequinol is used primarily for the treatment of hyperpigmented solar lentigines. With regard to hypo−/depigmentation, monobenzone has been used for extensive vitiligo (greater than

A. Burli (✉)
Department of Dermatology, Stanford University School of Medicine, Redwood City, CA, USA
e-mail: anukb@stanford.edu

C. Chiang
Department of Dermatology, University of Rochester Medical Center, Rochester, NY, USA
e-mail: chavyz@gmail.com

R. M. Law, H. I. Maibach (eds.), *Handbook of Topical Drug Treatment in Dermatology*,
https://doi.org/10.1007/978-3-031-93616-6_20

50% body surface area) to depigment normal skin. Methoxsalen has been used off-label for the treatment of depigmentation in vitiligo—to increase pigmentation in vitiligous skin. Methoxsalen is also used together with UVA for the treatment of psoriasis. There is also an oral formulation for methoxsalen.

Hydroquinone/Triluma

Classification and Mode of Action

- Hydroquinone: Depigmenting agent: Reversibly depigments the skin by inhibiting tyrosine hydroxylase which oxidizes tyrosine to DOPA (3,4-dihydroxyphenylalanine). Sun exposure however can reverse this, leading to repigmentation.
- Triluma: Depigmenting agent combined with topical corticosteroid and topical retinoid.

Indications and Dermatological Uses

- *Clinical indications (not FDA approved)*: Skin bleaching. This product has been banned for over the counter use as part of the Coronavirus Aid, Relief, and Economic Security (CARES) Act.
- *Comparative trials*
  - A double-blind randomized clinical trial showed that hydroquinone had a near 10% improvement of hyperpigmentation compared to skin whitening agents, but with 25% more side effects.

Formulations/Presentation

- US hydroquinone: 1.5% cream, 2% cream, 4% cream, 2% gel, 3% external solution
- Canada hydroquinone: 4% cream, 4% gel
- US Triluma: 0.01% cream, 4% cream, 0.05% cream

Dosages and Suggested Regimens

- Topical: Apply a thin layer to hyperpigmented areas and rub the cream in twice daily, both in the morning and at night before sleep.
- Patient can discontinue use if there is no depigmentation seen after 2 to 3 months of treatment.

Baseline Investigations and Considerations

- None

Pharmacokinetics

- Onset and duration of the depigmentation effect varies among individuals depending on genetic profile.

Use in Special Populations

- Approved for use in children. Adult dosing can be used for patients 12 years old and above.
- Listed as FDA pregnancy classification C (former classification system).
- Unknown whether hydroquinone is present in breast milk.
- Renal insufficiency: dose adjustment is not expected to be needed.
- Hepatic insufficiency: dose adjustment is not expected to be needed.

Monitoring

- Skin irritation

Contraindications and Cautions

- Certain individuals have hypersensitivity to hydroquinone or any component of the formulation in triluma.

Important Drug Interactions

- No known significant interactions

Adverse Effects and Their Management

- Patients can have allergic skin reaction or dermatitis in response to component of formulation.
- Erythema and inflammation as a result of excessive application.
- Mild stinging of the skin when initially applying.
- Xeroderma.
- Exogenous ochronosis: discontinue treatment if this occurs.

Patch Test Concentration

- 1% pet. (Chemotechnique, SmartPracticeEurope; SmartPracticeCanada); this test concentration may cause irritant reactions.

Essential Patient Information

- Sunscreen use is necessary to use during hydroquinone therapy, as sunlight can sustain melanocytic activity. To avoid repigmentation, during treatment and maintenance therapy, sun exposure on affected areas should be avoided by applying a broad spectrum sunscreen (SPF 15 or greater) or by using sun-protective clothing.
- Avoid contact with eyes and mucous membranes when applying.

- Keep hydroquinone out of reach of children. In the case of accidental ingestion, call a physician or a poison control center immediately.

Monobenzone

Classification and Mode of Action

- Depigmenting agent. Monobenzone is the monobenzyl ether of hydroquinone.
- The proposed mechanism of action is increasing the excretion of melanin from melanocytes where the melanin is then lost with normal loss and sloughing of stratum corneum.

Indications and Dermatological Uses

- Clinical indications (FDA): Help to permanently depigment normal skin surrounding vitiligious lesions, used only in patients with extensive disseminated vitiligo (greater than 50% body surface area)

Formulations/Presentation

- USA: Monobenzone cream 20%
- Canada: Monobenzone cream 20%

Dosages and Suggested Regimens

A thin layer of monobenzone cream 20% can be applied two or three times daily. Depigmentation can be seen after 1 to 4 months of topical treatment. If satisfactory results are not obtained after 4 months of treatment, the drug should be discontinued.

Pharmacokinetics

- Onset of the depigmentation effect varies among individuals

Use in Special Populations

- Pregnancy: Category C (former classification system).
- Lactation: It is not known whether this drug is excreted in human milk.
- Pediatric population: The safety and effectiveness of monobenzone cream 20% in pediatric patients below the age of 12 years have not been established.
- Renal insufficiency: No FDA guidance.
- Hepatic Insufficiency: No FDA guidance.

Monitoring

- Discontinue use if patient has severe irritation, burning sensation, or dermatitis.

Contraindications and Cautions

- Monobenzone cream 20% is contraindicated for any other conditions other than disseminated vitiligo (>50% body surface area).
- Monobenzone cream 20% can produce irreversible depigmentation and should not be a substitute for hydroquinone.
- Monobenzone cream 20% is contraindicated in individuals with a history of sensitivity or allergic reactions to monobenzone product, or any of the ingredients.

Important Drug Interactions

- Limited information

Adverse Effects and Their Management

- Mild, transient skin irritation and sensitization, such as erythematous and eczematous skin reactions.
- Discontinue use if patient has irritation, a burning sensation, or dermatitis.

Patch Test Concentration

- 1% pet. (Chemotechnique, SmartPractice Europe, SmartPractice Canada)

Essential Patient Information

- Monobenzone cream should only be used when having disseminated vitiligo (greater than 50%). Stop the use if no improvement after 4 months and pet. Stop severe irritation, burning, or dermatitis occur.

Mequinol (Solage = Mequinol + Tretinoin)

For the tretinoin monograph, please see Chap. 23.

Classification and Mode of Action

- Substrate for the enzyme tyrosinase acts as a competitive inhibitor of the formation of melanin precursors.

Indications and Dermatological Uses

- *Clinical indications (FDA)*: Treatment of solar lentigines

Formulations/Presentation

- USA: Solage: mequinol 2%, tretinoin 0.01% topical solution
- Canada: Solage: mequinol 2%, tretinoin 0.01% topical solution

Dosages and Suggested Regimens

- Apply Solage to solar lentigines using the applicator tip given with the topical solution while avoiding application to the surrounding non-affected skin. Use twice daily, morning and evening at least 8 hours apart, or as stated by the physician.
- Patients should not shower or wash with water the treatment areas for at least 6 hours after application of Solage.
- Special caution is needed when applying Solage to avoid the eyes, mouth, and mucous membranes throughout the body.

Pharmacokinetics

- The percutaneous absorption of tretinoin and mequinol in Solage was assessed in healthy subjects (n = 8) following 2 weeks of twice daily topical treatment of Solage for solar lentigines. Approximately 0.8 mL of Solage was applied to a 400 cm^2 area of the back, corresponding to a dose of 37.3 mg/cm^2 for mequinol and 0.23 mg/cm^2 for tretinoin.
- The percutaneous absorption of tretinoin was 4.4%, and systemic concentrations did not increase over baseline endogenous levels.
- The mean Cmax for mequinol was 9.92 ng/mL with a range 4.22 to 23.62 ng/mL, and the Tmax was 2 hours with a range 1 to 2 hours.

Use in Special Populations

- Pregnancy: Pregnancy category X (former classification). Teratogenic. Contraindicated in pregnancy.
- Lactation: It is not known to what extent mequinol and/or tretinoin is excreted in human milk.
- Children: The safety of this product have not been established in pediatric patients. Solage should not be used in the pediatric population.
- Renal insufficiency: Unknown.
- Hepatic insufficiency: Unknown.

Monitoring

If a drug sensitivity, chemical irritation, or a systemic adverse reaction occurs, patient should discontinue use of Solage

Contraindications and Cautions

- Absolutely contraindicated in pregnancy
- History of hypersensitivity to any of the ingredients.

Important Drug Interactions

- Topical products with a strong drying effect, high concentrations of alcohol, astringents, spices /lime, medicated soaps or shampoos, permanent wave solutions, electrolysis, hair depilatories or waxes, or various other products that might dry or irritate the skin should be used with caution in patients using Solage as they can increase irritation.

Adverse Effects and Their Management

- Erythema occurred in 49% of patients in a clinical trial; burning, stinging or tingling occurred in 26%; desquamation occurred in 14%; pruritus occurred in 12% of patients; and skin irritation occurred in 5%.
- Some patients experienced temporary hypopigmentation of treated lesions (5%) or of the unaffected skin surrounding the lesion. This hypopigmentation generally resolved after discontinuation of the product within 120 days.

Patch Test Concentration

- No data available (mequinol)
- 0.005 alcohol (tretinoin); if higher is used (0.01% or 0.02%), perform adequate controls.

Essential Patient Information

Solage should only be used as an adjunct treatment along with sun protection and sun avoidance for solar lentigos.

Methoxsalen

Classification and Mode of Action

- Psoralen: Methoxsalen covalently bonds to DNA, specifically the pyrimidine bases. This inhibits DNA synthesis and suppresses cell division. A sunburn reaction excites methoxsalen with UVA radiation, transferring energy to methoxsalen, allowing it to reach an excited state or a "triplet state." The molecule, in this "triplet state," then reacts with skin DNA. An erythematous reaction then is repaired with increased melanization of the epidermis and stratum corneum thickening.

Indications and Dermatological Uses

- *Clinical indications (FDA)*: Palliative treatment of cutaneous T-cell lymphoma
- *Off-label common uses*: Repigmentation of idiopathic vitiligo

Formulations/Presentation

- USA: Sterile solution 20 mcg/mL (this was difficult for me to find how it is actually dosed). 1% cream
- Canada
- Europe

Dosages and Suggested Regimens

Topical: Prior to UVA light exposure, methoxsalen location is applied. These sessions are done no more than once weekly, but the ultimate frequency is decided by the level of erythema.

Baseline Investigations and Considerations

Pharmacokinetics

Half-life of 2 hours and rapidly excreted in both humans and rats

Use in Special Populations

- Pregnancy Risk Factor C. (Former FDA pregnancy risk classification system)
- Lactation: Unknown if excreted in breast milk.
- Children: Dosing can be same as adults in children greater than 12 years old. Contraindicated less than 12 years old.
- Renal insufficiency: No specific guidelines regarding changes in dosing.
- Hepatic insufficiency: No specific guidelines regarding changes in dosing.

Monitoring

- Patients require sunlight precautions while using this drug.

Contraindications and Cautions

- Hypersensitivity to methoxsalen or any component of the drug formulation
- Photosensitivity and associated diseases such as porphyria, albinism, lupus erythematosus, or xeroderma pigmentosum
- Any kind of invasive skin cancer
- Active melanoma or a personal history of melanoma
- Contraindicated in children <12 years of age
- Use with caution in patients with basal cell carcinoma or history of basal cell carcinoma

Important Drug Interactions

- No known significant drug interactions. However, ensure sun protection if on concomitant medication with photosensitizing potential.

Adverse Effects and Their Management

- Burns: Wear protective clothing and sunscreen to prevent.
- Cataracts: Eyes should be shielded for 24 hours to prevent.
- Photosensitivity: Avoid sun exposure for 8 hours after methoxsalen, and sun protective clothing, eye wear, and sunscreen should be used for several days after treatment.
- Skin cancer: Use with caution in patients with sun damage, history of arsenic exposure, or history of radiation exposure

Patch Test Concentration

- 0.15% alcohol; for photopatch testing, a dilution series (0.15%, 0.015%, 0.0015%) may be necessary to differentiate photoallergy from phototoxicity.

Essential Patient Information

- Sun protection is essential when undergoing treatment with this medication.

References

Hydroquinone/Triluma

1. FDA Drug Monograph Hydroquinone/Triluma. Available from http://assets.openstudy.com/updates/attachments/4f0d5cb6e4b084a815fccd72-chmvijay-1326448458607-dipolemoment.pdf. Accessed 11/04/2021.
2. LexiComp drug monograph Hydroqinone/Triluma. Available from: LexiComp Online at online.lexi.com Copyright 2021 UpToDate, Inc.
3. Schwartz C, Jan A, Zito PM. Hydroquinone. [Updated 2021 May 10]. In: StatPearls [Internet]. Treasure Island: StatPearls Publishing; 2021. Available from: https://www.ncbi.nlm.nih.gov/books/NBK539693/.
4. Kim GH, Cheong KA, Lee AY. Increased skin irritation by hydroquinone and retinoic acid used in combination. Ann Dermatol. 2017;29(6):715–21. https://doi.org/10.5021/ad.2017.29.6.715. Epub 2017 Oct 30. PMID: 29200759; PMCID: PMC5705352.
5. Haddad AL, Matos LF, Brunstein F, Ferreira LM, Silva A, Costa D Jr. A clinical, prospective, randomized, double-blind trial comparing skin whitening complex with hydroquinone vs. placebo in the treatment of melasma. Int J Dermatol. 2003;42(2):153–6. https://doi.org/10.1046/j.1365-4362.2003.01621.x. PMID: 12709008.

Monobenzone

6. FDA Drug Monograph Monobenzone. Accessed from: https://www.accessdata.fda.gov/drugsatfda_docs/label/2003/08173slr015_benoquin_lbl.pdf. Accessed 11/04/2021.
7. van den Boorn JG, Melief CJ, Luiten RM. Monobenzone-induced depigmentation: from enzymatic blockade to autoimmunity. Pigment Cell Melanoma Res. 2011;24(4):673–9. https://doi.org/10.1111/j.1755-148X.2011.00878.x. Epub 2011 Jul 6. PMID: 21689385.
8. Catona A, Lanzer D. Monobenzone, Superfade, vitiligo and confetti-like depigmentation. Med J Aust. 1987;146(6):320–1. https://doi.org/10.5694/j.1326-5377.1987.tb120272.x. PMID: 3821640.

Mequinol (Solage = Mequinol + Tretinoin)

9. FDA Drug Monograph Mequinol. Accessed from: https://www.accessdata.fda.gov/drugsatfda_docs/label/2007/020922s003lbl.pdf. Accessed 11/04/2021.
10. Jarratt M. Mequinol 2%/tretinoin 0.01% solution: an effective and safe alternative to hydroquinone 3% in the treatment of solar lentigines. Cutis. 2004;74(5):319–22. PMID: 15605971.
11. Fleischer AB Jr, Schwartzel EH, Colby SI, Altman DJ. The combination of 2% 4-hydroxyanisole (Mequinol) and 0.01% tretinoin is effective in improving the appearance of solar lentigines and related hyperpigmented lesions in two double-blind multicenter clinical studies. J Am Acad Dermatol. 2000;42(3):459–67. https://doi.org/10.1016/s0190-9622(00)90219-6. PMID: 10688717.

Methoxsalen

12. FDA Drug Monograph Methoxsalen. Accessed from: https://www.accessdata.fda.gov/drugsatfda_docs/label/2007/020922s003lbl.pdf. Accessed 11/04/2021.
13. LexiComp drug monograph Methoxsalen. Available from: LexiComp Online at online.lexi.com Copyright 2021 UpToDate, Inc.
14. von Weymarn LB, Zhang QY, Ding X, Hollenberg PF. Effects of 8-methoxypsoralen on cytochrome P450 2A13. Carcinogenesis. 2005;26(3):621–9. https://doi.org/10.1093/carcin/bgh348. Epub 2004 Dec 3.

15. Recommendations for the Safe Handling of Parenteral Antineoplastic Drugs, NIH Publication No. 83–2621. For sale by the Superintendent of Documents, U.S. Government Printing Office, Washington, DC 20402.
16. AMA Council Report. Guidelines for Handling of Parenteral Antineoplastics. JAMA. 1985;2.53 (11):1590–2.
17. National Study Commission on Cytotoxic Exposure- Recommendations for Handling Cytotoxic Agents. Available from Louis P. Jeffrey, ScD., Chairman, National Study Commission on Cytotoxic Exposure, Massachusetts College of Pharmacy and Allied Health Sciences, 179 Longwood Avenue, Boston, Massachusetts 02115.
18. Clinical Oncological Society of Australia. Guidelines and recommendations for safe handling of reference ID: 4204794 antineoplastic agents. Med J Australia. 1983;1:426–8.
19. Jones RB, et al. Safe handling of chemotherapeutic agents: a report from the Mount Sinai Medical Center. CA Cancer J Clin. 1983;33:258–63.
20. American Society of Hospital Pharmacists Technical Assistance Bulletin of Handling Cytotoxic and Hazardous Drugs. Am J Hosp Pharm. 1990;47:1033–49.
21. Controlling Occupational Exposure to Hazardous Drugs. (OSHA Work-Practice Guidelines). Am J Health Syst Pharm. 1996;53:1669–85.

Psoriasis 21

Rebecca M. Law, Erin Bartholomew, Mimi Chung, Sarah J. Currie, Marwa Hakimi, Samuel Yeroushalmi, and Wilson Liao

Contents

R. M. Law (✉)
School of Pharmacy and Faculty of Medicine (Discipline of Family Medicine), Memorial University of Newfoundland, St. John's, NL, Canada
e-mail: rlaw@mun.ca; rlawUCSF@gmail.com

E. Bartholomew
Department of Dermatology, Eastern Virginia Medical School, Norfolk, VA, USA
e-mail: erin.bartholomew@ucsf.edu

M. Chung
University of Alabama at Birmingham, Birmingham, AL, USA
e-mail: mimi.chung@ucsf.edu

S. J. Currie
Faculty of Medicine, Memorial University of Newfoundland, St. John's, NL, Canada
e-mail: sarahjcurrie@gmail.com

M. Hakimi
Department of Dermatology, University of California San Francisco (UCSF), San Francisco, CA, USA
e-mail: marwa.hakimi@ucsf.edu

R. M. Law, H. I. Maibach (eds.), *Handbook of Topical Drug Treatment in Dermatology*,
https://doi.org/10.1007/978-3-031-93616-6_21

Introduction

Rebecca M. Law and Wilson Liao

Psoriasis is a progressive T-lymphocyte-mediated systemic inflammatory disease that results from a complex interplay between multiple genetic factors and environmental influences. Management involves nonpharmacologic and pharmacologic therapies, with attention to also manage any comorbid conditions (such as metabolic syndrome, depression), and other specific patient considerations such as hepatic or renal dysfunction [1].

Treatment of psoriasis is based on managing the underlying pathophysiology. Agents that modulate the abnormal immune response, such as topical corticosteroids (TCS) and biologic agents, are important treatment strategies for psoriasis. Topical therapies that affect cell turnover, such as retinoids, are also effective for psoriasis. In addition, nonpharmacologic therapies are effective adjuncts and should be considered for all patients with psoriasis. A treatment regimen should always be individualized, taking into consideration severity of disease, patient responses, and tolerability to various interventions. Furthermore, if comorbidities exist, they must be taken into treatment considerations and managed early. Optimal psoriasis care needs to maintain a focus on the patient's overall health-related quality of life [1].

Nonpharmacologic alternatives such as stress reduction and the liberal use of moisturizers may be beneficial and should always be considered and initiated when appropriate [1]. These will not be discussed in this chapter.

Pharmacologic alternatives for psoriasis include topical agents, phototherapy, and systemic agents (traditional, biologics, and newer nonbiologics, e.g., apremilast and deucravacitinib). There are also

S. Yeroushalmi
Department of Dermatology, University of California San Francosco, San Francisco, USA
e-mail: samuel.yeroushalmi@ucsf.edu

W. Liao (✉)
Department of Dermatology, University of California (UCSF), San Francisco, CA, USA
e-mail: wilson.liao@ucsf.edu

many more biologics on the horizon. Pharmacologic therapy is generally guided by the severity of disease and its impact on the patient's quality of life [1]. For limited or mild-to-moderate disease, topical treatments are the mainstay of care [1–3]. Phototherapy and photochemotherapy are used in moderate-to-severe cases [1, 4, 5]. For patients presenting with extensive or moderate-to-severe disease, systemic therapies (non-biologic and biologic) with or without the use of topical treatments are the usual standard of care.[1, 6.7] Newer systemic treatments such as biologic agents or targeted oral agents may be the treatments of choice, especially for patients with comorbidities such as PsA or if traditional systemic treatments (such as methotrexate or cyclosporine) are contraindicated [1, 7–9]. This chapter will only include drug monographs for topical agents.

Approximately 80% of patients with psoriasis have mild-to-moderate disease, and the majority of these patients can be treated with topical therapies alone [3]. Individualized approaches are essential because of the wide variation in patients' presentations, their psychosocial health, and their personal opinions as to what would be acceptable treatment [10, 11]. Traditional topical therapies include corticosteroids, vitamin D_3 analogs, retinoids, anthralin, and coal tar [1, 3]. In addition, topical calcineurin inhibitors may be useful for difficult-to-treat sites such as the intertriginous areas or the face. More biologic agents and targeted nonbiologic agents are on the horizon [1]. Topical agents are also used as adjunctive therapy for patients with more extensive disease, who are being treated concurrently with phototherapy or systemic agents [1].

Drug Monographs

Anthralin [12]

Rebecca M. Law

Classification and Mode of Action

- Anthralin has a direct antiproliferative effect on epidermal keratinocytes [12–14], normalizing keratinocyte differentiation [15].

- It has a direct effect on mitochondria [15, 16] and reduces the mitotic activity of epidermal cells [14]. It inhibits synthesis of nucleic protein from inhibition of DNA synthesis [17].
- It also prevents T-lymphocyte activation [15].
- Small placebo-controlled studies demonstrated efficacy for anthralin used continuously or as short contact (1 minute of treatment) [15].

Indications and Dermatologic Uses

- Clinical indication (FDA): Plague psoriasis. (Anthralin is not as commonly used as other topical therapies currently available for psoriasis; however, there are situations where its use is appropriate and efficacious.)

Formulations

- Anthralin 1% cream, anthralin 1% shampoo
  - USA: Drithocreme, Dithro-Scalp, Psoriatec, and Zithranol
  - Can: Anthraforte 2, Anthraforte 3, and Anthrascalp
- Extemporaneously compounded anthralin used in short-contact anthralin therapy (SCAT) (various formulations—see under dosages)

Dosages and Suggested Regimens

- Short-contact anthralin therapy (SCAT) is usually the preferred regimen, where the anthralin ointment is applied only to the thick plaque lesions for 2 hours or less and then wiped off [15, 18]. To minimize irritation, it can be applied for 5 to 10 minutes daily initially and then titrating up the application time to 20 to 30 minutes or more as tolerated [14]. Because lesions are generally well demarcated, zinc oxide ointment or a nonmedicated stiff paste should be applied to the surrounding normal skin to protect it from irritation and burning [15].
- Concentrations for SCAT range from 1% to 4% or as tolerated
- Concentrations for continuous anthralin therapy vary from 0.05% to 0.4%

Contraindications and Cautions

- Anthralin should be used with caution, if at all, on the face and intertriginous areas because of the risk of severe skin irritation [15].
- Anthralin powder causes skin irritation. People who handle the dry anthralin powder should avoid skin contact (e.g., by wearing gloves while compounding) [18].

Use in Special Populations

- Elderly skin is more fragile and friable. Be cautious if using anthralin in elderly patients, if used at all. Use otheralternative treatments.
- Anthralin should not be applied to broken skin.

Adverse Effects and Their Management

- Aside from significant and often severe skin irritation, other adverse effects include folliculitis and allergic contact dermatitis, but these are uncommon.

Calcipotriene (Calcipotriol) Drug Monograph [20, 21]

Samuel Yeroushalmi, Rebecca M. Law, and Wilson Liao

Classification and Mode of Action

- Vitamin D3 analog. Calcipotriene (calcipotriol) is a synthetic derivative of vitamin D3 (cholecalciferol) that binds to vitamin D receptors on keratinocytes in order to enhance both keratinocyte proliferation and differentiation.
- For patients with mild to moderate psoriasis, calcipotriene has been shown to be superior to fluocinonide 500ug/g twice daily and betamethasone valerate 1–1.2 mg/g twice daily [22] Kragballe, 1991).
- Calcipotriene has been shown to be effective and safe in combination with other topical, systemic, or phototherapy treatments for psoriasis, and its use can reduce the dosage of these treatments [23].

Indications and Dermatologic Uses

- *Clinical indications (FDA)*: Plaque psoriasis
- *Off label common uses*: Vitiligo, acantholytic disorders, ichthyoses, morphea/linear scleroderma, lichen planus, prurigo nodularis, and pityriasis alba

Formulations/Presentation

- USA: 0.005% cream, 0.005% foam, 0.005% ointment, 0.005% solution
- Canada: 0.005% ointment

Dosages and Suggested Regimens

- Apply to skin once to twice daily.
- No suggested dosing adjustments for renal or hepatic impairment as per manufacturer.

Baseline Investigations and Considerations

Pharmacokinetics

- Absorption when applied to psoriasis plaques: ointment: 6%; solution: <1%; cream and foam undetermined. Serum half-life in rats shown to be 4 minutes. Converted to inactive metabolites and excreted in bile.
- Onset of effect: About 2 weeks, with marked improvement after 8 weeks.

Carcinogenicity: No indications of increased carcinogenic risk

Use in Special Populations

- Approved for use in children, though higher risk of systemic adverse events.
- Severity of skin-related adverse events may be increased in the elderly.
- FDA pregnancy category C.
- No dosage adjustment for hepatic or renal impairment.

Breast Milk

- Unknown if excreted in human breast milk

Monitoring

- Hypercalcemia has been observed with excessive topical use.
- Rash, skin irritation.
- Pruritus.
- Signs of allergic reaction such as hives, swollen lips or mouth, wheezing, trouble breathing, etc.

Contraindications and Cautions

- Hypersensitivity to calcipotriene or any formulation component
- Vitamin D toxicity
- Hypercalcemia
- Cream and ointment contraindicated for face use
- Scalp solution contraindicated for acute eruptions

Important Drug Interactions

- Acidic topical agents may inactivate calcipotriene (e.g., topical hydrocortisone valerate, lactic acid, and salicylic acid). If used together, consider separating the administration time by 10–12 hours to minimize the interaction. *Do not* compound these agents with calcipotriene into a combination product.
- Aluminum hydroxide: Calcipotriene may increase serum concentration of aluminum hydroxide by increasing aluminum absorption, resulting in increased serum aluminum concentrations. Avoid chronic use of aluminum-containing agents. If used together, monitor serum aluminum and aluminum-related toxicities.
- Thiazide and thiazide-like diuretics: Greater risk of hypercalcemia when used with calcipotriene.
- Calcium salts; may enhance toxicity of calcipotriene.
- Cardiac glycosides; calcipotriene may increase arrhythmogenic effects.
- Multivitamins/fluoride with ADE, or multivitamins/minerals with ADEK, iron, and folate may enhance toxicity of calcipotriene. Avoid combination.
- Sucralfate; calcipotriene may increase serum concentration of sucralfate, resulting in an increase in serum aluminum concentration. (Sucralfate is an aluminum-containing agent). Manage as per aluminum hydroxide discussion above.

- Calcipotriene may potentiate the effects of other vitamin D analogs

Adverse Effects and Their Management

- Tingling, burning, itching, and skin irritation are most commonly reported with use.
- May cause erythema, dry skin, and peeling were less commonly reported.
- May cause worsening of psoriasis, including development of facial or scalp psoriasis.
- May cause skin atrophy, hyperpigmentation, or folliculitis.
- May cause allergic contact dermatitis or contact dermatitis.
- Hypercalcemia may occur with excessive use. Calcipotriene should be discontinued until serum calcium returns to normal.

Patch Test Concentration [24]

- 2mcg/ml in citrate-buffered isopropyl alcohol is recommended. Positive test should be repeated in >3 months to ensure consistency over time; a repeated open application test may be needed.

Essential Patient Information

- For external use only.
- Wash hands after each use.
- Avoid application to mucous membranes or eyes.
- If excessive irritation or sensitivity reaction occurs on uninvolved areas, discontinue use.
- Avoid exposure to natural or artificial sunlight in areas where drug is applied.
- Foam may be flammable, keep away from open flame.

Calcitriol

Mimi Chung, Rebecca M. Law, and Wilson Liao

Classification and Mode of Action

- Vitamin D analog. Calcitriol is a synthetic version of vitamin D3. The mechanism behind its effectiveness in psoriasis is unclear, but it has been suggested that calcitriol may inhibit inflammatory mediators and decrease keratinocytes proliferation [32].
- High potency and super-high potency topical corticosteroids are slightly more efficacious than calcitriol [33]; however, topical calcitriol has been reported in one study to have a greater proportion of psoriasis patients to remain in remission post-treatment compared to betamethasone [34].
- Topical calcitriol and calcipotriene appear equally effective for psoriasis [33]. One study showed mild skin irritation and perilesional irritation on sensitive areas such as the intertriginous areas occurred less often with calcitriol than calcipotriene [35].
- Combination treatment of topical corticosteroids with vitamin D analogs has been shown to be more effective than topical corticosteroids or vitamin D analogs alone [33].

Indications and Dermatological Uses

- Clinical indications (FDA): Mild-to-moderate plaque psoriasis
- Off label common uses: Vitiligo (in combination with corticosteroids and phototherapy), some acantholytic disorders, morphea, pityriasis alba, prurigo nodularis, and polymorphous light eruption [36]

Formulations/Presentation

- USA: 3 mcg/g ointment
- Canada: 3 mcg/g ointment

Dosages and Suggested Regimens

- Apply topically twice daily to affected areas. Two hundred grams weekly maximum for adults and children 7 years and older.
- No recommendations regarding suggested dosage adjustment for renal or hepatic impairment.

Baseline Investigations and Considerations

- Topical corticosteroids are the preferred initial topical treatment for psoriasis compared to vitamin D analogs alone like calcitriol and calcipotriene based on data showing better efficacy and lower price point [37].

Pharmacokinetics

- Minimal topical absorption. Topical absorption when applied twice daily for 21 days caused an increase of 36% geometric mean plasma concentration values and an increase of 44% in geometric mean value of $AUC_{(0-12\ hr)}$. Calcitriol is a minor substrate of CYP3A4. Terminal half-life was not determined, as plasma levels of calcitriol were relatively flat during pharmacokinetic studies. Excretion in urine and bile, via enterohepatic system [37].
- Onset of effect: Approximately 2 weeks [38].

Use in Special Populations

- Approved for use in children 2 years or older. Maximum use for children ages 2–7 years old should not exceed 100 g per week.
- Listed as FDA pregnancy classification C. Other topical agents other than calcitriol recommended for treatment in pregnant women, though the limited available data has not shown any drug-associated risk for major birth defects or adverse maternal outcomes.
- Unknown whether calcitriol is present in breast milk. Recommend against using topical calcitriol on the nipple and areola and avoidance of infant exposure if breastfeeding.
- Renal insufficiency: Not evaluated; monitoring of calcium and phosphorus levels is recommended in patients with renal failure with concurrent appropriate nutritional counseling.

- Hepatic insufficiency: Not evaluated.
- *Canadian labeling*: Contraindications for topical calcitriol use include severe renal impairment or end-stage renal disease. Hepatic impairment is also a contraindication for use.

Monitoring

- Consider monitoring for hypercalcemia and hypercalciuria per the drug interactions listed below
- Skin discomfort and irritation
- Pruritus
- Acute blistering dermatitis (reported postmarking)

Contraindications and Cautions

- Calcitriol should not be used in combination with other vitamin D analogs.
- Use caution in patients with known calcium disorders, including patients taking calcium supplementation, high doses of vitamin D, or other medications known to cause hypercalcemia.
- Calcitriol may enhance the photosensitizing effect of both systemic and topical aminolevulinic acid. Avoid combination therapy.
- Calcitriol may exacerbate the side effects of burosumab. Avoid combination therapy.
- *Canadian labeling*: Contraindications to treatment include the following: hypersensitivity to calcitriol or any of its components; disorders of calcium metabolism, history of hypercalcemia, or active treatment of calcium abnormalities; and hepatic impairment or significant renal impairment/end-stage renal disease (ESRD). Ophthalmic and internal use is contraindicated.

Important Drug Interactions

- *Other vitamin D analogs*: Adverse effects may be exacerbated by calcitriol. Avoid concomitant use.
- *Burosumab*: Adverse effects of burosumab may be exacerbated by vitamin D analogs like calcitriol. Avoid concomitant use.
- *Multivitamins with folate, iron, fluoride, and vitamin A, D, E, or K* may enhance adverse events related to calcitriol. Avoid combination therapy.

- *Aminolevulinic acid*: Calcitriol should not be used with systemic aminolevulinic acid due to enhanced photosensitivity. Use with topical aminolevulinic acid should be monitored.
- *Aluminum hydroxide and sucralfate*: Calcitriol may increase serum aluminum levels when used in combination with aluminum hydroxide and sucralfate. Alternative therapies should be considered; if used concurrently, monitoring of aluminum levels and signs of aluminum-related toxicities is recommended.
- *Thiazides and thiazide diuretics*: Effects on calcium homeostasis may be influenced by calcitriol. Monitoring therapy and response recommended.
- *Cardiac glycosides*: Antiarrhythmic effects may be enhanced with calcitriol. Monitoring treatment recommended.
- *Photosensitizing agents*: Calcitriol will potentially exacerbate photosensitizing effect of medications that cause photosensitivity (e.g., systemic methoxsalen, porfimer, and verteporfin). Therapy should be monitored.

Adverse Effects and Their Management

- *Hypercalcemia:* Alterations in calcium metabolism causing hypercalcemia were seen, though symptomatic elevations are extremely rare. Cases in postmarketing reporting were generally in older adults who used topical calcitriol on larger areas of the body. If lab abnormalities are noted, discontinue treatment until values normalize.
- *Hypercalciuria:* Urine lab abnormalities, specifically hypercalciuria, were reported to occur. Discontinue treatment until values normalize.
- *Skin discomfort and irritation*: Skin discomfort, erythema, acute blistering dermatitis, and skin burning sensation were reported to occur. Discontinue treatment with topical calcitriol.
- *Kidney stones*: Kidney stones were reported in a small number of patients during open label trial.

Patch Test Concentration

- Not available

Essential Patient Information

- Apply medication only to lesional skin. Do not apply to healthy skin.
- Do not ingest. For external use only. Avoid contact with face, eyes, lips, or other mucous membranes (e.g., inside nose).
- Avoid using photosensitizing medications. Calcitriol ointment may make skin more photosensitive.
- Do not use at the same time as multivitamins containing folate, iron, and fluoride. Do not take with multivitamins with vitamin A, vitamin D, vitamin E, and/or vitamin K.
- Do not use at the same time as vitamin D or other vitamin D analogs.

Corticosteroids

Kiha Kim, Taylor Skinner, and Rebecca M. Law

See Chap. 18 for a discussion of topical corticosteroids (TCS), the drug monographs of TCS, and a Corticosteroid Potency Table.

Crisaborole

Rebecca M. Law

See Chap. 17 for the crisaborole drug monograph.

Coal Tar & Tar Distillates

Sarah J. Currie and Rebecca M. Law

Classification and Mode of Action

Coal tar and tar distillates loosen and soften scales and crusts through their antiseptic, antibacterial, and antiseborrheic properties. Coal tar has been shown to be very effective for full-body psoriasis, although there is a lack of data regarding its efficacy in the scalp. One study demonstrated that use of a coal tar gel for 5 days was effective in improving scalp psoriasis. Another study showed the effectiveness of a topical coal tar foam combined with topical steroids for treatment-resistant scalp psoriasis. One prospective randomized study compared the application of a coal tar ointment overnight (on one side of the lesion) with calcipotriol ointment (on the other side of the lesion). The calcipotriol ointment showed superior cosmetic acceptability and faster initial response; however, coal tar ointment had comparable efficacy after a long period of treatment, i.e., a comparable reduction in the ESI (erythema, scaling, and induration) score after 12 weeks. There was no statistically significant difference in the relapse rates between the two treatments in this study.

Indications and Dermatological Uses

- *Clinical indications (FDA)*
  - *Scalp conditions (dandruff, psoriasis, seborrheic dermatitis)*: Shampoo. See under Chap. 23 monograph.
  - *Skin conditions (psoriasis, seborrheic dermatitis)*: Cream, foam, lotion, ointment, bath, and foot/hand soak. To relief symptoms (itching, scaling, flaking, redness, and irritation).
- *Off-label common uses*
  - *Atopic dermatitis in children and adolescents*: Two percent to 5% coal tar cream applied once daily or once every other day, to reduce inflammation. Limited data available.

Formulations/Presentation

- USA:
  - Emulsion, external: Cutar: 1.5% (177 mL) (contains methylparaben, polysorbate 80, propylparaben)
  - Foam, external: Scytera: 2% (100 g) (contains disodium edta)
  - Ointment, external: Psoriasin: 2% (113 g (DSC)) (contains alcohol, usp, polysorbate 80)

Dosages and Suggested Regimens

- *Scalp conditions (dandruff, psoriasis, seborrheic dermatitis)*: Topical shampoo. Rub shampoo onto wet hair and scalp, leave on for 5 minutes, and then rinse thoroughly. Repeat. Apply at least twice weekly or more often if needed. (See under Chap. 23 monograph).
- *Skin conditions (psoriasis, seborrheic dermatitis)*
  - *Cream, foam, lotion, ointment*: Apply to the affected area one to four times/day.
  - *Bath (Cutar)*: Add 60 to 120 mL to bath water and mix well. Soak for 10 to 20 minutes or as directed, and then pat dry.
  - *Foot/hand soak (Cutar)*: Add 30 to 60 mL of lotion to a sink or basin filled with water, and then mix well. Soak for 5 to 10 minutes or as directed.

Baseline Investigations and Considerations

- None documented

Use in Special Populations:

- *Pregnancy*: Limit application of coal tar during pregnancy in treating psoriasis to maximize safety in pregnant women.
- *Lactation*: Avoid direct contact by the infant if coal tar is used in a nursing mother, as one case report described the absorption of the components of coal tar containing ointment by a nursing infant. The components were not detected in breast milk, however were assumed to be absorbed by the infant following skin-to-skin contact with the mother while nursing.

- *Children*: For external use only; avoid contact with eyes. Do not apply in or near anogenital areas unless directed by a physician. Wash hands before and after application
- *Renal insufficiency*: There are no dosage adjustments provided in the manufacturer's labeling for renal impairment.
- *Hepatic insufficiency*: There are no dosage adjustments provided in the manufacturer's labeling for liver impairment.

Contraindications and Cautions

- *Concerns related to adverse effects*
  - Hair color changes: shampoo may cause discoloration of gray, blonde, tinted, or bleached hair.
  - Photosensitivity: May increase photosensitivity; avoid exposure to direct sunlight for 24 hours following application.
  - Staining: May stain light colored fabrics; do not use in plastic or fiberglass tubs, sinks, or basins.
- *Other warnings/precautions*
  - Polysorbate 80: Some dosage forms may contain polysorbate 80 (Tweens). Hypersensitivity reactions, usually delayed, have been reported following exposure to pharmaceutical products containing polysorbate 80 in certain individuals.
  - Self-medication (OTC use): for external use only; avoid the eyes. If the condition covers a large area of the body or is around the genital, groin, or rectal area, talk to your healthcare provider before application. Do not use this product with other forms of psoriasis therapy such as ultraviolet radiation or prescription drugs unless directed by healthcare provider. Overuse may make the condition worse; do not use more often or longer than recommended by your healthcare provider. Discontinue use and contact healthcare provider if condition worsens, does not improve after regular use as directed, or excessive irritation occurs.
- *Additional pediatric considerations*
  - Some dosage forms may contain propylene glycol; in neonates, large amounts of propylene glycol delivered orally, intravenously, or topically have been associated with poten-

tially fatal toxicities which can include metabolic acidosis, seizures, renal failure, and CNS depression.

Important drug interactions

There are no known significant interactions.

Adverse Effects and Their Management

- *Dermatologic*: dermatitis, folliculitis, skin irritation, skin photosensitivity.
- *Hair color changes*: shampoo may cause discoloration of gray, blonde, tinted, or bleached hair.
- *Photosensitivity*: may increase photosensitivity, avoid exposure to direct sunlight for 24 hours following application.
- *Staining*: may stain light colored fabrics. Do not use in plastic or fiberglass tubs, sinks, or basins.
- *Polysorbate 80*: some dosage forms contain polysorbate 30 (Tweens). In certain individuals, hypersensitivity reactions, usually a delayed reaction, have been reported following exposure to pharmaceutical products containing polysorbate 80.

Carcinogenicity

There have been cancer warnings on some coal tar products in California. This warning was added due to animal studies where the animals were exposed to a significantly higher amount of coal tar than is used to treat psoriasis. Studies, however, fail to demonstrate an increased risk of cancer in people using coal tar to treat psoriasis or atopic dermatitis. People who work with industrial coal tar have an increased risk of developing cancer of the lungs, scrotum, and skin, however.

Patch Test Concentration

- 5.0% pet. (Chemotechnique, SmartPracticeEurope, SmartPracticeCanada)

Essential Patient Information

- Prior to use, tell your doctor if you are allergic to this drug, any part of this drug, or any other drugs, foods, or substances. Tell your doctor if you have lupus, if your skin is sensitive to light, and if large areas need to be treated.

- Inform all your healthcare providers that you take this drug, including doctors, nurses, pharmacists, and dentists.
- May stain the fingernails, hair, and skin. Protect clothing and fabrics from staining.
- Avoid sun, sunlamps, and tanning beds. Use sunscreen and wear clothing and eyewear that protects you from the sun, as you may get sunburned more easily.
- Tell your doctor if you are pregnant, plan on getting pregnant, or are breastfeeding. You will need to discuss the benefits and risks to you and the baby.
- Tell your doctor or get medical help immediately if you have any of the following signs and symptoms of an allergic reaction that may be related to a bad side effect: rash, hives, itching, red, swollen, blistered, or peeling skin with or without fever, wheezing, chest or throat tightness, trouble breathing, swallowing, or talking, unusual hoarseness, or swelling of the mouth, face, lips, tongue, or throat.
- Topical use only: Use only on the skin. Do not take this drug by mouth. Keep out of your mouth, nose, and eyes (may burn). If this drug gets in the eyes, rinse with cool water.
- Wash your hands before and after use. If your hand is the affected area requiring treatment, do not wash your hand after use.
- Put a thin layer on the skin and rub in gently.
- This drug may catch on fire. Do not use near an open flame or while smoking.
- Store all products at room temperature in a dry place. Do not store in bathroom. Keep all drugs in a safe place and out of reach of children and pets.

Ruxolitinib

Marwa Hakimi and Wilson Liao

Note that at time of publication, ruxolitinib has FDA-labeled indications for atopic dermatitis and vitiligo. It is used off label for psoriasis.

Classification and Mode of Action

- Janus kinase (JAK) inhibitor. Ruxolitinib is a selective inhibitor of Janus kinase 1 (JAK1) and Janus kinase 2 (JAK2), key components of the JAK-STAT signaling pathway, which is involved in the pathogenesis of various inflammatory and autoimmune diseases. By inhibiting these kinases, ruxolitinib reduces the production and signaling of pro-inflammatory cytokines, thereby reducing inflammation and abnormal cell proliferation associated with skin disorders.
- Ruxolitinib has been shown to decrease the expression of inflammatory mediators and the hyperactivation of immune pathways implicated in conditions like atopic dermatitis and vitiligo. The cream is generally well-tolerated and has demonstrated efficacy in reducing the severity of these conditions.
  - TRuE-AD1 and TRuE-AD2 Trials: These two randomized, double-blind, vehicle-controlled phase 3 trials evaluated the efficacy and safety of ruxolitinib cream in patients with mild to moderate atopic dermatitis. The trials demonstrated that ruxolitinib cream was significantly more effective than the vehicle in reducing the severity of atopic dermatitis, as measured by the Investigator's Global Assessment (IGA) score and Eczema Area and Severity Index (EASI-75). The trials reported that approximately 50% of patients achieved an IGA score of 0 or 1 by week 8, compared to around 15% in the vehicle group.
  - TRuE-V1 and TRuE-V2 Trials: These phase 3, randomized, double-blind, vehicle-controlled studies assessed the efficacy and safety of ruxolitinib cream in patients with vitiligo. The studies found that ruxolitinib cream led to significant repigmentation of facial vitiligo, with about 30% of patients achieving at least 75% improvement in the facial Vitiligo Area Scoring Index (F-VASI75) at week 24 compared to about 10% with the vehicle. The trials also noted a favorable safety profile.

Indications and Dermatological Uses

- *Clinical indications (FDA)*
  - Atopic dermatitis (mild to moderate)
  - Nonsegmental vitiligo
- *Off-label common uses*
  - Alopecia areata
  - Lichen planus
  - Psoriasis

Formulations/Presentation

- USA: 1.5% cream in 5-g and 60-g tubes
- Canada: No data available
- Europe: 1.5% cream in 30-g and 60-g tubes

Dosages and Suggested Regimens

- Atopic dermatitis: Apply a thin layer to the affected areas twice daily. Application should be limited to less than 20% of body surface area (BSA). Discontinue use once signs and symptoms have resolved. If symptoms persist beyond 8 weeks, reassess the treatment plan.
- Vitiligo: Apply twice daily to affected areas until repigmentation occurs or as directed by a healthcare provider. Application should be limited to less than 20% of body surface area (BSA). Reevaluate the necessity of ongoing treatment if meaningful improvement with repigmentation has not occurred by 24 weeks.
- Maximum dosage: Do not exceed 60 g per week or 100 g per 2 weeks to minimize systemic absorption.

Baseline Investigations and Considerations

- Patient has a diagnosis of mild to moderate atopic dermatitis and meets one of the following:
  - Trial and failure (of at least a 30-day supply), contraindication, or intolerance to one prescription strength topical corticosteroid, unless the affected area is sensitive (i.e., face, axillae, and groin)

  - Trial and failure (of a minimum 30-day supply) or intolerance to one generic topical calcineurin inhibitor, unless the patient is not a suitable candidate for therapy
  - Patient has a diagnosis of nonsegmental vitiligo and trial and failure of a minimum 30-day supply, contraindication, or intolerance to ONE of the following:
    - Medium or higher potency topical corticosteroid
    - Pimecrolimus cream
    - Tacrolimus ointment
- Consideration of baseline complete blood count (CBC) with differential as clinically indicated to monitor for potential cytopenias during treatment, especially in long-term use.

Pharmacokinetics
- *Absorption*: Minimal systemic absorption observed with topical application. In clinical trials, plasma concentrations were low and not expected to lead to systemic immunosuppression.
- *Distribution*: Primarily stays localized to the site of application with minimal distribution to systemic circulation.
- *Metabolism*: Metabolized by hepatic CYP3A4 enzymes.
- *Excretion*: Predominantly excreted in the urine as metabolites.

Use in Special Populations:
- *Pediatrics*: Approved for use in children aged 12 years and older for atopic dermatitis and nonsegmental vitiligo. Safety and efficacy in younger children have not been established.
- *Pregnancy*: There is no adequate data on ruxolitinib use in pregnant women. Use only if the potential benefit justifies the potential risk to the fetus.
- *Lactation*: It is unknown whether ruxolitinib is present in human breast milk following topical application. The manufacturer advises against breastfeeding during therapy and for approximately 4 weeks following the last dose of ruxolitinib
- *Renal insufficiency*: No dose adjustment is necessary for patients with renal impairment.
- *Hepatic insufficiency*: No specific dose adjustments recommended; however, systemic exposure could be higher in these patients, and monitoring is recommended. Use is not advised in patients with active hepatitis B or C.

Monitoring

- Atopic dermatitis/segmental vitiligo: Monitor for signs of local skin reactions, including irritation or hypersensitivity.
- Periodic CBCs may be considered in patients on long-term therapy to monitor for potential cytopenias.
- Infection risk: Monitor for signs of infections, as ruxolitinib may increase the risk of bacterial, fungal, or viral infections, including herpes zoster.
- Malignancy risk: Periodic skin examinations for basal cell and squamous cell carcinoma.

Contraindications and Cautions

- *Contraindications*: Hypersensitivity to ruxolitinib or any of the components in the formulation.
- *Cautions*: Use with caution in patients with a history of skin malignancies or with active, untreated infections. Avoid use in immunocompromised patients unless the benefit outweighs the risks.
- *Serious infections:* Monitor for and promptly manage serious bacterial, mycobacterial, fungal, and viral infections.
- *Non-melanoma skin cancers:* Periodically examine the skin for basal cell and squamous cell carcinomas.
- *Thrombosis:* Be aware of the risk of thromboembolic events.
- *Hematologic issues:* Monitor for thrombocytopenia, anemia, and neutropenia with CBC tests as needed.

Important Drug Interactions

- CYP3A4 inhibitors: Concurrent use of strong CYP3A4 inhibitors (e.g., ketoconazole) may increase plasma concentrations of ruxolitinib, increasing the risk of systemic side effects.
- Immunosuppressants: Co-administration with other immunosuppressants (e.g., methotrexate and cyclosporine) may increase the risk of infections or exacerbate immunosuppression.
- Avoid using topical ruxolitinib concurrently with therapeutic biologics, other Janus kinase inhibitors, or potent immunosuppressants (e.g., azathioprine and cyclosporine).

Adverse Effects and Their Management

- *Local skin reactions*: Redness, itching, and irritation at the site of application. Usually mild and transient. Discontinue use if severe skin reactions occur.
- *Infections*: Increased risk of upper respiratory tract infections and herpes zoster. Discontinue treatment in the presence of a serious infection.
- *Hematological effects*: Rare cases of anemia and thrombocytopenia reported. Regular monitoring with CBC is recommended during prolonged therapy

Patch Test Concentration

- Not available

Essential Patient Information

- Apply only to affected areas and avoid healthy skin.
- Wash hands thoroughly after application unless the hands are the treatment area.
- Do not cover the treated area with occlusive dressings unless directed by a healthcare provider.
- Report any signs of infection or severe irritation to your healthcare provider.
- Do not use this medication if pregnant or planning to become pregnant without consulting a healthcare provider.

Salicylic Acid

Erin Bartholomew, Rebecca M. Law, and Wilson Liao

Classification and Mechanism of Action

Salicylic acid is an active ingredient intopical acne products. It is a keratolytic agent. It produces desquamation of hyperkeratotic epithelium by dissolution of the intercellular cement causing the cornified tissue to swell, soften, macerate, and desquamate.

Indications and Dermatological Use

- *Acne:* Topical management: often used in combination products. See Chap. 8 for a discussion of acne and other topical treatments for acne and the drug monographs.
- *Hyperkeratotic skin disorders:* Removal of excess keratin in various hyperkeratotic skin disorders and psoriasis (including affected areas of the scalp, skin, and feet; treatment and removal of common and plantar warts).

Off-Label Common Uses

- Seborrheic dermatitis. See Chap. 24 for a discussion of topical treatments and the drug monographs.

Formulations/Presentations

USA

Cream, External
Atrix medicated formula: 2% (59 mL) (contains disodium EDTA)

- Salimez: 6% (227 g)
- Salimez Forte: 10% (227 g)

Foam, External
- SalAc: 2% (100 g) (contains alcohol, usp)
- Salvax: 6% (70 g, 200 g) (contains ethylparaben, methylparaben, polysorbate 80, propylene glycol, propylparaben, trolamine (triethanolamine))
- Generic: 6% (70 g, 200 g)

Gel, External
- AcNesic: 0.5% (48 g) (contains benzalkonium chloride, butylparaben, eggshells, ethylparaben, isobutylparaben, methylparaben, propylene glycol, propylparaben, trolamine (triethanolamine))
- Keralyt: 3% (28.4 g) (contains alcohol, usp)
- Keralyt: 6% (40 g, 60 g, 100 g) (contains hydroxypropyl cellulose, propylene glycol, sd alcohol 40)

Kit, External

- Atrix system 1: 2% (contains disodium EDTA, menthol)
- Keralyt Scalp: 6% (contains edetate (EDTA) sodium (tetrasodium), propylene glycol, sd alcohol 40)
- Generic: 6%

Liquid, External

- DermacinRx Atrix Antibac Wash: 2% (118 mL) (contains disodium EDTA, menthol)
- DermacinRx Atrix Clarify Toner: 2% (118 mL) (contains benzalkonium chloride, benzyl alcohol, menthol)
- Neutrogena Oil-Free Acne Wash: 2% (124 mL) (contains benzalkonium chloride, disodium EDTA, FD&C red #40, propylene glycol)
- Psoriasin: 3% (177 mL) (dye free, fragrance free)
- Salicylic acid wart remover: 27.5% (10 mL) (contains isopropyl alcohol)
- Virasal: 27.5% (10 mL) (contains isopropyl alcohol, isopropyl-m-cresol)

Ointment, External

- Bensal HP: 3% (30 g)

Pad, External

- Clear Away 1-Step Wart Remover: 40% (14 ea)
- Corn Remover One Step: 40% (6 ea)

Shampoo, External

- Betasal: 3% (480 mL)
- Ionil: 2% (120 mL)
- Keralyt: 6% (160 mL) (contains cocamidopropyl betaine, edetate (EDTA) sodium (tetrasodium), propylene glycol)
- P & S: 2% (236 mL) (contains edetate (EDTA) sodium (tetrasodium), methylparaben, propylparaben, trolamine (triethanolamine))
- Salex: 6% (177 mL) (contains methylparaben, propylparaben, trolamine (triethanolamine))
- Generic: 6% (177 mL)

Solution, External

- Gordofilm: 16.7% (15 mL)
- UltraSal-ER: 28.5% (10 mL) (contains isopropyl alcohol, phenol, polysorbate 80)
- Xalix: 28% (10 g) (contains isopropyl alcohol)
- Generic: 26% (10 mL); 28.5% (10 mL)

Dosages and Suggested Regimens: Adult

Acne

Topical

- Salicylic acid 0.5% to 2%: OTC labeling: Apply thin layer to affected area one to time times daily. Products that are labeled for multiple daily doses should be initiated with 1 dose daily and increased gradually, because excessive drying may occur. Reduce to once daily or every other day if dryness or peeling occurs.
- Cream, gel, liquid, lotion, and pads: Salicylic acid ≤2%: Apply thin layer to affected area one to three times daily; reduce to once daily or every other day if dryness or peeling occurs.
- Cleansers: Salicylic acid ≤2%: Use to cleanse skin one to two times daily; reduce to once daily or every other day if dryness or peeling occurs.

Dandruff, Psoriasis, or Seborrheic Dermatitis

- Topical: *Note*: Product-specific indications may vary; refer to manufacturer's labeling.
- Cream, gel: Salicylic acid 2% or 3%: OTC labeling: Apply to affected area one to four times daily.
- Shampoo: Salicylic acid 3%: OTC labeling: Apply to wet hair and gently massage into scalp; work up lather; rinse thoroughly. Use at least twice weekly.

Pharmacokinetics

- *Onset of action:* Treatment of warts: 1 to 2 weeks; full resolution may take >4 to 6 weeks. Treatment of psoriasis: topical salicylic acid use for 8 to 16 weeks is recommended for the treatment of mild to moderate plaque psoriasis.

- *Absorption:* Salicylic acid gel 6%: >60% under occlusion. Percutaneous; systemic toxicity unlikely with normal use.
- *Protein binding:* 50% to 80% to albumin.
- *Time to peak, serum*: Salicylic acid gel 6%: Within 5 hours of application with occlusion.
- *Excretion:* Urine (salicyluric acid (52%), salicylate glucuronides (42%), and salicylic acid (6%)).

Use in special populations:

Pregnancy Considerations

- Salicylic acid crosses the placenta. Systemic absorption of topical salicylic acid occurs and varies depending on duration and vehicle (~9% to 25%) and is increased with occlusion.
- Current guidelines do not recommend salicylic acid for the treatment of psoriasis in pregnant women due to limited safety data and the potential for systemic absorption.
- For the topical treatment of acne or warts, salicylic acid can be used in pregnant women if the area of exposure and duration of therapy is limited, although other agents may be preferred due to limited safety data and the potential for systemic absorption.
- Consider maternal/fetal adverse events associated with aspirin if significant systemic exposure occurs.

Breastfeeding Considerations

- Salicylates are excreted in breast milk after oral administration.
- Systemic absorption of topical salicylic acid occurs and varies depending on duration and vehicle (~9% to 25%) and is increased with occlusion.
- Consider adverse events associated with aspirin in nursing infants if significant systemic exposure occurs.
- For the topical treatment of warts, salicylic acid can be used in breastfeeding women (systemic absorption is usually minimal).
- Breastfeeding women should avoid use around the chest area to prevent exposure to the nursing infant.

- Due to the potential for serious adverse reactions in the nursing infant, the manufacturer recommends making a decision whether to discontinue nursing or discontinue the drug, taking into account the importance of treatment to the mother.

Altered Kidney Function, Adult
There are no dosage adjustments provided in the manufacturer's labeling.

Hepatic Impairment: Adult
There are no dosage adjustments provided in the manufacturer's labeling.

Monitoring
Signs of salicylate toxicity

Contraindications and Cautions
- Hypersensitivity to salicylic acid or any component of the formulation
- Additional contraindications
  - Bensal HP: hypersensitivity to topical polyethylene glycols
  - Keralyt, Salex: children <2 years
  - UltraSal-ER, Virasal: impaired circulation or diabetes; moles and birthmarks; and warts with hair growth or on the face

OTC Labeling
- Corns/warts: When used for self-medication, do not use if you have diabetes or have poor blood circulation; do not use on irritated skin, on any area that is infected or reddened, on moles, birthmarks, warts with hair growing from them, genital warts, or warts on the face or mucous membranes.
- Documentation of allergenic cross-reactivity for salicylates is limited. However, because of similarities in chemical structure and/or pharmacologic actions, the possibility of cross-sensitivity cannot be ruled out with certainty.

Important Drug Interactions

- Calcipotriene: Salicylic acid may diminish the therapeutic effect of calcipotriene.
- Management: Monitor for reduced calcipotriene efficacy if combined with salicylic acid.
- Consider separating the administration of these agents by 10 to 12 hours to minimize the risk of this potential interaction.
- *Risk C: Monitor therapy.*

Adverse Effects and Their Management

The following adverse drug reactions and incidences are cited from product labeling. Frequency is not defined.

- Central nervous system: headache, dizziness, and localized burning at site of exposure on normal tissue
- Dermatologic: desquamation and exfoliation of the skin
- Local: irritation and burning at site of application on normal tissue
- Otic: tinnitus
- Respiratory: hyperventilation

Patch Test Concentration

- 5% pet. (SmartPracticeCanada)

Common Brand Names

AcNesic; Atrix medicated formula; Bensal HP; Betasal (OTC); Clear Away 1-Step Wart Remover (OTC); Corn Remover One Step (OTC); DermacinRx Atrix Antibac Wash (OTC); DermacinRx Atrix Clarify Toner (OTC); Exuviance Blemish Treatment (OTC) (DSC); Gordofilm; Ionil (OTC); Keralyt; Keralyt Scalp; Keralyt (OTC); Neutrogena Oil-Free Acne Wash (OTC); P & S (OTC); Psoriasin (OTC); SalAc (OTC); Salex; Salicylic Acid Wart Remover; Salimez; Salimez Forte; UltraSal-ER; Virasal; Xalix

References

Introduction

1. Law RM, Gulliver W. Chapter 118: Psoriasis. In: Dipiro's pharmacotherapy: a pathophysiologic approach. 12th ed. McGraw-Hill Medical; 2023. p. 1639–60.
2. Jeon C, Sekhon S, Bhutani T, Koo J. Topical treatments. In: Bhutani T, Liao W, Nakamura M, eds. Evidence-Based Psoriasis, Diagnosis and Treatment. (A textbook in the series Updates in Clinical Dermatology, with series editors Berth-Jones J, Gob CL, and Maibach HI, at http://www.springer.com/series/13203). Cham, Switzerland: Springer International Publishing AG; 2018, pp. 17–29.
3. Elmets CA, Korman NJ, Prater EF, et al. Joint AAD–NPF guidelines of care for the management and treatment of psoriasis with topical therapy and alternative medicine modalities for psoriasis severity measures. J Am Acad Dermatol. 2021;84:432–70.
4. Griffith JL, Zarbo AJ, Lim HW. Phototherapy and photochemotherapy. In: Bhutani T, Liao W, Nakamura M, eds. Evidence-Based Psoriasis, Diagnosis and Treatment. (A textbook in the series Updates in Clinical Dermatology, with series editors Berth-Jones J, Gob CL, and Maibach HI., at http://www.springer.com/series/13203). Cham: Springer International Publishing AG; 2018, pp. 31–53.
5. Elmets CA, Lim HW, Stoff B, et al. Joint American Academy of Dermatology–National Psoriasis Foundation guidelines of care for the management and treatment of psoriasis with phototherapy. J Am Acad Dermatol. 2019;81:775–804.
6. Menter A, Gelfand JM, Connor C, et al. Joint American Academy of Dermatology–National Psoriasis Foundation guidelines of care for the management of psoriasis with systemic nonbiologic therapies. J Am Acad Dermatol. 2020;82:1445–86.
7. Menter A, Strober BE, Kaplan DH, et al. Joint AAD-NPF guidelines of care for the management and treatment of psoriasis with biologics. J Am Acad Dermatol. 2019;80(4):1029–72.
8. Smith CH, Yiu ZZN, Bale T, et al. British Association of Dermatologists guidelines for biologic therapy for psoriasis 2020: a rapid update. Br J Dermatol. 2020;183(3):628–37. https://doi.org/10.1111/bjd.19039.
9. Elmets CA, Leonardi CL, Davis DMR, et al. Joint AAD-NPF guidelines of care for the management and treatment of psoriasis with awareness and attention to comorbidities. J Am Acad Dermatol. 2019;80(4):1073–113.
10. Basavaraj KH, Ashok NM, Rashmi R, Praveen TK. The role of drugs in the induction and/or exacerbation of psoriasis. Int J Dermatol. 2010;49:1351–61.

11. Papp KA, Gulliver W, Lynde CW, Poulin Y. Canadian Guidelines for the Management of Plaque Psoriasis. 1st Edition, June 2009. Available at: (Steering Committee). Also see: Canadian Psoriasis Guidelines Addendum Committee. Addendum to the Canadian Guidelines for the Management of Plaque Psoriasis, May 2016. *J Cutan Med Surg*. 2016;20(5):375–431. Available at: https://dermatology.ca/dermatologists/guidelines/psoriasis. Also see: Canadian Psoriasis Guidelines Addendum Committee. Addendum to the Canadian Guidelines for the Management of Plaque Psoriasis, May 2016. J Cutan Med Surg. 2016;20(5):375–431. Available at: https://www.ncbi.nlm.nih.gov/pmc/articles/PMC5014087/. Accessed 28 Feb 2022.

Drug Monographs

12. Law RM, Gulliver W. Chapter 118: Psoriasis. In: Dipiro's pharmacotherapy: a pathophysiologic approach. 12th ed. McGraw-Hill Medical; 2023. p. 1639–60.
13. Papp KA, Gulliver W, Lynde CW, Poulin Y. Canadian Guidelines for the Management of Plaque Psoriasis. 1st Edition, June 2009. Available at: (Steering Committee). Also see: Canadian Psoriasis Guidelines Addendum Committee. Addendum to the Canadian Guidelines for the Management of Plaque Psoriasis, May 2016. J Cutan Med Surg. 2016;20(5):375–431. Available at: https://dermatology.ca/dermatologists/guidelines/psoriasis. Also see: Canadian Psoriasis Guidelines Addendum Committee. Addendum to the Canadian Guidelines for the Management of Plaque Psoriasis, May 2016. J Cutan Med Surg. 2016;20(5):375–431. Available at: https://www.ncbi.nlm.nih.gov/pmc/articles/PMC5014087/. Accessed 29 Aug 2024.
14. Jeon C, Sekhon S, Bhutani T, Koo J. Topical treatments. In: Bhutani T, Liao W, Nakamura M, eds. Evidence-based psoriasis, diagnosis and treatment. (A textbook in the series Updates in Clinical Dermatology, with series editors Berth-Jones J, Gob CL, and Maibach HI, at http://www.springer.com/series/13203). Cham: Springer International Publishing AG; 2018, pp. 17–29.
15. Menter A, Korman NJ, Elmets CA, et al. 2009 Guidelines of care for the management of psoriasis and psoriatic arthritis—section 3. Guidelines of care for the management and treatment of psoriasis with topical therapies. J Am Acad Dermatol. 2009;60:643–59.
16. McGill A, Frank A, Emmett N, et al. The anti-psoriatic drug anthralin accumulates in keratinocyte mitochondria, dissipates mitochondrial membrane potential, and induces apoptosis through a pathway dependent on respiratory competent mitochondria. FASEB J. 2005;19:1012–4.

17. LexiComp drug monograph (anthralin). Available from: LexiComp Online at online.Lexi.com. Copyright 2024 UptoDate, Inc.
18. Law RM. Chapter 64: Psoriasis. In: Chisholm-Burns M, editor. Pharmacotherapy principles and practice. 3rd ed. New York: McGraw-Hill; 2013. p. 1127–41.
19. Mayo Clinic Drugs and Supplements: Anthralin (Topical Route). Last updated Feb. 1, 2024. Available at: https://www.mayoclinic.org/drugs-supplements/anthralin-topical-route/description/drg-20061896. Accessed 29 Aug 2024.

Calcipotriene (Calcipotriol) Drug Monograph

20. FDA drug monograph (calcipotriene). Available from (https://www.accessdata.fda.gov/drugsatfda_docs/label/2015/020273s013,020554s012lbl.pdf). Accessed 6 Jan 2022.
21. LexiComp drug monograph (calcipotriene). Available from: LexiComp Online at online.Lexi.com. Copyright 2021 UptoDate, Inc.
22. Kragballe K, Gjertsen BT, de Hoop D, van de Kerkhof PCM, Karlsmark T, Larko O, Nieboer C, Roed-Petersen J, Strand A, Tikjob G. Double-blind, right/left comparison of calcipotriol and betamethasone valerate in treatment of psoriasis vulgaris. Lancet. 1991;337(8735):193–6. https://doi.org/10.1016/0140-6736(91)92157-W.
23. Ashcroft DM, Li Wan Po A, Williams HC, Griffiths CEM. Combination regimens of topical calcipotriene in chronic plaque psoriasis: systematic review of efficacy and tolerability. Arch Dermatol. 2000;136(12):1536–43. https://doi.org/10.1001/archderm.136.12.1536.
24. De Groot AC. Monographs in contact allergy, volume 3 topical drugs. CRC Press; 2021.
25. Frosch PJ, Rustemeyer T. Contact allergy to calcipotriol does exist. Report of an unequivocal case and review of the literature. Contact Derm. 1999;40(2):66–71. https://doi.org/10.1111/j.1600-0536.1999.tb05993.x.
26. Kissmeyer AM, Binderup L. Calcipotriol (MC 903): pharmacokinetics in rats and biological activities of metabolites. A comparative study with 1, 25(OH)2D3. Biochem Pharmacol. 1991;41(11):1601–6. https://doi.org/10.1016/0006-2952(91)90160-7.
27. Pearce DJ, Camacho F, Balkrishnan R, Fleischer AB Jr, Feldman SR. Trends in on and off-label calcipotriene use. J Dermatolog Treat. 2006;17(5):308–13. https://doi.org/10.1080/09546630600813659.
28. Scott LJ, Dunn CJ, Goa KL, Calcipotriol ointment. A review of its use in the management of psoriasis. Am J Clin Dermatol. 2001;2(2):95–120. https://doi.org/10.2165/00128071-200102020-00008.
29. Elmets CA, Korman NJ, Prater EF, et al. Joint AAD-NPF Guidelines of care for the management and treatment of psoriasis with topical therapy

and alternative medicine modalities for psoriasis severity measures. J Am Acad Dermatol. 2021;84(2):432–70. https://doi.org/10.1016/j.jaad.2020.07.087.
30. Oranje AP, Marcoux D, Svensson A, et al. Topical calcipotriol in childhood psoriasis. J Am Acad Dermatol. 1997;36(2):203–8.
31. Zeichner JA, Lebwohl MG, Menter A, et al. Optimizing topical therapies for treating psoriasis: a consensus conference. Cutis. 2010;86(3 Suppl):5–31.

Calcitriol

32. Raychaudhuri S, Mitra A, Datta-Mitra A. Immunomodulatory mechanisms of action of calcitriol in psoriasis. Indian J Dermatol. 2014;59(2):116–22. https://doi.org/10.4103/0019-5154.127668.
33. Mason AR, Mason J, Cork M, Dooley G, Hancock H. Topical treatments for chronic plaque psoriasis. Cochrane Datab Syst Rev 2013;3:CD005028. https://doi.org/10.1002/14651858.CD005028.pub3.
34. Camarasa JM, Ortonne JP, Dubertret L. Calcitriol shows greater persistence of treatment effect than betamethasone dipropionate in topical psoriasis therapy. J Dermatolog Treat. 2003;14(1):8–13. https://doi.org/10.1080/09546630305545.
35. Ortonne JP, Humbert P, Nicolas JF, et al. Intra-individual comparison of the cutaneous safety and efficacy of calcitriol 3 microg g(−1) ointment and calcipotriol 50 microg g(−1) ointment on chronic plaque psoriasis localized in facial, hairline, retroauricular or flexural areas. Br J Dermatol. 2003;148(2):326–33. https://doi.org/10.1046/j.1365-2133.2003.05228.x.
36. Wat H, Dytoc M. Off-label uses of topical vitamin D in dermatology: a systematic review. J Cutan Med Surg. 2014;18(2):91–108. https://doi.org/10.2310/7750.2013.13109.
37. Food and Drug Administration Center for Drug Evaluation and Research. Application Number 22-087: Pharmacology Review. 30 Jun 2008. https://www.accessdata.fda.gov/drugsatfda_docs/nda/2009/022087s000_PharmR.pdf
38. Lebwohl M, Menter A, Weiss J, et al. Calcitriol 3 microg/g ointment in the management of mild to moderate plaque type psoriasis: results from 2 placebo-controlled, multicenter, randomized double-blind, clinical studies. J Drugs Dermatol. 2007;6(4):428–35.
39. Elmets CA, Korman NJ, Prater EF, et al. Joint AAD-NPF Guidelines of care for the management and treatment of psoriasis and alternative medicine modalities for psoriasis severity measures. J Am Acad Dermatol. 2021;84(2):432–70. https://doi.org/10.1016/j.jaad.2020.07.087.
40. Maul JT, Anzengruber F, Conrad C, Cozzio A, Häusermann P, Jalili A, Kolios AGA, Laffitte EH, Lapointe AK, Mainetti C, Schlapbach C, Trüeb

R, Yawalkar N, Dippel M, Navarini AA. Topical treatment of psoriasis vulgaris: the Swiss treatment pathway. Dermatology. 2021;237:166–78. https://doi.org/10.1159/000512930.
41. Maul JT, Anzengruber F, Conrad C, et al. Topical treatment of psoriasis vulgaris: the Swiss treatment pathway. Dermatology. 2021;237(2):166–78. https://doi.org/10.1159/000512930.
42. Silkis (calcitriol) [product monograph]. Thornhill: Galderma Canada Inc.; October 2017.
43. Simionescu AA, Danciu BM, Stanescu AMA. State-of-the-art review of pregnancy-related psoriasis. Medicina (Kaunas). 2021;57(8):804. https://doi.org/10.3390/medicina57080804.
44. Vectical (calcitriol) [prescribing information]. Fort Worth: Galderma Laboratories LP; September 2021.

Coal Tar and Tar Distillates

45. FDA drug monograph (Drug Products for the Control of Dandruff, Seborrheic Dermatitis, and Psoriasis for Over-the-Counter Human Use). Available from FDA weblink at https://www.accessdata.fda.gov/drugsatfda_docs/omuf/OTC%20Monograph_M032-Drug%20Products%20for%20the%20Control%20of%20Dandruff%20Seborrheic%20Dermatitis%20and%20Psoriasis%2012.16.2021.pdf. Accessed 19 Aug 2024.
46. LexiComp drug monograph (coal tar). Available from: LexiComp Online at online.Lexi.com. Copyright 2024 UptoDate, Inc. Available from: https://ssouptodatecom/contents/coal-tar-drug-information?search=coal%20tar&source=search_result&selectedTitle=1%7E18&usage_type=panel&kp_tab=drug_general&display_rank=1. Accessed 10 Aug 2024.
47. De Groot AC. Patch testing. 3rd edition. Vol. 3, Chapter 3.
48. De Groot AC. Patch testing, 4th Edition: Update 2018–2022. Wapserveen: Acdegroot Publishing, 2022 (37 pages). ISBN/EAN 978-90-813233-7-6.
49. Mosca M, Hong J, Hadeler E, Brownstone N, Bhutani T, Liao W. Scalp psoriasis: a literature review of effective therapies and updated recommendations for practical management. Dermatol Ther (Heidelb) [Internet]. 2021;11(3):769–97. https://doi.org/10.1007/s13555-021-00521-z.
50. Fargnoli MC, De Simone C, Gisondi P, Pellacani G, Calzavara-Pinton P. Topical treatment for the management of mild-to-moderate psoriasis: a critical appraisal of the current literature. Dermatol Ther (Heidelb) [Internet]. 2023;13(11):2527–47. https://doi.org/10.1007/s13555-023-01024-9.

Ruxolitinib

51. FDA drug monograph for Ruxolitinib cream. Available from: https://www.accessdata.fda.gov/drugsatfda_docs/label/2022/215309s001lbl.pdf. Accessed 25 Aug 2024.
52. LexiComp drug monograph (Ruxolitinib). Available from: LexiComp Online at online.Lexi.com. Copyright 2024 UptoDate, Inc.
53. Papp K, Szepietowski JC, Kircik L, et al. Efficacy and safety of ruxolitinib cream for the treatment of atopic dermatitis: results from 2 phase 3, randomized, double-blind studies. J Am Acad Dermatol. 2021;85(4):863–72. https://doi.org/10.1016/j.jaad.2021.04.085.
54. Rosmarin D, Passeron T, Pandya AG, et al. Two phase 3, randomized, controlled trials of Ruxolitinib cream for vitiligo. N Engl J Med. 2022;387(16):1445–55. https://doi.org/10.1056/NEJMoa2118828.
55. Blauvelt A, Kircik L, Papp KA, et al. Rapid pruritus reduction with ruxolitinib cream treatment in patients with atopic dermatitis. J Eur Acad Dermatol Venereol. 2023;37(1):137–46. https://doi.org/10.1111/jdv.18571.
56. Kashetsky N, Turchin I. Utilization of topical ruxolitinib in dermatology: a review. Skin Therapy Lett. 2023;28(3):8–13.

Salicylic Acid

57. LexiComp drug monograph Salicylic Acid. Available from: http://www.crlonline.com.ucsf.idm.oclc.org/lco/action/doc/retrieve/docid/patch_f/7647?cesid=ayXFh9Nrqni&searchUrl=%2Flco%2Faction%2Fsearch%3Fq%3Dsalicylic%252520acid%26t%3Dname%26va%3Dsalicylic%252520acid.
58. LexiComp Online at online.lexi.com Copyright 2021 UpToDate, Inc.
59. De Groot AC. Patch testing. 3rd edition. Volume 3 Chapter 3.
60. AcNesic (salicylic acid). Santa Fe Springs: Blaine Labs Inc; received May 2021.
61. Akhavan A, Bershad S. Topical acne drugs: review of clinical properties, systemic exposure, and Safety. Am J Clin Dermatol. 2003;4(7):473–92.
62. American Academy of Pediatrics Committee on Drugs. "Inactive" ingredients in pharmaceutical products: update (subject review). Pediatrics. 1997;99(2):268–78.
63. Bae YS, Van Voorhees AS, Hsu S, et al. National Psoriasis Foundation. Review of treatment options for psoriasis in pregnant or lactating women: from the Medical Board of the National Psoriasis Foundation. J Am Acad Dermatol. 2012;67(3):459–77.

64. Bensal HP (salicylic acid) [prescribing information]. Easley: 7 Oaks Pharmaceuticals; 2010.
65. Butler DC, Heller MM, Murase JE. Safety of dermatologic medications in pregnancy and lactation: part II. Lactation. J Am Acad Dermatol. 2014;70(3):417.e1–e10; quiz 427.
66. FDA Drug Safety Communication. FDA warns of rare but serious hypersensitivity reactions with certain over-the-counter topical acne products, June 25, 2014. http://www.fda.gov/Drugs/DrugSafety/ucm400923.htm.
67. Menter A, Korman NJ, Elmets CA, et al. American Academy of Dermatology. Guidelines of care for the management of psoriasis and psoriatic arthritis. Section 3. Guidelines of care for the management and treatment of psoriasis with topical therapies. J Am Acad Dermatol. 2009;60(4):643–59.
68. Elmets CA, Korman NJ, Prater EF, Wong EB, Rupani RN, Kivelevitch D, Armstrong AW, Connor C, Cordoro KM, Davis DMR, Elewski BE, Gelfand JM, Gordon KB, Gottlieb AB, Kaplan DH, Kavanaugh A, Kiselica M, Kroshinsky D, Lebwohl M, Leonardi CL, Lichten J, Lim HW, Mehta NN, Paller AS, Parra SL, Pathy AL, Siegel M, Stoff B, Strober B, Wu JJ, Hariharan V, Menter A. Joint AAD-NPF Guidelines of care for the management and treatment of psoriasis with topical therapy and alternative medicine modalities for psoriasis severity measures. J Am Acad Dermatol. 2021;84(2):432–70. https://doi.org/10.1016/j.jaad.2020.07.087. Epub 2020 Jul 30. PMID: 32738429.

Retinoids

22

Enzo Berardesca

Contents

Introduction

Retinoids may be classified into two different categories based on their pharmacologic actions and uses [1, 2, 3]. Retinoids with anti-inflammatory activities are used to modulate the inflammatory conditions acne, rosacea, and psoriasis. Retinoids with antineoplastic activities are used in the treatment of various neoplastic conditions.

Topical retinoids for inflammatory conditions include adapalene, tretinoin, and tazarotene,

Please refer to Chaps. 8, 9, 14, and 21 for discussions of other topical antineoplastic agents.

E. Berardesca (✉)
Dr. Phillip Frost Department of Dermatology and Cutaneous Surgery, Miller School of Medicine, University of Miami, Miami, FL, USA
e-mail: Berardesca@berardesca.it

R. M. Law, H. I. Maibach (eds.), *Handbook of Topical Drug Treatment in Dermatology*,
https://doi.org/10.1007/978-3-031-93616-6_22

Anti-inflammatory Retinoids

Adapalene

Classification and Mode of Action

- Retinoic acid derivative. Adapalene is a retinoid-like substance that modulates cellular differentiation, keratinization, and inflammation. Adapalene is better than tretinoin or tazarotene in reducing inflammatory acne lesions and total lesion count and causes less irritation.

Indications and Dermatological Uses

- *Clinical indications (FDA)*: acne vulgaris
- *Off-label common uses*: Rosacea (level of evidence: C)

Formulations/Presentation

- USA: 0.1% gel, 0.1% cream, 0.1% lotion, 0.1% pad, and 0.1% solution
- Canada: 0.1% cream and 0.1% gel
- Europe: 0.1% cream and 0.1% gel

Dosages and Suggested Regimens

- Apply once daily before bedtime.
- No suggested dosage adjustment for renal or hepatic impairment due to low systemic absorption.

Baseline Investigations and Considerations

Pharmacodynamics/Kinetics

- Minimal topical absorption, even after chronic use (trace amounts measured in serum). Elimination half-life between 7 and 51 hours (gel). Excreted in bile.
- Onset of effect: Between 8 and 12 weeks.

Use in Special Populations

- Approved for use in children. May cause mild hyperglycemia which is more common in children. Avoid internal use.

- Listed as FDA pregnancy classification C (former classification system).
- Unknown whether adapalene is present in breast milk.
- Renal insufficiency: Not evaluated; dose adjustment is not expected to be needed.
- Hepatic insufficiency: Not evaluated; dose adjustment is not expected to be needed.

Monitoring

- Skin irritation/dryness
- Initial acne flare
- Severe skin reactions (exfoliation, desquamation)
- Allergy (angioedema, lip swelling, facial edema—reported postmarketing with gel)

Contraindications and Cautions

- Accidental ingestion especially of large amounts of products containing propylene glycol may result in toxicity (metabolic acidosis/lactic acidosis, hyperosmolality, respiratory depression, seizures). Fatalities have been reported in neonates given large amounts of propylene glycol internally (po or IV).

Important Drug Interactions

- Other topical medications which may cause skin irritation will potentially exacerbate the skin irritation (e.g., benzoyl peroxide, medicated soaps, and cleansers).
- Other topical medications (or cosmetics) containing alcohol, acetone, or astringents may exacerbate adapalene's drying effect.
- Adapalene may increase the levels/effects of aminolevulinic acid (topical or systemic). Avoid concomitant use.
- Levels/effects of adapalene may be increased by concomitant use of multivitamins with minerals (i.e., ADEK, folate, or iron).

Adverse Effects and Their Management

- Skin irritation can occur. Less skin irritation than other retinoids, i.e., tretinoin. Erythema, stinging/burning, dryness, or

pruritus may occur especially during the initial 2–4 weeks of use. These may lessen with continued use.
- May cause initial exacerbation of acne.
- May cause increased sensitivity to UV rays. Use sunscreen and avoid sunlamp use.
- Hypersensitivity reactions including facial and eyelid edema and swelling have been reported. Use must be discontinued immediately as anaphylactoid/anaphylactic reactions may occur.

Patch Test Concentration

- 0.1% and 0.01% pet.

Essential Patient Information

- Avoid contact with broken, sunburned, eczematous, or abraded skin.
- Avoid contact with eyes, lips, or other mucous membranes (e.g., inside nose).
- Avoid using products including cosmetics which contain alpha hydroxyl or glycolic acid, as they may further irritate the skin.
- Do not ingest. For external use only.
- Use sun protection. Apply sunscreen with SPF 30 daily. If there is a sunburn, discontinue use until sunburn has healed.

Tretinoin

Classification and Mode of Action

- Retinoic acid derivative. Tretinoin is a retinoid-like substance that modulates cellular differentiation, keratinization, and inflammation. Improves stratum corneum turnover and dermal fibroblast differentiation. Tretinoin is more irritating than adapalene even though more effective in reducing the count of inflammatory lesions in acne. It is also used to improve keratinocyte turnover in the treatment of early signs of photoaging, thus improving skin texture and wrinkles.

Indications and Dermatological Uses

- *Clinical indications (FDA)*: acne vulgaris, photoaging, wrinkles, and hyperpigmentation

Formulations/Presentation

- USA: 0.01%–0.1% gel, 0.025%–0.05% cream, and 0.01% lotion
- Canada: 0.01%–0.1% cream and 0.01%–0.1% gel
- Europe: 0.05% cream, 0.025% gel, and 0.05% solution

Dosages and Suggested Regimens

- Apply once daily before bedtime.
- No suggested dosage adjustment for renal or hepatic impairment due to low systemic absorption.

Baseline Investigations and Considerations

Pharmacodynamics/Kinetics

Onset of action: Acne: ≥2 weeks, may take ≥7 weeks. Facial wrinkles: Up to 6 months

Absorption: Minimal

Bioavailability: Avita cream and gel: <0.3%; Retin A Micro 0.1% gel: ~1%

Metabolism: Hepatic; forms metabolites

Excretion: Urine and feces

Use in Special Populations

- Approved for use in children. Some dosage forms may contain propylene glycol; in neonates large amounts of propylene glycol delivered topically have been associated with potentially fatal toxicities which can include metabolic acidosis, seizures, renal failure, and CNS depression; toxicities have also been reported in children and adults including hyperosmolality, lactic acidosis, seizures, and respiratory depression; use caution (AAP 1997; Shehab 2009).
- Adverse events were observed in some animal reproduction studies following topical application of tretinoin. Teratogenic

effects were also observed in pregnant women following topical use; however, a causal association has not been established. When treatment for acne is needed during pregnancy, other agents are preferred (Chien 2016; Kong 2013; Leachman 2006). These products should not be used in women who are pregnant.

- Unknown whether tretinoin is present in breast milk.
- Renal insufficiency: Not evaluated; dose adjustment is not expected to be needed.
- Hepatic insufficiency: Not evaluated; dose adjustment is not expected to be needed.

Monitoring

- Skin irritation/dryness
- Photosensitivity
- Severe skin reactions (exfoliation, desquamation)
- Allergy (angioedema, lip swelling, facial edema, reported postmarketing with gel)

Contraindications and Cautions

- Accidental ingestion especially of large amounts of products containing propylene glycol may result in toxicity (metabolic acidosis/lactic acidosis, hyperosmolality, respiratory depression, seizures). Fatalities have been reported in neonates given large amounts of propylene glycol internally (po or IV).

Important Drug Interactions

- Other topical medications which may cause skin irritation will potentially exacerbate the skin irritation (e.g., benzoyl peroxide, medicated soaps, and cleansers).
- Other topical medications (or cosmetics) containing alcohol, acetone, or astringents may exacerbate tretinoin's drying effect.
- Tretinoin may interact with aminolevulinic acid (topical or systemic). Avoid concomitant use.
- Levels/effects of tretinoin may be increased by concomitant use of multivitamins with minerals (i.e., ADEK, folate, or iron).

Adverse Effects and Their Management

- Skin irritation can occur.
- Erythema, stinging/burning, dryness, or pruritus may occur especially during the initial 2–4 weeks of use. These may lessen with continued use.
- May cause initial exacerbation of acne.
- May cause increased sensitivity to UV rays. Use sunscreen and avoid sunlamp use.
- Hypersensitivity reactions including facial and eyelid edema and swelling have been reported. Use must be discontinued immediately as anaphylactoid/anaphylactic reactions may occur.

Patch Test Concentration

- 0.005% alcohol; if higher (0.01% or 0.02%), perform adequate controls; petrolatum is not suitable for patch testing tretinoin.

Essential Patient Information

- Avoid contact with broken, sunburned, eczematous, or abraded skin.
- Avoid contact with eyes, lips, or other mucous membranes (e.g., inside the nose).
- Avoid using products including cosmetics which contain alpha hydroxyl or glycolic acid, as they may further irritate the skin
- Do not ingest. For external use only.
- Use sun protection. Apply sunscreen with SPF 30 daily. If there is a sunburn, discontinue use until sunburn has healed.

Tazarotene

Classification and Mode of Action

- Retinoic acid derivative. Tazarotene is a retinoid-like substance that modulates cellular differentiation, keratinization, and inflammation. Improves stratum corneum turnover and dermal fibroblast differentiation. Tazarotene is slightly irritating. It is used to improve keratinocyte turnover in the treatment of psoriasis and other disorders of keratinization. Like other retinoids can be used to treat early signs of photoaging and to improve white and black comedones.

Indications and Dermatological Uses

- *Clinical indications (FDA):* psoriasis, acne vulgaris, photoaging, wrinkles, and hyperpigmentation

Formulations/Presentation

- USA: 0.05%–0.1% cream/gel
- Canada: 0.05%–0.1% cream/gel
- Europe: 0.05% gel and 0.1% gel

Dosages and Suggested Regimens

- Apply once daily before bedtime.
- No suggested dosage adjustment for renal or hepatic impairment due to low systemic absorption.
- In patients experiencing excessive pruritus, burning, skin redness, or peeling, discontinue until integrity of the skin is restored, or reduce dosing to an interval the patient is able to tolerate.

Baseline Investigations and Considerations

Pharmacodynamics/Kinetics

Onset of action: psoriasis: 1 week

Duration: therapeutic: psoriasis: Effects have been observed for up to 3 months after a 3-month course of topical treatment.

Absorption: Minimal following cutaneous application (≤6% of dose).

Distribution: Retained in the skin for prolonged periods after topical application.

Protein binding: >99% (tazarotenic acid).

Metabolism: Prodrug, rapidly metabolized via esterase hydrolysis to an active metabolite (tazarotenic acid) following topical application and systemic absorption; tazarotenic acid undergoes further hepatic metabolism.

Excretion: Urine and feces.

Use in Special Populations

- Approved for use in children. Some dosage forms may contain propylene glycol; in neonates large amounts of propylene glycol delivered topically have been associated with potentially fatal toxicities which can include metabolic acidosis, seizures, renal failure, and CNS depression; toxicities have also been reported in children and adults including hyperosmolality, lactic acidosis, seizures, and respiratory depression; use with caution (AAP 1997; Shehab 2009).
- Tazarotene products should not be used in women who are pregnant.
- Unknown whether tretinoin is present in breast milk.
- Renal insufficiency: Not evaluated; dose adjustment is not expected to be needed.
- Hepatic insufficiency: Not evaluated; dose adjustment is not expected to be needed.

Monitoring

- Skin irritation/dryness
- Photosensitivity
- Severe skin reactions (exfoliation, desquamation)
- Allergy (angioedema, lip swelling, facial edema)

Contraindications and Cautions

- Accidental ingestion especially of large amounts of products containing propylene glycol may result in toxicity (metabolic acidosis/lactic acidosis, hyperosmolality, respiratory depression, seizures). Fatalities have been reported in neonates given large amounts of propylene glycol internally (po or IV).

Important Drug Interactions

- Other topical medications which may cause skin irritation will potentially exacerbate the skin irritation (e.g., benzoyl peroxide, medicated soaps, and cleansers).
- Other topical medications (or cosmetics) containing alcohol, acetone, or astringents may exacerbate tretinoin's drying effect.

Adverse Effects and Their Management

- Skin irritation can occur.
- Erythema, stinging/burning, dryness, or pruritus may occur especially during the initial 2–4 weeks of use. These may lessen with continued use.
- May cause initial exacerbation of acne.
- May cause increased sensitivity to UV rays. Use sunscreen and avoid sunlamp use.
- Hypersensitivity reactions including facial and eyelid edema and swelling have been reported. Use must be discontinued immediately as anaphylactoid/anaphylactic reactions may occur.

Essential Patient Information

- Avoid contact with broken, sunburned, eczematous, or abraded skin.
- Avoid contact with eyes, lips, or other mucous membranes (e.g., inside nose).
- Avoid using products including cosmetics which contain alpha hydroxyl or glycolic acid, as they may further irritate the skin.
- Do not ingest. For external use only.
- Use sun protection. Apply sunscreen with SPF 30 daily. If there is a sunburn, discontinue use until sunburn has healed.

Trifarotene

Classification and Mode of Action

- Trifarotene is a new fourth-generation topical retinoid. Trifarotene is a strong and selective agonist of RAR-γ, with lower activity on RAR-β and RAR-α (16- and 65-fold, respectively), and has no activity on RXRs. Trifarotene exerts anti-inflammatory, comedolytic, and depigmenting actions.

Indications and Dermatological Uses

- *Clinical indications (FDA):* acne of the face and the trunk

Formulations/Presentation

- USA: cream, 0.005%
- Canada: cream, 0.005%
- Europe: cream, 0.005%

Dosages and Suggested Regimens

- Apply once daily before bedtime.
- No suggested dosage adjustment for renal or hepatic impairment due to low systemic absorption.

Pharmacodynamics/Kinetics

- Protein binding: ~99.9%
- Metabolism: Primarily metabolized by CYP2C9, CYP3A4, and CYP2C8
- Half-life elimination: Terminal: 2 to 9 hours
- Excretion: Feces

Use in Special Populations

- Patients exposed to photosensitizing agents may have an increased riskof a phototoxic skin reaction. Despite these local adverse effects and photosensitization, trifarotene is safer than other retinoids due to its hepatic instability and degradation.
- Due to its RAR-γ selectivity, it could be hypothesized that trifarotene is safer than other retinoids in pregnancy as the placenta presents a lower expression of RAR-γ (4.739 ± 0.399), with consequent minor absorption of the drug compared to other topical retinoids
- Trifarotene may share the characteristic of teratogenicity with other retinoids, other agents may be preferred. Avoid applying large amounts over prolonged periods of time to decrease the potential for systemic absorption.
- It is not known if trifarotene is present in breast milk following topical application.
- According to the manufacturer, the decision to breastfeed during therapy should consider the risk of infant exposure, the benefits of breastfeeding to the infant, and benefits of treatment to the mother.

Important Drug Interactions

- Other topical medications which may cause skin irritation will potentially exacerbate the skin irritation (e.g., benzoyl peroxide, medicated soaps, and cleansers).
- Other topical medications (or cosmetics) containing alcohol, acetone, or astringents may exacerbate trifarotene's drying effect.

Monitoring

- Skin irritation/dryness
- Skin reactions (exfoliation, desquamation)

Essential Patient Information

- Patients using trifarotene cream may experience erythema, scaling, dryness, and stinging/burning. Use a moisturizer from the initiation of treatment, and, if appropriate, depending upon the severity of these adverse reactions, reduce the frequency of application of trifarotene cream, suspend, or discontinue use. Avoid application of trifarotene cream to cuts, abrasions, or eczematous or sunburned skin. Use of "waxing" as a depilatory method should be avoided on skin treated with trifarotene cream. Minimize exposure to sunlight and sunlamps. Use sunscreen and protective clothing over treated areas when exposure cannot be avoided.

Antineoplastic Retinoids

Alitretinoin

Classification and Mode of Action

- Retinoic acid derivative. It is used as antineoplastic (topical) and anti-inflammatory (oral) agent. Alitretinoin is a naturally occurring endogenous retinoid that binds to and activates intracellular retinoid receptors (RAR and RXR subtypes); this results in altered expression of the genes controlling cellular differentiation and proliferation in normal and neoplastic cells, inhibiting the growth of Kaposi sarcoma.

Indications and Dermatological Uses

- *Clinical indications*: Topical: Kaposi sarcoma, pyogenic granuloma. Oral: chronic hand dermatitis

Formulations/Presentation

- USA: 0.1% cream/gel (topical)
- Canada:
- Europe: Tablets 10 mg and 30 mg (Oral)

Dosages and Suggested Regimens

- Topical: Apply several times a day on the skin affected.
- Oral: 10 mg to 30 mg once a day
- No suggested dosage adjustment for renal or hepatic impairment due to low systemic absorption.

Baseline Investigations and Considerations

Pharmacodynamics/Kinetics

Onset of action: Oral: 2 weeks

Duration: Therapeutic: Hand dermatitis 12 to 24 weeks

Absorption: Minimal following cutaneous application

Distribution: Retained in skin for prolonged periods after topical application

Excretion: Urine and feces

Use in Special Populations: Pregnancy (FDA Guidance), Lactation, Children, Renal Insufficiency, and Hepatic Insufficiency

- Alitretinoin should not be used in women who are pregnant.
- Unknown whether alitretinoin is present in breast milk.
- Renal insufficiency: Not evaluated; dose adjustment is not expected to be needed.
- Hepatic insufficiency: Not evaluated; dose adjustment is not expected to be needed.

Monitoring

- Skin irritation
- Dermal irritation

- Photosensitivity
- Severe skin reactions (exfoliation, desquamation)
- Allergy (angioedema, lip swelling, facial edema)

Contraindications and Cautions

Products containing DEET: Do not use concurrently with topical products containing DEET (e.g., insect repellant); an increase in DEET toxicity has been observed.

Important Drug Interactions

Aminolevulinic acid (systemic): Photosensitizing agents may enhance the photosensitizing effect of aminolevulinic acid (systemic). Risk X: Avoid combination.

Aminolevulinic acid (topical): Photosensitizing agents may enhance the photosensitizing effect of aminolevulinic acid (topical). Risk C: Monitor therapy.

Multivitamins/fluoride (with ADE): May enhance the adverse/toxic effect of retinoic acid derivatives. Risk X: Avoid combination.

Multivitamins/minerals (with ADEK, folate, iron): May enhance the adverse/toxic effect of retinoic acid derivatives. Risk X: Avoid combination.

Multivitamins/minerals (with AE, no iron): May enhance the adverse/toxic effect of retinoic acid derivatives. Risk X: Avoid combination.

Porfimer: Photosensitizing agents may enhance the photosensitizing effect of Porfimer. Risk C: Monitor therapy.

Verteporfin: Photosensitizing agents may enhance the photosensitizing effect of verteporfin. Risk C: Monitor therapy.

Adverse Effects and Their Management

- Skin irritation can occur.
- Erythema, stinging/burning, dryness, or pruritus may occur especially during the initial 2–4 weeks of use. These may lessen with continued use.
- May cause initial exacerbation of acne.
- May cause increased sensitivity to UV rays. Use sunscreen and avoid sunlamp use.

- Hypersensitivity reactions including facial and eyelid edema and swelling have been reported. Use must be discontinued immediately as anaphylactoid/anaphylactic reactions may occur.

Essential Patient Information

- Avoid contact with broken, sunburned, eczematous, or abraded skin.
- Avoid contact with eyes, lips, or other mucous membranes (e.g., inside nose).
- Avoid using products including cosmetics which contain alpha hydroxyl or glycolic acid, as they may further irritate the skin.
- Use sun protection. Apply sunscreen with SPF 30 daily. If there is a sunburn, discontinue use until sunburn has healed.

Bexarotene

Classification and Mode of Action

Bexarotene binds to and activates retinoid X receptor subtypes. Once activated, these receptors function as transcription factors that regulate the expression of genes which control cellular differentiation and proliferation, resulting in decreased cell proliferation, apoptosis of some cancer cell types, and tumor regression.

- *Clinical indications*: Topical or oral: cutaneous T-cell lymphoma

Formulations/Presentation

- USA: 1% cream/gel (topical)
- Canada
- Europe: tablets 75 mg (oral)

Dosages and Suggested Regimens

- Topical: Apply to lesions once every other day for the first week, and then increase on a weekly basis to once daily, two times daily, three times daily, and finally four times daily, according to individual lesion tolerance.

- Oral: 300 mg/sq meter/day.
- No suggested dosage adjustment for renal or hepatic impairment due to low systemic absorption.

Baseline Investigations and Considerations

Pharmacodynamics/Kinetics

Onset: Response may be seen at 4 weeks, although longer application may be required for response (range: up to 56 weeks).

Absorption: Systemically absorbed following topical application (1% gel: generally less than 5 ng/mL and did not exceed 55 ng/mL).

Protein binding: >99% to plasma proteins.

Metabolism: Oral bexarotene metabolism is primarily hepatic via CYP450 3A4 to form oxidative metabolites, which may then be glucuronidated.

Use in Special Populations: Pregnancy (FDA Guidance), Lactation, Children, Renal Insufficiency, and Hepatic Insufficiency

- Bexarotene is contraindicated in women who are pregnant.
- Unknown whether bexarotene is present in breast milk.
- Due to the potential for serious adverse reactions in a breastfeeding infant, a decision should be made to discontinue bexarotene gel or to discontinue breastfeeding during therapy, considering the importance of treatment to the mother.
- Renal insufficiency: Not evaluated; dose adjustment is not expected to be needed.
- Hepatic insufficiency: Not evaluated; dose adjustment is not expected to be needed.

Monitoring

- In females of reproductive potential, obtain a pregnancy test 1 week before initiation and then monthly while on bexarotene; monitor for signs/symptoms of hypersensitivity.
- Skin irritation.
- Dermal irritation.
- Photosensitivity.

- Severe skin reactions (exfoliation, desquamation).
- Allergy (angioedema, lip swelling, facial edema).

Contraindications and Cautions

Products containing DEET: Do not use concurrently with topical products containing DEET (e.g., insect repellant); an increase in DEET toxicity has been observed.

Important Drug Interactions

Aminolevulinic acid (systemic): Photosensitizing agents may enhance the photosensitizing effect of aminolevulinic acid (systemic). Risk X: Avoid combination.

Aminolevulinic acid (topical): Photosensitizing agents may enhance the photosensitizing effect of aminolevulinic acid (topical). Risk C: Monitor therapy.

Multivitamins/fluoride (with ADE): May enhance the adverse/toxic effect of retinoic acid derivatives. Risk X: Avoid combination.

Multivitamins/minerals (with ADEK, folate, iron): May enhance the adverse/toxic effect of retinoic acid derivatives. Risk X: Avoid combination.

Multivitamins/minerals (with AE, no iron): May enhance the adverse/toxic effect of retinoic acid derivatives. Risk X: Avoid combination.

Porfimer: Photosensitizing agents may enhance the photosensitizing effect of Porfimer. Risk C: Monitor therapy.

Verteporfin: Photosensitizing agents may enhance the photosensitizing effect of verteporfin. Risk C: Monitor therapy.

Adverse Effects and Their Management

- Skin irritation can occur.
- Erythema, stinging/burning, dryness, or pruritus may occur especially during the initial 2–4 weeks of use. These may lessen with continued use.
- May cause initial exacerbation of acne.
- May cause increased sensitivity to UV rays. Use sunscreen and avoid sunlamp use.

- Hypersensitivity reactions including facial and eyelid edema and swelling have been reported. Use must be discontinued immediately as anaphylactoid/anaphylactic reactions may occur.

Essential Patient Information

- Burning
- Itching
- Redness
- Peeling
- Loss of strength and energy
- Sweating a lot
- Headache
- Infection
- Burning or numbness feeling
- Swelling
- Swollen glands
- Severe skin irritation

References

1. FDA drug monographs for each of the drugs. Available from Accessdata. fda.gov
2. Lexicomp drug monographs for each of the drugs. Available from: LexiComp/lexidrug Online at online.Lexi.com. Copyright 2024 UptoDate, Inc.
3. De Groot AC. Patch testing. 3rd edition. Volume 3 Chapter 3

Anti-inflammatory Retinoids

4. Brogden R, Goa K. Adapalene: a review of its pharmacological properties and clinical potential in the management of mild to moderate acne. Drugs. 1997;53(3):511–9.
5. Altinyazar HC, Koca R, Tekin NS, et al. Adapalene vs metronidazole gel for the treatment of rosacea. Int J Dermatol. 2005;44(3):252–5.

6. Autret E, Berjot M, Jonville-Bera AP, et al. Anophthalmia and agenesis of optic chiasma associated with adapalene gel in early pregnancy. Lancet. 1997;350(9074):339.
7. Shehab N, Lewis CL, Streetman DD, et al. Exposure to the pharmaceutical excipients benzoyl alcohol and propylene glycol among critically ill neonates. Pediatr Crit Care Med. 2009;10(2):256–9.
8. Kong YL, Tey HL. Treatment of acne vulgaris during pregnancy and lactation. Drugs. 2013;73(8):779–87.
9. Eichenfield LF, Krakowski AC, Piggott C et al. Evidence-based recommendations for the diagnosis and treatment of pediatric acne. Pediatrics 2013 (131 Suppl 3):S163–86.
10. Asai Y, Baibergenova A, Dutil M, et al. Management of acne: Canadian clinical practice guideline. CMAJ. 2016.
11. Maguiness S. Acne. 5-minute video available from the Society for Pediatric Dermatology Website at https://tinyurl.com/saa9t4s

Tretinoin

12. Shehab N, Lewis CL, Streetman DD, Donn SM. Exposure to the pharmaceutical excipients benzyl alcohol and propylene glycol among critically ill neonates. Pediatr Crit Care Med. 2009;10(2):256–9.
13. Chien AL, Qi J, Rainer B, Sachs DL, Helfrich YR. Treatment of acne in pregnancy. J Am Board Fam Med. 2016;29(2):254–62.
14. Kong YL, Tey HL. Treatment of acne vulgaris during pregnancy and lactation. Drugs. 2013;73(8):779–87. https://doi.org/10.1007/s40265-013-0060-0.
15. Leachman SA, Reed BR. The use of dermatologic drugs in pregnancy and lactation. Dermatol Clin. 2006;24(2):167–97.
16. Vitamin A Acid (tretinoin) [product monograph]. Laval, Quebec, Canada: Bausch Health, Canada Inc; September 2020.

Tazarotene

17. Arazlo (tazarotene) [prescribing information]. Bridgewater: Bausch Health US. LLC; December 2019.
18. Avage (tazarotene) [prescribing information]. Irvine: Allergan, Inc; July 2017.
19. Bae YS, Van Voorhees AS, Hsu S, et al; National Psoriasis Foundation. Review of treatment options for psoriasis in pregnant or lactating women:

from the Medical Board of the National Psoriasis Foundation. J Am Acad Dermatol. 2012;67(3):459–77. https://doi.org/10.1016/j.jaad.2011.07.039.
20. Butler DC, Heller MM, Murase JE. Safety of dermatologic medications in pregnancy and lactation: Part II. Lactation. J Am Acad Dermatol. 2014;70(3):417.e1–10; quiz 427. https://doi.org/10.1016/j.jaad.2013.09.009.
21. Centers for Disease Control (CDC). Neonatal deaths associated with use of benzyl alcohol—United States. MMWR Morb Mortal Wkly Rep. 1982;31(22):290–1. http://www.cdc.gov/mmwr/preview/mmwrhtml/00001109.htm.
22. Chien AL, Qi J, Rainer B, Sachs DL, Helfrich YR. Treatment of acne in pregnancy. J Am Board Fam Med. 2016;29(2):254–62. https://doi.org/10.3122/jabfm.2016.02.150165.

Trifarotene

23. Aklief (trifarotene) [prescribing information]. Fort Worth: Galderma Laboratories LP; January 2022.
24. Aklief (trifarotene) [product monograph]. Fort Worth: Galderma Laboratories LP; November 2019.
25. American Academy of Pediatrics Committee on Drugs. "Inactive" ingredients in pharmaceutical products: update (subject review). Pediatrics.1997;99(2):268–78.
26. Kong YL, Tey HL. Treatment of acne vulgaris during pregnancy and lactation. Drugs. 2013;73(8):779–87. https://doi.org/10.1007/s40265-013-0060-0.
27. Naik PP. Trifarotene: a novel therapeutic option for acne. Dermatol Res Pract 2022; 2022:1504303. https://doi.org/10.1155/2022/1504303.
28. Shehab N, Lewis CL, Streetman DD, Donn SM. Exposure to the pharmaceutical excipients benzyl alcohol and propylene glycol among critically ill neonates. Pediatr Crit Care Med. 2009;10(2):256–9.
29. Tan J, Thiboutot D, Popp G, et al. Randomized phase 3 evaluation of trifarotene 50 μg/g cream treatment of moderate facial and truncal acne. J Am Acad Dermatol. 2019;80(6):1691–9. https://doi.org/10.1016/j.jaad.2019.02.044.

Antineoplastic Retinoids

30. Panretin (alitretinoin) [prescribing information]. Concordia Pharmaceuticals; May 2020.

31. Walmsley S, Northfelt DW, Melosky B, Conant M, Friedman-Kien AE, Wagner B. Treatment of AIDS-related cutaneous Kaposi's sarcoma with topical alitretinoin (9-cis-retinoic acid) gel. Panretin Gel North American Study Group. J Acquir Immune Defic Syndr. 1999;22(3):235–46.

Bexarotene

32. Breneman D, Duvic M, Kuzel T, Yocum R, Truglia J, Stevens VJ. Phase 1 and 2 trial of bexarotene gel for skin-directed treatment of patients with cutaneous T-cell lymphoma [published correction appears in Arch Dermatol. 2002;138(10):1386]. Arch Dermatol. 2002;138(3):325–32. https://doi.org/10.1001/archderm.138.3.325
33. Heald P, Mehlmauer M, Martin AG, Crowley CA, Yocum RC, Reich SD; Worldwide Bexarotene Study Group. Topical bexarotene therapy for patients with refractory or persistent early-stage cutaneous T-cell lymphoma: results of the phase III clinical trial. J Am Acad Dermatol. 2003;49(5):801–15. https://doi.org/10.1016/s0190-9622(03)01475-0
34. Targretin (bexarotene) [prescribing information]. Bridgewater, NJ: Valeant; October 2016.

Seborrheic Dermatitis

23

Aileen Feschuk and Nadia Kashetsky

Contents

A. Feschuk (✉)
Faculty of Medicine, Memorial University of Newfoundland, St. John's, NL, Canada
e-mail: afeschuk@mun.ca

N. Kashetsky
Department of Dermatology and Skin Science, Faculty of Medicine, University of British Columbia, Vancouver, BC, Canada
e-mail: nkashetsky@mun.ca

R. M. Law, H. I. Maibach (eds.), *Handbook of Topical Drug Treatment in Dermatology*,
https://doi.org/10.1007/978-3-031-93616-6_23

Introduction

Seborrheic dermatitis, a common condition, affects the seborrheic areas of the body and causes, scaling, flaking, inflammation, pruritus, and erythema [1, 2]. Sebaceous glands are present all over the body sparing only the palms and soles [1] and are particularly dense on the scalp, face, and body folds [2]. The central third of the face, central forehead, eyebrows, postauricular area, and the external ear canal are particularly vulnerable to this condition [2].

Dandruff, a form of seborrheic dermatitis, involves itchy, flaky skin, but unlike seborrheic dermatitis, it is restricted to the scalp [1]. Both seborrheic dermatitis and dandruff are characterized by an inflammatory genomic signature [3].

Seborrheic dermatitis affects about 5% of the population worldwide; however, almost 50% of the population are affected by dandruff [2]. Furthermore, seborrheic dermatitis has a bimodal age distribution, most commonly affecting infants and adults [2]. Infants commonly present with seborrheic dermatitis around the scalp, or "cradle cap" [1]. This usually occurs during the first three months of life, is mild, and self-limiting [2]. Unfortunately, in adults, seborrheic dermatitis is chronic, relapsing and remitting [2].

The main hypothesis regarding the pathophysiology of seborrheic dermatitis includes the interplay of individual susceptibility, the yeast *Malassezia* spp., and inflammatory processes [1, 2]. Therefore, the most common treatments for seborrheic dermatitis include anti-fungals and/or anti-inflammatories [1]. It is important these patients receive treatment, as seborrheic dermatitis can have emotional symptoms (e.g., embarrassment) as well as a negative effect on overall quality of life (e.g., pruritis) [4].

Betamethasone Valerate Foam

Betamethasone valerate foams contains betamethasone valerate—a synthetic topical corticosteroid, which has anti-inflammatory, antipruritic and vasoconstrictive actions.

It is indicated as treatment for inflammatory and pruritic manifestations of dermatoses of the scalp (including seborrheic dermatitis) that are corticosteroid responsive. For further details, see Chap. 18.

Coal Tar Shampoo

Classification and Mode of Action

- Coal tar shampoos are classified as dandruff, seborrheic dermatitis, and psoriasis controlling agents. Coal tar's mode of action is related to its keratoplastic and mild local irritant properties. Although the exact mechanism is currently unknown, it is thought that coal tar abstracts oxygen from the skin which in turn inhibits mitosis causing a decrease in the number of stratum germinativum and stratum corneum cells.
- In addition, coal tar is thought to possibly remove the scales produced by the abovementioned skin disorders.
- Coal tar possibly reacts with epidermal sulfhydryl groups, affecting the skin in a similar way to when it is exposed to sunlight, which theoretically decreases epidermal mitosis and dermal infiltration.
- Coal tar is thought to have weak antiseptic and antipruritic effects. Additionally, coal tar is thought to be a vasoconstrictor and astringent. Specific coal tar shampoos have not been evaluated by the FDA. However, the active ingredient, coal tar, has been approved by the FDA for over-the-counter use in the treatment of seborrheic dermatitis.

Indications and Dermatological Uses

- *Clinical indications:* Coal tar shampoos have not been approved by the FDA but are informally indicated for the temporary relief of symptoms associated with dandruff, psoriasis, and seborrheic dermatitis including itching, flaking, scaling, redness, and irritation of the scalp.
- *Off-label common uses:* Common off-label uses of coal tar and its preparations include for the treatment of eczema, atopic dermatitis, chronic exudative, or lichenoid dermatitis and used in conjunction with ultraviolet therapy (UVA) for psoriasis (Goeckerman therapy).

Formulations/Presentation (Table 23.1)

According to the CPS, coal tar is also available in Canada as an emulsion, gel, liquid, ointment, and shampoo. Specifically, the shampoo is available in various concentrations between 0.05 and 10%.

Table 23.1 Coal tar shampoos available in the United Sates according to Lexicomp

Strengths (equivalent to coal tar)	Brand names	Manufacturer
Coal tar (crude coal tar, pix carbonis)		
Equivalent to coal car 0.5%	DHS ® Tar	Person an Covey
equivalent to coal tar 2%	Ionil T® Plus	Healthpoint
Coal tar combinations		
Equivalent to coal tar 0.5% (4.5% Polytar® consisting of a solution of crude coal tar and coal tar solution)	Polytar® Shampoo	Stiefel
0.5% with salicylic acid 2% and sublimed sulfur 2%	Sebutone® (cream or lotion)	Bristol-Myers Squibb
Coal tar distillate		
3% (equivalent to coal tar 1.2%)	Doak® Tar	Doak

(continued)

Table 23.1 (continued)

Strengths (equivalent to coal tar)	Brand names	Manufacturer
Coal tar extract		
2% (equivalent to coal tar 0.5%)	Neutrogena® T/Gel® (with Neutar®, a solubilized coal tar extract)	Neutrogena
4% (equivalent to coal tar 1%)	Neutrogena® T/Gel Extra Strength (with Neutar®, a solubilized coal tar extract)	Neutrogena
Coal tar topical solution (liquid carbonis detergens, liquor picis carbonis)		
5% (equivalent to coal tar 1%)	Ionil T® (with SD alcohol 40 12% and isopropyl alcohol 4%)	Healthpoint
10% (equivalent to coal tar 2%)	X-Seb® T Plus	Teva
15% (equivalent to coal tar 3%)	MG 217® Medicated Tar Extra Strength with Conditioners	Triton
Coal tar solution combinations		
10% (equivalent to coal tar 2%) with salicylic acid 2%	Tarsum®	Summers

Dosages and Suggested Regimens

- The exact dosages and suggested regimens for using a coal tar shampoo vary depending on the specific preparation and strength used. However, it is generally suggested that the coal tar shampoo is applied thoroughly to wet hair and massaged into the scalp. The shampoo should be left on the hair and scalp to lather for several minutes before rinsing.
- For best results, car tar shampoos should be used at least twice weekly.

Pharmacokinetics

- No data available.

Use in Special Populations

- No data available.

Monitoring: No data available

Contraindications and Cautions

- Coal tar shampoos are for external use only and are contraindicated in those with a history of hypersensitivity to it, and should not be applied to acutely damaged, inflamed, or infected skin.
- The use of a coal tar shampoo should be discontinued if the condition worsens or does not improve after using this product as directed.
- Coal tar shampoos should be kept out of reach of children, and if swallowed, one should seek medical attention or contact a poison control center immediately.
- This product should also be kept away from the eyes, and if the eyes are affected, they should be rinsed thoroughly with water.

Important Drug Interactions

- Coal tar has no known drugs interactions. However, it is recommended that coal tar is not used with other phototoxic/photoactive agents.

Adverse Effects and Their Management

- Coal tar may produce dermatitis which may be allergic or irritant in nature. In hypersensitive patients, coal tar may cause a pustular eruption keratocystic response.
- Additionally, prolonged use of coal tar may result in chronic folliculitis, also called tar acne. This is generally painless and clears following discontinuance or reduction in application frequency.

- Coal tar preparations may also stain hair and clothing.
- Coal tar preparation use results in photosensitivity and therefore exposure to sunlight should be avoided.

NOTE: Coal tar contains chemicals (PAH dibenzo[a,h]anthracene and benzo[a]pyrene (B[a]P) recognized by the State of California to cause cancer (California Proposition 65 Warning), and is classified as a Group 1 carcinogen by the International Agency for Research on Cancer. Animal and occupational studies have shown a clear increased risk of cancer following exposure to coal tar. There are case reports attributing skin cancer to the use of coal tar, most of which occurred in the anogenital region. Therefore, it is recommended to avoid using coal tar in the genital, groin, or rectal area. However, studies on patients treated with coal tar for dermatological conditions such as dandruff have not shown an increased risk of skin cancer. Shampoos have very limited contact time with the skin before they are rinsed off and are therefore generally considered safe. However, other preparations of coal tar that are to be left on the skin for prolonged periods should be used with caution. The combined risk of the carcinogenicity of coal tar in addition to the increased risk of UV damage due to its photoactivating potential has yet to be determined.

Patch Test Concentration

- 5% pet. (Chemotechnique, SmartPracticeeurope, SmartPracticeCanada)

Essential Patient Information

- Contact with the eyes should be avoided. If contact with the eyes does occur, they should be rinsed thoroughly with water.
- Use caution when in the sun, as coal tar shampoos may cause an increased vulnerability to sunburns for up to 24 hours following use.

- Do not use this product with other psoriasis therapies, including ultraviolet radiation or prescription medications unless directed by a physician. Do not use this product for prolonged periods of time unless directed by a physician.
- Although rare, temporary discoloration of bleached, tinted, blonde, or grey hair may occur.

Fluocinolone Acetonide

Classification and Mode of Action

- Fluocinolone acetonide (6α,9-Difluoro-11β,16α, 17,21- tetrahydroxypregna-1,4-diene-3, 20-dione cyclic 16,17-acetal with acetone) comes as both a scalp oil and a shampoo, sold under the name Capex. It is indicated for seborrheic dermatitis but has not been proven effective in other corticosteroid-responsive dermatoses.
- For further details see Chap. 18.

Ketoconazole Gel, Cream, Kit, Foam, and Shampoo

Note: Ketoconazole is also discussed in Chap. 13. Please see the discussion in that chapter for additional information about ketoconazole.

Classification and Mode of Action

- Ketoconazole ((±)-cis-1-acetyl-4-[p-[[2-(2,4-dichlorophenyl)-2-(1Himidazol-1-ylmethyl)-1,3-dioxolan-4-yl]methoxy]phenyl]piperazine) is commonly used as a topical antifungal agent. The proposed mode of action of ketoconazole is the reduction of a yeast—*Malassezia furfur* (also known as *Pityrosporum ovale*)—by inhibiting the synthesis of ergosterol (a key sterol in the membrane of *M. furfur/P. ovale*) resulting in the death of the yeast. Note that this mode of action has yet to be proven.

- In vehicle-controlled studies, 25.3% of those using Xolegel gel (ketoconazole USP at 2% in a topical anhydrous gel vehicle) were considered to have been effectively treated, whereas only 13.9% of those using vehicle gel were considered to have been effectively treated. Effective treatment in this case was defined based on Investigator's Global Assessment Score of ≤1 (completely or almost completely clear), and an Erythema and Scaling score of 0 (none) or 1 (mild) if baseline scores were 2 or 3, respectively.

Indications and Dermatological Uses

- *Clinical indications (FDA):* Ketoconazole creams are indicated for the treatment of tinea corporis, tinea cruris, tinea pedis, tinea versicolor, cutaneous candidiasis, and seborrheic dermatitis. Foams and gels are indicated for the treatment of seborrheic dermatitis in immunocompetent individuals over 12. According to US labelling, ketoconazole shampoos are indicated for the treatment of tinea versicolor caused by *P. orbiculare* (*M. furfur* or *Malassezia orbiculare*). According to Canadian labelling, ketoconazole shampoos are indicated for prophylaxis and treatment of dandruff and seborrheic dermatitis.
- *Off-label common uses:* There is a level of evidence C for the use of ketoconazole in tinea manuum.

Formulations/Presentation (Table 23.2)

Table 23.2 Ketoconazole gel, foam, and shampoo available in the United States and Canada according to Lexicomp

Strength	Brand
Dosage forms: United States	
Cream, external	
2% (15 g, 30 g, 60 g)	Generic
Foam, external	
2% (50 g (DSC), 100 g (DSC)) (contains alcohol, usp, cetyl alcohol, propylene glycol)	Extina
2% (50 g, 100 g) (cfc free; contains alcohol, usp, cetyl alcohol, propylene glycol)	Extina
2% (100 g) (contains alcohol, usp, cetyl alcohol, propylene glycol)	Ketodan
2% (50 g, 100 g)	Generic
Gel, external	
2% (45 g) *contains alcohol, usp, fd&c yellow #10 (quinoline yellow), fd&c yellow #6 (sunset yellow), propylene glycol)	Xolegel
Kit, external	
2% (contains cetyl alcohol, edetate (edta) disodium, propylene glycol)	Ketodan
Shampoo, external	
2% (120 mL (DSC)) [contains fd&c red #40]	Nizoral
1% (125 mL, 200 mL (DSC))	Nizoral A-D
1% (125 mL (DSC), 200 mL (DSC)) (contains brilliant blue fcf (fd&c blue #1), edetate (edta) sodium (tetrasodium))	Nizoral A-D
2% (120 mL)	Generic
Dosage forms: Canada	
Cream, external	
2% (30 g) (contains cetyl alcohol, polysorbate 80, propylene glycol)	Ketoderm

Dosages and Suggested Regimens

- For seborrheic dermatitis, creams and foams should be applied to the affected area twice a day for 4 weeks. Gels should be applied once daily for 2 weeks. Two percent shampoos (products only in Canada) should be used twice daily for 2–4 weeks by lathering 5–10 mL into wet hair, leaving for 3–5 minutes and rinsing.
- For dandruff, 1% shampoo can be applied to wet hair, lathered and rinsed every 3–4 days for up to 8 weeks. Two percent shampoo can be used prophylactically once every 1–2 weeks, or as a treatment twice a week for 2–4 weeks.

Pharmacokinetics

- In a pharmacokinetic absorption study of Xolegel gel (ketoconazole USP at 2% in a topical anhydrous gel vehicle), 18 individuals (both male and female) with between 1 and 14% of body surface area affected by seborrheic dermatitis used Xolegel gel once daily for 14 days. Daily doses ranged from 0.05 to 3.47 g, giving a median total amount of 4.6 g of gel applied over the 2 weeks. The mean ± standard deviation of peak plasma levels was 1.35 ± 3.18 ng/mL on day 7 and was 0.80 ± 1.22 ng/mL on day 14. The median time taken to reach maximum concentration (Tmax) was 8 hrs on day 7 and 7 hrs on day 14. The mean ± standard deviation area under the plasma concentration time curve over the last 24-hour dosing interval (AUC_{0-24}) were 20.8 ± 44.7 (ng)(hr)/mL on day 7 and 15.6 ± 26.4 (ng)(hr)/mL on day 14.

Use in Special Populations

- Chronic use of ketoconazole shampoo does not result in detectable plasma levels, and Vestergaard (2019) showed that topical ketoconazole is safe for the treatment of atopic dermatitis in pregnant individuals.

- When used orally, ketoconazole has been detected in the breastmilk. However, when ketoconazole is used as a gel, it has a plasma concentration less than 250 times that of when it is given orally. Therefore, it is suggested that breastfeeding individuals weigh the risk to the fetus and the benefit of treatment. The nipple, area surrounding the nipple, and direct contact with the child should all be avoided in breastfeeding individuals.
- Of 933 subjects who have participated in safety and efficacy studies of Xolegel gel (ketoconazole USP at 2% in a topical anhydrous gel vehicle), 20.7% were 65 and older, and 6.5% were 75 and older. Differences in safety of effectiveness of Xolegel in those patient populations were not found.

Monitoring: No data available

Contraindications and Cautions

- Hypersensitivity reactions have been reported (contact sensitization, photoallergenicity, and rarely, anaphylaxis). Discontinue use if hypersensitivity or irritation occurs.
- Refer to Chap. 13 for additional contraindications and cautions.

Important Drug Interactions

- There are no known significant drug interactions.

Adverse Effects and Their Management

- Adverse effects that affect 1–10% include dermatological reactions such as application site pruritus, skin stinging, and xeroderma and local reactions such as application site reactions, local irritation, and application site burning.
- The following adverse reactions have been reported in less than 1% of users and are listed alphabetically directly from the

Lexicomp drug monograph: "abnormal texture of hair, acne vulgaris, alopecia, anaphylaxis, angioedema, application site dermatitis, application site discharge, application site erythema, application site pain, cheilitis, contact dermatitis, dizziness, dry eye syndrome, eye irritation, facial swelling, hair discoloration, headache, hypersensitivity reaction, impetigo, localized warm feeling, nail discoloration, paresthesia, pustules, pyogenic granuloma, skin irritation, skin rash, swelling of eye, and urticaria."

- Although the adverse reaction rates observed in clinical trials may not reflect rates observed in clinical practice, they do provide a basis for identifying adverse effects that appear to be related to the use of a treatment. In safety and efficacy studies of Xolegel gel (ketoconazole USP at 2% in a topical anhydrous gel vehicle) to date, 65/933, or 7%, of users experienced at least one treatment-related adverse effect, the most common being application site burning. Other treatment-related adverse reactions occurring at the application site included dermatitis, dryness, irritation, discharge, erythema, pustules, pain, and pruritus. Treatment-related adverse effects which did not occur at the application site included eye irritation and swelling, keratoconjunctivitis, impetigo, granuloma, sicca, pyogenic, headache, dizziness, paresthesia, acne, facial swelling, and nail discoloration.
- Although long-term studies assessing carcinogenicity of Xolegel gel (ketoconazole USP at 2% in a topical anhydrous gel vehicle) have not be conducted, a long-term feeding study in Swiss albino mice and Wistar rats was conducted. There was no evidence of carcinogenicity from this study. Additionally, 5 mg/kg/dose of ketoconazole gel was topically applied to hairless mice 5 days a week for 40 weeks, and no evidence of photocarcinogenicity was found. When ketoconazole was given as a single oral dose up to 80 mg/ kg to mice, no evidence of mutagenicity in the dominant lethal mutation test was found. An Ames assay (an assay which is used bacteria to determine if a compound can cause DNA mutations) was conducted and ketoconazole was not found to cause mutation in *Salmonella typhimurium*, both in the presence and absence of metabolic activation.

Patch Test Concentration

- 1% alcohol

Essential Patient Information

- Xolegel gel (ketoconazole USP at 2% in a topical anhydrous gel vehicle)
  - Should be used as directed by a healthcare provider.
  - Is for external use only.
  - May irritate mucous membranes, and therefore, contact with the nostrils, mouth, and eyes should be avoided.
  - Should not be used for anything other than that for which it was prescribed.
  - Warrants handwashing after use.
  - Adverse health effects to a healthcare provider.

Selenium Sulfide Shampoo

Classification and Mode of Action

- Selenium sulfide shampoo is classified as an antiseborrheic and antifungal, although the exact mode of action is unknown. However, selenium sulfide shampoo appears to have a cytostatic effect on epidermal and follicular epithelial cells, resulting in a reduction of corneocyte production. The active ingredient, selenium sulfide, has been approved by the FDA for over-the-counter treatment of seborrheic dermatitis, although specific selenium sulfide shampoos have not been approved.
- Danby et al. (1993) investigated the use of ketoconazole 2% shampoo versus selenium sulfide 2.5% shampoo for the treatment of dandruff. They found that both were effective treatments, with the mean total adherent dandruff scores declining throughout the treatment period. Ketoconazole was statistically superior to selenium sulfide on day 8 only.

Indications and Dermatological Uses

- *Clinical indications (FDA)*: Selenium sulfide is approved for over-the-counter use by the FDA, and selenium sulfide shampoos are indicated for use in those with seborrheic dermatitis of the scalp, dandruff, and tinea versicolor.
- *Off-label common uses*: No data available.

Formulations/Presentation (Table 23.3)

Dosages and Suggested Regimens

- The exact dosages and suggested regimens for using this product may vary depending on the specific brand used. Generally, after wetting the hair and skin, gently massage into the skin working into a full lather, and then rinse thoroughly and pat dry. This should be repeated twice per week for 2 weeks. The shampoo should not be used more frequently than what is necessary for managing the condition.

Pharmacokinetics

- No information available

Table 23.3 Selenium sulfide shampoos available in the United States according to Lexicomp

Strengths	Brand names
1% (207 mL) (contains brilliant blue fcf (fd&c blue #1), menthol)	Anti-Dandruff
2.3% (180 mL (DSC)) (contains fd&c red #40, methylparaben, propylene glycol, propylparaben)	SelRx
2.25% (180 mL); 2.3% (180 mL)	Generic

Use in Special Populations

- Whether this product is safe to use during pregnancy or while nursing is unknown. No animal reproductive studies with this product have been conducted, and its effect on fertility is unknown. Safety and effectiveness in children under the age of 12 is also unknown.

  Monitoring: No information available

Contraindications and Cautions

- Selenium sulfide shampoos are contraindicated in those with known or suspected hypersensitivity to any ingredients in the shampoo. The product should be kept out of reach of children and is for external use only. Selenium sulfide shampoos are not for ophthalmic use. The product should only be used as directed by a physician and should not be used to treat anything other than that for which it was prescribed. In the event of redness or irritation, discontinue use and consult a physician.

  Important drug interactions: No known interactions

Adverse Effects and Their Management

- The following adverse effects, in decreasing order of sensitivity, may occur: skin irritation, occasional increased hair loss, and discoloration of the hair (although this can be minimized through thorough rinsing of hair after use).
- Systemic toxicity has been reported. Selenium sulfide lotion was used topically on an open scalp lesion, resulting in tremors, hyperhidrosis, garlicky breath, lower abdominal pain, weakness, lethargy, anorexia, and occasional emesis. Symptoms resolved within 10 days of discontinuation. Therefore, it is important to ensure selenium sulfide is not used on damaged skin.

- When 25–50% solutions of 2.5% selenium sulfide were dermally applied to mice over an 88-week period, no carcinogenic effects were observed.

Patch Test Concentration

- 2% pet. Perform controls.

Essential Patient Information

- This product should be discontinued if a rash develops in the treated area or elsewhere, or if the condition worsens. Contact with the eyes, lips, and mucous membranes should be avoided. If contact with any of these areas occurs, they should be rinsed thoroughly with water. The product should not be used on broken or inflamed skin.

Zinc Pyrithione Shampoo

Classification and Mode of Action

- Zinc pyrithione shampoo is classified as an anti-dandruff shampoo. The active ingredient, zinc pyrithione, has been approved for over the counter treatment of seborrheic dermatitis; however, specific zinc pyrithione shampoos have not been approved by the FDA.
- In a comparative study by Shin et al. (2009), patients with dandruff were randomly assigned to a treatment of topical betamethasone, topic tacrolimus, or zinc pyrithione. After 4 weeks, all treatment groups displayed significant improvements on clinical assessment. Interestingly though, the cohort of patients receiving zinc pyrithione continued to improve, even after treatment cessation.

Indications and Dermatological Uses

- *Clinical indications (FDA):* Zinc pyrithione shampoos have not been approved by the FDA but are informally indicated for the relief of symptoms such as scalp itch, irritation, redness, and flaking associated with seborrheic dermatitis, dandruff, and other hyperkeratotic skin conditions.
- *Off-label common uses*: None found.

Formulations/Presentation (Table 23.4)

Dosages and Suggested Regimens

- Zinc pyrithione should be applied to wet hair and scalp. The product should be massaged to a lather, and then let sit for 2–3 minutes before rinsing thoroughly. This should be done at least twice a week or as directed by a physician.

Pharmacokinetics (percutaneous absorption, distribution, metabolism, excretion) as relevant: No data available

Use in special populations: Pregnancy (FDA guidance), lactation, children, renal insufficiency, hepatic insufficiency: No data available

Monitoring: No data available

Table 23.4 Zinc pyrithione shampoos available in the United States according to Lexicomp

Strengths	Brand names
2% (480 mL)	Beta Med
2% (240 mL, 480 mL) (contains fd&c yellow #6 (sunset yellow))	DHS Zinc
2% (240 mL)	Theraplex Z

Contraindications and Cautions

- Zinc pyrithione shampoo is for external use only, and contact with the eyes should be avoided. If contact with the eyes does occur, they should be rinsed thoroughly with water. This product should not be used on wounded areas and should be kept out of reach of children. If any redness, swelling, itching, or other symptom occurs following the use of a zinc pyrithione shampoo, consult a physician.

Important drug interactions: No significant interactions known

Adverse effects and their management: Zinc pyrithione has been classified as a category 1B carcinogen, meaning that based on animal studies, the substance presumably has carcinogenic effects in humans. In March of 2020, The European Commission's Scientific Committee on Consumer Safety (SCCS) determined that zinc pyrithione was safe for use as a rinse- off anti-dandruff ingredient at a concentration of 1%. However, because there are suitable anti-dandruff alternatives, the SCCS concluded that zinc pyrithione will be removed from Annex III (where is was listed as permitted for use in leave-on hair products up to a concentration of 0.1%) and Annex V (where is was listed as permitted in concentrations up to 1% and 0.5% in rinse off hair products and other products, respectively). In addition, zinc pyrithione will be added to the SCCS's list of prohibited cosmetic products in Annex II in March of 2022.

Patch Test Concentration

- No data available

Essential Patient Information: No data available

References

Introduction

1. Borda LJ, Wikramanayake TC. Seborrheic dermatitis and dandruff: a comprehensive review. J Clin Investig Dermatol. 2015; https://doi.org/10.13188/2373-1044.1000019.
2. Tucker D, Masood S. Seborrheic dermatitis. Treasure Island: StatPearls Publishing; 2021.
3. Mills KJ, Hu J, Henry M, Tamura M, Tiesman JP, Xu J. Dandruff/ seborrhoeic dermatitis is characterized by an inflammatory genomic signature and possible immune dysfunction: transcriptional analysis of the condition and treatment effects of zinc pyrithione. Br J Dermatol. 2012; https://doi.org/10.1111/j.1365-2133.2012.10863.x.
4. Xuan M, Lu C, He Z. Clinical characteristics and quality of life in seborrheic dermatitis patients: a cross-sectional in China. Health Qual Life Outcomes. 2020; https://doi.org/10.1186/s12955-020-01558-y.

Betamethasone Valerate Foam

5. https://fda.report/DailyMed/801BAC90-2ED7-4F68-9FA4-BE1705B1F98C.pdf. Revised: July 2020. Accessed 22 Oct 2021.

Coal Tar Shampoo

6. https://fda.report/DailyMed/7CAFB511-0AB7-F3B4-E053-2991AA0A2E0B.pdf. Revised: October 2018. Accessed 22 Oct 2021.
7. https://fda.report/DailyMed/DB9941FD-8861-4E8C-B564-CC01CF3ABB82.pdf. Revised: May 2020. Accessed 22 Oct 2021.
8. https://fda.report/DailyMed/35F3C56D-CC4C-4A0C-866B-8D4133D8FCE6.pdf. Revised: May 2021. Accessed 22 Oct 2021.
9. https://www.fda.gov/media/75758/download. Revised: April 2010. Accessed 28 Oct 2021.
10. Van Schooten F-J, Godschalk R. Coal tar therapy. Drug Saf. 1996;15(6):374–7. https://doi.org/10.2165/00002018-199615060-00002.
11. Roelofzen JHJ, Aben JKH, Oldenhof UTH, Coenraads P-J, Alkemade HA, van de Kerkhof PCM, van der Valk PGM, Kiemeney LALM. No increased risk of cancer after coal tar treatments in patients with psoriasis or eczema. J Invest Dermatol. 2010;130(4):953–61. https://doi.org/10.1038/jid.2009.389.

12. https://www.drugs.com/mtm/coal-tar-topical.html. Revised: March 2021. Accessed: 01 Jan 2022.
13. Lexicomp Monograph: Coal Tar Preparations (Topical). http://online.lexi.com.qe2a-proxy.mun.ca/lco/action/doc/retrieve/docid/complete_ashp/413896?cesid=0qF7a5Ssy0V&searchUrl=%2Flco%2Faction%2Fsearch%3Fq%3DCoal%252520Tar%252520Shampoo%26t%3Dname%26va%3DCoal%252520Tar%252520Shampoo#preps-nested. Revised: June 2021. Accessed 10 Jan 2022.
14. CPS Monograph: Coal Tar. https://www-myrxtx-ca.qe2a-proxy.mun.ca/search. Revised: June 2018. Accessed 15 Jan 2022.

Fluocinolone Acetonide

15. https://fda.report/DailyMed/A52763D0-7024-48A8-9CCA-3127333DFB01.pdf. Revised: June 2018. Accessed 22 Oct 2021

Ketoconazole Gel, Cream, Kit, Foam, and Shampoo

16. https://www.accessdata.fda.gov/drugsatfda_docs/label/2008/021946s002lbl.pdf. Revised: August 2008. Accessed 22 Oct 2021.
17. https://fda.report/DailyMed/EFBC6388-90CE-11DE-B92C-8B7156D89593.pdf. Revised April 2020. Accessed 22 Oct 2021.
18. https://fda.report/DailyMed/63840ff7-d447-4f4e-a05b-1fbed2da8a25. Accessed 22 Oct 2021.
19. Lexicomp Monographs: Ketoconazole (Topical). http://online.lexi.com.qe2a-proxy.mun.ca/lco/action/doc/retrieve/docid/patch_f/1797827?cesid=6sltmghPUfn&searchUrl=%2Flco%2Faction%2Fsearch%3Fq%3Dketoconazole%252520topical%26t%3Dname%26va%3Dketoconazole%252520topical#foc. Revised: January 2022. Accessed 10 Jan 2022.
20. Vestergaard C, Wollenberg A, Barbarot S, Christen-Zaech S, Deleuran M, Spuls P, Flohr C, Trzeciak M, von Kobyletzki L, Seneschal J, Paul C, Bieber T, Werfel T, Folster-Holst R, Darsow U, Gieler U, Svensson A, Corl M, Stalder J-F, De Raeve L, Kunz B, Simon D, Chernyshov P, Hijnen D, Gelmetti C, Ring J, Taieb A, de Bruin-Weller M, Thyssen JP. European task force on atopic dermatitis position paper: treatment of parental atopic dermatitis during preconception, pregnancy and lactation period. J Eur Acad Dermatol Venereol. 2019;33(9):1644–59. https://doi.org/10.1111/jdv.15709.

Selenium Sulfide Shampoo

21. https://fda.report/DailyMed/CA97B19F-2195-4F9C-A6C1-14161B026231.pdf. Revised: February 2020. Accessed 22 Oct 2021.
22. https://www.fda.gov/media/75758/download. Revised: April 2010. Accessed 28 Oct 2021.
23. Danby FW, Maddin WS, Margesson LJ, Rosenthal D. A randomized, double-blind, placebo-controlled trial of ketoconazole 2% shampoo versus selenium sulfide 2.5% shampoo in the treatment of moderate to severe dandruff. J Am Acad Dermatol. 1993;129(6):1008–12. https://doi.org/10.1016/0190-9622(93)70282-x.
24. Lexicomp Monographs: Selenium Sulfide (Topical). http://online.lexi.com.qe2a-proxy.mun.ca/lco/action/doc/retrieve/docid/complete_ashp/413464?cesid=9EXjTQDPbpk&searchUrl=%2Flco%2Faction%2Fsearch%3Fq%3Dselenium%252520sulfide%26t%3Dname%26va%3Dselenium%252520sulfide#uses-nested. Revised February 2021. Accessed 10 January 2022.
25. Lexicomp Monographs: Selenium Sulfide. http://online.lexi.com.qe2a-proxy.mun.ca/lco/action/doc/retrieve/docid/patch_f/7657?cesid=9EXjTQDPbpk&searchUrl=%2Flco%2Faction%2Fsearch%3Fq%3Dselenium%252520sulfide%26t%3Dname%26va%3Dselenium%252520sulfide#. Revised: December 2021. Accessed 10 Jan 2022.

Zinc Pyrithione Shampoo

26. https://fda.report/DailyMed/373692F9-A056-4333-BCF9-EA9B1553D17C.pdf. Revised: March 2021. Accessed 22 Oct 2021.
27. https://fda.report/DailyMed/984780FD-4969-150B-E053-2995A90AED77.pdf Revised: November 2020. Accessed 22 Oct 2021.
28. https://www.fda.gov/media/75758/download. Revised: April 2010. Accessed 28 Oct 2021.
29. Shin H, Kwon OS, Won CH, Kim BJ, Lee YW, Choe YB, Ahn KJ, Eun HC. Clinical efficacies of topical agents for the treatment of seborrheic dermatitis of the scalp: a comparative study. J Dermatol. 2009;36:131–7. https://doi.org/10.1111/j.1346-8138.2009.00607.x.
30. https://chemicalwatch.com/208245/european-commission-to-ban-more-cmrs-in-cosmetics January 2021. Accessed 01 Jan 2022.
31. Lexicomp Drug Monographs: Pyrithione Zinc. http://online.lexi.com.qe2a-proxy.mun.ca/lco/action/doc/retrieve/docid/patch_f/7596?cesid=9eND8QPiEHX&searchUrl=%2Flco%2Faction%2Fsearch%3Fq%3DZinc%252520Pyrithione%26t%3Dname%26va%3DZinc%252520Pyrithione#. Revised: January 2021. Accessed 10 Jan 2022.

Sinecatechins

24

Victoria Nguyen, Linda B. Ou,
and Rebecca M. Law

Contents

V. Nguyen (✉)
School of Pharmacy, University of Waterloo, Kitchener, ON, Canada
e-mail: vtpnguye@uwaterloo.ca

L. B. Ou
Sunnybrook Health Sciences Centre, Toronto, ON, Canada
e-mail: lindaou25@gmail.com

R. M. Law
School of Pharmacy and Faculty of Medicine (Discipline of Family Medicine), Memorial University of Newfoundland, St. John's, NL, Canada
e-mail: rlaw@mun.ca; rlawUCSF@gmail.com

R. M. Law, H. I. Maibach (eds.), *Handbook of Topical Drug Treatment in Dermatology*,
https://doi.org/10.1007/978-3-031-93616-6_24

Classification and Mode of Action

- Sinecatechins 10% and 15% (Veregen®) is a botanical drug product indicated in the treatment of genital and perianal warts.
- Sinecatechins, the active ingredient in Veregen® ointment, is a water extract of green tea leaves from *Camellia sinensis.*
- The mechanism of action of Veregen® is not fully elucidated. In vitro studies have shown that sinecatechins inhibit the activation of keratinocytes. Sinecatechins also exhibit anti-oxidative and anti-inflammatory activity which block kinases involved in tumor cell signaling and induce apoptosis.
- Comparative efficacy:
  - In a pooled analysis of two randomized, double-blind, multicenter studies, Veregen®-treated patients had a higher clearance rate than placebo-treated patients at 60.7% and 44.2%, respectively.

Indications and Dermatological Uses

- *Clinical indications (FDA):* external genital and perianal warts
- *Off-label common uses:* No data available

Formulations/Presentation

- USA: Veregen® ointment (15%)
- Canada: Veregen® ointment (10%)
- Europe: Veregen® ointment (10%, 15%)

Dosages and Suggested Regimens

- External genital and perianal warts: Apply a thin film, around a 0.5 cm strand of ointment, three times daily to each wart until they have been cleared or for a maximum of 16 weeks.

Pharmacokinetics

- Has not been characterized. Data suggests that systemic exposure after repeated topical application of Veregen® is minimal and likely to be less than after a single oral intake of 400 mL of green tea.

Use in Special Populations

- Pregnancy: No data on use of Veregen® in pregnant women. Veregen® should not be used in pregnancy unless benefits outweigh potential risks to the fetus.
- Lactation: Unknown whether Veregen® is secreted into breast milk but manufacturer recommends use with caution in breastfeeding patients.
- Children: Safety and efficacy of Veregen® not established in children under 18 years of age.
- Renal insufficiency: No dose adjustments on manufacturer's labelling.
- Hepatic insufficiency: No dose adjustments on manufacturer's labelling.

Monitoring

- Intense application site reactions, including severe discomfort, desquamation, or association with lymph nodes may occur. Dosing interruption may be warranted. Treatment can be resumed after resolution of skin reaction. In the event of a vesicular local reaction, genital herpes infections should be ruled out before resuming treatment.
- Signs and symptoms of hypersensitivity.

Contraindications and Cautions

- Known sensitivity to extract from green tea leaves or to any ingredients in formulation.

Important Drug Interactions

- No drug interactions on manufacturer's labelling.
- Concomitant use of alternative local treatments for warts should be avoided.

Adverse Effects and Their Management

- Application site reactions like erythema, pruritus, vesicular eruption, bleeding, discharge, localized burning, and discomfort. Acute cases can be managed by temporary dosing interruption and use of cold compresses. The frequency of reactions should decrease with continued use.
- Application of ointment on genital warts in vulvar region are associated more often with severe local reactions. Accidental application into vagina should be immediately rinsed with warm water and mild soap. If patient uses tampons, advise inserting tampon prior to application of ointment.
- Phimosis is a risk when uncircumcised patients treat warts under the foreskin. The foreskin should be retracted, and the affected area should be cleaned daily for prevention.
- Type IV hypersensitivity reaction observed in 2% of patients.

Carcinogenicity (If Known (Including Mouse Painting Studies)

- Treatment with oral sinecatechins administered daily for 26 weeks to p53 transgenic mice was not associated with increased carcinogenicity. Dermal carcinogenicity studies have not been conducted.

Patch Test Concentration

- No data available

Essential Patient Information

- Do not apply to open wounds, broken, or inflamed skin.
- For topical use only. Do not administer orally, intravaginally, or intra-anally.
- Avoid contact with the eyes, nostrils, lips, and mouth. Rinse immediately if contact occurs.
- Avoid use of occlusive dressings over treatment area.
- Avoid exposure of treated areas to sun/UV light.
- Tampons should be inserted prior to application of Veregen® to prevent accidental application into vagina.
- Uncircumcised patients treating warts beneath the foreskin should retract foreskin, and clean the affected area daily.
- Veregen® is not a cure. New warts may develop during or after treatment.
- Sexual contact should be avoided while ointment is on the skin.
- Veregen® may weaken condom and vaginal diaphragms. Alternative methods of contraception are recommended.
- Veregen® may stain clothes and bedding.

References

1. FDA drug monograph Veregen® (sinecatechins) ointment, for topical use. Available from https://www.accessdata.fda.gov/drugsatfda_docs/label/2018/021902s033lbl.pdf. Accessed 30 Apr 2023.
2. LexiComp drug monograph Sinecatechins. Available from: LexiComp Online at online.Lexi.com. Copyright 2023 UptoDate, Inc.
3. Deeb M, Levy R, Pope E, Lara-Corrales I. Sinecatechins ointment for the treatment of warts in children. Pediatr Dermatol. 2019;36(1):121–4.

4. Gross G, Meyer KG, Pres H, Thielert C, Tawfik H, Mescheder A. A randomized, double-blind, four-arm parallel-group, placebo-controlled Phase II/III study to investigate the clinical efficacy of two galenic formulations of Polyphenon E in the treatment of external genital warts. J Eur Acad Dermatol Venereol. 2007;21(10):1404–12.
5. Health Canada drug monograph Veregen® (sinecatechins) ointment 10% w/w. Available from https://www.paladin-labs.com/our_products/Veregen-PM-En.pdf?ver=3.0. Accessed 30 Apr 2023.
6. Singh BN, Shankar S, Srivastava RK. Green tea catechin, epigallocatechin-3-gallate (EGCG): mechanisms, perspectives and clinical applications. Biochem Pharmacol. 2011;82(12):1807–21.
7. Stockfleth E, Beti H, Orasan R, Grigorian F, Mescheder A, Tawfik H, Thielert C. Topical Polyphenon E in the treatment of external genital and perianal warts: a randomized controlled trial. Br J Dermatol. 2008;158(6):1329–38.
8. Stockfleth E, Meyer T. Sinecatechins (Polyphenon E) ointment for treatment of external genital warts and possible future indications. Expert Opin Biol Ther. 2014;14(7):1033–43.
9. Tatti S, Swinehart JM, Thielert C, Tawfik H, Mescheder A, Beutner KR. Sinecatechins, a defined green tea extract, in the treatment of external anogenital warts: a randomized controlled trial. Obstet Gynecol. 2008;111(6):1371–9.
10. Tyring SK. Sinecatechins: effects on HPV-induced enzymes involved in inflammatory mediator generation. J Clin Aesthet Dermatol. 2012;5(1):19.
11. Tyring SK. Effect of sinecatechins on HPV-activated cell growth and induction of apoptosis. J Clin Aesthet Dermatol. 2012;5(2):34.

Sirolimus for Facial Angiofibroma Associated with Tuberous Sclerosis Complex

25

Arian Farahani, Michael Pham,
Sreedevi Boggarapu, and Eric Beresford

Contents

Introduction

Facial angiofibroma are small swellings consisting of fibrous dermal tissue and blood vessels typically appearing on the malar, nasal dorsum, nasolabial fold, forehead, and chin areas that progressively enlarge and multiply over time [1–3]. They are one of the predominant cutaneous manifestations of tuberous sclerosis

A. Farahani · M. Pham · S. Boggarapu (✉) · E. Beresford
Nobelpharma America, LLC, Bethesda, MD, USA
e-mail: arian.farahani@nobelpharma-us.com;
michael.pham@nobelpharma-us.com;
Sreedevi.boggarapu@nobelpharma-us.com;
Eric.beresford@nobelpharma-us.com

R. M. Law, H. I. Maibach (eds.), *Handbook of Topical Drug Treatment in Dermatology*,
https://doi.org/10.1007/978-3-031-93616-6_25

complex (TSC), an autosomal dominant genetic rare disorder caused by mutations in tumor-suppressor genes, *TSC1* or *TSC2*, leading to dysfunction of hamartin or tuberin, respectively [4]. Hamartin and tuberin are critical negative regulators of mechanistic target of rapamycin (mTOR), which has a central role in the regulation of cell growth and tumorigenesis [2, 4, 5]. Dysfunction in hamartin and tuberin leads to chronic activation of mTOR pathway, resulting in tumor growth in multiple organs, including the skin, brain, eyes, heart, and kidneys.[2, 5].

TSC affects 1 in 6000 to 10,000 live births [3]. Over one million people worldwide may have TSC with ~50,000 in the USA. No difference in the prevalence has been observed by gender, race, or ethnicity [3].

TSC is a complex and highly variable disease, with differing intra- and inter-individual topical and systemic clinical presentations that may change over time [3, 6]. This necessitates a multidisciplinary approach involving dermatologists, neurologists, pulmonologists, urologists, cardiovascular specialists, pediatricians, and geneticists [3, 5]. TSC typically first appears in infancy or early childhood; >60% of patients are diagnosed under 2 years of age [7]. Skin manifestations (including facial angiofibromas, hypomelanotic macules, shagreen patches, and cephalic plaques) are common and appear in >90% of TSC [1, 2].

Germline mutations cause TSC in about 30% of cases, while sporadic (or somatic) mutations, frequently in *TSC2,* cause the majority of cases [2]. TSC can be diagnosed via molecular identification, or by using TSC clinical diagnostic criteria [4], which yields a positive result in ~75–90% of TSC cases [2, 4]. There is an International TSC Consensus Group clinical diagnostic criteria [4].

There are currently no US-specific guidelines for the management of TSC-related skin manifestations, including facial angiofibroma. Updated International TSC Consensus Group recommendations suggest that more evidence is necessary to guide the choice of treatment for TSC-related skin lesions but recognize existing evidence supporting several approaches [4]. Pharmacological (topical or oral mTOR inhibitors) and non-pharmacological (surgical or excision) treatment options are currently in clinical practice [4]. Physical removal using methods such as laser therapy, dermabrasion, radiofrequency ablation, cryotherapy, and electrocoagulation potentially yield good results, however, may be associated with the risk of adverse effects such as pain, scarring, pigmentation disorders, skin texture changes, postoperative infections, and high recurrence rates, often making follow-up treatment necessary.[4, 8] The International TSC Consensus Group does not recommend systemic therapy for the exclusive treatment of facial angiofibroma due to the risk of systemic side effects [4].

Topical mTOR inhibitors was suggested as a safe and effective approach for treating facial angiofibroma.

Topical sirolimus 0.2% gel was approved in Japan in 2018 for the treatment of skin lesions and in the USA in 2022 for the treatment of facial angiofibroma associated with TSC. A placebo-controlled phase III randomized clinical trial showed the efficacy and safety of topical sirolimus 0.2% gel for the management of facial angiofibroma over 12 weeks [9], which was maintained over 52 weeks [10].

In a postmarketing surveillance [11], topical sirolimus 0.2% gel showed improvement in overall cutaneous manifestations (facial angiofibroma, hypomelanotic macules, shagreen patches, fibrous plaque, and periungual fibroma) in 74.8% of patients over 52 weeks, and the responder rate was the highest for facial angiofibroma (86.2%). Topical sirolimus 0.2% gel was generally well tolerated with major drug-related AEs were application site irritation, dry skin, acne, eye irritation, pruritus, erythema, dermatitis acneiform, and contact dermatitis [10].

Sirolimus 0.2% Gel

Drug Monograph [12, 13]

Classification and Mode of Action

- Sirolimus, a macrocyclic lactone produced by *Streptomyces hygroscopicus* [14] is a mechanistic target of rapamycin (mTOR) inhibitor immunosuppressant.[13]

- The mechanism of action of sirolimus in the treatment of tuberous sclerosis complex (TSC)-related facial angiofibroma is unknown. TSC is associated with genetic defects in *TSC1* and *TSC2* which leads to chronic activation of mTOR. Sirolimus inhibits mTOR activation.
- In a multicenter, placebo-controlled, stratified, randomized, double-blind phase 3 trial [9] treatment with topical sirolimus 0.2% gel resulted in improvement in the size and color of facial angiofibroma, which was further confirmed in the long-term extension study [10].
- Postmarketing surveillance (conducted in Japan) further confirmed the findings from clinical studies [11].

Indications and Dermatologic Uses

- *Clinical indications (FDA)*: Indicated for the treatment of facial angiofibroma associated with TSC in adults and pediatric patients 6 years of age and older in the USA [12].
- Clinical indications (Japan): Skin lesions associated with TSC [15].
- *Off-label common uses*: Vascular anomalies, cutaneous lymphatic malformations, pachyonychia congenita, lingual microcystic lymphatic malformations, epidermolysis bullosa simplex, epidermolysis bullosa simplex Kobner, and Weber-Cockayne syndrome.

Formulations/Presentation

- USA and Japan: Hyftor (topical sirolimus 0.2% gel).

Dosages and Suggested Regimens

- Apply to the skin of the face affected with angiofibroma twice daily.
  - The maximum daily dosage is as follows:
    - 600 mg (2 cm) for patients 6 to 11 years of age
    - 800 mg (2.5 cm) for patients 12 years of age and older.

Baseline Investigations and Considerations

Pharmacokinetics

- Blood concentrations ranged from undetectable to 0.50 ng/mL after multiple doses.
- Maximum sirolimus concentration measured at any time was 3.27 ng/mL in adults and 1.80 ng/mL in pediatric subjects.
- No evidence on the systemic accumulation of sirolimus upon topical application in patients with tuberous sclerosis for periods of up to 1 year.

Carcinogenicity

Oral Carcinogenicity Studies

Mice Studies

- Once daily oral administration for 86 weeks was associated with a statistically significant increase in malignant lymphoma.
- Sirolimus-related hepatocellular adenoma and carcinoma were induced.

Rat Study

- There were no significant findings.

Use in Special Populations

- Approved for use in children >6 years old.
- No sufficient numbers of subjects aged 65 years old.
- *Pregnancy*: Based on animal studies, oral sirolimus may cause fetal harm when administered to pregnant women. The available data from case reports on HYFTOR use in pregnant women are insufficient to evaluate for a drug-associated risk of major birth defects, miscarriage, or adverse maternal or fetal outcomes.
- Oral sirolimus may compromise the male and female fertility based on animal studies.
- *Breastfeeding*: Breastfeeding not recommended.
- *Renal insufficiency*: No dosage adjustment needed.
- *Hepatic insufficiency*: No dosage adjustment needed.

Monitoring

- Oral sirolimus has been associated with increased serum cholesterol and triglycerides.
- Concomitant use of topical sirolimus gel with CYP3A4 inhibitors require monitoring for potential adverse reactions.

Contraindications and Cautions

- History of hypersensitivity to sirolimus or any other component.
- Oral sirolimus has been associated with hypersensitivity reactions, including anaphylactic/anaphylactoid reactions, angioedema, exfoliative dermatitis, and hypersensitivity vasculitis.
- Serious infection: Serious infections, including opportunistic infections and latent viral infections, such as progressive multifocal leukoencephalopathy, have been reported with oral sirolimus.
- Oral sirolimus has been associated with malignancy, including lymphoma and skin cancer.

Important Drug Interactions

- Concomitant use of topical sirolimus gel with CYP3A4 inhibitors require monitoring for potential drug interactions.

Adverse Effects and Their Management

- Most common adverse reactions ($\geq$1%) are dry skin, application site irritation, pruritus, acne, acneiform dermatitis, ocular hyperemia, skin hemorrhage, and skin irritation.

Patch Test Concentration

- 0.1% oral solution; also patch test with excipients; test controls.

Essential Patient Information

- Apply to affected skin of the face in the morning and at bedtime.
- Do not use with occlusive dressings. Do not cover treated skin with bandages, dressings, or wraps.

- Wash hands before and after application.
- For topical use only; not for oral, ophthalmic, or intravaginal use.
- For pediatric patients limit exposure to natural or artificial sunlight; protective clothing should be worn.

References

1. Cardis MA, DeKlotz CMC. Cutaneous manifestations of tuberous sclerosis complex and the paediatrician's role. Arch Dis Child. 2017;102(9):858–63. https://doi.org/10.1136/archdischild-2016-312001.
2. Portocarrero LKL, Quental KN, Samorano LP, Oliveira ZNP, Rivitti-Machado MCDM. Tuberous sclerosis complex: review based on new diagnostic criteria. An Bras Dermatol. 2018;93(3):323–31. https://doi.org/10.1590/abd1806-4841.20186972.
3. Northrup H, Krueger DA, Group ITSCC. Tuberous sclerosis complex diagnostic criteria update: recommendations of the 2012 International Tuberous Sclerosis Complex Consensus Conference. Pediatr Neurol. 2013;49(4):243–54. https://doi.org/10.1016/j.pediatrneurol.2013.08.001.
4. Northrup H, Aronow ME, Bebin EM, et al. Updated international tuberous sclerosis complex diagnostic criteria and surveillance and management recommendations. Pediatr Neurol. 2021;123:50–66. https://doi.org/10.1016/j.pediatrneurol.2021.07.011.
5. Schwartz RA, Fernández G, Kotulska K, Jóźwiak S. Tuberous sclerosis complex: advances in diagnosis, genetics, and management. J Am Acad Dermatol. 2007;57(2):189–202. https://doi.org/10.1016/j.jaad.2007.05.004.
6. Zöllner JP, Franz DN, Hertzberg C, et al. A systematic review on the burden of illness in individuals with tuberous sclerosis complex (TSC). Orphanet J Rare Dis. 2020;15(1):23. https://doi.org/10.1186/s13023-019-1258-3.
7. Boggarapu S, Roberds SL, Nakagawa J, Beresford E. Characterization and management of facial angiofibroma related to tuberous sclerosis complex in the United States: retrospective analysis of the natural history database. Orphanet J Rare Dis. 2022;17(1):355. https://doi.org/10.1186/s13023-022-02496-2.
8. Salido-Vallejo R, Garnacho-Saucedo G, Moreno-Giménez JC. Current options for the treatment of facial angiofibromas. Actas Dermosifiliogr. 2014;105(6):558–68. https://doi.org/10.1016/j.ad.2012.11.020.

9. Wataya-Kaneda M, Ohno Y, Fujita Y, et al. Sirolimus gel treatment vs placebo for facial angiofibromas in patients with tuberous sclerosis complex: a randomized clinical trial. JAMA Dermatol. 2018;154(7):781–8. https://doi.org/10.1001/jamadermatol.2018.1408.
10. Wataya-Kaneda M, Nagai H, Ohno Y, et al. Safety and efficacy of the Sirolimus gel for TSC patients with facial skin lesions in a long-term, open-label, extension, uncontrolled clinical trial. Dermatol Ther (Heidelb). 2020;10(4):635–50. https://doi.org/10.1007/s13555-020-00387-7.
11. Egami A, Takahashi S, Kokubo T, Boggarapu S, Beresford E. Topical sirolimus 0.2% gel for the management of tuberous Sclerosis complex-related cutaneous manifestations: an interim analysis of postmarketing surveillance in Japan. Dermatol Ther (Heidelb). 2023.
12. FDA drug monograph (Hyftor). Available from https://www.accessdata.fda.gov/drugsatfda_docs/label/2022/213478s000lbl.pdf. Accessed 27 Mar 2023.
13. Sirolimus (Topical) (Lexi-drugs). LexiComp drug monograph Available from: LexiComp Online at online.Lexi.com. Copyright 2023 UptoDate, Inc.
14. Kahan BD, Chang JY, Sehgal SN. Preclinical evaluation of a new potent immunosuppressive agent, rapamycin. Transplantation. 1991;52(2):185–91. https://doi.org/10.1097/00007890-199108000-00001.
15. Rapalimus Gel 0.2%. Information for people using this medication. https://www.rad-ar.or.jp/siori/english/search/result?n=44731. Accessed 27 Mar 2023.

Trichogenic and Antitrichogenic Agents

26

Sheeva Shahinfar, Rebecca M. Law, and Howard I. Maibach

Contents

S. Shahinfar (✉)
Texas A&M University College of Medicine, Bryan, TX, USA
e-mail: Sheeva.Shahinfar@tamu.edu

R. M. Law
School of Pharmacy and Faculty of Medicine (Discipline of Family Medicine) Memorial University of Newfoundland, St. John's, NL, Canada
e-mail: rlaw@mun.ca; rlawUCSF@gmail.com

H. I. Maibach
Department of Dermatology, University of California San Francisco (UCSF), San Francisco, CA, USA
e-mail: howard.maibach@ucsf.edu

R. M. Law, H. I. Maibach (eds.), *Handbook of Topical Drug Treatment in Dermatology*,
https://doi.org/10.1007/978-3-031-93616-6_26

Bimatoprost

It contains benzalkonium chloride.

Classification and Mode of Action

- Bimatoprost is a prostaglandin analog that increases the thickness, darkness, and length of eyelashes.
- Mechanism of action is unknown, although it is thought to be due to an increased number of hairs in the anagen phase along with melanogenesis stimulation.

Indications and Dermatological Uses

- *Clinical indications (FDA):* Hypotrichosis of eyelashes, elevated intraocular pressure
- *Off-label common uses*: Hair thinning on the scalp and eyebrows

Formulations/Presentation

- USA: 0.03% ophthalmic solution
- Canada: 0.03% ophthalmic solution
- Europe: 0.03% ophthalmic solution

Dosages and Suggested Regimens

- Remove make-up and contact lenses before application. Ensure a clean face. Place one drop of solution on provided applicator, and apply evenly on the skin of the upper eyelid at the base of eyelashes once daily at night. Perform on both eyes, using a separate clean applicator for each eye. Do not use other applicators or brushes; do not reuse applicators. May re-insert contacts 15 mins post application.

- No suggested dosage adjustment for renal or hepatic impairment due to low systemic absorption.

Baseline Investigations and Considerations

Pharmacokinetics (Percutaneous Absorption, Distribution, Metabolism, Excretion) as Relevant

- Minimal topical absorption. Oxidation, N-demethylation, and glucuronidation occur after entering systemic circulation with subsequent metabolite formation.
- Excreted primarily in urine; also excreted in feces.
- Onset of effect: 4–6 months.

Use in Special Populations: Pregnancy (FDA Guidance), Lactation, Children, Renal Insufficiency, and Hepatic Insufficiency

- Approved for use in children ≥5 years old. The same dosage and regimen as adults.
- There are no studies in pregnant women. In animal studies, at doses more than 41 times the maximum intended human use, fetal abortion was noted. Bimatoprost should be administered in pregnancy only when benefits outweigh the potential risks.
- Unknown if bimatoprost is present in breast milk, although animal studies show its excretion in breast milk. Due to short half-lives, bimatoprost may be considered safe in breastfeeding; application after breastfeeding may help decrease possible exposure to infant during lactation.
- Contact lens users: Topical solution contains benzalkonium chloride, which can potentially result in change in coloration of soft contact lenses. Remove prior to application, and reinsert contact lenses 15 minutes postapplication.

Monitoring

- Intraocular pressure
- Ocular pigmentation changes

Contraindications and Cautions

- Consult physician prior to using if simultaneously using medications to reduce intraocular pressure.

Important Drug Interactions

- Latanoprost: Simultaneous use may cause increased intraocular pressure.
- Latanoprostene bunod: Simultaneous use may cause increased intraocular pressure
- Nonsteroidal anti-inflammatory agents (oral and ophthalmic): May decrease or increase the proposed effects of prostaglandins (e.g., bimatoprost).

Adverse Effects and Their Management

- Eye irritation. Notify physician if bothersome or does not go away.
- Dark eyelids. Notify physician if bothersome or does not go away.
- Serious side effects warrant seeking medical help and immediately discontinuing drug: change in eyesight, eye pain, very bad eye irritation, photophobia, eye discharge, and eye color changes.
- Allergic reactions include rash, hives, itching, redness, swelling, blistered/peeling skin, wheezing, chest/throat tightness, difficulty breathing, difficulty swallowing, difficulty talking, unusual hoarseness, and swollen mouth/face/lips/tongue/throat. Discontinue medication and seek immediate help if experiencing an allergic reaction.
- May cause bacterial keratitis and change in pigmentation of iris/eyelid skin/periorbital skin/eyelashes. May increase thickness, length, or number of eyelashes. Long-term effects of increased pigmentation are possible, but unknown.
- May cause eyelid erythema, periorbital erythema, hypertrichosis, local skin hyperpigmentation of the skin/eyelashes/eyelid/iris, blurred vision, conjunctival edema, conjunctival hemorrhage, decreased visual acuity, dry eye syndrome, eye irritation, eye pain, eye pruritus, eyelid pruritus, punctate keratitis, foreign body sensation in the eye, hypotony of the eye, allergic dermatitis, erythematous rash, periocular dryness of the skin, macular eruption, trichorrhexis, eyelid xeroderma, madarosis,

blepharoptosis, deepening of the eyelid sulcus, eye discharge, eyelid edema, eyelid entropion, hordeolum, intraocular inflammation, increased lacrimation, macular edema, misdirected growth of eyelashes, ocular allergy, ocular edema, periorbital swelling, photophobia, and scaling of the eyelid.
- May cause hypertension, dizziness, headache, dyspnea, or pulmonary complications.

Carcinogenicity
- Mice studies of bimatoprost used as an antiglaucoma agent have not shown carcinogenic potential. Studies have not been performed for the carcinogenicity of bimatoprost used for hypotrichosis.

Patch Test Concentration
- N/A

Essential Patient Information
- Eyelash growth will return to baseline if therapy is discontinued.
- May cause unwanted hair growth if applied to unintended areas repeatedly. When using, only apply to upper eyelid and remove excess.

Relative efficacy to innovator drug: None

Minoxidil (Topical)

Classification and Mode of Action

- Minoxidil is a mitogenic agent that was first used as an antihypertensive medication. Side effects of hypertrichosis helped in the development of a topical version that now is known to promote hair growth.
- Mechanism of action is not entirely understood, but it is thought to be due to a combination of factors including vasodilation, increased blood flow to the skin, and hair follicle stimulation.

- Minoxidil is also recognized as an agonist for potassium channels, causing cell membrane hyperpolarization.
- It is believed that the synergistic effect of vasodilation and hyperpolarization allows more blood, nutrients, and oxygen into the hair follicle.
- Some clinical trials suggest that the 5% formulation has a higher efficacy and earlier treatment response than 2% for both men and women.
- Continuous therapy of at least 4 months may be needed for visible results.

Indications and Dermatological Uses

- *Clinical indications (FDA):* Androgenetic alopecia.
- *Off-label common uses*: Used for other hair loss conditions including telogen effluvium, scarring alopecia, alopecia areata, chemotherapy-induced alopecia, monilethrix, and eyebrow hypotrichosis.
- Oral minoxidil is not FDA approved for hair loss, but clinical trials show efficacy.

Formulations/Presentation

- USA: 2% solution, 5% solution, 5% aerosol foam
- Canada: 2% solution, 5% solution, 5% aerosol foam
- Europe: 2% solution, 5% solution, 5% aerosol foam

Dosages and Suggested Regimens

- Apply directed amount topically to hair-thinning areas of the scalp, and massage in with fingers. Wash hands after use.
- No suggested dosage adjustment for renal or hepatic impairment due to low systemic absorption.

Pharmacokinetics (Percutaneous Absorption, Distribution, Metabolism, Excretion) as Relevant

- Metabolism/transport effects are unknown.

Use in Special Populations: Pregnancy (FDA Guidance), Lactation, Children, Renal Insufficiency, and Hepatic Insufficiency

- Adverse effects have been seen in pregnancy.
- Present in breast milk after oral administration.
- Not approved for use in children <18 years old.
- For renal insufficiency or hepatic insufficiency, no dosage adjustments have been provided by the manufacturer.

Monitoring

- Allergic dermatitis
- Change in hair texture
- Hair discoloration

Contraindications and Cautions

- Caution for those with heart disease: Due to the possibility of systemic absorption followed by fluid/electrolyte changes, risk-vs-benefit analysis should be done in patients with heart disease.

Adverse Effects and Their Management

- Change in hair texture. Notify physician if bothersome or does not go away.
- Hair discoloration. Notify physician if bothersome or does not go away.

- Allergic reactions include rash, hives, itching, red/swollen/blistered/peeling skin, wheezing, chest/throat tightness, difficulty breathing/swallowing/talking, unusual hoarseness, and swollen mouth/face/lips/tongue/throat. Discontinue medication, and seek immediate medical help if experiencing an allergic reaction.
- Local erythema or pruritus may occur.
- Allergic reaction may occur to propylene glycol, which is a nonactive ingredient present in some formulations.

Carcinogenicity

- Minoxidil is a mitogenic agent, which are a class of drugs that induce cell division and thus have the increased risk for inducing DNA damage. Mice studies have shown that topical administration of high minoxidil doses can induce DNA damage without producing cytotoxicity.

Patch Test Concentration

- 5% alcohol

Essential Patient Information

- OTC Labeling: Do not use if amount of hair loss differs from that displayed on product label, if you do not have a family history of hair loss, if you have sudden/patchy hair loss, if your hair loss is triggered by childbirth, if you are unaware of the reason for your hair loss, if you are <18 years old, if your scalp is red/inflamed/painful/irritated/infected, or if you use other topical scalp medications.
- Do not use products on women intended for men.
- Avoid contact with the eyes, lips, or other mucous membranes. In the event of contact with eyes, wash eyes with a large amount of cool, filtered water.

- Not formulated for receding hairline or frontal baldness.
- Continued use is needed in order to maintain hair growth.
- Discontinue use if you experience chest pain, rapid heartbeat, faintness, dizziness, unexplained weight gain, swollen hands/feet, scalp irritation/redness, unwanted facial hair growth, or no hair growth results seen after 4–6 months.
- Flammable product. Avoid fire, flame, or smoking immediately after application.

Eflornithine

Classification and Mode of Action

- Eflornithine irreversibly inhibits ornithine decarboxylase. This process is thought to inhibit cell division and synthetic functions, which, in turn, affects the rate of hair growth.

Indications and Dermatological Uses

- *Clinical indications (FDA):* Facial hair reduction
- *Off-label common uses*: West African trypanosomiasis with CNS involvement (level of evidence: B)

Formulations/Presentation

- USA: 13.9% cream
- Canada: 13.9% cream
- Europe: 11.5% cream

Dosages and Suggested Regimens

- Apply a thin layer of cream to affected areas of face and chin two times a day, at least 8 hours apart. Massage in with fingers.

- Wait at least 5 minutes after hair removal to apply cream. Hair removal techniques can still be used concomitant with eflornithine.
- Do not wash affected area at least 4 hours after application.

Baseline Investigations and Considerations

Pharmacokinetics (Percutaneous Absorption, Distribution, Metabolism, Excretion) as Relevant

- Onset of effect: 4–8 weeks.
- Continued results until about 8 weeks after discontinuing treatment.
- Elimination half-life is 8 hours.
- Excreted primarily in urine as unchanged drug.

Use in Special Populations: Pregnancy (FDA Guidance), Lactation, Children, Renal Insufficiency, and Hepatic Insufficiency

- Unknown if eflornithine is present in breast milk. Caution should be exercised if using eflornithine while breastfeeding.
- Pregnancy category C (former). Eflornithine should be administered in pregnancy only when benefits outweigh the potential risks; although, it is recommended to not be used or discontinued due to unknown effects.
- Approved in children ≥12 years old.
- Renal insufficiency: Not evaluated; dose adjustment is not expected to be needed.
- Hepatic insufficiency: Not evaluated; dose adjustment is not expected to be needed.

Monitoring

- Hypersensitivity reaction

Contraindications and Cautions

- Hypersensitivity to eflornithine or any part of formula
- For topical facial use for females only

Important Drug Interactions

- None known

Adverse Effects and Their Management

- May cause pimples, burning or stinging sensation, redness, skin tingling, or hair bumps. Notify physician if bothersome or does not go away.
- Immediately discontinue and seek medical help if experiencing very bad skin irritation.
- Allergic reactions include rash, hives, itching, redness, swelling, blistered/peeling skin, wheezing, chest/throat tightness, difficulty breathing, difficulty swallowing, difficulty talking, unusual hoarseness, and swollen mouth/face/lips/tongue/throat. Discontinue medication and seek immediate help if experiencing an allergic reaction.
- May cause acne vulgaris, pseudofolliculitis barbae, headache, skin tingling, dizziness, stinging of skin, burning skin sensation, pruritus, rash, xeroderma, erythema, alopecia, skin irritation, folliculitis, ingrown hair, dyspepsia, anorexia, acne rosaces, cheilitis, contact dermatitis, dermal hemorrhage, facial edema, herpes simplex infection, nausea, numbness, swollen lips, vertigo, and weakness.

Carcinogenicity

- Animal studies do not show carcinogenicity comparable to the maximum recommended dosage in humans. Eflornithine inhibits ornithine decarboxylase, which is an enzyme active in the cell cycle and thought to play a role in carcinogenesis. It can be postulated that eflornithine may even have anticarcinogenetic properties, although this has not been tested in clinical trials.

Patch Test Concentration

- N/A

Essential Patient Information

- Do not wash area for at least 4 hours after application.
- Makeup and sunscreen can be applied on treated areas after topical cream has dried.

Relative efficacy to innovator drug: None

References

Bimatoprost

1. FDA drug monograph Latisse® (bimatoprost ophthalmic solution). Available from https://www.accessdata.fda.gov/drugsatfda_docs/label/2012/022369s005lbl.pdf. Accessed 05/01/2022.
2. LexiComp drug monograph Bimatoprost. Available from: LexiComp Online at online.Lexi.com. Copyright 2021 UptoDate, Inc.
3. Vergilis-Kalner IJ. Application of bimatoprost ophthalmic solution 0.03%; for the treatment of eyebrow hypotrichosis: series of Ten cases. Dermatol Online J. 2014;20
4. Elias MJ, Weiss J, Weiss E. Bimatoprost Ophthalmic Solution 0.03% for eyebrow growth. Dermatologic Surg. 2011;37:1057–9.
5. Harii K, Arase S, Tsuboi R, Weng E, Daniels S, VanDenburgh A. Bimatoprost for eyelash growth in Japanese subjects: two multicenter controlled studies. Aesth Plast Surg. 2014;38:451–60.
6. Smith S, Fagien S, Whitcup SM, Ledon F, Somogyi C, Weng E, Beddingfield FC. Eyelash growth in subjects treated with Bimatoprost: a multicenter, randomized, double-masked, vehicle-controlled, parallel-group study. J Am Acad Dermatol. 2012;66:801–6.
7. Glaser DA, Hossain P, Perkins W, Griffiths T, Ahluwalia G, Weng E, Beddingfield FC. Long-term safety and efficacy of bimatoprost solution 0·03% application to the eyelid margin for the treatment of idiopathic and chemotherapy-induced eyelash hypotrichosis: a randomized controlled trial. Br J Dermatol. 2015;172:1384–94.
8. Centofanti M, Oddone F, Chimenti S, Tanga L, Citarella L, Manni G. Prevention of dermatologic side effects of bimatoprost 0.03% topical therapy. Am J Ophthalmol. 2006;142:1059–60.

9. Woodward DF, Phelps RL, Krauss AH-P, Weber A, Short B, Chen J, Liang Y, Wheeler LA. Bimatoprost: a novel antiglaucoma agent. Cardiovasc Drug Rev. 2006;22:103–20.
10. Patil AJ, Vajaranant TS, Edward DP. Bimatoprost—a review. Expert Opin Pharmacother. 2009;10:2759–68.

Minoxidil (Topical)

11. FDA drug monograph Minoxidil. Available from https://www.accessdata.fda.gov/drugsatfda_docs/anda/2001/75-839_Minoxidil.pdf. Accessed 05/01/2022.
12. LexiComp drug monograph Minoxidil. Available from: LexiComp Online at online.Lexi.com. Copyright 2021 UptoDate, Inc.
13. Naranjo-Vázquez E, Sánchez-Parada MG, Gómez-Meda BC, Zamora-Perez AL, Gallegos-Arreola MP, González-Santiago AE, Zúñiga-González GM. Effect of high-dose topical minoxidil on erythrocyte quality in SKH1 hairless mice. Animals. 2020;10:731.
14. Suchonwanit P, Thammarucha S, Leerunyakul K. Minoxidil and its use in hair disorders: a review. Drug Des Dev Ther. 2019;13:2777–86.
15. Randolph M, Tosti A. Oral Minoxidil treatment for hair loss: a review of efficacy and safety. J Am Acad Dermatol. 2021;84:737–46.
16. Stoehr JR, Choi JN, Colavincenzo M, Vanderweil S. Off-label use of Topical Minoxidil in alopecia: a review. Am J Clin Dermatol. 2019;20:237–50.
17. Rossi A, Cantisani C, Melis L, Iorio A, Scali E, Calvieri S. Minoxidil use in dermatology, side effects and recent patents. Recent Patents Inflamm Allergy Drug Discov. 2012;6:130–6.
18. Gupta AK, Talukder M, Venkataraman M, Bamimore MA. Minoxidil: a comprehensive review. J Dermatol Treat. 2021:1–11.
19. Olsen EA, Dunlap FE, Funicella T, Koperski JA, Swinehart JM, Tschen EH, Trancik RJ. A randomized clinical trial of 5% topical minoxidil versus 2% topical minoxidil and placebo in the treatment of androgenetic alopecia in men. J Am Acad Dermatol. 2002;47:377–85.
20. Lucky AW, Piacquadio DJ, Ditre CM, Dunlap F, Kantor I, Pandya AG, Savin RC, Tharp MD. A randomized, placebo-controlled trial of 5% and 2% topical minoxidil solutions in the treatment of female pattern hair loss. J Am Acad Dermatol. 2004;50:541–53.
21. Ramos PM, Sinclair RD, Kasprzak M, Miot HA. Minoxidil 1 mg oral versus minoxidil 5% topical solution for the treatment of female-pattern hair loss: a randomized clinical trial. J Am Acad Dermatol. 2020;82:252–3.

Eflornithine

22. FDA drug monograph Vaniqa™ (eflornithine hydrochloride) cream 13.9%. Available from https://www.accessdata.fda.gov/drugsatfda_docs/label/2000/21145lbl.pdf. Accessed 05/01/2022.
23. LexiComp drug monograph (name of monograph). Available from: LexiComp Online at online.Lexi.com. Copyright 2021 UptoDate, Inc.
24. Wolf JE, Shander D, Huber F, Jackson J, Lin C-S, Mathes BM, Schrode K. Randomized, double-blind clinical evaluation of the efficacy and safety of topical eflornithine hcl 13.9% cream in the treatment of women with facial hair. Int J Dermatol. 2006;46:94–8.
25. Jackson J, Caro JJ, Caro G, Garfield F, Huber F, Zhou W, Lin C-S, Shander D, Schrode K. The effect of eflornithine 13.9% cream on the bother and discomfort due to hirsutism. Int J Dermatol. 2007;46:976–81.
26. Hamzavi I, Tan E, Shapiro J, Lui H. A randomized bilateral vehicle-controlled study of eflornithine cream combined with laser treatment versus laser treatment alone for facial hirsutism in women. J Am Acad Dermatol. 2007;7:54–9.
27. Vissing AC, Taudorf EH, Haak CS, Philipsen PA, Haedersdal M. Adjuvant eflornithine to maintain IPL-induced hair reduction in women with facial hirsutism: a randomized controlled trial. J Eur Acad Dermatol Venereol. 2015;30:314–9.
28. Barman Balfour JA, McClellan K. Topical eflornithine. Am J Clin Dermatol. 2001;2:197–201.
29. Ramot Y, Pietilä M, Giuliani G, Rinaldi F, Alhonen L, Paus R. Polyamines and hair: a couple in search of perfection. Exp Dermatol. 2010;19:784–90.

Miscellaneous Agents

27

Rebecca M. Law, Victoria Nguyen,
Linda B. Ou, Sheeva Shahinfar,
and Howard I. Maibach

Contents

R. M. Law (✉)
School of Pharmacy and Faculty of Medicine (Discipline of Family Medicine), Memorial University of Newfoundland, St. John's, NL, Canada
e-mail: rlaw@mun.ca; rlawUCSF@gmail.com

V. Nguyen
School of Pharmacy, University of Waterloo, Kitchener, ON, Canada
e-mail: vtpnguye@uwaterloo.ca

L. B. Ou
Sunnybrook Health Sciences Centre, Toronto, ON, Canada
e-mail: lindaou25@gmail.com

S. Shahinfar
Texas A&M University, College of Medicine, Bryan, TX, USA
e-mail: Sheeva.Shahinfar@tamu.edu

R. M. Law, H. I. Maibach (eds.), *Handbook of Topical Drug Treatment in Dermatology*,
https://doi.org/10.1007/978-3-031-93616-6_27

Becaplermin

Rebecca M. Law

Classification and Mode of Action

- Becaplermin is a recombinant B-isoform homodimer of human platelet-derived Growth Factor (rPDGF-BB). It helps in the formation of new granulation tissue, induces fibroblast proliferation and differentiation, thus promoting wound healing. It also promotes angiogenesis.

Indication & Dermatological Use

- Diabetic ulcers (lower extremity) in adults and adolescents 16 years of age and older. It is indicated as an adjunctive treatment of lower extremity diabetic neuropathic ulcers that extend into the subcutaneous tissue or beyond and there is an adequate blood supply.
- Efficacy has not been established for other other ulcers (ie. Pressure and venous stasis ulcers) and has not been evaluated in diabetic neuropathic ulcers that do not extend into subcutaneous tissue or in diabetic ischemic ulcers.

H. I. Maibach
Department of Dermatology, University of California San Francisco (UCSF), San Francisco, CA, USA
e-mail: howard.maibach@ucsf.edu

- Not for use in wounds that close by primary intention. Effects on exposed joints, tendons, ligaments and bone have not been established.
- No overall differences in efficacy or safety were seen between patients <60 vs >65 years of age.

Formulation/Presentation

- 0.01% gel

Dosages & Suggested Regimens

- Apply once daily as a coating over the ulcer. Squeeze appropriate amount of gel onto a clean measuring surface and spread onto the entire ulcer area in a thin, continuous layer about 1/16 inch thick. Cover with saline moistened dressing and leave dressing in place for about 12 hours. After 12 hrs, remove dressing and rinse with saline or water and cover with saline moistened dressing without becaplermin gel for the remainder of the day. Continue use once daily until the ulcer is healed.
- The amount to be applied will vary depending on the size of the ulcer area. To estimate the gel requirement: measure the greatest length of the ulcer by the greatest width of the ulcer; and recalculate the amount needed every 1-2 weeks, as the ulcer heals. If the ulcer does not reduce in size by about 30% after 10 weeks of treatment, or if complete healing has not occurred by 20 weeks, continued treatment with becaplermin gel should be reassessed.

Pharmacokinetics

- Low systemic absorption

Use in Special Populations

- No dosage adjustment provided for altered kidney function or altered hepatic function in the manufacturer's labelling. Dosement adjustment is unlikely due to low systemic absorption.
- No overall differences in safety or effectiveness were observed between patients <65 and >65 years of age.
- Safety in pregnancy has not been established.
- Unknown whether becaplermin is present in breast milk.

Monitoring

- Monitor for adverse effects as described below under Warnings/Precautions and Adverse Reactions.
- Monitor for effectiveness: ulcer volume, wound area, evidence of closure, drainage.

Warnings/Precautions

- Monitor for application site reactions: Sensitization or irritation of skin may occur. This may be due to preservatives parabens or m-cresol. If seen, interruption or discontinuation of treatment should be considered, and further evaluation (e.g. via patch testing) may be necessary.
- Malignancies of varying types have been reported. These were all remote from the becaplermin treatment site. Use with caution in patients with known malignancy. Becaplermin should only be used with benefits can be expected to outweigh the risks.

Adverse Reactions

- Erythematous rash
- Application site burning, application-site erythema

Drug Interactions

- None known

Carcinogenicity

- See under Warnings/Precautions for discussion.
- Use with caution in patients with known malignancy.

Patch Test Concentration

- Not available

Hydrogen Peroxide

Rebecca M. Law

Classification and Mode of Action

- Hydrogen peroxide is an oxidizing agent with antiseptic properties. It is an antiseptic oxidant that slowly releases oxygen and water upon contact with tissue catalase or serum (i.e., catalase decomposes hydrogen peroxide to protect cells and tissues.) The mechanism of action for the treatment of seborrheic keratosis is unknown.

Indications and Dermatological Uses

- *Clinical indications (FDA)*: Antiseptic for minor dermal abrasions; oral rinse for mouth, gum or dental irritation; topical solution for removal of oral secretions; a potent topical solution (40%) for treatment of raised seborrheic keratoses

Formulations/Presentation

- USA: Topical solution (3%), topical solution (40%), topical spray (3%), oral rinse (1.5%), oral gel (1.7%).

Dosages and Suggested Regimens

- As antiseptic: Clean the affected area and apply the 3% solution/spray. May cover the area with a sterile bandage after the solution has dried. Solutions >3% are irritants and must be diluted prior to application.
- As treatment of raised seborrheic keratoses: Use the 40% solution—not for oral, ophthalmic, or intravaginal use. Apply to lesion four times during a single in-office treatment session. If the treated lesions have not completely cleared after 3 weeks, may repeat. However, do not start a second treatment course until the skin has recovered from any reaction caused by the previous treatment.
- As oral rinse: Use 1.5% solution to swish over the affected for one or more minutes and then spit out. Do not swallow.
- As oral gel: Use 1.7% spray on affected area, leave on for at least 1 min, and then spit out. Do not swallow.

Pharmacokinetics

- Duration of action: only while bubbling action occurs
- Absorption: none

Use in Special Populations

- Some dosage forms may include propylene glycol. In neonates, large amounts of propylene glycol (IV, orally, or topically) have been associated with fatal toxicities including seizures, metabolic acidosis, renal failure, and CNS depression. Toxicities

have also been reported in children and adults including hyperosmolality, lactic acidosis, seizures, and respiratory depression.
- Renal insufficiency: No dose adjustments on manufacturer's labelling.
- Hepatic impairment: No dose adjustments on manufacturer's labelling.

Monitoring

- For adverse effects as discussed below. Repeated/frequent uses may increase the risk of irritation and other adverse effects.

Contraindications and Cautions

- Not to be used in the eyes or over large areas of the body.
- Not to be used for longer than a week.
- Bandages should not be applied too quickly after using hydrogen peroxide.
- Ten percent and 30% solutions must be diluted prior to use.
- Topical solution 40%: Do not apply to eyes or mucous membranes. Avoid treating seborrheic keratoses within the orbital rim.

Important Drug Interactions

- Avoid using with taurolidine: Concomitant use of taurolidine and hydrogen peroxide may increase the risk of metabolic acidosis. Risk X: Avoid combination.

Adverse Effects and Their Management

- Irritation may occur at the site of application (for all uses of hydrogen peroxide).
- Other adverse effect for use in seborrheic keratoses: Stinging, red and blistered or swollen skin, crusting, scaling, and change in skin color may occur.

- Avoid the eyes. Direct contact with the eye can cause corneal injury (erosion, scarring, ulceration, perforation), chemical conjunctivitis, eyelid edema, and severe eye pain. And there may be permanent eye injury including blindness. For accidental exposure, immediately flush with water for 15–30 min, and further evaluate as appropriate.
- Repeat use as a mouthwash or gargle may cause irritation of the buccal mucous membrane or "hairy tongue."

Carcinogenicity

- Unknown

Patch Test Concentration

- Not available

Essential Patient Information

- Hydrogen peroxide may cause skin irritation, redness, itching, stinging, blistering or swelling, and change in skin color. Avoid using in or near the eye. If drug accidentally gets in the eye, immediately flush with water for 15–30 min, and contact a health care professional.
- Do not use the 10% or 30% solution undiluted.
- If using as a mouth rinse or gargle, must spit out. Do not swallow.
- Repeated/frequent uses of hydrogen peroxide may cause increased irritation.

Sodium Hypochlorite and Hypochlorous Acid

Rebecca M. Law

Classification and Mode of Action

- Topical antiseptic with activity against bacterial, viral, and fungal microorganisms.

Indications and Dermatological Uses

- *Clinical indications (FDA)*: Antiseptic for prevention and treatment of skin and tissue infections and treatment of cuts, abrasions, and skin ulcers (e.g., stage I to IV pressure ulcers, diabetic foot and leg ulcers, postsurgical wounds).

Formulations/Presentation

- USA
  - Gel: Anasept antimicrobial 0.057% (latex free); H-Chlor Wound 0.062%
  - Liquid: Anasept 0.057% (two formulations with one being latex free)
  - Solution: Avenova 0.01% (as hypochlorous acid). Various formulations available from 0.012% to 0.5% from various manufacturers including generic products
  - Spray solution: Avenova 0.01%

Dosages and Suggested Regimens

- Gel can be applied as a thin layer for ostomy or skin care and as a thick layer (1/4–½ inch) to entire wound bed for wound care, with a thin layer to periwound skin areas.
- Liquid/solution/spray can be poured on or sprayed onto entire wound bed, including margins (avoid pooling), or saturate sterile gauze, and apply to wound site. Cover with sterile gauze/wound dressing, and ensure that the wound bed remains moist between dressing changes.

Pharmacokinetics

- Not available

Use in Special Populations

- Renal insufficiency: no dose adjustments on manufacturer's labelling.
- Hepatic impairment: no dose adjustments on manufacturer's labelling.
- Use in older adults, children and pregnancy are similar to use in adults.

Monitoring

- For signs of redness, swelling, or irritation

Contraindications and Cautions

- Contraindication: Hypersensitivity to sodium hypochlorite, chlorine compounds, or any component of the formulations

Important Drug Interactions

- Avoid using with taurolidine: Concomitant use of taurolidine and hydrogen peroxide may increase the risk of metabolic acidosis. Risk X: Avoid combination.

Adverse Effects and Their management

- No adverse reactions listed in the manufacturer's labeling.
- Irritation, swelling, and redness would be signs of a hypersensitivity reaction.

Carcinogenicity

- Unknown

Patch Test Concentration

- Not available

Essential Patient Information

- When used for self-medication (OTC use): Patients should be instructed to discontinue use and consult a health care professional if irritation, swelling, redness, or pain persists or increases.
- The products may bleach clothing.

Imiquimod

Victoria Nguyen, Linda Ou, and Rebecca M. Law

Classification and Mode of Action

- Imiquimod is an immune response modulator from the imidazoquinolinamines drug class.
- It is a Toll-like receptor 7 (TLR-7) agonist that stimulates the innate immune system. Consequently, this leads to the production of cytokines, like IFN-α, IL-6, and TNF-α, which modulate immune responses.
- Topically applied imiquimod has been found to activate Langerhans cells, which then migrate to local lymph nodes to stimulate the adaptive immune system.
- A randomized, double-blind, Phase III trial found that 3.5% imiquimod cream was superior to placebo in the clearance of genital warts at 24.9% and 9%, respectively.

Indications and Dermatological Uses

- *Clinical indications (FDA)*—actinic keratosis, superficial basal cell carcinoma, external genital, and perianal warts
- *Off-label common uses*—cutaneous flat wart, acyclovir resistant genital herpes simplex virus infection, nongenital warts, epidermodysplasia verruciformis, keratoacanthoma, keratoacanthoma, oral leukoplakia, verrucous carcinoma, mycosis fungoides, pyogenic granuloma, and keloid, follicular mucinosis
  - Level of evidence for cutaneous flat wart: C
  - Level of evidence for acyclovir resistant genital herpes simplex virus infection: C, G

Formulations/Presentation

- USA: Zyclara® cream (2.5%, 3.75%)
- Canada: Cream (2.5%, 3.75%, 5%)
- Europe: Cream (3.75%, 5%)

Dosages and Suggested Regimens

- Actinic keratosis
  - 2.5% and 3.5% cream: Apply a thin film to affected areas once daily for 2 weeks. Leave on for 8 h and then remove with mild soap and water.
  - 5% cream: Apply to affected areas two times per week for 16 weeks. Leave on for 8 h and then remove with mild soap and water.
- Superficial basal cell carcinoma
  - 5% cream: Apply to tumor and 1 cm of skin surrounding tumor once daily 5 times per week for 6 weeks. Leave on for 8 h and then remove with mild soap and water. Tumor treatment area, including 1 cm of surrounding skin, should not be greater than 3 cm.
- External genital and perianal warts
  - 3.75% cream: Apply a thin film once daily. Leave on for 8 h and then remove with mild soap and water. Continue treatment until clearance of warts or for a maximum of 8 weeks.
  - 5% cream: Apply a thin film three times per week. Leave on for 6–10 h and then remove with mild soap and water. Continue treatment until clearance of warts or for a maximum of 16 weeks.
- Cutaneous flat warts (off-label use)
  - 5% cream: Apply once daily until clearance of warts or for a maximum of 12 weeks.
- Acyclovir resistant genital herpes simplex virus (off-label)
  - 5% cream: Apply to affected areas three times per week. Leave on skin for 8 h. Continue treatment until resolution.

Pharmacokinetics

- Minimal systemic absorption across affected skin. Systemic absorption is more dependent on the body surface area of application than dose. Peak plasma concentrations range from 0.1 to 3.5 ng/mL. Half-life is approximately 30 h. Peak effect occurs at 9–12 h. Excreted in urine.

Use in Special Populations

- Pregnancy: Listed as pregnancy category C. Appears to be low risk when used topically for anogenital warts but manufacturer's caution against use during pregnancy unless potential benefits outweigh risks.
- Lactation: Unknown whether imiquimod is secreted into breast milk, but the manufacturer recommends use with caution in breastfeeding patients.
- Children: Safety and efficacy not established in patients less than 18 years of age.
  - Actinic keratosis and superficial basal cell carcinoma: These conditions are not often seen in children. Safety and efficacy not established in children less than 18 years of age.
  - External genital/perianal warts: Safety and efficacy not established in patents less than 12 years of age.
- Renal insufficiency: No dose adjustments on manufacturer's labelling.
- Hepatic impairment: No dose adjustments on manufacturer's labelling.

Monitoring

- Intense local inflammatory reactions may occur. Dosing interruption may be warranted.
- Severe local inflammatory reaction can lead to vulvar swelling and, consequently, urinary retention. Dose should be interrupted or discontinued.

- Flu-like symptoms including malaise, fever, and myalgias may occur. Dosing interruption may be warranted.
- Increased serum glucose.
- Signs and symptoms of hypersensitivity.

Contraindications and Cautions

- Hypersensitivity to imiquimod or any ingredient in formulation

Important Drug Interactions

- No drug interactions on manufacturer's labelling.
- Not recommended for concomitant use with immunosuppressive drugs like tacrolimus, cyclosporine, or methotrexate.
- Concomitant use with corticosteroids may limit efficacy.

Adverse Effects and Their Management

- Local skin reaction (50–96%) like crusting, edema, flaking, itching, scaling, and ulceration. Acute cases can be managed by temporary dosing interruption and the use of cold compresses. Imiquimod increases the risk of sun-induced skin damage. Minimizing exposure to UV light and use of sunscreens is advised.
- Gastrointestinal symptoms like nausea, diarrhea, vomiting, and dyspepsia may occur
- May increase incidence of infections like herpes simplex, lymphadenopathy, urinary tract infection, upper respiratory tract infections, and fungal infections.
- May cause respiratory symptoms like cough, pharyngitis, and rhinitis.

Carcinogenicity

- Not teratogenic in animal studies

Patch Test Concentration

- Not available

Essential Patient Information

- Medication should not be administered orally, intravaginally, or intra-anally.
- Avoid getting medication in the eyes, lips, and nostrils. If contact occurs, immediately rinse with water.
- Apply cream at bedtime and leave on skin for 8 h. Do not bathe or get treated area wet until the next morning.
- Avoid using occlusive dressings. If desired, cotton gauze dressings can be used.
- Imiquimod increases risk of sunburns. Use sun protection including sunscreen and sunglasses.
- Imiquimod may decrease efficacy of condoms and diaphragms. Use other forms of contraception while on therapy.
- Seek immediate medical attention if you experience signs of an allergic reaction like rash, hives, peeling skin with or without fever, and difficulty breathing.

Podofilox (Podophyllotoxin)

Rebecca M. Law and Howard I. Maibach

Classification and Mode of Action

- Podofilox (podophyllotoxin) is a keratolytic agent. It binds to a protein subunit of spindle microtubules (tubulin) to arrest mitosis in the epithelial cell, thus causing wart necrosis.
- Podofilox is *not* podophyllum resin—also a keratolytic agent with a similar mechanism of action. Although both are available commercially in the USA, podophyllum resin is not recommended in the CDC sexually transmitted diseases guidelines due to reports of significant systemic toxicity when applied incorrectly. (Podophyllin resin, if used, must be administered by a physician—see podophyllin as a separate drug monograph below.)

Indications and Dermatological Uses

- *Clinical indications (FDA)*: External genital warts (solution or gel); perianal warts (gel only)
- *Off-label common uses*: Molluscum contagiosum

Formulations/Presentation

- USA: 0.5% solution or gel
- Canada: 0.5% solution

Dosages and Suggested Regimens

- Apply to warts using either the supplied applicator or with finger (gel only) while minimizing contact with surrounding normal tissue. Do not apply to mucous membrane warts.

Pharmacokinetics

- In systemic absorption studies in 52 patients
  - topical application of 0.05 mL of 0.5% podofilox solution to external genitalia did not result in detectable serum levels.
  - Applications of 0.1–1.5 mL resulted in peak serum levels of 1–17 ng/mL 1–2 h after application.
  - The elimination half-life ranged from 1.0 to 4.5 h.
  - The drug was not found to accumulate after multiple treatments.

Use in Special Populations

- Should not be used during pregnancy.
- Unknown if podofilox is present in breast milk.
- Renal insufficiency: no dose adjustments on manufacturer's labelling.
- Hepatic impairment: no dose adjustments on manufacturer's labelling.
- Use in older adults is similar to use in adults.

Monitoring

- Efficacy and adverse effects: Monitor treated areas for adequate healing and for tolerability of treatment.

Contraindications and cautions

- Not for use in pregnancy or breastfeeding.
- Do not use concurrently with other podophyllin-containing products.
- Do not use if open wounds or inflamed or bleeding lesions exist.

- Do not use in children <12 years old.
- Severe skin reactions can occur, most frequently within the first 2 weeks of treatment.

Important Drug Interactions

- Any other podophyllin-containing product should not be used concurrently.

Adverse Effects and Their Management

- >10%: Localized burning and pain, skin erosion, local hemorrhage, inflammation, and pruritus.
- Others: dermal ulcer, desquamation, skin blister/tenderness, skin discoloration, and xeroderma.
- Although most skin reactions are mild to moderate, severe skin reactions can occur—most frequently within the first 2 weeks of treatment.

Carcinogenicity

- Published animal studies, in general, have not shown the drug substance, podofilox, to be carcinogenic.
- There are published reports that, in mouse studies, crude podophyllin resin (containing podofilox) applied topically to the cervix produced changes resembling carcinoma in situ [15]. These changes were reversible at 5 weeks after cessation of treatment. In one reported experiment, epidermal carcinoma of the vagina and cervix was found in 1 out of 18 mice after 120 applications of podophyllin [16] (the drug was applied twice weekly over a 15-month period).

Patch Test Concentration

- Not available

Essential Patient Information

- Avoid contact with eyes. If drug accidentally gets in eyes, flush eyes with water and get medical help.
- The gel and solution are flammable. Keep away from fire or flame.
- Wash hands before and after application.
- Do not apply to mucous membrane warts.
- Storage: Avoid excessive heat. Do not freeze.

Podophyllum Resin

Rebecca M. Law and Howard I. Maibach

Classification and Mode of Action

- Podophyllum is a keratolytic agent. It directly affects epithelial cell metabolism by binding to tubulin (a protein subunit of spindle microtubules). It arrests mitosis in metaphase (i.e., cytotoxic). This is *not* podofilox.
- Podophyllum resin is not recommended in the CDC sexually transmitted diseases guidelines due to reports of significant systemic toxicity when applied incorrectly.

Indications and Dermatological Uses

- *Clinical indications (FDA)*: For removal of genital warts. However, it is no longer recommended in the CDC sexually transmitted diseases guidelines due to significant systemic toxicity reported. It is to be used by physician only; it is *not* to be dispensed to the patient.

Formulations/Presentation

- USA: Podophyllin 25% solution (Podocon-25 external). The podophyllin resin used in this product is exclusively the American podophyllin (rather than the Indian resin). American podophyllin typically has a reduced level of podophyllotoxin (see drug monograph above).
- Canada: Podofilm.

Dosages and Suggested Regimens

- Use a toothpick or a cotton-tipped or glass applicator to apply the podophyllin solution. Apply 1 drop at a time, allowing time for drying between drops, until the affected area is covered. Allow solution to remain on wart as directed, and then remove by washing with soap and water.
- Do not touch adjacent normal skin.
- Avoid contact with eyes and other mucous membranes, e.g., the inside of the nose, mouth, or vagina.
- If contact with eyes occur, immediately flush the eyes with water for 15 min.
- If contact with normal skin occurs, thoroughly wash the skin with soap and water.

Pharmacokinetics

- Oral absorption: Podophyllum is very well and rapidly absorbed after accidental ingestion. *Avoid* route.
- Dermal absorption: Systemic poisoning was reported after topical application in some cases. Symptoms were delayed between 2 and 24 h.

Use in Special Populations

- Use in breastfeeding is contraindicated by the manufacturer. Unknown whether it is present in breast milk.
- Contraindicated in pregnancy. Fetal abnormalities, fetal death, and stillbirth have been reported following the use of podophyllin resin in pregnant patients.

Monitoring

- Efficacy and adverse effects: Monitor treated areas for adequate healing and for tolerability of treatment.

Contraindications and Cautions

- Not for use on bleeding warts, birthmarks, moles, or warts with hair growth
- Not for use in patients with diabetes or poor circulation
- Not to be used in patients on concurrent steroids
- Contraindicated in pregnancy or if breastfeeding

Important Drug Interactions

- Any other podophyllin-containing product should not be used concurrently.

Adverse Effects and Their Management

- May cause severe skin irritation.
- The use of topical podophyllin has been known to result in paresthesia, polyneuritis, paralytic ileus, pyrexia, leukopenia, thrombocytopenia, coma, and death.

Carcinogenicity

- There are published reports that, in mouse studies, crude podophyllin resin (containing podofilox) applied topically to the cervix produced changes resembling carcinoma in situ [21]. These changes were reversible at five weeks after cessation of treatment. In one reported experiment, epidermal carcinoma of the vagina and cervix was found in 1 out of 18 mice after 120 applications of podophyllin [22] (the drug was applied twice weekly over a 15-month period).

Patch Test Concentration

- Not available

Essential Patient Information

- This product is to be used *only* by a physician.
- Podophyllum is a poison. It is harmful if swallowed.
- Avoid contact with eyes and other mucous membranes, e.g., the inside of the nose, mouth, or vagina.
- May cause severe irritation.
- If contact with eyes occur, immediately flush the eyes with water for 15 min.
- If contact with normal skin occurs, thoroughly wash the skin with soap and water.

Propylene Glycol

Sheeva Shahinfar, Rebecca M. Law, and Howard I. Maibach

Classification and Mode of Action

- Propylene glycol is a product that has humectant properties. Its mechanism of action is simple in that, when applied topically, it attracts and retains water in the skin layers to increase the moisture and improve hydration in the skin. It can also be used as a vehicle or solvent, in combination with lipophilic drugs that are not stable in water.

Indications and Dermatological Uses

- *Clinical indications (FDA)*: dry skin
- *Off-label common uses*

Formulations/Presentation

- USA: Not sold individually for dermatologic use. Combined with pharmaceutical and cosmetic products for increased moisture
- Canada: Not sold individually for dermatologic use. Combined with pharmaceutical and cosmetic products for increased moisture
- Europe: Not sold individually for dermatologic use. Combined with pharmaceutical and cosmetic products for increased moisture

Dosages and Suggested Regimens

- N/A—not applied individually as dermatological therapy. Follow dosage and regimen guidelines for labeled drugs that propylene glycol is combined with.

Pharmacokinetics

- Absorption of propylene glycol may be quick, although much research has not been performed on it.
- Of note, a case was reported of an infant with burns who was instructed to apply cream with propylene glycol as one of the ingredients. The patient skipped 2 days of application. Subsequent use resulted in cardiopulmonary arrest within 1 h of re-exposure to the cream [33].
- Half-life was described as 16.9 h in an infant [33].
- Propylene glycol is metabolized into pyruvic acid, lactic acid, acetic acid, and propionaldehyde via liver oxidation.
- Elimination of the drug depends on the dosage used. Most undergoes urinary excretion as the glucuronide conjugate, but up to 45% of the drug may be excreted unchanged.

Use in Special Populations

- No studies have been done on the use of topical propylene glycol in pregnancy
- No studies have been done on the use of topical propylene glycol in lactation
- No recommendations have been given on the use of topical propylene glycol in children.
- No dose adjustments for renal insufficiency noted in research, although adverse effect of renal impairment noted in animal studies.
- No dose adjustments for hepatic insufficiency noted in research, although adverse effect of hepatic impairment noted in animal studies

Monitoring

- Product should not be ingested. Ingestion may result in drowsiness, stupor, unconsciousness, or coma. Serum hyperosmolality, hypoglycemia, and lactic acidosis may also be noted.
- Skin absorption into systemic system is minimal.
- Monitor for local irritations or hypersensitivity.
- System effects unlikely, although may be increased with repeated use.
- Monitor for eye irritation if product comes into contact with eye.

Contraindications and Cautions

- Do not use on open wounds, irritated skin, or burns.

Important Drug Interactions

- No data available

Adverse Effects and Their Management

- Skin irritation and hypersensitivity reactions may occur. Discontinue drug and treat irritation in the event of an allergic reaction.
- Application into the ear may result in cochlear toxicity in patients with tympanic membrane damage.
- System adverse effects are highly unlikely due to the low systemic absorption of the drug. Immediately discontinue drug if patient experiences shortness of breath, chest pain, fever, allergic reaction, or anaphylaxis after product use.
- If dosage is high resulting in high systemic concentration, the primary adverse effect is CNS depression, particularly in children.

- Other adverse effects include hyperosmolarity, hepatic impairment, renal impairment, arrhythmias, cardiorespiratory arrest, seizures, and intravascular hemolysis, and lactic acidosis.
- Toxicity should be managed symptomatically. If patients do not respond to supportive management, alcohol or fomepizole may be used to inhibit the metabolism of propylene glycol. Hemodialysis may also be considered as an alternative treatment.
- Chronic use of propylene glycol may have increased skin irritation if impermeable pads are used to cover the application site.

Carcinogenicity

- No data available

Patch Test Concentration

- Not available

Essential Patient Information

- Discontinue use and contact your health provider if skin irritation occurs.
- Do not apply to open wounds, irritated skin, or burns. Do not apply to eye or inner ear.
- Immediately discontinue medication and seek medical attention if you experience shortness of breath, chest pain, fever, allergic reaction, or anaphylaxis after product use.
- It is recommended to not cover the application site with an impermeable pad, as this may increase the chance of skin irritation.

Urea

Victoria Nguyen, Linda Ou, and Rebecca M. Law

Classification and Mode of Action

- Urea is a hygroscopic substance naturally occurring in the epidermis. It improves skin barrier function and maintains hydration.
- Urea-containing formulations are commonly used in dermatology as moisturizers and keratolytic agents.
- Urea induces the expression of genes involved in keratinocyte differentiation, like filaggrin, loricrin, and transglutaminase 1, which are important for skin barrier function. Also, urea exhibits its keratolytic action on hyperkeratotic areas by dissolving the intercellular matrix of cells in the stratum corneum.
- Urea has been shown to increase skin and nail penetration which can improve the therapeutic action of topical drugs.
- While urea has historically been used to improve skin hydration and treat hyperkeratotic conditions, the FDA has not given approval for this indication. Generally, at low concentrations, urea is used as moisturizers and keratolytics. At higher concentrations ($\geq$30%), urea is used for conditions like psoriasis, xerosis, eczema, and for the debridement of necrotic tissue.

Indications and Dermatological Uses

- *Clinical indications (FDA)*—no labelling has been approved by the FDA.
- *Off-label common uses*—hyperkeratotic conditions.

Formulations/Presentation

- USA: Cream (10–40%), foam (30–35%), gel (45%), lotion (10–40%), ointment (10–20%), solution (25%), suspension (40–50%)
- Canada: Cream (10–40%)
- Europe: Cream (10–40%)

Dosages and Suggested Regimens

- Hyperkeratotic conditions (off-label): Apply topically to affected area one to three times daily.

Pharmacokinetics

- No published studies on pharmacokinetics

Use in Special Populations

- Pregnancy: Studies have not been conducted with all products. Animal studies have not demonstrated adverse effects on the fetus.
- Lactation: Unknown whether urea is secreted into breast milk. Caution is warranted when used by nursing women.
- Children: Not assessed; use not recommended in children under 2 years of age
- Renal insufficiency: Not assessed; dosage adjustments likely unnecessary.
- Hepatic insufficiency: Not assessed; dosage adjustments likely unnecessary.

Monitoring

- Intense application site reactions may occur. Dosing interruption may be warranted.
- Signs and symptoms of hypersensitivity like rash, urticaria, dyspnea, and angioedema

Contraindications and Cautions

- Known hypersensitivity to urea or any ingredients of formulation.
- Contraindicated to use on open wounds and irritated and infected skin.

Important Drug Interactions

- No documented significant interactions

Adverse effects and Their Management

- Local skin reactions including transient itching, burning, and/or stinging sensation. Symptoms generally resolve upon discontinuing therapy.
- Some formulations contain tartrazine (FD&C yellow #5 or E102), an aniline dye. Allergic reactions to tartrazine-containing products include anaphylactic reactions, like urticaria and angioedema, and asthmatic reactions. Patients with a known hypersensitivity should avoid the product. There is no conclusive evidence about whether tartrazine can cause asthma exacerbations. Patients with aspirin-sensitive or insensitive asthmatics are not contraindicated to tartrazine-containing drugs unless they have had a proven sensitivity.
- Some formulations contain ammonium lactate or lactic acid which can increase sensitivity to UV light and increase the risk of sunburns. The use of sunscreen and protective clothing while outdoors is advised.

Carcinogenicity

- No published studies on carcinogenicity

Patch Test Concentration

- Not Available

Essential Patient Information

- For topical use only.
- Avoid contact with the mouth, nose, and eyes. Contact may cause burning sensation.
- Do not apply to open wounds, irritated, or infected skin.
- Seek immediate medical attention if you experience signs of an allergic reaction like rash, hives, peeling skin with or without fever, and difficulty breathing.
- If using foam or lotion, shake well before use.
- Some products may stain clothing.

References

Becaplermin

1. Lexidrug/LexiComp drug monograph (Becaplermin). Available from: LexiComp Online at online.Lexi.com. Copyright 2025 UptoDate, Inc.

Hydrogen Peroxide

2. FDA drug monograph (name of monograph). Available from (FDA weblink). Accessed (date).
3. Lexidrug/LexiComp drug monograph (hydrogen peroxide). Available from: LexiComp Online at online.Lexi.com. Copyright 2024 UptoDate, Inc.

Sodium Hypochlorite and Hypochlorous Acid

4. FDA drug monograph (name of monograph). Available from (FDA weblink). Accessed (date).
5. LexiComp drug monograph (name of monograph). Available from: LexiComp Online at online.Lexi.com. Copyright 2024 UptoDate, Inc.

Imiquimod

6. FDA drug monograph Zyclara® (imiquimod) Cream, 3.75%. Available from https://www.accessdata.fda.gov/drugsatfda_docs/label/2011/201153s000,022483s001lbl.pdf. Accessed 30 Apr 2023.
7. LexiComp drug monograph (imiquimod). Available from: LexiComp Online at online.Lexi.com. Copyright 2023 UptoDate, Inc.
8. Hadley G, Derry S, Moore RA. Imiquimod for actinic keratosis: systematic review and meta-analysis. Journal of Investig Dermatol. 2006;126(6):1251–5.
9. Hanna E, Abadi R, Abbas O. Imiquimod in dermatology: an overview. Int J Dermatol. 2016;55(8):831–44.
10. Korman N, Moy R, Ling M, Matheson R, Smith S, McKane S, Lee JH. Dosing with 5% imiquimod cream 3 times per week for the treatment of actinic keratosis: results of two phase 3, randomized, double-blind, parallel-group, vehicle-controlled trials. Arch Dermatol. 2005;141(4):467–73.
11. National Library of Medicine (U.S). (2008–2011) Phase 3 Study of Imiquimod Creams in the Treatment of External Genital Warts. Identifier NCT00735462. https://clinicaltrials.gov/ct2/show/results/NCT00735462
12. Miller RL, Gerster JF, Owens ML, Slade HB, Tomai MA. Review article imiquimod applied topically: a novel immune response modifier and new class of drug. Int J Immunopharmacol. 1999;21(1):1–14.
13. Moore RA, Edwards JE, Hopwood J, Hicks D. Imiquimod for the treatment of genital warts: a quantitative systematic review. BMC Infect Dis. 2001;1(1):1–9.
14. Navi D, Huntley A. Imiquimod 5 percent cream and the treatment of cutaneous malignancy. Dermatol Online J. 2004;10(1)
15. Stockfleth E, Meyer T, Benninghoff B, Salasche S, Papadopoulos L, Ulrich C, Christophers E. A randomized, double-blind, vehicle-controlled study to assess 5% imiquimod cream for the treatment of multiple actinic keratoses. Arch Dermatol. 2002;138(11):1498–502.

Podofilox (Podophyllotoxin)

16. FDA drug monograph (podofilox topical solution 0.5%). Available from https://dailymed.nlm.nih.gov/dailymed/fda/fdaDrugXsl.cfm?setid=6af07697-5203-43e0-ba35-83683af851c3. Assessed 15 Nov 2024.
17. FDA drug guidance (podofilox topical gel 0.5%). Oct 2022. Available from https://www.accessdata.fda.gov/drugsatfda_docs/psg/PSG_020529.pdf. Accessed 15 Nov 2024.
18. LexiComp drug monograph (podofilox). Available from: LexiComp Online at online.Lexi.com. Copyright 2024 UptoDate, Inc.
19. Podofilox (Condylox) product monograph. Health Canada. Available at: https://pdf.hres.ca/dpd_pm/00062150.PDF. Accessed 13 Nov 2024.
20. Kaminetzky HA, McGrew EA, Phillips RL. Experimental cervical epithelial dysplasia. J Obst Gyn. 1959;14:1–10.
21. Kaminetzky HA, McGrew EA. Podophyllin and mouse cervix: effect of long term application. Arch Path. 1962;73:481–5.

Podophyllum Resin

22. Podocon-25 drug monograph (podophyllin). Available from Drugs.com at: https://www.drugs.com/pro/podocon-25.html. Accessed 17 Nov 2024.
23. FDA drug monograph (podofilox topical solution 0.5%). Available from https://dailymed.nlm.nih.gov/dailymed/fda/fdaDrugXsl.cfm?setid=6af07697-5203-43e0-ba35-83683af851c3. Assessed 15 Nov 2024.
24. LexiComp drug monograph (podophyllin resin). Available from: LexiComp Online at online.Lexi.com. Copyright 2024 UptoDate, Inc.
25. Podophyllum resin (topical route). Mayo Clinic Drugs & Supplements. Available at: https://www.mayoclinic.org/drugs-supplements/podophyllum-resin-topical-route/description/drg-20065566. Accessed 17 Nov 2024.
26. Podophyllum resin. PubChem. Available at: https://pubchem.ncbi.nlm.nih.gov/compound/Podophyllum-Resin#section=ATC-Code. Accessed 17 Nov 2024.
27. Kaminetzky HA, McGrew EA, Phillips RL. Experimental cervical epithelial dysplasia. J Obst Gyn. 1959;14:1–10.
28. Kaminetzky HA, McGrew EA. Podophyllin and mouse cervix: effect of long term application. Arch Path. 1962;73:481–5.

Propylene Glycol

29. FDA drug monograph CFR – Code of Federal Regulations Title 21. Sec. 184.1666 Propylene glycol. Available from https://www.accessdata.fda.gov/scripts/cdrh/cfdocs/cfcfr/cfrsearch.cfm?fr=184.1666. Accessed 20 Nov 2024.
30. Propylene glycol. In: Propylene glycol (PIM 443). https://inchem.org/documents/pims/chemical/pim443.htm#SectionTitle:7.6%20%20Interactions. Accessed 20 Nov 2024.
31. Adams RM, Maibach HI, Adams RM, et al. A five-year study of cosmetic reactions. J Am Acad Dermatol. 1985;13:1062–9.
32. Bekeris L, Baker C, Fenton J, Kimball D, Bermes E. Propylene glycol as a cause of an elevated serum osmolality. Am J Clin Pathol. 1979;72:633–6.
33. Bizjak M, Adamič K, Bajrovič N, Eržen R, Jošt M, Kopač P, Košnik M, Lalek N, Zidarn M, Dinevski D. Patch testing with the European Baseline Series and 10 added allergens: Single-centre study of 748 patients. Contact Dermat. 2022;87:439–46.
34. Fligner CL. Hyperosmolality induced by propylene glycol. JAMA. 1985;253:1606.
35. Goldsmith LA. Propylene glycol. Int J Dermatol. 1978;17:703–5.
36. Hannuksela M, Förström L. Reactions to peroral propylene glycol. Contact Dermat. 1978;4:41–5.
37. Kaur G, Woodruff CM, Botto N. Life after patch testing: allergic contact dermatitis caused by propylene glycol in Vivelle transdermal estradiol patch. JAAD Case Rep. 2021;9:34–5.
38. Kulik MI, Lewis NS, Bansal V, Warpeha R. Hyperosmolality in the burn patient. J Trauma Injury Infect Crit Care. 1980;20:223–8.
39. Lalla SC, Nguyen H, Chaudhry H, Killian JM, Drage LA, Davis MDP, Yiannias JA, Hall MR. Patch testing to propylene glycol: the Mayo Clinic experience. Dermatitis. 2018;29:200–5.
40. Martin G, Finberg L. Propylene glycol: a potentially toxic vehicle in liquid dosage form. J Pediatr. 1970;77:877–8.
41. Miller ON, Bazzano G. Propanediol metabolism and its relation to lactic acid metabolism*. Annals NY Acad Sci. 2006;119:957–73.
42. Ruddick JA. Toxicology, metabolism, and biochemistry of 1,2-propanediol. Toxicol Appl Pharm. 1972;21:102–11.
43. Soni H. Martindale: The Complete Drug Reference Brayfield alison (ED) martindale: The Complete Drug Reference £459 4,688pp pharmaceutical press 9780857111395 0857111396. Emerg Nurse. 2014; 22:12
44. Silverberg JI, Chaubal M, Warshaw EM, et al. Prevalence and trend of allergen sensitization in patients with cheilitis referred for patch testing, North American contact dermatitis group data, 2001–2018. Contact Dermat. 2022; https://doi.org/10.1111/cod.14265.

45. Trancik RJ, Maibach HI. Propylene glycol: irritation or sensitization? Contact Dermat. 1982;8:185–9.
46. Yu DK, Elmquist WF, Sawchuk RJ. Pharmacokinetics of propylene glycol in humans during multiple dosing regimens. J Pharm Sci. 1985;74:876–9.
47. Zhu YY, Liang J, Xiao W. Enhancing effects of chemical permeation enhancer propylene glycol and ultrasonic technology on transdermal permeation of Baimai Ointment. Zhongguo Zhong Yao Za Zhi. 2022;24:6607–14.

Urea

48. LexiComp drug monograph Urea (Topical). Available from: LexiComp Online at online.Lexi.com. Copyright 2024 UptoDate, Inc.
49. Bissonnette R, Maari C, Provost N, Bolduc C, Nigen S, Rougier A, Seite S. A double-blind study of tolerance and efficacy of a new urea-containing moisturizer in patients with atopic dermatitis. J Cosmet Dermatol. 2010;9(1):16–21.
50. Emtestam L, Kaaman T, Rensfeldt K. Treatment of distal subungual onychomycosis with a topical preparation of urea, propylene glycol and lactic acid: results of a 24-week, double-blind, placebo-controlled study. Mycoses. 2012;55(6):532–40.
51. Hagemann I, Proksch E. Topical treatment by urea reduces epidermal hyperproliferation and induces differentiation in psoriasis. Acta Dermato-Venereologica. 1996;76(5):353–6.
52. Lodén M. Urea-containing moisturizers influence barrier properties of normal skin. Arch Dermatol Res. 1996;288:103–7.
53. Pan M, Heinecke G, Bernardo S, Tsui C, Levitt J. Urea: a comprehensive review of the clinical literature. Dermatol Online J. 2013;19(11)
54. Piquero-Casals J, Morgado-Carrasco D, Granger C, Trullàs C, Jesús-Silva A, Krutmann J. Urea in dermatology: a review of its emollient, moisturizing, keratolytic, skin barrier enhancing and antimicrobial properties. Dermatol Ther. 2021;11(6):1905–15.

Index

R. M. Law, H. I. Maibach (eds.), *Handbook of Topical Drug Treatment in Dermatology*,
https://doi.org/10.1007/978-3-031-93616-6

Q

R

S

MIX
Papier aus verantwortungsvollen Quellen
Paper from responsible sources
FSC® C105338
FSC
www.fsc.org

If you have any concerns about our products,
you can contact us on
ProductSafety@springernature.com

In case Publisher is established outside the EU,
the EU authorized representative is:
Springer Nature Customer Service Center GmbH
Europaplatz 3, 69115 Heidelberg, Germany

Printed by Libri Plureos GmbH
in Hamburg, Germany

Pocket Dermatology

Sara Hylwa · Elisabeth Hurliman
Jing Liu · Erin Luxenberg
Christina Boull

Pocket Dermatology

A Practical, High-Yield Guide

Springer

Sara Hylwa
Dermatology
University of Minnesota/
Hennepin Health Care Systems
Minneapolis, MN
USA

Elisabeth Hurliman
Dermatology
University of Minnesota/
Hennepin Health Care Systems
Minneapolis, MN
USA

Jing Liu
Dermatology
University of Minnesota/
Hennepin Health Care Systems
Minneapolis, MN
USA

Erin Luxenberg
Dermatology
University of Minnesota/
Hennepin Health Care Systems
Minneapolis, MN
USA

Christina Boull
Dermatology, Division of
Pediatric Dermatology
University of Minnesota
Minneapolis, MN
USA

ISBN 978-3-030-83601-6 ISBN 978-3-030-83602-3 (eBook)
https://doi.org/10.1007/978-3-030-83602-3

This Springer imprint is published by the registered company Springer Nature Switzerland AG
The registered company address is: Gewerbestrasse 11, 6330 Cham, Switzerland

Preface

Purpose of this Book

We hope that this book will be like having an experienced dermatologist with you in clinic helping to guide you or offering advice and reminders.

Disclaimer

These are just recommendations to guide you. You should always double-check these approaches and use your own clinical judgment in an approach to a patient.

How this Book Should Be Used

- As a resource in clinic when seeing patients or when on call for reminders on work-ups, diagnostic pearls, and therapeutic algorithms

How this Book Should Not Be Used

- This book is not a substitute for a formal dermatology residency.
- This not a substitution for reading textbooks or journal articles.

Information in the Text

We created this text while finishing our residency and preparing for attending life to make an easy-to-read guide for ourselves to use in clinic to hit high points of things to remember or refreshers of important information. While we tried to be as thorough as possible and had many eyes read over these suggestions over the course of several years, there may be errors or other approaches that we may have missed or overlooked. Additionally, this book represents our approach to clinical practice; other approaches or information can be equally valid. We encourage you to email us at pocketdermatology@gmail.com with any errors noted or suggestions.

Helpful Dermatology Web Pages

For General Derm

AAD.org
Emedicine.com (good information for drugs, general derm things)
DermnetNZ: http://www.dermnetnz.org/
NCCN Guidelines for Oncology: http://www.nccn.org/professionals/physician_gls/f_guidelines.asp
Visual Dx

Patient Education Resources

Up-to-date patient ed sections
Mayoclinic.com – patient care and health info link
VisualDx patient education sections

For Medications

Litt's Drug Eruption online: http://www.drugeruptiondata.com/
Information on all drugs: http://dailymed.nlm.nih.gov (lists ALL drug ingredients including excipients)
Drug interaction checks: Medscape (emedicine.com) or Micromedex
Primary literature: Pubmed (pubmed.gov)

For Contact Derm

- American Contact Dermatitis CAMP Database (contactderm.org)
- For ingredients in medications: https://dailymed.nlm.nih.gov/dailymed/
- Vaccine excipients: https://www.cdc.gov/vaccines/pubs/pinkbook/downloads/appendices/B/excipient-table-2.pdf
- Skin Deep online cosmetic database maintained by the Environmental Working Group (https://www.ewg.org/skindeep/)
- Label Insight – online food product database contains ingredient and nutritional information for more than 22,000 items sold in American grocery stores. (https://www.labelinsight.com/)
- Household product database: https://hpd.nlm.nih.gov/ or Householdproducts.nlm.nih.gov
- Botanical Dermatology Database: http://www.botanical-dermatology-database.info/
- Voluntary Cosmetic Registration Program – can be queried (https://www.fda.gov/Cosmetics/RegistrationProgram/default.htm)
- For ingredients in make-up: https://www.makeupalley.com/also Walgreens web pages lists all ingredients easily
- https://whatsinsidescjohnson.com/us/en/brands
- Nickel-free belts: Nicklefreebelts.com
- Which gloves protect from certain chemicals: www.ansellpro.com/specware/
- p-tert free shoes: http://shoeallergies.50webs.com/ptbp.htm#Do
- Dermnetnz for clothing dermatitis and other good sources of information: https://www.dermnetnz.org/topics/textile-contact-dermatitis

For Derm Products

- Dermstore.com
- Regimenmd.com

For Reporting

- FDA medication reactions: https://www.accessdata.fda.gov/scripts/medwatch/

Boards

- AAD recommended tools for boards
- https://www.aad.org/members/residents-fellows-resource-center/boards-study-tools/more-boards-resources

Contents

Chapter 1
Biopsy Kits, Methods, and Guidelines

Punch Biopsy

- Alcohol swabs
- 30-gauge needles for injecting
- 25 or 26 gauge needles for drawing up medication
- 1–3cc syringes
- Goggles (*always* wear goggles when injecting)
- Lidocaine 1% with epinephrine 1:100,000 +/– bicarbonate 8.4% in a 10:1 ratio
- 4 mm (or other sized) punch
- Forceps, scissors, needle driver
- 4-0 Prolene, Nylon, or Vicryl Rapide (6-0 if on face)
  - Consider clear 5-0 Monocryl for face
- Surgifoam/gelfoam (in case you are unable to place a stitch)
- Vaseline
- Band-Aid
- 4 × 4 gauze pads
- Formalin container (with patient label, site, + your initials)
- Zeus/Michael Media for DIF – if not available, can place in sterile saline-soaked gauze and rush to lab (<6 h from collection for processing ideally)

S. Hylwa et al., *Pocket Dermatology*,
https://doi.org/10.1007/978-3-030-83602-3_1

Shave Biopsy

- Alcohol swabs
- 30-gauge needles for injecting
- 25- or 26-gauge needles for drawing up medication
- 1–3cc syringes
- Goggles (*always* wear when injecting!)
- Lidocaine 1% with epinephrine 1:100,000 +/– bicarbonate 8.4% in a 10:1 ratio
- Razor (Gillette) blade or Dermablade
- Aluminum chloride (Drysol) or ferric subsulfate solution (Monsel's solution)
  - Monsel's solution is good if the lesion is in an area prone to bleeding. Note that it can permanently stain the skin a brown color
- Cotton applicators
- Vaseline
- Band-Aids
- 4 × 4 gauze pads
- Formalin container (with patient label, site, + your initials)
- Optional: heat cautery – *do not use if pt on oxygen*

Sterile Biopsy for Culture

- Good video for review: https://www.youtube.com/watch?v=vEoS1oMaHGw.
- Punch biopsy above with the following changes:
  - Sterile container (like for urine specimen) with sterile 2 × 2 gauze placed with sterile technique in the bottom of the cup which is then moistened with non-bacteriostatic saline on the bottom (NOT drenched).
- Note that some use normal clean gloves and procedures for sterile biopsies. Others use:

  - Sterile gloves (if possible)
  - Sterile drapes
  - Mask +/– gown
  - Chlorhexidine instead of alcohol swabs
  - Non-bacteriostatic lidocaine without epinephrine

- If you believe the sites is infected, do not close with suture; instead place gelfoam/surgifoam.
- Cover specimen(s) with the moistened gauze once placed in container and bring immediately to the microbiology laboratory.
- Send three more pieces (sterile) to microbiology for aerobic and anaerobic bacterial, fungal (at 25° and 37°), and mycobacterial cultures.
- Send one piece to pathology H&E processing with special stains (for fungi, mycobacteria, and conventional bacteria).

  - For the piece going in formalin to pathology, can do a touch preparation for Gram, acid-fast, and fungal stains if needed based on the clinical presentation
  - *If coccidioidomycosis is suspected, MUST MAKE LAB AWARE as the organism is extremely infectious in the mycelial form and may infect laboratory workers.*

Biopsy for Flow Cytometry

- Use RPMI media.
- Do a punch/deep shave of the concerning area and place specimen in RPMI.
- If busy in clinic, can do the biopsy and place the specimen in a sterile urine cup with moistened saline gauze until the RPMI media can be procured.

Non-biopsy diagnostic procedures: *Information on scraping a bullae* from Lindy Fox.

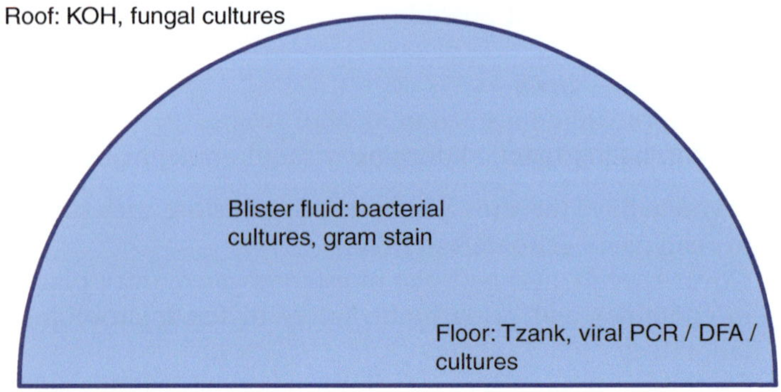

Adjunctive Tests

- Galactomannan – ELISA test which can help aid in the diagnosis of invasive aspergillosis. Can be tested in the blood, bronchoalveolar lavage fluid, or CSF.
  - Negative test rules out disease.
  - Positive test requires confirmation with a second Galactomannan test.
  - False positives occur with loss of integrity of the gut mucosa and piperacillin-tazobactam abx.
- Beta-D-glucan assay – nonspecific marker for invasive fungal infection; detects the glucan component of the cell wall of various fungi including *Aspergillus*, *Fusarium*, *Trichosporon*, and *Candida*.
- Complement fixing IgG antibodies to coccidioidomycosis – will become positive 2–3 weeks after infection.
- Cryptococcal antigen titer by latex agglutination – will always be positive in disseminated disease.
  - Will also be positive in disseminated trichosporonosis.
- Histoplasmosis antigen detection by radioimmunoassay in urine – positive in up to 90% of patients with disseminated histoplasmosis.
  - Can also perform a blood smear in patients with disseminated disease and find intracellular yeast forms, which can aid in diagnosis.

Biopsy Guidelines

Always confirm site and patient name on the sticker when performing biopsies.

Always take a picture of the lesion (for location identification purposes, see photodocumentation guideline section for common views to take per anatomic site) before taking any biopsy.

Always confirm the patient has no allergy to anesthesia/epinephrine before injecting.

General Guidelines

- If patient is pregnant, use lidocaine withOUT epinephrine.
- If patient is allergic to lidocaine or epinephrine, can subcutaneously inject sterile diphenhydramine or saline – must create good wheal for anesthesia.
- Make sure your label site and initial EXACTLY match those on your requisition form.
- 6 mm punch or greater will require subcutaneous stitches with 4-0 Vicryl with 4-0 Prolene over top

General Biopsy Recommendations

For Keratinocyte Carcinomas (NMSC) and Pigmented Lesions

- Shave biopsy preferred over punch biopsy.
- In general, try to biopsy the entire lesion if possible.
  - If cannot, it is okay to sample a section of a suspected NMSC.
  - For pigmented lesions, whole lesion should be removed with minimum depth of 1 mm.
  - For pigmented lesions, excisional biopsy preferred to partial biopsy.

- For large lentiginous lesions of the face, a broad shave of the darkest, most popular, or most atypical area is preferred. Information to the pathologist on the size of the lesion +/– picture is preferable.

For Rashes

- Punch biopsy is usually preferred, typically 4 mm biopsy, but on special locations (face), smaller diameters may be used for cosmetic purposes.
- Special considerations – see Table below for full details. Highlights are below.
  - Chronic lupus: biopsy the oldest lesion (if doing DIF, see below).
  - Blistering lesions: biopsy the edge of the blister.
  - For any ulcerated lesions, biopsy the edge with a tiny bit of the ulcer floor.
  - For hair loss, biopsy an active site, not a scarred site.
  - For vasculitic lesions, biopsy the newest lesion.
  - For other rashes, try to avoid any secondarily manipulated sites.

For Cultures

- Include areas with necrosis, eschar, or other skin breakdown as this is where the most pathogens are likely to be found.

Biopsy Guidelines for Direct Immunofluorescence

- Collect specimen in Michel's medium (also called Zeus medium).
- Alternative is to collect on sterile saline-soaked gauze, but specimen must get to the laboratory within 24 h (ideally <6 h).
- The saline split IIF technique can be performed on specimens transported in saline, Michel, or Zeus media.

Biopsy Guidelines Based on Disease/Diagnosis

See Table 1.1.

Tips for biopsy re: morphea, sclerodactyly, amyloidosis, vitiligo, extragenital LS&A: It may be helpful to biopsy most involved and noninvolved skin for dermatopathologist to compare.

Table 1.1 Biopsy guidelines

Disease	**Recommended biopsy technique**	**Comments**
Bullous disease	H&E – shave removal of intact bulls if possible or broad saucerization of periphery of bulla. Punch biopsy is an alternative at edge DIF – perilesional skin <1 cm from bulla	Avoid lower extremities when possible because of delayed healing, infection risk, and greater risk of false-negative results Nonbullous lesional or perilesional skin from the trunk is preferred for pemphigoid Brief immersion in formalin produces false-negative results in pemphigus but not in most other bullous diseases Saline is superior to liquid nitrogen, Michel medium, Zeus medium for DIF specimens delivered to the lab within 48 h (ideally within <6h) False-positive DIF for pemphigoid can be seen in bullous scabies

(continued)

TABLE 1.1 (continued)

Disease	Recommended biopsy technique	Comments
Epidermolysis bullosa	H&E & DIF: shave removal if possible or broad saucerization of periphery of bulla. Avoid palms/soles if possible If blister is induced, the biopsy should include the border of erythematous and nonerythematous skin so that the split is clearly shown	Blisters >12 h old should be avoided; a fresh blister can be induced in clinically uninvolved skin near a site where the patient usually blisters: You can induce a blister by rotating the skin with a moist Q-tip or gloved finger with firm downward pressure and then twisting 180° in each direction until erythema is produced. For patients with mild skin fragility, <2 min of friction is usually necessary Topical anesthetics should be avoided because they induce artificial blistering Be sure to send for DIF, which can be more helpful than H&E For electron microscopy, the specimen should be placed in 2% glutaraldehyde solution (glutaraldehyde buffered by 0.1 M sodium cacodylate, pH 7.4) and stored at 4 °C before overnight shipping at ambient temperature or with a cold pack if ambient temperatures are <37 °C

Table 1.1 (continued)

Disease	Recommended biopsy technique	Comments
Vasculitis	H&E – punch biopsy of well-established purpuric lesion (>72 h old) DIF – punch of acute lesion (<24 h old) Biopsy yield for temporal arteritis increases with Doppler localization and harvesting of a 2 cm segment - generally needs general surgery/opthalmology/ENT consultation	IgA vasculitis is more likely to retain positive DIF findings in established lesions The biopsy should be obtained from the center of the lesion. In patients with livedo racemosa, a biopsy should be obtained from the pale center of an erythematous ring (this is where the occluded vessels are most likely to be seen). When ulceration is present, take biopsy from the edge. If vasculitis involving large muscular vessel is suspected, a deep incisional biopsy with step sections may be appropriate

(continued)

Table 1.1 (continued)

Disease	Recommended biopsy technique	Comments
Panniculitis	Deep incisional biopsy or double punch technique with larger punch done first to gain access to fat and then (minimum 6 mm) punch performed inside of this within the fat to obtain a column of fat for analysis	Punch biopsy specimens tend to fracture, leaving inflamed or necrotic fat behind. An electric rotary power punch should be helpful
Sterile culture	Punch biopsy – at the edge of necrotic focus (if there is necrosis)	A 6-mm punch is the smallest size that should be performed if the specimen is divided for culture and H&E. The edge of a necrotic focus provides high yield for culture and special stains. Skin surface should be prepped with alcohol and allowed to evaporate. Deliver the culture specimen in a sterile urine cup with sterile gauze and sterile saline directly to the desk that handles microbiology
Lupus and dermatomyositis	H&E – punch biopsy of an established lesion (>6 months) that is still active. Minimum 4 mm size DIF – Punch of lesional skin; choose an established lesion (>6 months old) that is still active	On DIF, the lupus band is usually present in normal sun-protected skin in patients with active systemic lupus who are at high risk of renal disease For lupus panniculitis, a deep incisional biopsy may be required

Table 1.1 (continued)

Disease	Recommended biopsy technique	Comments
Morphea	Punch biopsy (minimum 4 mm), go deep into the dermis	Biopsy of the lilac border reveals the characteristic lymphoplasmacytic aggregates of the superficial and deep vascular plexus. More advanced lesions show the fibrosis and square biopsy sign
SJS/TEN vs SSSS	Shave of the epidermis or punch biopsy including the full thickness of the epidermis. Avoid areas that are already desquamated.	The desquamated sheets are an alternative to biopsy
Alopecia	Scarring or non-scarring: H&E – TWO 4 mm punches (one for vertical and one for horizontal sectioning) of an established lesion/active area (>6 months old if scarring)	For all forms of alopecia, avoid the active advancing border. Established lesions are preferred - although avoid frank scar. Place the punch at the same angle as the emerging hairs in order to avoid transecting hair follicles
BCC/SCC	Shave or punch biopsy to show the invasive pattern and detect perineural invasion if present	In convex sites or thin facial skin, more superficial shave biopsy specimens may be appropriate. The skin should be pulled taught to provide greater control of depth. Avoid creating contour defects in sebaceous skin

(continued)

TABLE 1.1 (continued)

Disease	Recommended biopsy technique	Comments
Suspected melanoma	Must get at least 1 mm of depth. Attempt for full removal either by shave or excisional biopsy (shave/saucerization preferred to limited disruption to lymphatics)	For a large lentigo maligna, preference is a broad thin shave. Pick areas that are most atypical under the dermatoscope or are palpable/ulcerated. Smaller scouting biopsies are possible but not preferred. If you do perform an incisional biopsy, aim for doing so along a naturally occurring skin crease for cosmesis Acral lesions should be bisected perpendicular to the dermatoglyphics. If you cannot trust your laboratory to do this, you should do it yourself
DFSP	Deep incisional biopsy	
CTCL	Broad shave biopsy below the depth of the DEJ	Biopsy specimens from different anatomic sites that show an identical clone are helpful to establish the diagnosis in indeterminate cases
Primary cutaneous B-cell lymphoma	Deep incisional biopsy whenever possible	In general, a punch biopsy specimen or shave does not allow assessment of architecture
Ulcerative disorders	Punch biopsy at the edge of the lesion	Avoid sampling frank necrosis

TABLE 1.1 (continued)

Disease	Recommended biopsy technique	Comments
Mastocytosis	Shave or punch biopsy	Inject lidocaine adjacent to the lesion and not through it and avoid epi in order to prevent mast cell degranulation. Ideal would be to biopsy a vesicle as mast cells collect below the vesicle

Adapted from: Elston et al. [1]; Stratman et al. [2]

Post-biopsy Instructions for Patients

Place these in patient chart when doing inpatient biopsies.

- Leave Band-Aid in place for 24 h. Then, can remove.
- Wash with soap and water, and then apply Vaseline and a new Band-Aid; repeat daily.
- Avoid use of Neosporin or other topical over-the-counter topical antibiotics unless there are developing signs of infection.
- Signs of infection include increasing rather than decreasing pain, pus, fever, redness >1 cm from the incision margin, and fluctuance.
- If any sign of infection, call the service immediately.
- Sutures on the head are removed in 1 week; from neck down in 2 weeks.
  - Give specific date in inpatient chart.
  - Ask to put these instructions into the patient discharge summary.

Photodocumentation of the Skin

Important for Biopsies and Pre-/Post-Procedures

Frankfurt plane = line from superior auditory canal to inferior infraorbital rim should be parallel to ground; line the patient up with this in mind for standardization of photos. See Fig. 1.1.

Tips for photographing specific areas:

- Scalp: take bird's eye view, nose in front, left superior helix, and right superior helix in picture; in addition measure

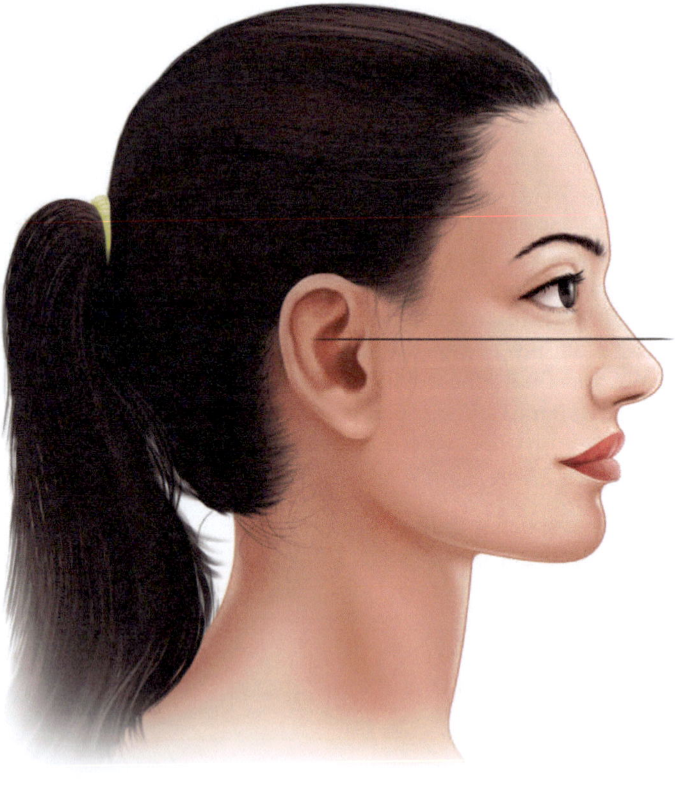

FIGURE 1.1 Frankfurt plane

triangulation: biopsy site to L superior helix, biopsy site to right superior helix, and biopsy site to nasal tip. Include these measurements in your note.

- Ears: lateral face view, full face view, back of the head.
- Nose: lateral face view, full face view, lateral oblique (45°) face view, base/swimmers view.
- Eyelids: full face eyes open, full face eyes closed, full face eyes looking up, lateral oblique face view.
- Cheeks: Full face view, lateral oblique face view.
- Forehead: Full face upper half, lateral oblique upper half face.
- Lips/chin: full face lower half mouth closed, lateral oblique face view lower half mouth closed, full face smiling, lateral oblique face view smiling.
- Hands: flat fingers/thumb lateral and include the wrist.
- Arms: flat fingers/thumb lateral and include wrist and elbow.
- Legs: standing, include ankle and knees.
- Foot: standing, include toes and ankles.

References

1. Elston DM, et al. Skin biopsy: biopsy issues in specific diseases. J Am Acad Dermatol. 2016;74(1):1–16.
2. Stratman EJ, et al. Skin biopsy: identifying and overcoming errors in the skin biopsy pathway. J Am Acad Dermatol. 2016;74(1):19–25.

Chapter 2
Anatomy

S. Hylwa et al., *Pocket Dermatology*,
https://doi.org/10.1007/978-3-030-83602-3_2

Anatomic Landmarks (Figs. 2.1, 2.2, and 2.3)

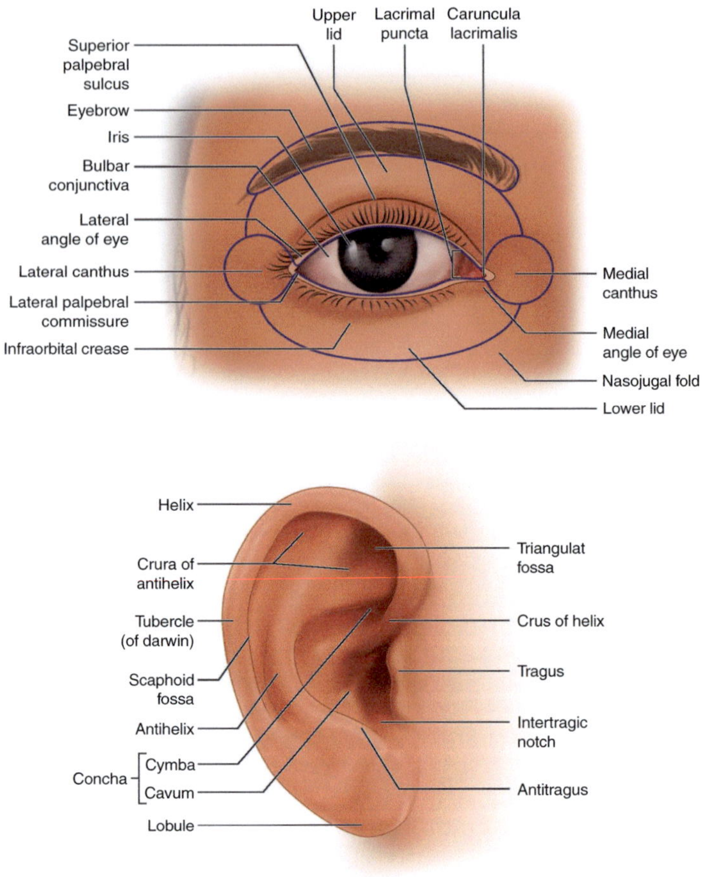

FIGURE 2.1 Anatomic landmarks of the eye and ear

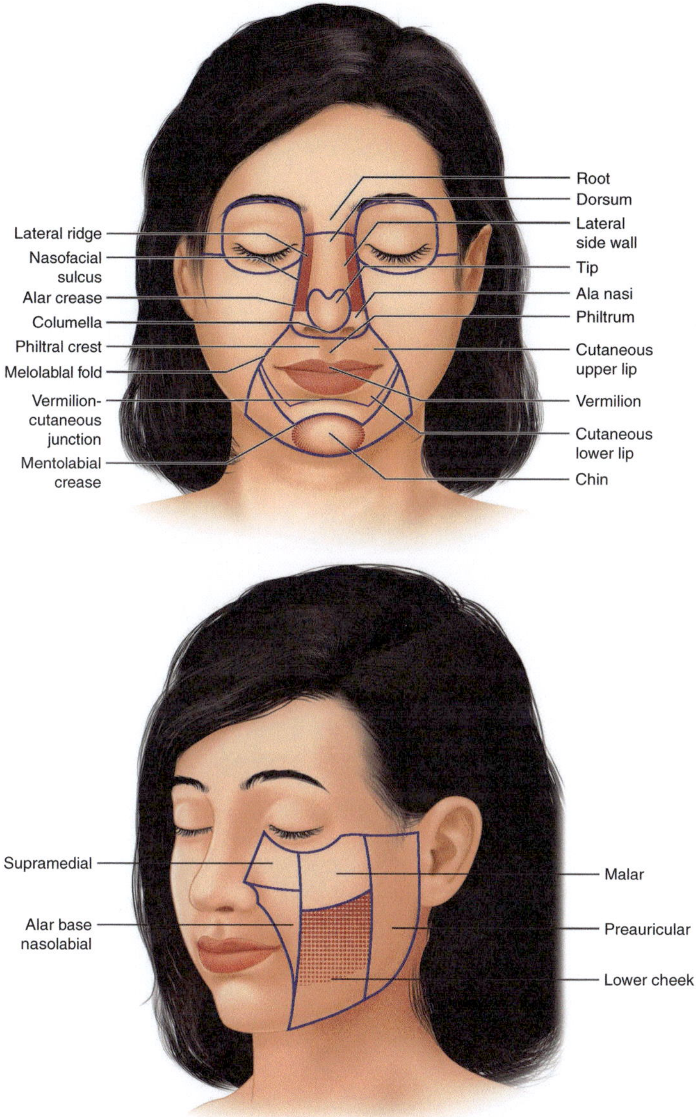

FIGURE 2.2 Anatomic landmarks of the face

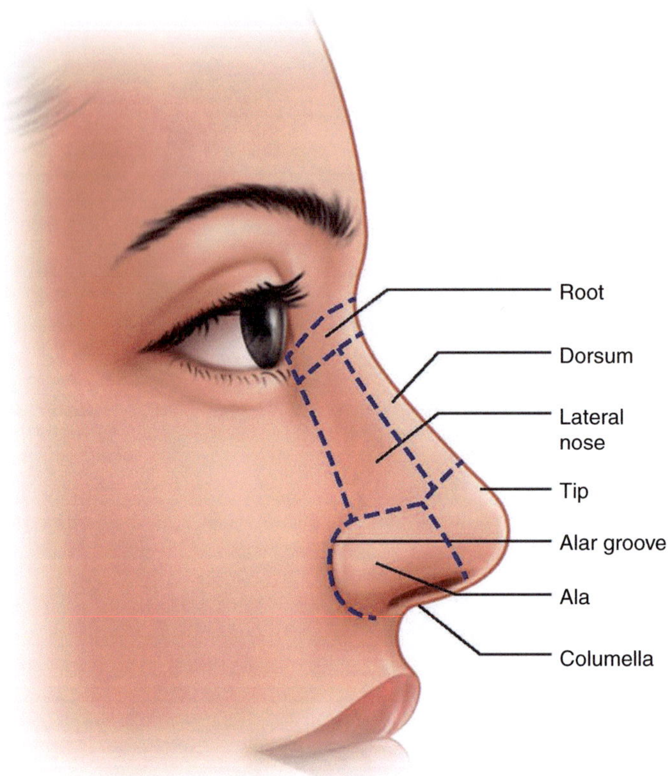

FIGURE 2.3 Anatomic landmarks of the nose

Arteries and Nerves of the Face (Figs. 2.4, 2.5, 2.6, 2.7, 2.8, and 2.9)

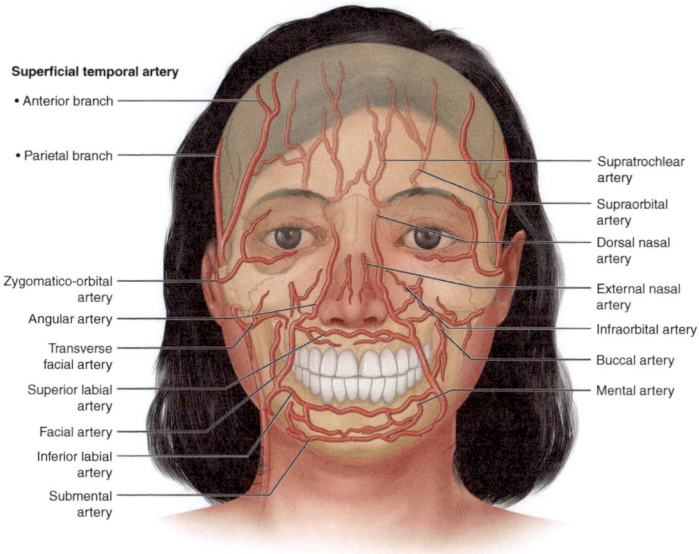

FIGURE 2.4 Major arteries of the face

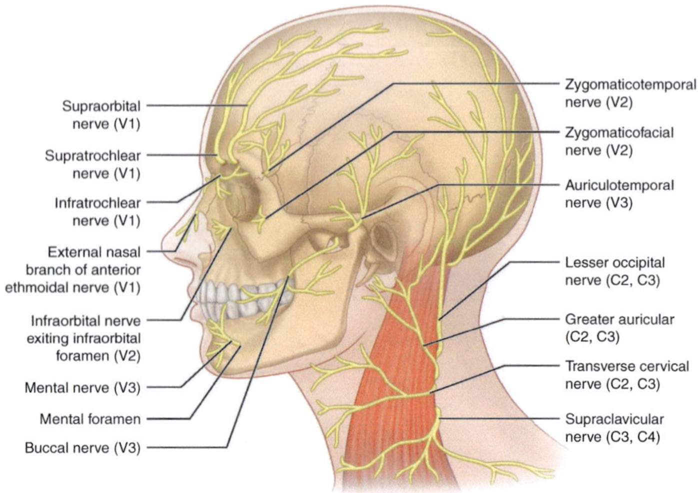

FIGURE 2.5 Cranial nerve V (trigeminal nerve)

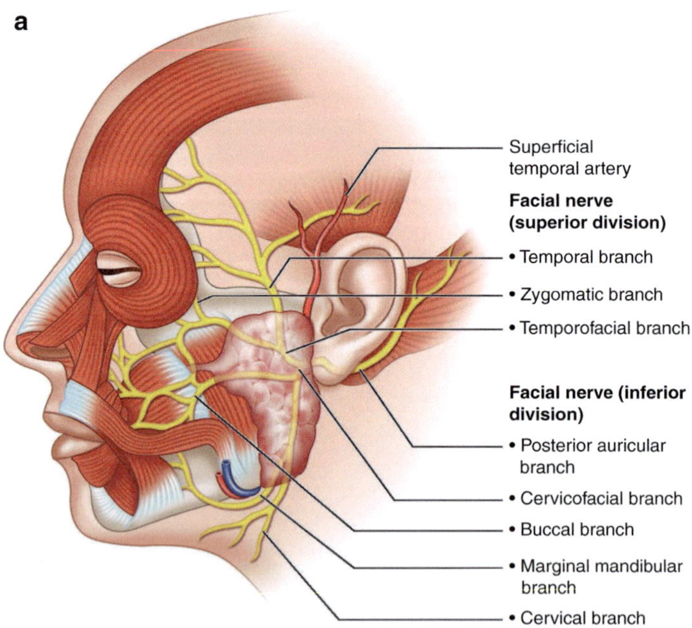

FIGURE 2.6 Cranial nerve VII (facial nerve) (**a**) and its danger zones (**b**)

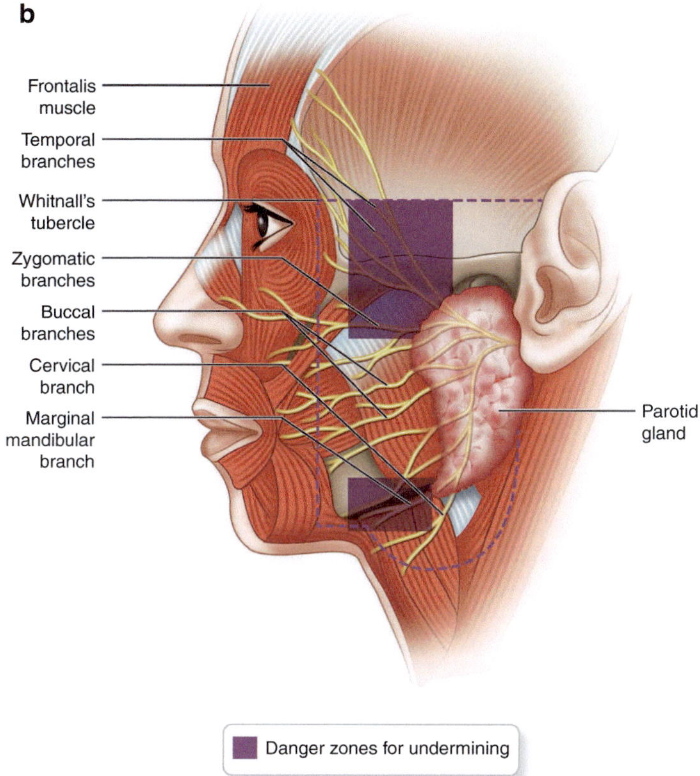

FIGURE 2.6 (continued)

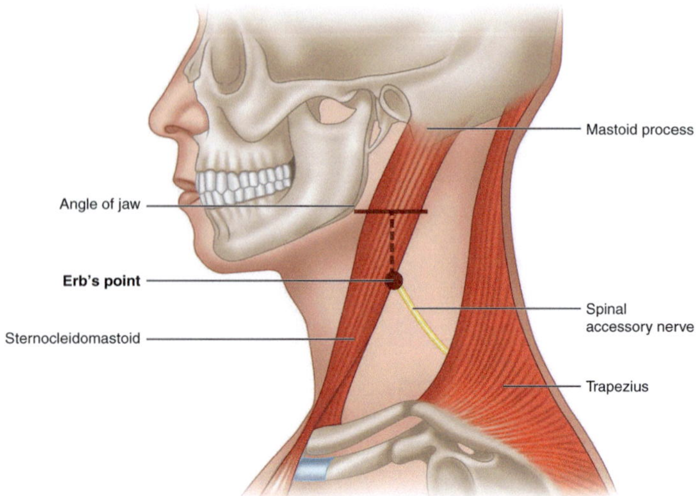

FIGURE 2.7 Cranial nerve XI danger zone

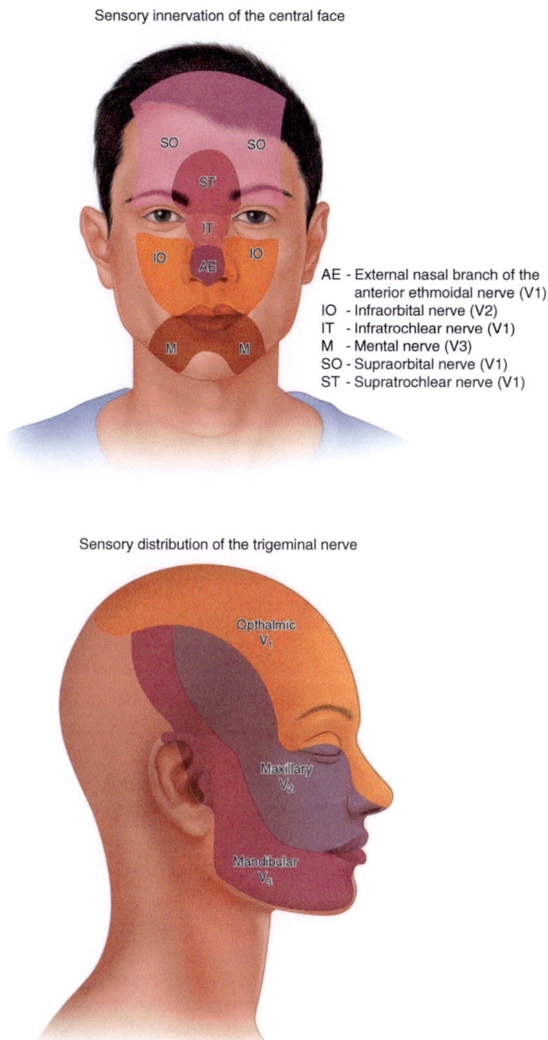

FIGURE 2.8 Sensory innovation of the face

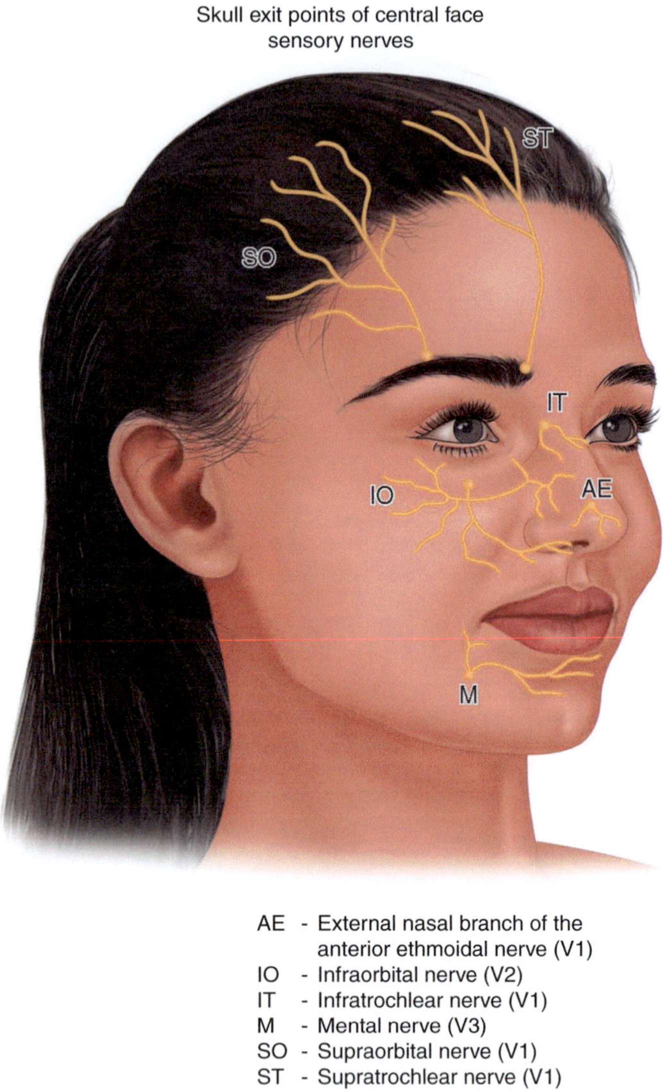

FIGURE 2.9 Sensory nerve exit points on the face. (From Bolognia, Jorizzo & Rapini: Dermatology, 2nd ed. © 2008 Elsevier, Ltd.)

Muscles of Facial Expression (Fig. 2.10)

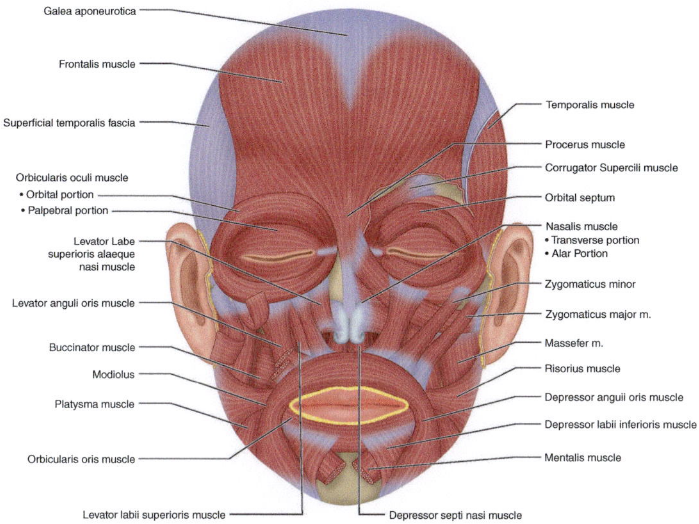

FIGURE 2.10 Muscles of the face

Relaxed Skin Tension Lines (Figs. 2.11 and 2.12)

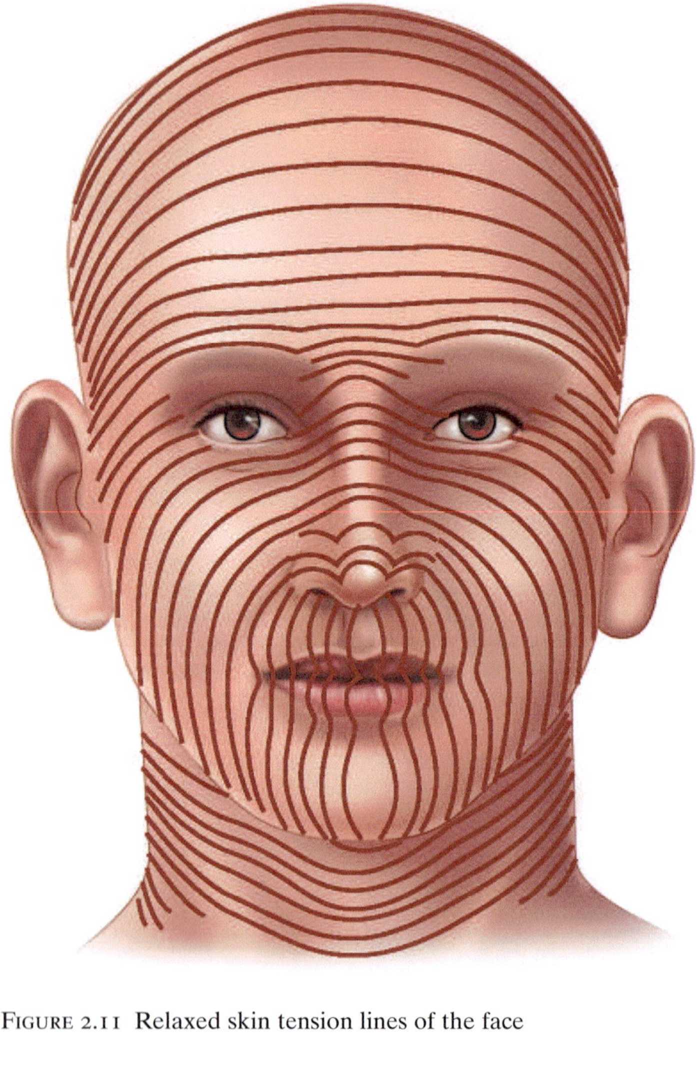

FIGURE 2.11 Relaxed skin tension lines of the face

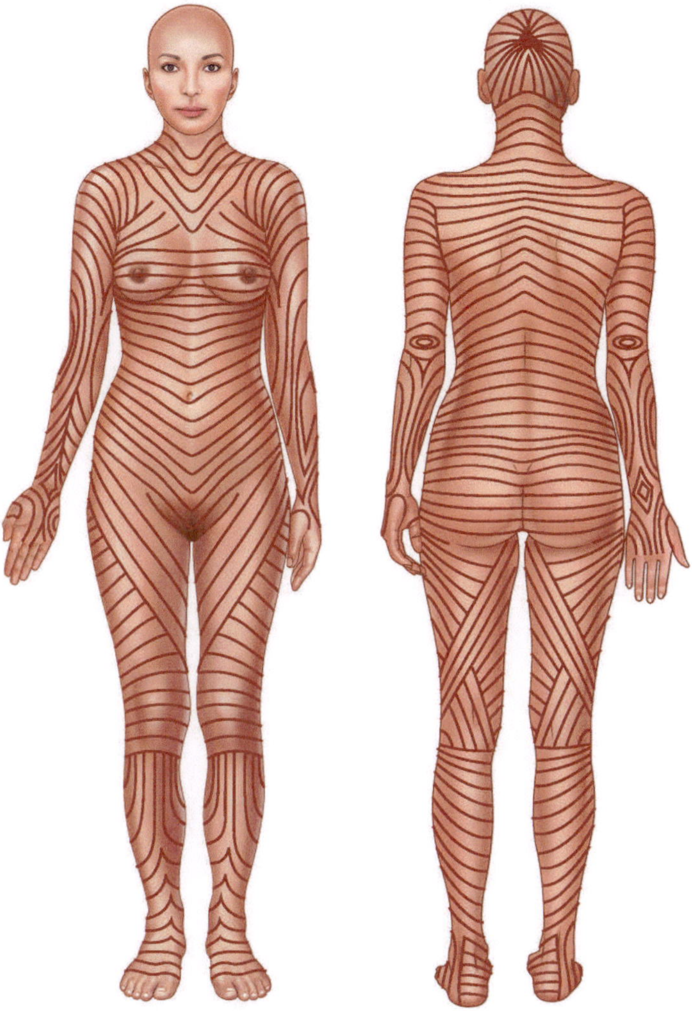

FIGURE 2.12 Relaxed skin tension lines of the body

Dermatomes

See Fig. 2.8 for sensory innovation of the face/facial dermatomes; Fig. 2.13 for body dermatomes.

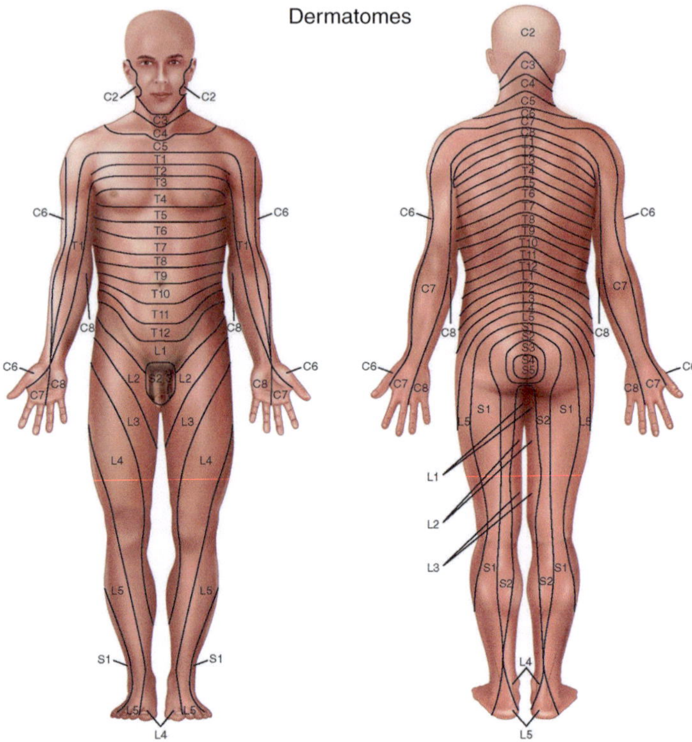

FIGURE 2.13 Dermatomes of the body

Blaschko's Lines (Fig. 2.14)

See surgical danger zones in surgical section.

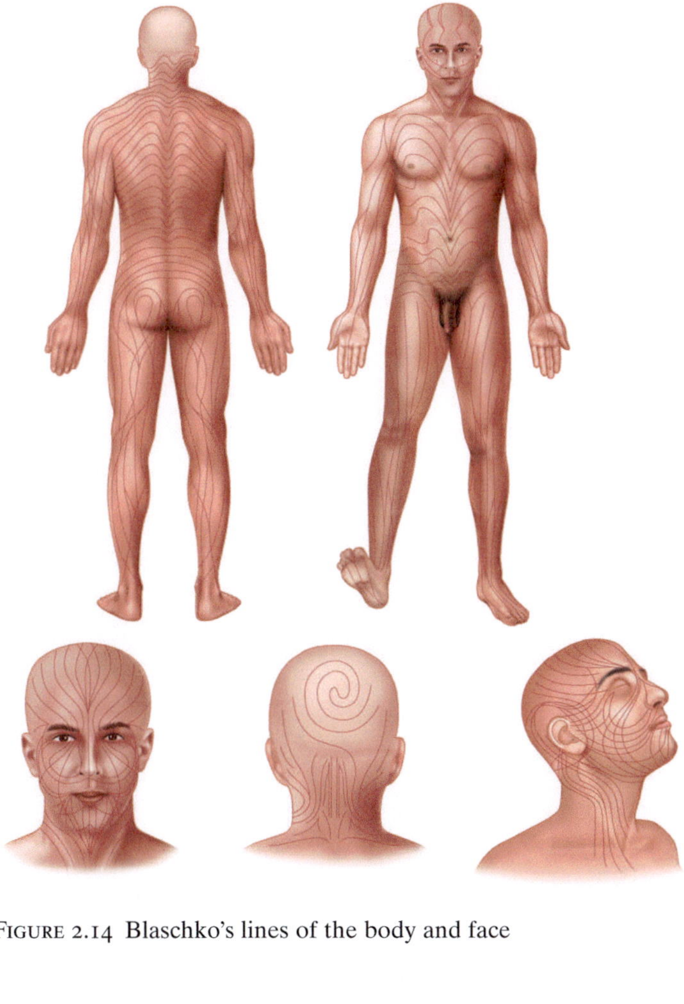

FIGURE 2.14 Blaschko's lines of the body and face

Chapter 3
General Dermatology

Pruritus Without Skin Lesions

Additional reading: http://www.ucsfcme.com/2009/slides/MDM09M07/16FoxCommonDermatologicDisordersTipsForDiagnosisAndMgmt.pdf

History

Attempt to rule out itch *with* rash.

Suggestions of itch + rash: acute onset (days), related to exposure or recent travel, household members affected, and localized itch.

Itch is almost always worse at night (nonspecific).

Aquagenic pruritus suggests polycythemia vera.

Itch without rash (neurogenic itch) should have *no* primary lesions present.

Etiologies of Itch Without Rash

Forty percent will have an underlying cause:

- Xerosis
- Liver disease (especially cholestatic/obstructive liver disease)
- Renal failure/uremia
- Iron deficiency
- Low or high calcium
- HIV

S. Hylwa et al., *Pocket Dermatology*,
https://doi.org/10.1007/978-3-030-83602-3_3

- Thyroid disease (hyperthyroidism and hypothyroidism)
- Diabetes
- Cancer: especially lymphoma (Hodgkin's), leukemia, myeloma, carcinoma, and polycythemia vera
- Medications (see below)
- Parasites (scabies, pediculosis, hookworm, ascariasis)
- Multiple sclerosis
- Neuropsychiatric conditions
- Illicit drugs
- Pregnancy-related disorders

Medications that Induce Pruritus
Opioids
Chemotherapeutic agents
Chloroquine (especially in patients of African ancestry)
Antimicrobials

- Penicillin G
- Amoxicillin/clavulanate
- Ampicillin
- Cefotaxime
- Ceftazidime
- Erythromycin
- Ciprofloxacin
- Vancomycin
- Clindamycin
- Tetracyclines
  - Minocycline
- Rifampin
- Trimethoprim/sulfamethoxazole
- Oral antifungals
  - Terbinafine
- Antimalarials
  - Chloroquine
  - Amodiaquine

Cardiovascular Medications

- ACE inhibitors

  - Captopril
  - Enalapril
  - Lisinopril

- Calcium channel blockers

  - Amlodipine
  - Diltiazem
  - Verapamil

- ARBs

  - Candesartan
  - Irbesartan

- Clonidine
- Methyldopa
- Amiodarone

Diabetic Medications

- Metformin
- Gliclazide

Neuropsychiatric Medications

- Amitriptyline
- Citalopram
- Fluoxetine
- Paroxetine
- Sertraline
- Carbamazepine
- Phenytoin
- Topiramate
- Chlorpromazine
- Phenothiazine
- Risperidone

Opioids
Non-opioid analgesics

- Aspirin

Steroids and Hormones

- Danazol

- Some oral contraceptive pills

Chemotherapeutics and Immunological Agents

- Chlorambucil
- Gemcitabine
- Nilotinib
- Vemurafenib
- Temsirolimus
- Ipilimumab
- Cetuximab
- Rituximab
- Panitumumab
- Gefitinib

Other Medications

- Allopurinol
- Alcohol
- Dextran
- Enoxaparin
- Hydroxyethyl starch
- Radiopaque contrast agents
- Scopolamine

Evaluation
- CBC with differential
- TSH and free T4
- Liver function tests (total and direct bilirubin, AST, ALT, alk phos, GGT; consider fasting total plasma bile acids)
- Amylase/lipase
- BUN/creatinine
- Iron/ferritin/TIBC
- Calcium
- HIV
- ESR/CRP
- LDH
- UA
- Fasting glucose/HgbA1c
- SPEP
- CXR

- Pemphigoid antibodies
- Skin biopsy ± DIF: may reveal microscopic dermatitis or other etiologies
- Age-appropriate malignancy screening: with more advanced testing as indicated by symptoms

  Consider based on history:

- Stool O&P
- SPEP/UPEP
- Ultrasound of the abdomen
- CT scan

Erythroderma

Reading: Rothe MJ. *Clinics in Dermatology* (2005) 23, 206–217

Definition: 90%+ of skin involved with erythema and scale.

Etiology

See pediatrics section for specific differential of erythroderma in a newborn.

For half of the patients, the underlying cause is exacerbation of preexisting dermatosis:

- Caused by one of four etiologies: (1) flare of a preexisting skin disorder, (2) drug eruption, (3) leukemia/lymphoma, and (4) idiopathic
- Cutaneous diseases (10–40%)
  - Eczematous disorders (dermatitis: seborrheic, atopic, stasis, contact dermatitis, id reaction/autoeczematous reactions, dermatitis of immunosenescence)
  - Blistering (PF, BP, Hailey-Hailey)
  - Connective tissue disease (lupus erythematosus, dermatomyositis)
  - Infections (dermatophytosis, scabies, toxoplasmosis, histoplasmosis, HIV, TB)
  - Psoriasis

- Reactive arthritis
- Sarcoidosis
- Lichen planus
- Histiocytosis
- Congenital ichthyosis
- Pityriasis rubra pilaris

- Systemic diseases (10–40%)
  - Malignancies (really any malignancy)

    Lymphoma (CTCL, Hodgkin's, B-cell lymphoma, anaplastic large cell lymphoma)
    Leukemia
    Multiple myeloma/myelodysplasias
    Solid tumors (lung, prostate, colon, thyroid, liver, breast, ovarian, fallopian tube, rectal, esophageal, gastric, melanoma)

  - Acute GVHD
  - Immunodeficiency (HIV, CVID, SCID, etc. – see pediatrics section)
  - Thyrotoxicosis

- Drugs (3–10%)
  - Top suspects: allopurinol, antiepileptics, antihypertensives, antibiotics, calcium channel blockers
  - Allopurinol
  - Aminoglycosides
  - Amiodarone
  - Arsenic
  - Aztreonam
  - Barbiturates
  - Calcium channel blockers
  - Captopril
  - Carbamazepine
  - Cephalosporins
  - Chloroquine
  - Chlorpromazine
  - Chlorpropamide
  - Cimetidine

  - Clofazimine
  - Codeine
  - Dapsone
  - Dimercaprol
  - Gold
  - Hydroxychloroquine
  - Iodine
  - Isoniazid
  - Isotretinoin
  - Lithium
  - Mephenytoin
  - Mercurials
  - Mercury
  - Mexiletine
  - Minocycline
  - Neomycin
  - Paracetamol
  - Penicillins
  - Phenothiazines
  - Phenylbutazone
  - Phenytoin
  - Quinacrine
  - Quinidine
  - Ranitidine
  - Rifampin
  - Streptomycin
  - Sulfadiazine
  - Sulfonamides
  - Sulfonylureas
  - Terbutaline
  - Thiacetazone
  - Thiazides
  - Trimethoprim
  - Vancomycin

- Idiopathic (15–45%)

Reference

- Wilson DC, Jester, JD, et al. Erythroderma and exfoliative dermatitis. *Clinics in Dermatology*. 1993;11(1):6–72.

Diagnostic Evaluation/Algorithm (Rothe et al. Clin Derm. 2005;23:206–17)

History

- PMH, family history, medications

- Full skin examination + lymph nodes.
- *Multiple* skin biopsies (2–3) with DIF.
- Skin scale scrapings and culture if exudate.
- Labs: CBC, CD4/CD8 ratio, ANA, peripheral smear, IgE level
  - Flow cytometry, B- and T-cell gene rearrangement analysis as indicated
- CXR.
- Consider patch testing.
- Consider re-biopsy.
- Refer to PCP to rule out systemic disease (age-appropriate screenings (mammogram, colonoscopy, PSA, PAP, UA, CT, MRI)).

Treatment of Erythroderma

- Admit to hospital
  - Strict Is/Os.
  - Minimize fluid loss.
  - Maximize nutrition (nutrition consult).
  - Warm, humidified environment.
- Gentle skin care: oatmeal baths, wet dressings, sauna suits.
- Bland emollients.
- Low-potency topical steroids.
  - Higher potency not recommended d/t systemic absorption.
  - Avoid tacrolimus.
- Sedating H1 antihistamines (hydroxyzine) for pruritus.
- Treat underlying pathology.
- If idiopathic, consider systemic immunosuppression only once malignancy is ruled out.
- Monitor for infections and treat appropriately.

See further information in referenced reading.

References

- Rothe MJ, Bernstein ML, Grant-Kels JM. Life-threatening erythroderma: diagnosing and treating the "red man". *Clinics in Dermatology*. 2005;23:206–17.
- Rym BM, Mourad M, et al. Erythroderma in adults: a report of 80 cases. *International Journal of Dermatology*. 2004;44(9):731–5.
- Wilson DC, Jester, JD, et al. Erythroderma and exfoliative dermatitis. *Clinics in Dermatology*. 1993;11(1):67–72.

Acne

Medications that Exacerbate Acne

Corticosteroids, androgenic steroids (danazol, stanozolol, nandrolone, testosterone), progesterone-only OCPs and hormonal (levonorgestrel-containing) IUDs, lithium, barbiturates, DHEA, halogens (bromines/iodides), cyclosporine, antiepileptics (carbamazepine, phenytoin, phenobarbital), anti-TB meds (ethionamide, isoniazid, rifampin), amoxapine, B vitamins (B6, B12), azathioprine, phenytoin, ACTH, psoralens, disulfiram.

EGFR inhibitors (acneiform pustular reaction – see section "Drug Reactions" for more details).

Acne as a Sign of Endocrine Disease

- In prepubertal children, these features include acne, early-onset body odor, axillary or pubic hair, accelerated growth, advanced bone age, and genital maturation. Growth charts and a hand film for bone age are good screening tools before specific hormonal testing.
- In postpubertal females, clinical signs include infrequent menses, hirsutism, androgenetic alopecia, infertility, polycystic ovaries, clitoromegaly, and truncal obesity.

Signs of Virilization

- Deepened voice
- Decreased breast size
- Clitoromegaly

- Alopecia
- Oligomenorrhea
- Hirsutism (hair on jaw and around nipples, umbilicus, and inner thigh)

Polycystic Ovarian Syndrome

Hirsutism (especially truncal) and acanthosis nigricans are the most reliable cutaneous markers of PCOS. Acne and androgenetic alopecia are prevalent but unreliable markers of biochemical hyperandrogenism among this population.

Rotterdam Criteria

Requires two of the following:

- Androgen excess (clinical or biochemical)
  - Clinical: presence of cutaneous features of hyperandrogenism (acne, hirsutism, acanthosis nigricans, androgenetic alopecia, seborrheic dermatitis)
  - Biochemical: presence of at least one serum androgen
- Ovulatory dysfunction (oligo- or anovulation)
  - Oligo-anovulation: fewer than eight menstrual cycles per year
- Polycystic ovaries (based on ultrasound findings)

Hormonal Lab Work-Up

Perform in patients with clinical features/a history of hyperandrogenism.

Lab work-up should occur during the menstrual period or 1 week prior. The patient should not be on an oral contraceptive or have been on one within the last 6 weeks of testing.

- Serum total and free testosterone (values below 150 ng/dL [5.2 nmol/L] exclude ovarian or adrenal tumors)
- DHEA-S (concentrations >700 mcg/dL [13.6 mol/L] raise suspicion for an adrenal androgen-secreting tumor)
- Androstenedione
- Prolactin (rule out hyperprolactinemia: hirsutism and irregular menstrual cycles)

- Luteinizing hormone and follicle-stimulating hormone
- Estrogen and progesterone
- Growth hormone and insulin-like growth factor-1
- 17-OH progesterone (for late-onset CAH: acne, hirsutism, and menstrual irregularity [identical to PCOS])
- 24-hour urine cortisol (for Cushing's: obesity, hypertension, striae, moon face, buffalo hump)
- TSH and free T4
- Fasting lipid levels
- Insulin
- Sex hormone-binding globulin
- Free androgen index

Treatment Protocol Guidelines
General Guidelines

- Acne warrants early and aggressive treatment.
- Maintenance therapy often needed for optimal outcomes.
- Always prescribe a topical antibiotic with benzoyl peroxide (wash-off or leave-on) in order to minimize resistance and increase efficacy. Antibiotics can be used concomitantly or pulsed.
- Combine topical retinoid + antimicrobial (oral or topical): these have complementary modes of action that can increase the speed or response and result in greater clearing of lesions.
- Oral antibiotics
  - Combine with topical regimen (BP + retinoid).
  - Tetracycline class is typically first line to be used.
  - Limit use of antibiotics: oral antibiotics should ideally be used for ≤3 months.

    Limitation is not only for antibiotic stewardship but also because of reports of associations with inflammatory bowel disease, pharyngitis, collagen vascular disease, *C. difficile* infections, and induction of *Candida* vulvovaginitis. There may be an association between the use of oral tetracycline-class antibiotics and breast and colon cancer.

- Oral and topical antibiotics should not be used as monotherapy.
- Concurrent use of topical and oral antibiotics should be avoided.
- Do not switch antibiotics without adequate justification.
- Use topical retinoids as maintenance with BP added for an antimicrobial effect if needed.
- Avoid use of antibiotics as maintenance therapy.

See Tables 3.1 and 3.2 for further recommendations and algorithms. See Table 3.3 for more specifics on topical and oral medications available for acne.

Comedolytic agents: retinoids, benzoyl peroxide, azelaic acid.

Mild Comedonal Acne
- Topical retinoid once daily
- Salicylic acid cleanser once or twice daily
- Combination products
  - Retinoid/BP combo
  - Antibiotic/retinoid/BP combo

Moderate Combined Acne (Inflammatory + Comedonal)
- BP cleanser twice daily and topical retinoid once daily
- BP/topical antibiotic combination in AM and topical retinoid in PM
- Topical retinoid/topical antibiotic combination product once daily
- Consider topical dapsone

If the above regimen is not working, substitute a combo product, add missing component to the regimen (BP, topical abx, retinoid), and consider hormonal therapy for females.

Moderate-Severe Combination Acne (Inflammatory and Comedonal Lesions)
- Oral antibiotics and topical retinoid once daily
- Oral antibiotic and topical retinoid/BP combination product once daily
- Females: oral antibiotic and spironolactone (female patient) *or* OCP + oral antibiotic and topical retinoid once daily

TABLE 3.1 Global alliance acne treatment algorithm

Global Alliance Acne Treatment Algorithm

Acne Severity	MILD		MODERATE		SEVERE
	Comedonal	Mixed and Papular/pustular	Mixed and Papular/pustular	Nodular(2)	Nodular/Conglobate
1ST Choice	Topical Retinoid	Topical Retinoid + Topical Antimicrobial	Oral Antibiotic + Topical Retinoid +/- BPO	Oral Antibiotic + Topical Retinoid + BPO	Oral Isotretinoln(2)
Alternatives(1)	Alt Topical Retinoid or Azalaic acid* or Salkylic acid	Alt Topical Retinoid Antimicrobial Agent + Alt. Topical Retinoid or Azelaic Acid*	Alt Oral Antibiotic + Alt. Topical Retinoid +/- BPO	Oral Isotretinoln or Alt. Oral Antibiotic + Alt. Topical Retinoid +/- BPO/Azelaic Acid*	High Dose Oral Antibiotic + Topical Retinoid + BPO
Alternatives for Females(1,4)	See 1st Choice	See 1st Choice	Oral Antiandrogen(3) + Topical Retinoid/ Azelaic acid +/-Topical Antimicrobial	Oral Antiandrogen(2) + Topical Retinoid/ +/- Alt.Topical Antimicrobial	High Dose Oral Antiandrogen(5) + Topical Retinoid/ +/- Alt.Topical Antimicrobial
Maintenance Therapy	Topical Retinoid		Topical Retinoid +/- BPO		

1. Consider physical removal of comedones. 2. With small nodules (<0.5 cm). 3. Second course in case of relapse. 4. For pregnancy, options are limited. 5. For full discussion, see Gollnick H, et al. JAAD, 2003.49 (Suppl):1-37.

(1) Consider physical removal of comedones. (2) With small nodules (<0.5 cm). (3) Second course in case of relapse. (4) For pregnancy, options are limited. (5) For full discussion, see Gollnick H, et al. *JAAD*. 2003;49(Suppl):1–37

Table 3.2 Approach to acne in adolescents and young adults

	Mild	**Moderate**	**Severe**
First-line treatment	Benzoyl peroxide (BP) or topical retinoid -or- Topical combination therapy** BP + antibiotic or retinoid + BP or retinoid + BP + antibiotic	Topical combination therapy** BP + antibiotic or retinoid + BP or retinoid + BP + antibiotic -or- Oral antibiotic + topical retinoid + BP -or- Oral antibiotic + topical retinoid + BP + topical antibiotic	Oral antibiotic + Topical combination therapy** BP + antibiotic or retinoid + BP or retinoid + BP + antibiotic -or- Oral isotretinoin
Alternative treatment*	Add topical retinoid or BP (if not on already) -or- Consider alternate retinoid -or- Consider topical dapsone -or- Consider blue light therapy	Consider alternate combination therapy -or- Consider change in oral antibiotic -or- Add combined oral contraceptive or oral spironolactone (females) -or- Consider oral isotretinoin	Consider change in oral antibiotic -or- Add combined oral contraceptive or oral spironolactone (females) -or- Consider oral isotretinoin -or- Consider photodynamic therapy

From: *JAAD*. 2016;74(5):948

*See below for other alternative therapies in table

The *double asterisks (**)* indicate that the drug may be prescribed as a fixed combination product or as separate component, *BP* Benzoyl peroxide

TABLE 3.3 Topical and oral medications for acne

	Medication	Concentrations and vehicle	Notable side effects
Topical agents			
	Salicylic acid	0.5–2% both wash-off and leave-on	Irritation
	Clindamycin	1% solution, gel, pledgets, lotion 1% pledgets 1% foam	Must be used in combination with BP Low risk of *C. diff* with topical application
	Clindamycin/BP combo	1% (5% BP) gel 1.2% (2.5%) gel 1% (3.75%) gel	Dryness, irritation, bleaching of fabrics
	Dapsone	5%, 7.5% gel	Works primarily for inflammatory lesions. Most benefits in F > M *May be oxidized by the coapplication of benzoyl peroxide causing an orange-brown coloration of the skin which can be brushed or washed off*

(continued)

Table 3.3 (continued)

Medication	Concentrations and vehicle	Notable side effects
Erythromycin	2% gel, cream, ointment, solution, pledget 1.5–2% 2% solution + zinc acetate	Reduced efficacy in comparison with clindamycin due to resistance by *Staph.* and *P. acnes*
Meclocycline	1% cream	Not available in the USA (discontinued) May cause yellowing of the skin
Erythromycin/BP combo	3% (5% BP) gel	Dryness, irritation, bleaching of fabrics. Note reduced efficacy due to bacterial resistance
Sulfacetamide	10% lotion 10% emulsion	
Azelaic acid	20% cream 15% foam	Can lighten dyspigmentation
Benzoyl peroxide	Can be leave-on or wash-off Wash, lotion, liquid, foam, bar, cream, gels all available in strengths 2.5–10%	Dryness, irritation, bleaching of fabrics Uncommon contact allergen Results can be noted in as soon as 5 days
Sodium sulfacetamide	10% wash, lotion	Irritation

	Niacinamide (nicotinamide)	2–4% gel	Flushing
Retinoids			Dryness, peeling, erythema, irritation All are contraindicated in pregnancy
	Adapalene	0.1%, 0.3% cream 0.1% lotion	
	Adapalene/BP combo	0.1% (2.5% BP) gel	
	Tretinoin	0.025, 0.05, 0.1% cream 0.01, 0.025 0.04, 0.1% gel or microsphere gel	Not photostable and should be applied in the evening *Tretinoin (not microsphere formulation) may be inactivated by coadministration of benzoyl peroxide* Increased risk of photosensitivity
	Tretinoin/clindamycin	0.025% (1.2% clindamycin) gel	
	Tazarotene	0.05%, 0.1% gel, cream, or foam	Pregnancy category X

(continued)

Table 3.3 (continued)

	Medication	Concentrations and vehicle	Notable side effects
Oral antibiotics			
	Tetracycline	250–500 mg q12h	Dental staining <9 years Dairy products decrease absorption GI upset, photosensitivity, teratogenic, pseudotumor cerebri, vulvovaginal candidiasis Contraindicated in pregnancy
	Minocycline	50–200 mg daily (often 100 mg BID) 45, 90, 135 mg ER daily	Dental staining <9 years Dairy products decrease absorption Vertigo, GI upset, blue-gray skin pigmentation, severe drug/lupus-like reactions, teratogenic, autoimmune hepatitis, pseudotumor cerebri, tinnitus, SJS/TEN, DRESS, vulvovaginal candidiasis Contraindicated in pregnancy

Doxycycline	50–200 mg daily (usually 100 mg BID) 20, 75, 100, 150 mg ER daily Submicrobial: 20 mg BID or 40 mg daily	Dental staining <9 years Dairy products decrease absorption Photosensitivity, photo-onycholysis, GI upset, teratogenic, pseudotumor cerebri (less than mino), vulvovaginal candidiasis Contraindicated in pregnancy Metabolized by the liver, so safer for patients with renal disease
Sarecycline	<54 kg: 60 mg PO qDay 55–84 kg: 100 mg PO qDay 85–136 kg: 150 mg PO qDay	Nausea Vulvovaginal candidiasis
Erythromycin	250–500 mg daily	GI upset (common), cardiac conduction abnormalities, rare hepatotoxicity, vulvovaginal candidiasis Can increase cyclosporine levels
Trimethoprim/sulfamethoxazole (TMP/SMX)	80/400, 160/800 mg	Severe drug reactions (SJS/TEN), DRESS/DIHS, bone marrow suppression/blood dyscrasias, fulminant hepatitis, respiratory hypersensitivity, GI upset, vulvovaginal candidiasis

(continued)

TABLE 3.3 (continued)

Medication	Concentrations and vehicle	Notable side effects
Clindamycin	75–150 mg daily	Pseudomembranous colitis (*C. diff*), GI upset, drug reactions, vulvovaginal candidiasis
Cephalexin	250–500 mg daily	GI upset, drug reactions, vulvovaginal candidiasis
Azithromycin	500 mg PO once and then 250 mg PO daily × 4 days. Repeat q3–4 weeks Alternate: 250–500 mg three times per week for 8–12 weeks	Diarrhea, nausea, abdominal pain, loose stool Hepatitis (rare) Use with caution in patients with abnormal liver function as hepatic failure has been reported Contraindicated with pimozide Can increase cyclosporine levels Note increased risk of ventricular tachyarrhythmias or sudden cardiac death w/ macrolides (118 cases/1 million) FDA warning for increased risk of tendon ruptures (Achilles) and aortic tears and aortic rupture

Hormonal treatments			
	Combo oral contraceptive pill	See below for further information	See prescribing/medication section for details
	Spironolactone	50–200 mg/day	See prescribing/medication section for details
	Prednisone	5–15 mg/day 0.5–1 mg/kg/day	Long-term side effects prohibit use as primary therapy Used for acne fulminans or isotretinoin-induced flare; tapered over several months
Oral retinoids			
	Isotretinoin	Conventional dosing: 0.5 mg/kg/day starting, increasing to 1.0 mg/kg/day as tolerated Goal: 120–220 mg/kg final dose (many dermatologists now aiming for ~200 mg/kg goal)	Requires consent and registration with FDA's iPledge program. See prescribing/medication section for details Dry skin, nose, eyes, and lips, photosensitivity, decreased night vision, corneal opacities, alopecia, headache, pseudotumor cerebri (esp. with tetracyclines), hyperostosis, musculoskeletal pain, elevated triglycerides/cholesterol, hepatitis, (inflammatory bowel disease), rhabdomyolysis, teratogenic, depression/suicidal ideation

Adapted from Hurwitz

If the above regimen is not working, consider hormonal therapy for appropriate females or isotretinoin.

Severe or Scarring Acne
- Isotretinoin.
- If isotretinoin does not work, consider retreating or hormonal therapy for females and/or photodynamic therapy.

Goal for all types of acne should eventually be able to be maintained with a topical retinoid or benzoyl peroxide/retinoid combo.

Combination Oral Contraceptive Pills
Ethinyl estradiol *plus* either:

- First-generation progestins (estranges): norethindrone and ethynodiol diacetate
- Second-generation progestin (gonanes): levonorgestrel and norgestimate
- Third-generation progestin (less androgenic gonanes): desogestrel and gestodene
- Fourth generation (antiandrogen): drospirenone

Four approved OCPS for treatment of acne:

- Ethinyl estradiol/norgestimate
- Ethinyl estradiol/norethindrone acetate/ferrous fumarate
- Ethinyl estradiol/drospirenone/levomefolate
- Ethinyl estradiol/drospirenone

See Chap. 8 section in oral contraceptive pills for recommendations on OCP prescribing.

Alternative Acne Therapies (Table 3.4)

Others
- Comedone extraction
- Injection with intralesional triamcinolone into cysts/nodules
- Resurfacing lasers (useful for scarring)
- Dermabrasion (useful for scarring)
- Microneedling (useful for scarring)
- Collagen or saline injections (useful for scarring)

TABLE 3.4 Light-based therapies for acne

Energy device	Wavelength (nm)	Target acne type	Mechanism of action	Dose, timing, efficacy
Intense pulsed light (IPL)	400–1200	Mild-severe inflammatory	Absorption of red and blue light causes porphyrin activation > destruction of *P. acnes* (*bacteriacidal*), thermal destruction of sebaceous glands	Performed up to every 3 weeks >90% (inflam)
IPL with suction (photopneumatic technology)	400–1200	Mild-severe inflammatory	Broadband light with mechanical clearance of sebaceous duct	Up to 80% (inflam)
Blue LED[a]	400–500	Inflammatory	Penetrates the upper epidermis Porphyrins (coproporphyrin III and protoporphyrin IX) absorb light wavelengths between 400 and 700 nm with 415 nm wavelength within the blue light spectrum being most effectively absorbed which decreases Propionibacterium acnes (bacteriacidal); reduces pilosebaceous unit size and function level; Normalizes keratinocytes	Up to 77% (inflam)

(continued)

Table 3.4 (continued)

Energy device	Wavelength (nm)	Target acne type	Mechanism of action	Dose, timing, efficacy
Red LED[a]	620–600	Inflammatory and non-inflammatory	Penetrates to level of sebaceous glands in the dermis. Activates protoporphyrin IX leading to destruction of *P. acnes (bactericidal). Reduces inflammatory macrophage cytokine release*	More efficacious than blue light in the treatment of acne Up to 66% (inflam); 59% (non-inflam)
Blue-red LED[a]	400–500; 620–660 Home-use: illuMask Acne Light Therapy (La Lumiere), Omnilux Clear-U (Photherapeutics Ltd), OCimple Light Therapy System (Ceragem Medisys, Inc.)	Inflammatory and non-inflammatory	Keratinocyte normalization and porphyrin activation leading to destruction of *P .acnes*	More effective than either blue or red light alone Up to 90% (inflam); 54% (non-inflam)
Infrared lasers	700 nm to 1 mm	Inflammatory	Penetrates deeper into the dermis than red light with minimal impact on the epidermis Targets water in sebaceous gland > decreased sebum output	Up to 84%

Pulsed dye laser	595	Inflammatory	Unknown, possible effect on sebum production	Up to 53% reduction Can be used as light source for PDT with increased efficacy
KTP (potassium titanyl phosphate)	532	Inflammatory	*P. acnes* bactericidal; sebaceous gland disruption	Performed 1–2×/week Up to 26% Increased efficacy if applied with ALA (aminolevulinic acid) before treatment
PDT	N/A	Inflammatory and non-inflammatory	Application of 5-aminolevulinic acid (ALA) (1-3-hour incubation) Commonly used photosensitizers include ALA or MAL. New photosensitizers include indocyanine green (ICG) and indole-3-acetic acid. A photosensitizer is absorbed by pilosebaceous units and upon activation by light of an appropriate wavelength, is converted via the heme biosynthetic pathway to protoporphyrin IX and subsequently produces reactive oxygen species that exert bactericidal effects on P. acnes and damage the pilosebaceous units	Up to 100% Note: all light sources used in PDT may lead to erythema, stinging, peeling, pruritus, oozing, and pustules after treatment. Red light may have less side effects

(continued)

TABLE 3.4 (continued)

Energy device	Wavelength (nm)	Target acne type	Mechanism of action	Dose, timing, efficacy
Radiofrequency	N/A	Moderate inflammatory and non-inflammatory	Thermal destruction of sebaceous glands (energy coagulates the glands)	Up to 90% (inflam) Acute erythema can last up to 2 weeks after treatment Can pair with microneedling
Particle assisted + diode	800	Inflammatory	Exogenous particles (gold/silver) are placed inside the pilosebaceous units via massage, vibration, or ultrasound; the laser then destroys the pilosebaceous infundibulum and glands	Up to 61% (inflam)

[a] *LED* light-emitting diode. Both in-office and home-use blue LEDs are available. Blue light's efficacy is highest when paired with PDT. Red light is more efficacious than blue light in the treatment of acne, but blue-red combination works the best. Adapted from Handler NZ et al. Energy-Based Devices in Treatment of Acne Vulgaris Pei S, et al. Dermatol Surg. 2016;42(5):573–85. and Light-based therapies in acne treatment Indian Dermatol Online J. 2015;6(3):145–157.

- Chemical peels (useful for scarring, hyperpigmentation and comedones; less so for inflammatory lesions)
- Punch grafts, tissue augmentation (useful for scarring)

Diets that Are Helpful in Acne
- Low glycemic diet.
- Low dairy diets (avoid especially skim milk).
- Supplementation with probiotics may be tried.

References

- Thiboutot D. *J Am Acad Dermatol*. 2009 May;60(5 Suppl):S1–50.
- Kapadia N and Talib A. Acne treated successfully with azithromycin. *Int J Dermatol*. 2004;43(10):766–7.
- Zaenglein AL et al. *JAAD*. 2016;74:945–73.
- Handler M et al. Energy based devices in treatment of acne vulgaris. *Derm Surgery*. 2016;42(5):573–85.
- Barbieri J et al. Approaches to limit systemic antibiotic use in acne: Systemic alternatives, emerging topical therapies, dietary modification, and laser and light-based treatments. *JAAD*. 2019;80:538–49.

Hyperhidrosis

Primary focal hyperhidrosis: focal visible excessive sweating occurring in at least one site (axilla, palms, soles, or craniofacial region) for at least 6 months without apparent secondary causes (e.g., medications, endocrine disease, neurologic disease), plus two or more of the following characteristics:

- Bilateral and relatively symmetric
- Age of onset <25 years old
- Frequency of episodes at least once per week
- Positive family history
- Cessation of excessive sweating upon sleep
- Impairment of daily activities

Secondary causes of hyperhidrosis: diabetes mellitus, hyperthyroidism, hyperpituitarism, neurologic disease

(Parkinson's, complex regional pain syndrome, spinal injury), pheochromocytoma, respiratory disease, psychiatric disease.

Palmoplantar hyperhidrosis seen in patients with chronic alcoholism.

Asymmetric hyperhidrosis suggests a neurologic disease.

Work-Up for Secondary Hyperhidrosis
- Neurological exam
- Blood pressure
- CBC
- Fasting glucose
- Thyroid function
- Urinary catecholamines (for pheo)
- PPD/T-SPOT for TB (nocturnal hyperhidrosis)
- Med list: propranolol, physostigmine, pilocarpine, TCAs, SSRIs, venlafaxine

Treatment

<u>Topical Therapies (First Line)</u>

- OTC anti-perspirants
- Aluminum chloride hexahydrate 10–35% (generally 20%) in sal acid gel (2–4) or absolute alcohol
  - Apply to dry skin at night and wash off in the morning.
  - Start applying nightly for 1–2 weeks, and then the frequency can be reduced once response is noted.
  - Irritancy is the major side effect. It is usually mild. Hydrocortisone 1% cream applied in the AM after washing off may help.
  - Often compound with the salicylic acid in order to decrease the amount of aluminum chloride needed and thus decrease irritation.
- Topical glycopyrrolate 0.5–2%
- Tap water iontophoresis (in clinic or at home, time and equipment intensive) for palmar/plantar hyperhidrosis
  - Patient places the hand/feet into electrode-containing plastic trays of tap water with the water level just above the skin of the tops of the fingers/hands.

  - Treatment performed daily for 10 minutes, initially every 2–3 days with the energy intensity increased over time to a therapeutic range of 10–18 mA. After a therapeutic effect is achieved with daily treatments (usually about 2 weeks), the treatment interval may be reduced to once every 1–2 weeks.
  - Adverse effects: burning, stinging, erythema

- Botulinum toxin

  - Botox: dilute 100u with 5 mL of saline (concentration = 2u/0.1 cc)
  - Axilla: 50–100 units of Botox (200 units of Dysport) per axilla. Twenty injections are distributed evenly 1–2 cm apart in the hyperhidrotic area. Duration of anhidrosis is 4–14 months.
  - Palmo-plantar: response to therapy varies more than with axillary disease. 100–240 units of Botox injected intradermally per palm. Two to three units of Botox placed every 1–2 cm. Duration of action: 6 months. SE include pain and transient weakness of the muscles of the hands (finger pinch > hand grip). **Ref**: Saadia D. *Neurology.* 2001;57(11):2095–9.

Systemic Therapies

- Anticholinergics

  - Glycopyrrolate 1–2 mg BID/TID

    Adverse effects: xerostomia, urinary hesitancy, blurred vision/increased ocular pressure, dizziness, tachycardia, constipation, rarely confusion
    Contraindicated in patients with myasthenia gravis, pyloric stenosis, and paralytic ileus

  - Oxybutynin 10 mg/day: dosing should be based on individualized response and tolerability of patients

    Adverse effects: xerosis
    Contraindications: allergy, bladder or intestinal obstruction, severe ulcerative colitis, toxic megacolon, glaucoma, or myasthenia gravis

In kids, at least one study advocating first-line treatment for multifocal or generalized hyperhidrosis and second-line treatment for craniofacial and palmoplantar hyperhidrosis (del Boz Peds Derm 2016)

- Clonidine 0.1 mg BID or 0.2 mg/day transcutaneous patch
  - Alpha-adrenergic receptor agonist that reduces sympathetic outflow
  - Adverse effects: dry mouth, dizziness, constipation, sedation, decreased BP
  - May be good for craniofacial hyperhidrosis/generalized hyperhidrosis

Laser Therapies

- Radiofrequency thermotherapy
  - Shave skin, anesthetize, and spray disinfectant. Treatment given in two rounds 6 weeks apart with penetration depth of 3 mm, emission duration of 250 ms, and intensity of 70 and one round at penetration depth of 2 mm, duration of 200 ms, and intensity of 60. Device was applied to overlapping areas of the skin, and roughly 150 pulses were performed per session. After treatment, area is disinfected again and covered with sterile dressing for 12 hours.
  - Side effect: petechial bleeding during procedure, erythema, post-anesthesia pain, exudation/scab, superficial ulceration, needle puncture sites visible after 6 months.
  - See Schick CH et al. *Derm Surgery*. 2016;42(5):624–630.
- Microwave thermal ablation

Surgical Therapies

- Local axillary surgery – complete en block removal of axillary skin. Scarring and functional impairment noted. Relapse rates of 10–25%.
- Local axillary liposuction/axillary curettage – improved sweating in 80–90%.
- Sympathectomy.

- Note that compensatory sweating can develop in new/other areas after surgical therapy.

Reference: Walling HW and Swich BL. Treatment options of hyperhidrosis. *Am J Clin Dermatol.* 2011: 12(5):285–95.

Hair

Recommended Reading

- For cicatricial alopecias, *CME JAAD* Dec 2016;75(6)

Normal

- Growth: 0.37 mm/day (1 cm per month, 6 inches per year)
- 100,000 hairs ± 10,000 for blondes, redheads
- 85% anagen, 10–15% telogen, 1% catagen
- Lose roughly 50–150 hairs per day

Hair Anatomy

See Fig. 3.1.

Infundibulum is from sebaceous gland to opening on the epidermis.

Isthmus is from arrector pili muscle to sebaceous gland.

Bulb is from dermal papilla to arrector pili muscle.

Bulb is where hair matrix cells reside. Bulge is where the stem cells are located.

In alopecia areata, immune cells swarm the bulb; in cicatricial alopecias, immune cells swarm the bulge.

Hair Loss Examination

- Examine hair fibers and scalp: any redness, perifollicular accentuation, scale, pustules, bogginess of the scalp? Where is the hair loss? What is the pattern (e.g., thinning of the frontal hairline, part width, vertex, temples, or ophiasis (occipital scalp pattern)? Is there loss of the follicular openings/scarring? Tufting (i.e., doll's hair)? Are other hairy areas affected (eyebrows, eyelashes, arm/leg hair, axillary hair)? Excess hair in places (jawline, umbilicus, inner thighs, nipples)?

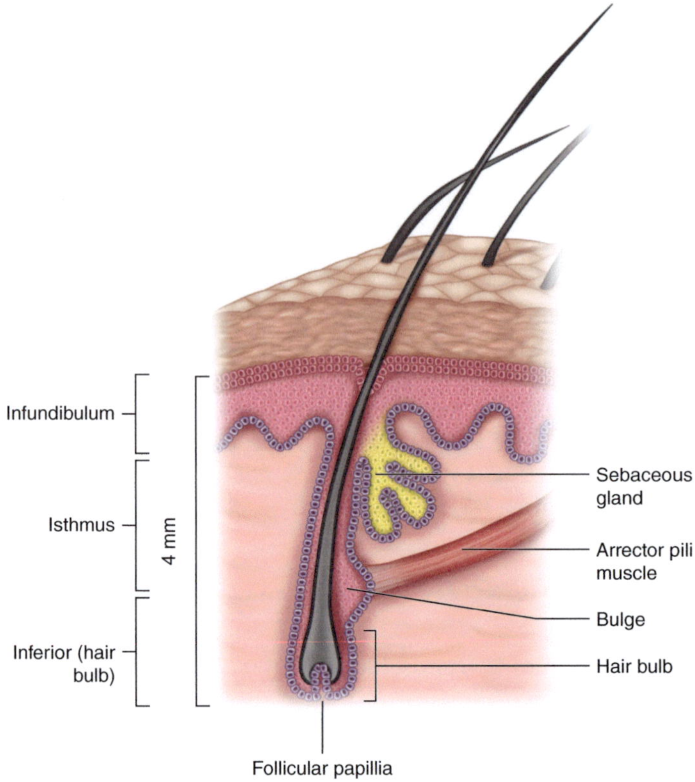

FIGURE 3.1 Anatomy of the hair follicle

- Examine nails for dystrophy (e.g., pitting with alopecia areata).
- Hair pull test. Positive if pull 40 hairs and >2 are removed (if patient has not showered that day).

Hair Loss Work-Up (As Indicated by History)

- Total and free testosterone, DHEA-S
- CBC, ferritin, transferrin, TIBC
- Vitamin D levels
- TSH

TABLE 3.5 Differentials for scarring alopecias and diffuse (non-scarring) hair loss

Scarring alopecia DDx	Diffuse (non-scarring) hair loss DDx
Lichen planopilaris (LPP)	Telogen effluvium
Discoid lupus	Chronic telogen effluvium
Central centrifugal scarring alopecia	Anagen effluvium (e.g., chemotherapy)
Folliculitis decalvans	Early androgenetic alopecia
Tufted folliculitis	Diffuse alopecia areata
Follicular degeneration syndrome	Hypothyroidism and hyperthyroidism
Acne keloidalis	Acute lupus
Dissecting cellulitis	Syphilis
Frontal fibrosing alopecia	Mechanical (traction, trichotillomania) - can progress to scarring if long-term
Infectious (syphilis, kerion)	
Unclassified (pseudopelade)	
Brunsting-Perry cicatricial pemphigoid	

- ESR
- Zinc
- ANA

For scarring and non-scarring diagnoses, see Table 3.5.

General Treatment Options

- Alopecia Areata
- Dilution: triamcinolone (Kenalog) 2.5–10 mg/cc; total volume, usually 3–4 cc. Inject to areas of active disease.
- Topical regimen: topical high to strong potency steroid lotions, gels, and solutions; Latisse, Rogaine., topical tofacitinib 2%.

- Regimen: repeat q1 month (if active) or q2 months (if quiescent).
- Systemic therapies: prednisone (if abruptly losing hair), cyclosporine, methotrexate, Vytorin, tofacitinib

Scarring Alopecias

- Dilution: triamcinolone (Kenalog) 10 mg/cc to areas of active disease
- Lymphocytic subtypes: hydroxychloroquine 200 mg daily and then BID (must get ophtho exam and ensure no other contraindications). For frontal fibrosing, consider dutasteride in patients without contraindications.
  - See dermatopharmacology section for more information.
- Neutrophilic subtypes: antibiotics (doxycycline, minocycline), dapsone

Telogen Effluvium

- Ask when hair loss started, and then inquire about stressors 3 months prior to start of hair loss.
- Treatment: Rogaine × 6–12 months; reassurance.
- Consider labs
  - Goal: ferritin >75 (at least >40–50), vitamin D, TSH, CBC, ± zinc
- Optimize scalp (i.e., control seb derm).

Androgenetic Alopecia

- Treatment: men's Rogaine foam nightly (if irritating, get formula without propylene glycol)
- Propecia 1 mg daily (or 1/4 of 5 mg tablet) (ladies: spironolactone 50–200mg daily)
  - See prescribing section for more information
- Platelet-rich plasma injections

Causes of Hypertrichosis

- Metabolic disorders (thyroid)
- Anorexia nervosa
- Porphyria
- Medications: oral (or topical) minoxidil, diazoxide, phenytoin, cyclosporine, streptomycin, penicillamine, cortico-

steroids, danazol and anabolic steroids, psoralens, PUVA, androgens, streptomycin, acetazolamide

- Eyelashes: IFN, AZT, cyclosporine, bimatoprost

- Malignancies (malignant down)
- Endocrine: adrenal, ovary/testicle (menopause), pituitary, hypothalamus

SALT Score = Severity of Alopecia Tool (Fig. 3.2)

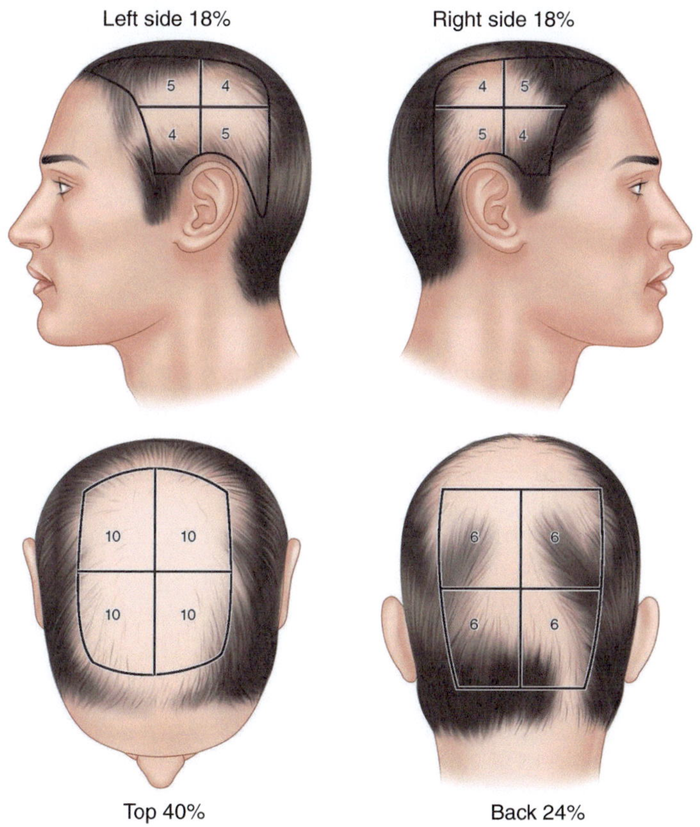

FIGURE 3.2 SALT score distributions on the scalp. (From: Olsen E and Canfield D. *JAAD*. 2015;75(6):1268–9)

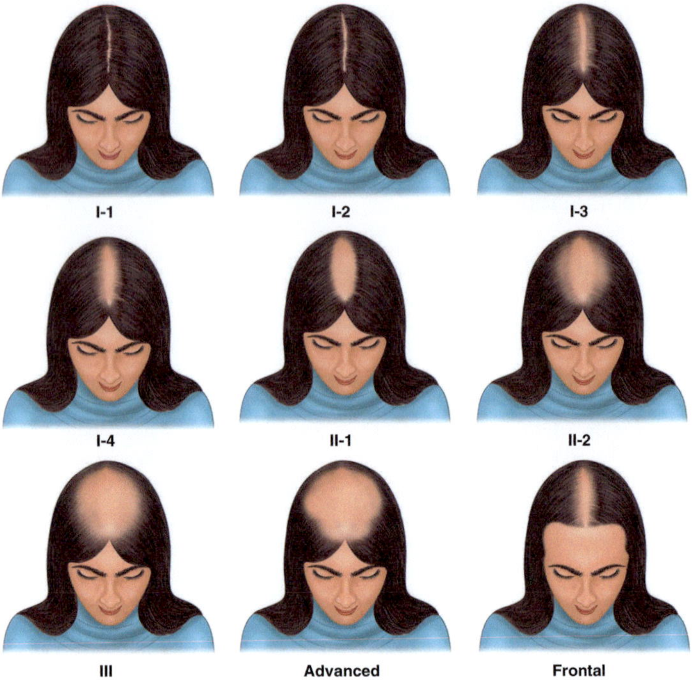

FIGURE 3.3 Ludwig part width schematic

Sum of percentage of hair loss in four views

Left lateral = 18%, right lateral = 18%, vertex = 40%, posterior = 24%

Female pattern hair loss is scored with the Ludwig part width (Fig. 3.3).

Ulcers and Wounds

Good reading: Powers et al. *JAAD* April 2016;74(4) CME. Alvari et al. *JAAD* April 2015;74(4) CME

Chronic wound usually affects the legs.

Common Causes and Work-Up

Chronic Venous Insufficiency (45–80%)

- Due to calf muscle pump dysfunction. High pressure > fibrin deposits in vessels > less diffusion of oxygen and nutrients > ischemia/necrosis. High association with h/o DVT.
- Signs: chronic edema, brawny stippled pigmentation, stasis dermatitis, varicose veins, lipodermatosclerosis, verrucous epidermis (elephantiasis nostra verrucosa), atrophie blanche.
- Medial malleolus is the most common location (L > R).
- Work-up
  - Check pulses.
  - Venous system analysis (both superficial and deep plexus investigations)
    Color duplex Doppler ultrasonography: provides anatomic and flow data (reflux/patency within veins)
    Air plethysmography: assesses reflux, obstruction, and calf muscle pump function
    Venography – invasive: uses contrast information on thrombus age and valve damage and helps provide information for future stenting
  - Assess DVT risk.
- Treatment
  - Compression, elevation
  - Control any surrounding stasis change
- Failure of venous leg ulcer healing correlated with larger initial area of wound, longer duration of wound, history of venous ligation/vein stripping, history of hip/knee replacement surgery, ABI <0.8, and 50% of the wound covered by fibrin.
- If wound is not 30% smaller by week 4, it is unlikely to heal by week 12; patient should be reassessed.

<u>Arterial Insufficiency (5–20%)</u>

- Due to arteriosclerosis (most commonly)
  - Risk factors: smoking, hyperlipidemia, hypertension, diabetes, obesity, history of vascular disease (MI, CVA, PVD)

- Arterial ulcers are painful and most often arise over bony prominences between toes, on heels, and in lateral malleolus area. Begins as a well-demarcated patch progressing to blackened slough or dry gangrene. Slough sheds to reveal a punched-out ulcer with a sharp border.
- Signs
  - Intermittent claudication (pain on exercise), progressing often to pain at rest with leg elevation that is relieved with placing leg in a dependent position (sign of advanced disease)
  - Cyanosed pale skin (especially on elevation, often with livedo-pattern vasculature, loss of hair of the legs, and shiny thin skin)
- Work-up: arterial studies of both the micro- and macrocirculation
  - Microcirculation studies

    Transcutaneous oxygen saturation
    Laser Doppler flowmetry
    Transcutaneous carbon dioxide saturation
    Capillaroscopy
  - Macrocirculation studies

    Ankle brachial pressure index
    Doppler arterial waveforms
    Duplex ultrasonography
    Angiography
    MRI
- *Ankle brachial index* (Fig. 3.4)
- ABI > 1.4 = calcification/vessel hardening → refer to vascular specialist.
- ABI 1–4 normal, 0.9–1.0 acceptable, NTD.
- ABI 0.8–0.9: some arterial disease → treat risk factors.
- ABI < 0.8: arterial disease → refer to vascular specialist.
  - 0.5–0.8: modify compression as well.
  - <0.4: high risk of limb ischemia

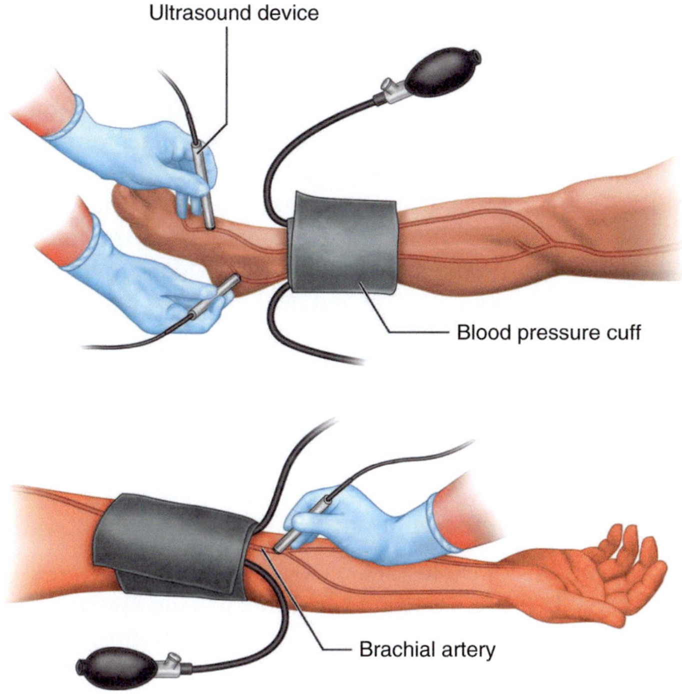

FIGURE 3.4 How to obtain an ankle brachial index (ABI)

- Treatment
  - Referral to vascular surgery for angioplasty, endarterectomy, bypass, debridement, and amputation as needed
  - Referral to primary care to help encourage/manage stopping smoking, exercise to increase collateral circulation, correct hyperlipidemia, treatment of hypertension, analgesics for pain

Neurogenic Ulcers (15–20%)

- Almost all due to diabetes.

- Mal perforans ulcers: deep ulcer, usually on toes or sole of foot that has a surrounding callus. Due to repeated trauma to an insensate area of the foot.
- Clues to diagnose include a warm, dry foot with adequate pulses, but with reduced response to light touch or painful stimulation and loss of ankle jerk reflexes.
- These are due to chronic/wear-and-tear on the skin in absence of pain reflex to stop the movement/trauma. Get callus formation that then breaks down and ulcerates. Soles, metatarsal head, great toe, and heel are often involved.
- Often can become infected.
- Referral to podiatry/orthopedics/general surgery.

Other Causes of Ulcers

- Necrobiosis lipoidica
- Panniculitis
- Pyoderma gangrenosum
  - Diagnosis of exclusion.
  - Over half are associated with underlying systemic disease (IBD, seronegative RA, lymphoproliferative diseases).
- Malignancy
  - Basal cell carcinoma
  - Marjolin ulcer (SCC arising in longstanding ulcerations) – often have rapid enlargement of a lesion despite treatment
  - Metastasis
- Infection
  - Bacterial
  - Atypical microbacterial
  - Viral
  - Fungal
  - Protozoan
- Radiation
- Medications
  - Lower extremity ulceration: hydroxyurea, sunitinib

- Penile erosions: foscarnet, lamivudine
- Scrotal erosions: all-trans-retinoic acid
- Methotrexate (at psoriatic sites)
- IFN-beta (at inoculation sites)
- Skin popping of illicit drugs
- BCG vaccination
- Medications that impair wound healing: cytotoxic, antineoplastic, and immunosuppressive agents, corticosteroids, NSAIDs, anticoagulants

• Vessel inflammation

- Thromboangiitis obliterans
- Small vessel vasculitis (leukocytoclastic vasculitis)
- Small-medium vasculitis/ANCA vasculitis

• Vasculopathy

- Hypercoagulable disorders
- DIC/purpura fulminans
- Sneddon syndrome (usually presenting as livedo reticularis)
- Calciphylaxis
- Warfarin- and heparin-induced necrosis
- Livedoid vasculopathy
- Degos disease (malignant atrophic papulosis)

• Others

- Hypertension (Martorell ulcer – d/t diastolic hypertension > anterolateral leg ulcers with pain out of proportion to the size of the ulcer)
- Malnutrition
- Blood dyscrasias
- Autoimmune conditions

  Scleroderma
  Autoimmune conditions (RA, CLE)
  IBD (metastatic Crohn's disease)

Substance abuse (skin popping, toxic and irritant nature of illicit drugs and adulterants, vasoactive cocaine)
Embolism (cholesterol, bacterial, other)
Trauma
Facticial

DDx of a painful wound: pyoderma gangrenosum, vasculitis, Martorell ulcer, calciphylaxis, sickle cell ulcer, arterial leg ulcer, hydroxyurea ulcer, antiphospholipid antibody syndrome

General Work-Up

- Photo wound at each visit.
- Get measurements: greatest length, perpendicular width, and depth of wound.
- Biopsy atypical wounds
  - Two 6 mm punch biopsies: one at wound edge and one in wound bed
- If the bone is seen or felt, need eval for osteo (bone scan, X-ray).
- Labs
  - CBC with diff
  - Albumin/prealbumin (assess nutritional status)
  - ESR/CRP
  - HgbA1c
  - Wound cultures/tissue cultures: deeper tissue and sent for quantification of colony count per gram. $>10^5$ = impede wound healing
  - Work-up for underlying systemic symptoms as needed

    ANA, RF, ANCAs, D-dimer
  - Venous/arterial flow studies as indicated
  - CT angiography/MR angiography as indicated
  - Referrals as per above

Principles of Wound Care

- TIME = tissue, infection, moisture imbalance, edge advancement: important barriers to wound care

- Tissue – remove necrotic/devitalized tissue and fibrinous slough through some type of debridement.
- Infection – pain, malodor, excessive exudate, friable tissue, and undermined borders are signs.
- Moisture – ensure adequate moisture of wound and reduce excess exudate
- Edge advancement – creates a wound bed environment that promotes healing at the cellular level.

- Wounds heal in a moist environment. Excessive moisture though may cause maceration (soft, white, friable skin). Ideal wound dressing should thus absorb exudate without excessively drying the wound.
- Debridement: removing slough, eschar, exudate, bacterial biofilms, and callus from wound bed in order to permit healing. Debridement can be surgical, mechanical, autolytic, or enzymatic (collagenases). Do not debride arterial ulcers or heel eschar!!
- Compression is a first-line treatment for venous leg ulcers. Must rule out arterial insufficiency before application. ABI or TBI of 0.9–1.2 is normal and can be safely treated with compression. If ABI <0.6 or TBI is <0.4, or either index >1.2, must get vascular consult prior to compression. Also, uncompensated CHF is a relative contraindication. (Note: ABI >1.4 usually means medial calcification due to diabetes and therefore ABI is unreliable.)
- Topical negative pressure devices (VAC): tube embedded in a dressing and covered in airtight dressing; tube is attached to a vacuum, and 100–125 mm Hg is applied in a continuous or intermittent manner. Not appropriate for ischemic wounds.
- Compression recommendations based on ABI in Table 3.6.

Debridement Options: Do Not Debride Arterial Ulcers or Heel Eschar!

- Surgical/mechanical – scissors, curette, scalpel. Should be performed by a skilled practitioner only. Gets faster results. May require local anesthesia. Should be avoided in ischemic limbs and heel ulcers.

TABLE 3.6 Compression recommendations based on ABI

ABI	Compression recommendations
0.8–1.2	High compression therapy
0.5–0.8	Modified compression (≤20 mmg Hg)
<0.5	NO compression

- Mechanical – saline gauze "wet to dry" – less painful than surgical but may hurt viable tissue.
- Autolytic – endogenous enzymes (e.g., proteolytic, fibrinolytic, and collagenic) interact with the moisture-retentive dressings to debride. Often pain-free but slower than other methods. Avoid in septic/immunocompromised patients. Done with a hydrocolloid dressing (DuoDERM, Restore).
- Proteolytic/enzymatic – collagenase ointment applied (Accuzyme, Santyl) (papain has been discontinued); faster than autolytic, selective, easy to use; may crosshatch over eschar with no. 11 or 15 blade and then add. Okay to use on infected wounds but may cause allergy/stinging. Avoid silver dressings.
- Protease-modulating matrix – a protease inhibitor (Promogran) used on diabetic and venous ulcers.
- Biological – maggots/larvae *Lucilia sericata*, *Phaenicia sericata*, and *Lucilia cuprina* (good for debriding very painful wounds as they only eat the dead tissue – but they can be painful, and you have to apply and remove them in the correct timeline).

Offloading Footwear: Refer to Podiatry

- Darko – for digital ulcers and dorsal foot ulcers
- Open heel Darko
- Wedge Darko – especially for distal foot (MT heads). Difficult to walk on.
- Felted foam – MT heads (not as good as total contact), but you can use Darko with it; has Vaseline on the inside. Change q5–7 days.
- PRAFO: posterior relief ankle foot orthosis; offloads the heel, especially in the nursing home – leave on until

TABLE 3.7 Types of compression systems

Compression type	Examples	Advantages	Disadvantages
Elastic (long-stretch) bandages	ACE, SurePress, Dauerbinde, and Biflex Thuasne	Base of the toes to the knees, low working pressure, high resting pressure, >140% extensibility, can be applied spiral or figure of 8	Tend to unravel, do not provide sustained compression, risk of incorrect application
Inelastic (short-stretch) bandages	Unna boot (zinc paste), Comprilan, Circaid (Velcro), FarrowWrap (Velcro), Action, Panelast, Porelast	Comfortable/better tolerance, minimal interference with daily activities, high working pressure, certain bandages with Velcro, enhance fibrinolytic activities	Gauze impregnated with different products, such as zinc oxide, not good for highly exudative wounds, need to be applied well by trained staff
Intermittent compression devices	Pneumatic pump	Enhance fibrinolytic activities	Expensive Require immobility for a few hours per day

(continued)

Table 3.7 (continued)

Compression type	Examples	Advantages	Disadvantages
Multicomponent bandages	Coban 2 (and Coban 2 Lite), Profore, Actico, Softban, "Duke Boot"	Higher compression Graduated compression Sustain a high compression Lite is for patients with mixed venous and arterial disease	Need to be applied by well-trained staff
Compression devices	Variable	Adjustable compression Easy to put on and remove	Expensive Bulky
Support system	Tubigrip	Easy to use Double layer to increase compression	Low compression

healed. Can use saline or Vaseline to heel ulcers; do not use DuoDERM because they get macerated – change daily.

- Total contact cast (gold standard) – change at 1 week and then every 2 weeks.
- Bledsoe Walking Boot – like a contact cast, but removable, which means patients may not wear them.

Compression Systems for Stasis Control (Table 3.7)

Compression Stockings

Compression stockings should be replaced about every 6 months.

Be sure that a patient has palpable arterial pulses and the ABI is appropriate for compression before advising/prescribing compression stockings.

See Table 3.8 for recommendations for how much pressure to recommend in a compression stocking.

- ACE wraps – variable compression
- TED hose – 10 mmg Hg
- Jobst/Advantra – prescription compression hose: need measurements from floor to the knee; shoe size is sometimes used for lighter compression; variety of pressures, up to 40 mm Hg, but these are impossible to put on; custom-made available, but pricey

Table 3.8 Pressure recommendations for compression stockings based on clinical findings

Class	Pressure at ankle	Indication
I	20–30 mm Hg	Mild edema, varicose veins, venous ulcers
II	30–40 mm Hg	Moderate edema, moderate venous disease, varicose veins, venous ulcers
III	40–50 mm Hg	Severe edema, severe venous disease, venous ulcers, lymphedema
IV	50–60 mm Hg	Lymphedema

Boots/Inelastic Compression

- Unna – zinc oxide, glycerin, acacia, castor oil impregnated wrap covered with Coban or ACE to hold in place
- Duke Boot – an Unna boot with DuoDERM over an open area
- Profore – for heavier compression. Four layers: cotton mesh, cotton batting, light compression, and cohesive. Up to 40 mm Hg
  - Better for more exudative wounds
- 3 M compression wrap – dual layer compression; no zinc; uses foam inside for absorption

Orthotic Shoes

- Orthotic shoes – one pair covered yearly by Medicare. Provide extra depth, custom insole; available from orthotics
- Custom-molded shoes – more pricey – made by making cast of the foot; good for Charcot feet

Classes of Dressings (Table 3.9)

Bacterial Control in Wounds

- Topical and/or systemic antibiotics.
  - Metronidazole gel – for odor reduction in malignant or necrotic wounds (works on anaerobes that create the smell)
  - Gram-positive control – e.g., neomycin, bacitracin, and mupirocin
  - Gram-negative control – e.g., gentamicin
- Solution soaks (see below).
- Cadexomer iodine ointment – for ulcers/wounds: spread 1/8–1/4 inch to dry sterile gauze; apply gauze to wound. No more than 50 g per application; no more than 150 g/week. Change 3×/week or when color turns yellow/gray. Can apply a small amount to minor cuts, scrapes, and burns daily – q8h as needed.

TABLE 3.9 Categories of wound dressings

Type of dressing	Notes	When and how to use	Disadvantage	Brand names
Gauze Vaseline-impregnated gauze Regular gauze	Good for packing deep wounds and drying. Used in wet-to-dry dressings. Vaseline gauze good for drier, more painful wounds. Inexpensive, accessible	Only use on minor wounds or as secondary dressings Apply to wound, change every 12 hours. Need secondary dressing.	Painful to remove; exudate can stick and remove healthy keratinocytes in addition to any debris in the wound	
Films	Thin layers of elastic polyurethane that are semi-occlusive. Allow exchange of oxygen and water vapor but impermeable to liquid and bacteria. Dressing does not stick to wound surface Provide barrier against bacteria, permeable to gases, allow for visualization of the wound	Shallow wounds with minimal exudate	Poor drainage of fluid and removal may be potentially damaging to newly formed epithelium	Tegaderm, Polyskin, Bioclusive, Blisterfilm, Omniderm, Proclude, Mefilm, Carrafilm, Transeal

(continued)

Table 3.9 (continued)

Type of dressing	Notes	When and how to use	Disadvantage	Brand names
Hydrogels	Cross-linked hydrophilic polymer holding significant amount of water – composed of mainly water in a complex network or fibers that keep the polymer gel intact. Water is released to keep the wound moist. Low absorption, water based, pain relief, usually good on painful wounds. Excelled for dry, necrotic wounds	Stimulates autolytic debridement and is comfortable for the patient Used for necrotic/sloughy wound beds to rehydrate and remove dead tissue Do not use in exudative wounds Good for painful, drier wounds without much exudate Change every 1–3 days	Low absorption May cause maceration	Vigilon, Nu-Gel, Tegagel, Curagel, Clearsite, Curafil, Curasol, Carrasyn, Hypergel, Normalgel, 2nd Skin, and TransiGel

Hydrocolloids	Malleable sheets composed of carboxymethylcellulose, gelatin, pectin, elastomers, and adhesives that turn into a gel when exudate is absorbed. This creates a warm, moist environment that promotes debridement and healing. Moderate absorption, occlusive, long wear time. Good for mildly exudative wounds. Can stimulate granulation tissue	Use in wounds with light to heavy exudate, sloughing, or granulating wounds Apply to wound, leave in place for up to 3 days, and then remove. No secondary dressing required Avoid in infected wounds	Can cause excess granulation tissue. Malodorous upon removal Gel formation upon removal. Not suitable for cavities Avoid in infected wounds	Most commonly used as self-adhesive pads: DuoDERM, Tegasorb, NuDerm, Comfeel, Cutinoval, Repolicare
Alginates and hydrofibers	Polysaccharides derived from kelp and algae with a component of calcium alginate. When in contact with wound, calcium is exchanged with sodium from wound fluid, and this turns the dressing into a gel that maintains a moist environment. Highly absorbent, hemostatic	Good for exudative wounds and helps debridement in sloughing wounds Exudative wounds (can macerate nearby skin, so only place in wound bed) Non-adherent, so require secondary dressing Hemostatic	Can macerate surrounding skin Not appropriate for dry wounds May need wetting before removal or removal can be painful if too dry	Algiderm, Algisite, Algisorb, Algosteril, Kalostatt, Curasorb, Sorbsan, Melgisorb, SeaSorb

(continued)

TABLE 3.9 (continued)

Type of dressing	Notes	When and how to use	Disadvantage	Brand names
Foams	Bilaminate dressings with hydrophobic polyurethane foam sheets with a hydrophilic surface, designed to absorb large amounts of exudates. Maintain a moist environment but are not as useful as alginates or hydrocolloids for debridement Moderately absorptive, semi-occlusive; provides thermal insulation, protection from shear forces. Good for wounds over bony surfaces and in body cavities and mild to moderately exudative wounds	Use for moderate exudates. Prevents leakage of drainage. Easily shaped to accommodate size of the wound Change every 3 days	Adhere to wound if the drainage dries	Allevyn, Mepilex, PolyMem, BioPatch, CuraFoam, Flexzan, Hydrasorb, Lyofoam

Collagens	Scaffold for new collagen fibers and granulation tissue; porcine, avian, or bovine type I collagen. Comes in gels, powders, and sheets		Cellerate, Fibracol, Puracol
Contact layers	Low adherence to wound prevents trauma and allows exudates to pass through		Mepitel

- Silver-impregnated gauze – used on deep burns and skin sloughing disorders to prevent/treat infection. Good for gram negative, gram positives, and fungi. Can cause localized argyria. Change every 5–7 days (e.g., Acticoat, Aquasel, Actisorb).
- Medihoney – manuka honey that contains natural waxes and oils (in addition to some other "natural" products like aloe vera, vitamin E, and chamomile flower extract depending on the product) and has antimicrobial properties (Medihoney wound gel, Medihoney gel sheet, Medihoney tulle dressing, Medihoney barrier cream). Sterilized with gamma irradiation. Touted to promote a moist wound environment and reduce inflammation, bioburden, and odor.
- Hydrofera Blue – foam dressing impregnated with methylene blue and gentian violet for antimicrobial control. Useful for MRSA, VRE, and *Candida*. Absorptive. Dressing can be left in place up to 7 days. No secondary dressing is required.

Solutions

- Acetic (vinegar) 0.25–0.5%. Boil 1 quart of water, and add 1/2 cup white vinegar or 1 tablespoon of vinegar in 8 ounces of water – good for *Pseudomonas* > Staph
- Dakin – sodium hypochlorite (1/4 cup bleach in 1 gallon of water) – good for staph/maggots
- Domeboro – aluminum sulfate and calcium acetate (1 tab/packet in 1 pint of water) – astringent for weepy/wet areas (Fig. 3.5)

Biologic Dressings and Re-epithelialization Options

- Need to connect wound edges, can use hydrocolloid (DuoDERM, Restore) or biologic dressing
- Biologic dressings
  - Oasis – an extracellular matrix derived from porcine small intestine with collagen, elastin, glycoproteins, proteoglycans, and glycosaminoglycans
  - Apligraf – bilayered bioengineered skin substitute. Constructed by culturing human foreskin-derived neonatal fibroblasts in a bovine type I collagen matrix over which human foreskin-derived neonatal epidermal

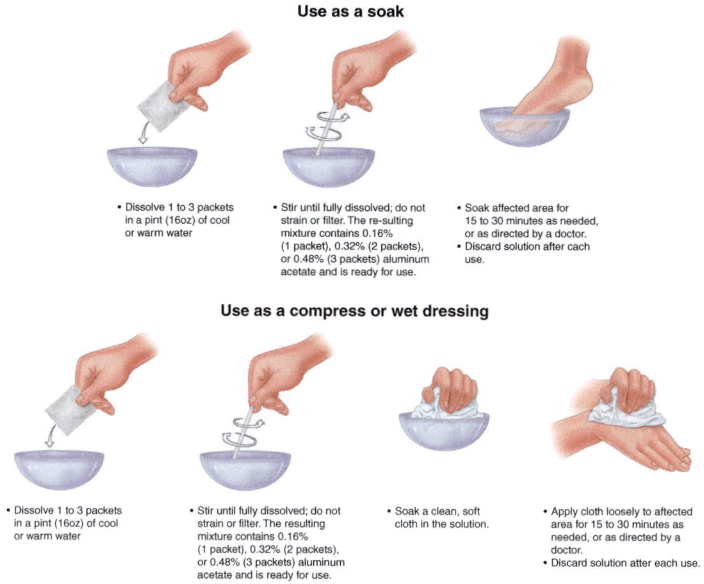

FIGURE 3.5 How to make Domeboro solution for a soak or wet dressing

keratinocytes are then cultured and allowed to stratify. FDA approved for venous leg ulcers >1-month duration and diabetic foot ulcers <3-week duration

Harder to apply than EpiFix

- EpiFix – dehydrated human amnion/chorion tissue that is derived from placental and then dehydrated. Contains cytokines/growth factors known to promote wound healing
- Skin grafting
- Others (see Table 3.10)

Other Options

- Hyperbaric oxygen therapy
- Horse chestnut extract – venodilator, useful in venous ulcers
- Hyperoxygenated fatty acid cream (Mepentol) for pressure ulcers

TABLE 3.10 Types of tissue-based biologic dressings

Type	Description	Uses	Advantages	Disadvantages	Brand names
Epidermal	Cultured epidermal allograft from patient's own skin	Full-thickness burns	Autograft	Expensive, requires pre-ordering, and is a humanitarian use device	Epicel
Dermal	Nylon mesh with porcine allogenic and human fibroblasts attached to silicone membrane Bilayered with matrix of type I bovine collagen and chondroitin 6-sulfate beneath a silicone epidermal sheet Matrix derived from porcine small intestine submucosa Dermal matrix with human fibroblasts seeded onto a bioabsorbable polyglactin mesh scaffold	Superficial burns Partial- and full-thickness chronic ulcers and surgical burns Variety of chronic wounds; contraindicated in third-degree burns Full-thickness diabetic foot ulcers	Transparent permitting visualization, different sizes available, pores allow for drainage Immediately available (2-year shelf life) and can use a variety of wounds Excellent for diabetic wounds	Adherent to wound and risk of infection Requires a two-step operation and is expensive Cannot be used in third-degree burns Must be stored at –75 °C until use and is expensive	Biobrane Integra bilayer wound matrix Oasis Dermagraft

Multilayer	Upper epidermal layer with differentiated keratinocytes; lower dermal layer with bovine type I collagen and human fibroblasts	Venous ulcers lasting for >4 weeks and diabetic foot ulcers lasting >3 weeks	Has occlusive properties	Requires advanced ordering, must be specifically applied	Apligraf

- Topical lidocaine for pain reduction in arterial and venous ulcers
- Negative pressure wound therapy – can promote granulation tissue
- Granulocyte-monocyte colony-stimulating factor by intralesional injection into the VLU wound bed
- Platelet-rich plasma injections

Urticaria and Angioedema

Recommended Reading: Kanani A, et al. *Allergy, Asthma, and Clinical Immunology*. 2001;7(Suppl 1):59 (https://aacijournal.biomedcentral.com/articles/10.1186/1710-1492-7-S1-S9)

Be sure to differentiate urticaria without angioedema from urticaria with angioedema (see section "Angioedema" for additional work-up and treatment considerations).

Also be sure to differentiate acute from chronic urticaria (different causes usually).

Aspirin and NSAIDs are contraindicated in urticaria.

Urticarial vasculitis : usually the lesions are painful or burning and last longer than regular hives per outbreak (>24–48 hours) and can leave residual hyperpigmentation on the skin. Need biopsy to diagnose this condition.

Chronic Urticaria

1. *Can be idiopathic*
2. *Physical urticarias* (Table 3.11)
3. *Drug-induced urticaria*

   - PCN (most common – even PCN in dairy products), NSAIDs (ibuprofen, naproxen, diclofenac), TMP-SMX, cephalosporins, tetracyclines, griseofulvin, opiates (morphine/codeine), radiocontrast agents, ACE inhibitors salicylates (aspirin, especially with nasal polyps, asthma, and food-induced anaphylaxis) but MANY
   - Others: macrolides, aminoglycosides, vancomycin, polymyxin B, tubocurarine, fluoroquinolones, anticoagulants, anticonvulsants, alkylating agents, taxanes, methotrexate, betadine/iodine, dextrans, dextrometho-

Table 3.11 Types of physical urticarias

Physical urticaria	Precipitating factors	Clinical manifestations	Diagnosis
Dermatographism	Rubbing the skin	Wheals with linear distribution appearing minutes after stimulus	Stroking uninvolved skin with pen, wooden tongue plade, or Fric test/ the friction test dermographometer
Pressure urticaria	Pressure	Dermal and subQ swelling appearing 4–6 hours after a pressure stimulus. Remains for 8–72 hours	Pressure challenge on shoulder (7 kg for 15 minutes)
Solar urticaria	UVA, UVB, or visible rays	Wheals within minutes of sun exposures lasting 30 minutes to 2 hours	Phototest (with emergency response equipment nearby)
Cold urticaria	Low temperature	Urticarial plaques can be generalized or confined to areas exposed to cold	Ice cube test (contact for 20 minutes; observe on rewarming)
Heat urticaria	High temperature	Well-defined urticarial lesions confined to sites of heat exposure	Warming of the skin (43 °C for 5 minutes)
Aquagenic urticaria	Water	Small wheal developing within minutes at the sites of contact regardless of temperature or source	Water compresses at 36 °C for 10 minutes
Cholinergic urticaria	Heat, exercise, stress	Pinpoint wheals surrounded by a red flare after sweating	Exercise, hot baths provoke
Vibrational urticaria	Vibration	Angioedema and urticaria on exposed sites	Vibration with a kitchen mixer, Buzzy, or other vibrator on forearm

rphan, trypsin, streptokinase, chymopapain, hydantoins, hydralazine, mannitol, atracurium, vecuronium, succinylcholine, curare, insulin, corticotrophin, vasopressin, progesterone, quinidine, sorbitol, corticosteroids, alteplase, urokinase, vaccines, tubocurarine

4. *Chronic autoimmune urticaria*: anti-FcεRI and less frequently, by anti-IgE autoantibodies that lead to mast cell and basophil activation, thereby giving rise to the release of histamine and other proinflammatory mediators.

   In older patients, also consider urticarial phase of bullous pemphigoid.

   Acute urticaria is often medication or infection related; the rest are idiopathic. Questions to consider in work-up

   - Any systemic involvement/angioedema (dyspnea, throat tightness/closing, trouble swallowing, abdominal pain)
   - Infections: recent sore throat, tooth/sinus infection/diarrhea/travel?
   - Medications: new or OTC Rx? Changing in brand or formulation? Recent exposure to contact material? New aspirin, NSAID, opiate, or ACE inhibitor?
   - Recent vaccinations?
   - Foods: ingestion of new or non-routine foods, esp. tomatoes, strawberries, melons, cheese, wine/alcohol, garlic, onions, eggs, milk, spices, shellfish, or processed/packaged foods?
   - Hepatitis – history of abdominal pain, jaundice, hepatitis, or IVDA?
   - Paraneoplastic – up to date on recommended cancer screening?
   - Chronic Urticaria - see tables 3.11 and 3.12 for consideration

Work-Up

History is important to diagnose urticaria and differentiate acute from chronic and establish a potential cause.

See Table 3.12 *for laboratory work-up recommendations.*

Urticaria Treatment Algorithm (Fig. 3.6)

Prescribe an EpiPen to all patients with urticaria with angioedema, anaphylaxis history, or symptoms.

Table 3.12 Laboratory work-up considerations for chronic urticaria

Lab evaluation	Indications
CBC with differential	Increased eos: parasitic infection, drug reaction, hypereosinophilic syndrome
ESR	Elevated with chronic inflammation (urticarial vasculitis)
CMP with LFTs	Hepatic and renal dysfunction may indicate underlying disease
Throat culture	If history suggestive of strep throat
Urinalysis	If history suggestive of UTI
Stool ova and parasites	Indicated if eosinophilia or travel, history of GI complaints
Hepatitis B and C titers	May be positive in chronic urticaria and cryoglobulin-associated cold urticaria
Serum cryoglobulins	May be positive in cold urticaria and urticarial vasculitis
Thyroid function tests and anti-thyroid Abs	Strong association with chronic autoimmune urticaria
ANA titers	Indicated in urticarial vasculitis
Complement studies (C3, C4, C1q)	Low C4 in C1-INH deficiency; low C3 in systemic vasculitis)
RAST and prick test	Indicated with history of food allergy or contact urticaria
Dental/sinus films	To assess for occult/chronic infection
Stool *H. pylori*	Associated with chronic urticaria
SPEP/UPEP	Can be used to ID increases in IgG and thus can help confirm the dx of chronic autoimmune disease
Anti IgE-IgG	

(continued)

TABLE 3.12 (continued)

Lab evaluation	Indications
Optional: basophil activation test, autologous serum skin test (ASST), allergy consultation	The ASST is currently one of the most useful tests for confirming a diagnosis of chronic autoimmune urticaria (sensitivity, 65–81%; specificity, 71–78%). It involves intradermal injection of the patient's own serum (collected while the patient is symptomatic) into uninvolved skin. A positive wheal and flare reaction is considered indicative of circulating autoantibodies to the high-affinity IgE receptor on mast cells
Biopsy	To rule out vasculitis or bullous pemphigoid

Angioedema

Angioedema in absence of urticaria should lead to investigation for diagnoses such as hereditary or acquired angioedema (HAE, AAE).

Angioedema associated with ACE inhibitors; bradykinin (which is regulated by the C1 inhibitor) appears to play a role.

Idiopathic angioedema is most common.

Arthropod bites may also trigger hypersensitivity rxn type I.

<u>Angioedema work-up</u>: must rule out C1-INH deficiency

- C1 inhibitor level
- C1 inhibitor function
- C1q
- C4
- + urticaria work-up (esp. CBC with diff, *H. pylori*, and SPEP)
- Lymph node examination

Comparison of HAE and AAE

HAE and AAE are characterized by recurrent episodes of angioedema without urticaria or pruritus, usually of the skin, mucosal tissues, GI, or upper respiratory tracts.

HAE usually presents in late childhood/adolescence (75%). May have + family history (in approx. 75%).

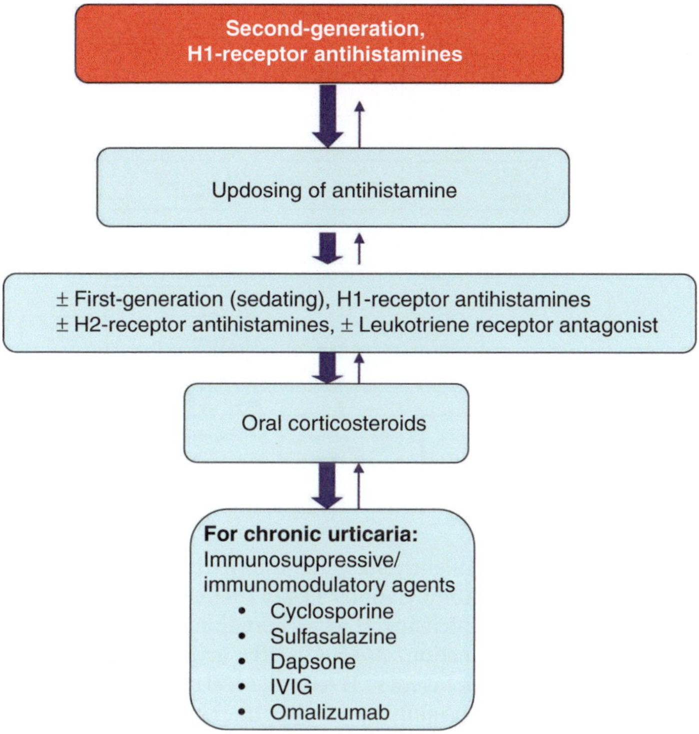

FIGURE 3.6 Therapeutic approach to treatment of chronic urticaria

AAE develops in patients in their 30s–40s with underlying lymphoproliferative d/o (especially B-cell) or autoimmune disease; no family history.

Diagnostic Algorithm for HAE and AAE (Fig. 3.7)

Laboratory Differences Between HAE1, HAE2, and AAE (Table 3.13)

HAE type I: C1q nl, C4 low, C1-INH low level and fxn
HAE type II: C1q nl, C4 low, C1-INH nl/high level, low fxn
AAE: C1q low, C4 low, C1-INH nl/low level, low fxn

Treatment of Angioedema

- Avoid ASA, NSAIDs, and alcohol.
- Patients must carry cards notifying of their conditions/ MediAlert bracelets

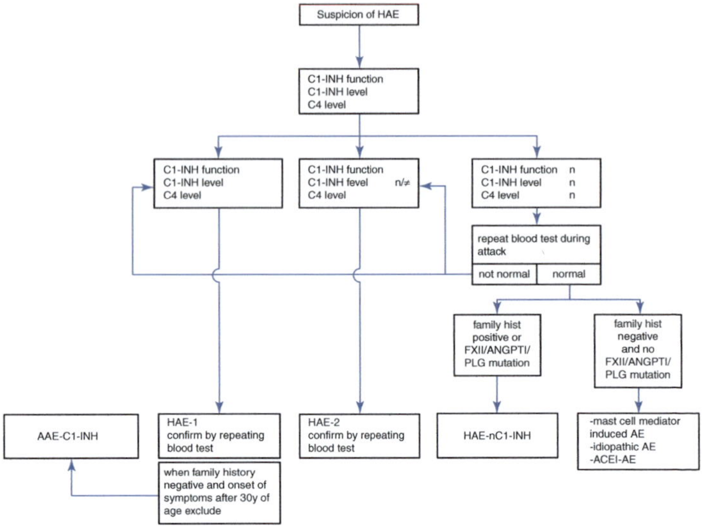

FIGURE 3.7 Diagnostic algorithm by the International WAO/EAACI for HAE and AAE. Abbreviations: HAE-1 hereditary angioedema due to C1-inhibitor deficiency, HAE-2 hereditary angioedema due to C1-inhibitor dysfunction, AAE-C1-INH acquired angioedema due to C1-inhibitor deficiency, HAE nC1-INH hereditary angioedema with normal C1-inhibitor levels, either due to mutation in factor XII (FXII) angiopoetin (ANGPTI) or plasminogen (PLG), ACEI-AE angiotensin converting enzyme inhibitor-induced angioedema. (From: *World Allergy Organization Journal*, volume 11, Article number: 5 (2018))

TABLE 3.13 Laboratory profile in HAE type I and II patients

	C1-INH function	**C1-INH protein level**	**C4 protein level**
HAE1	↓	↓	↓
HAE2	↓	Normal/↑	↓

- Develops in patients in their 30s–40s with underlying lymphoproliferative d/o (especially B-cell) or autoimmune disease.

Overview of Therapeutic Interventions for HAE and AAE
Prophylactic Steps for Patients with Angioedema

Trigger avoidance
- Mild trauma
- Anxiety/stress
- *H. pylori* infection
- ACE inhibitors
- Estrogen-containing medications

Attenuated androgens (danazol, stanozolol)
Tranexamic acid
C1 inhibitor replacement therapy

Treatment Algorithm for Hereditary Angioedema (As Recommended by the International WAO/EAACI)
- In HAE types I and II, the treatment of choice in acute attacks consists of replacement with commercially available C1 inhibitor (C1-INH) concentrates [12] or kallikrein inhibitor or, if those are unavailable, fresh-frozen plasma. In HAE with normal C1 inhibitor levels, infusion of C1-INH has proven to be ineffective.

Anaphylaxis
- *Life-threatening*
- *Occurs within minutes of drug administration/contact*
- *Most common to medications, especially antibiotics, latex, and radiocontrast*
- *Treatment: epinephrine, IV/PO steroids, and PO steroids*
- *Need to hospitalize serious cases. Hereditoary Angioedema should have fresh-frozen plasma administered.*

Prescribe an EpiPen to all patients with urticaria with angioedema, anaphylaxis history, or symptoms.

Blistering Diseases

Pemphigus

- Autoimmune blistering disease resulting in destruction of keratinocyte cell-to-cell adhesion above the basement membrane
- Groups
  - Pemphigus vulgaris (PV) (and pemphigus vegetans)
  - Pemphigus foliaceus (PF) (pemphigus erythematosus, fogo selvagem)
  - Paraneoplastic pemphigus
  - IgA pemphigus
  - Drug-induced (see dermatopharmacology section)
- Antibodies
  - PV: desmoglein 3
  - PF: desmoglein 1
  - IgA pemphigus: desmocollin 1
- Compensation theory
  - Desmogleins 1 and 3 are not evenly distributed in the skin (Fig. 3.8): desmoglein 1 higher up in the epidermis; desmoglein 3 lower in the epidermis.
  - In mucous membranes: more desmoglein 3 than 1 (thus why PV often with oral lesions, but PF lacks them)
  - Both anti-Dsg1 and anti-Dsg3: blisters in the skin and mucous membrane
- Important clinical features
  - All patients with PV have mucosal erosions.

    Esophagus, conjunctivae, and genital mucosa may be involved and can cause significant morbidity.
  - >50% have cutaneous involvement (erosions and flaccid bullae, + Nikolsky, + Asboe-Hansen sign).
  - PF: crusted "corn flakes," often in seb derm distribution; usually no mucosal involvemnet

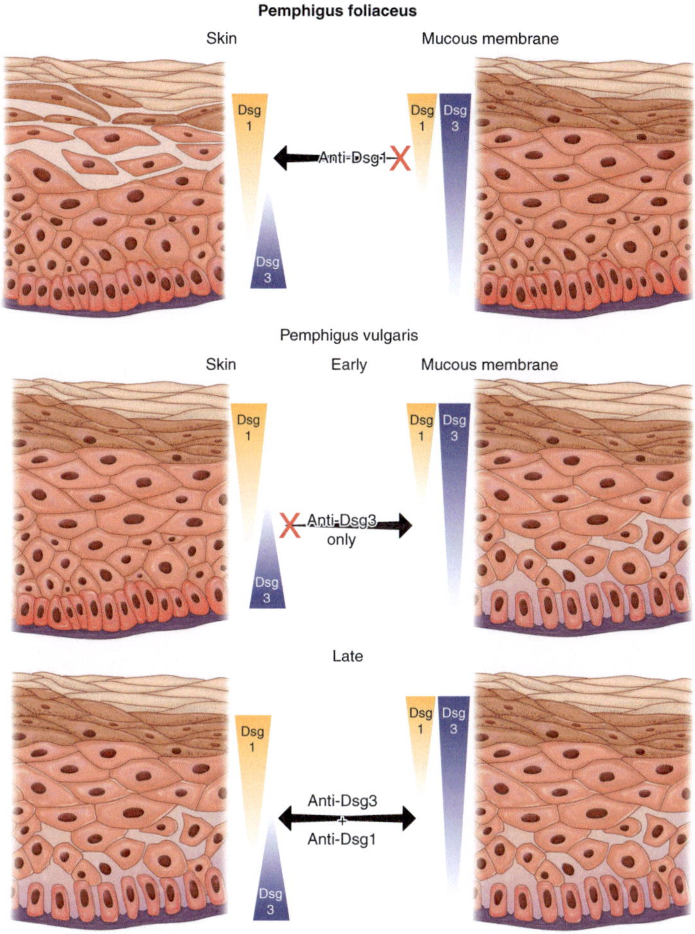

FIGURE 3.8 Distribution of desmogleins 1 and 3 in the skin and mucous membranes

- Pemphigus foliaceus subtypes
  - Fogo selvagem

    Type of endemic PF in Brazil
    Worsened by sun exposure and ionizing radiation
    May be due to an environmental trigger (*Simulium* black flies?)
  - Pemphigus erythematosus (Senear-Usher): PF + SLE overlap, in seborrheic areas

    ANA + in 30%
    DIF intercellular and linear IgG at basement membrane zone (BMZ)

IgA Pemphigus

- Two types:
  - Subcorneal pustular dermatosis (SPD)
  - Intraepidermal neutrophilic dermatosis (IEN)
- Clinical presentations
  - Flaccid vesicles or pustules on the skin; pustules tend to coalesce to form annular or circinate pattern with crusts in center.
  - Sunflower configuration is classic for IEN.
  - Axilla, groin, trunk, and proximal extremities most common; rarely have mucous membrane involvement.
- Work-up
  - Biopsy for H&E and DIF
    (a) SPD cannot be distinguished from Sneddon-Wilkinson; need DIF.
    (b) IgA deposits intracellularly in SPD.
    (c) May be associated with underlying IgA gammopathy.

Drug-Induced Pemphigus

Penicillamine & captopril (most common two), pyritinol, penicillin, ampicillin, rifampin (may be drug-triggered; rash does not resolve with stopping medication), cephalosporins, ACE inhibitors (likely to cause vegetans), piroxicam, gold, phenylbutazone, propranolol, carbamazepine, thiopurine, thiamazole, pyrazolone derivatives (phenylbutazone, aminopyrine, azapropazone, oxyphenbutazone), levodopa, heroin, progesterone, phenobarbital, lysine, N-acetylsalicylate

- Usually goes into remission once medication is stopped (except for rifampin)

Paraneoplastic Pemphigus (PNP)

- Antibodies attacking the plakins (basement membrane zone (BMZ) + inter-epithelial targets)
  - BP 230 (BP Ag1)
  - Desmoplakin I and II
  - Periplakin, envoplakin, plectin
- 1/3 of patients have no underlying malignancy at the time of first mucocutaneous eruption.
  - NHL 40% > CLL 30% > Castleman 10% > malignant/benign thymoma 6%; sarcomas 6%; Waldenstrom's macroglobulinemia 6%
- Clinical features
  - Intractable stomatitis; affects all oropharynx and extends to vermillion lip
  - Severe pseudomembranous conjunctivitis; GI and genital mucosa
  - Cutaneous: polymorphic vesicles, flaccid blisters, lichenoid or EM-like eruptions; can involve palms/soles (unlike PV)
- Bronchiolitis obliterans: most common cause of death.

Overall Work-Up for Pemphigus

Biopsy for H&E and DIF (see biopsy section)

- DIF: intercellular IgG4 > C3 (net-like, chicken wire)

  Indirect immunofluorescence

- Monkey esophagus: +80–90% PV
- Rat bladder: PNP
- Guinea pig: PF

Serum antibody (ELISA) correlates with disease activity and is helpful for clinical monitoring and more sensitive than IIF.

Malignancy screenings for PNP

Treatment of Pemphigus

- Rituximab – can be first-line therapy. No clear consensus on dosing schedule
  - 375 mg/m^2 body surface area once weekly for 4 weeks (lymphoma protocol) OR
  - Two infusions of 1000 mg 2 weeks apart (RA protocol)
  - Two infusions of 500 mg 2 weeks apart (low-dose RA protocol)
  - "The RA protocol produced a higher response rate, relapse rate, number of infections, but lower mortality rate, and lacked nonresponders." Zakka Labib. *Dermatol Ther*. 2012;2(1):17
  - "Patients who received lymphoma vs rheumatoid arthritis dosing were 2.70-fold more likely to achieve complete remission off therapy" (odds ratio [OR], 2.70; 95% CI, 1.03–7.12; $P = 0.04$). Kushner CJ. *JAMA Derm*. 2019;155(12):1404–9
- Oral prednisone/prednisolone 1 mg/kg/day to start WITH
- Azathioprine (40 mg/day up to 3 mg/kg/day), mycophenolate mofetil (2–3 g/day), or IVIG (400 mg/kg/day × 5 days followed by 400 mg/kg/day every 6 weeks for 6 months–1 year)
- Second line: methotrexate (12.5 mg/week on average), cyclophosphamide, plasmapheresis
- Dapsone for IgA pemphigus

Ref: Cholera M et al. *Adv Ther*. 2016;33:910–58.

Bullous Pemphigoid

- The most common autoimmune subepidermal blistering disease

- Usually a chronic disease with spontaneous exacerbations and remissions, which may be accompanied by significant morbidity
- Types
  - Bullous pemphigoid
  - Mucous membrane pemphigoid (MMP)/cicatricial pemphigoid
  - Pemphigoid gestationis
  - Childhood BP
  - Drug-induced (see below)
- Antibodies
  - BP antigen 1 (230)
  - BP antigen 2 (180)
  - Integrin and laminin 5 (MMP)
- Epidemiology
  - Onset usually after 60 years old (elderly)
  - Higher risk in patients with neurologic disease: stroke, Parkinson's disease, dementia
- Important clinical features
  - Prodrome stage can be characterized by intensely pruritic urticarial plaques.
  - Large tense blisters are common (vs flaccid bullae in PV).
  - 10–35% with oral involvement; eyes, nose, oropharynx, and anogenital region are rarely affected.
  - Fifty percent may have peripheral eosinophilia, correlated with disease severity.
  - Poorly controlled bullous pemphigoid can be associated with a transient palmoplantar keratoderma which goes away (generally over 4–6 months) with treatment.

Mucous Membrane/Cicatricial Pemphigoid

- Predominant involvement of external mucosal surfaces and tendency for scarring.
- Scarring and fibrosis affect conjunctivae, which can lead to blindness.

- Antibodies
  - $\beta 4$ subunit of a6$\beta 4$ integrin; predominantly ocular involvement.
  - BP 180, distal carboxyl terminus.
  - *Laminin 5 (332)*
    Associated with malignancy risk (adenocarcinoma, solid organ tumors)
  - Serum antibody is not predictive of disease activity.
- Important clinical features
  - 2× as common in females.
  - Oral mucosa (1) and conjunctivae (2) are the most commonly involved sites.
  - Can affect any mucosal surface (upper airway, esophagus, anogenital)
  - Eighty-five percent have oral involvement: often involve gingiva, buccal mucosa, palate, alveolar ridges > tongue, and lips.
  - Desquamative gingivitis and loss of teeth.
  - Conjunctivitis, symblepharon, and blindness.
  - Nasopharyngeal: voice hoarseness, strictures, and dysphagia.
  - Skin lesions in 25–30%; most frequently involve the scalp, face, neck, and upper trunk; erythematous plaques; may have blisters, erosions.
- Brunsting-Perry variant
  - Limited to the head and neck; mucosal involvement is absent; causes scarring alopecia

Pemphigoid Gestationis/Herpes Gestationis

- Occurs late in pregnancy (second or third trimester) or immediately postpartum
  - Starts periumbilically; abrupt onset with rapid progression to a generalized pemphigoid-like eruption.
  - Pruritic urticarial plaques/papules with tense bullae.
  - Usually spares mucous membranes.

- Most disease activity remits spontaneously weeks to months following delivery; flares/recurrences can happen during menses, OCP use, and subsequent pregnancies (very common).
- ~10% newborns develop mild skin involvement due to passive transfer of maternal antibodies; it usually resolves within days to weeks.
- *Increase prematurity in neonates and small for gestational age*
  Due to chronic placental insufficiency.
  Risk correlates with disease severity.
- Mom at risk for developing Grave's disease.

Childhood Bullous Pemphigoid

- Similar to adults, but sites may differ.
  - Genital involvement in about 1/2 of patients
- Infants: bullae first appear on acral sites > generalize.
- Disease may be self-limited.

Drug-Induced Pemphigoid

- Beta-blockers, furosemide, NSAIDs (ibuprofen), sulfa-containing drugs (sulfasalazine), terbinafine, estrogen (OCPs), PCN, penicillamine, captopril, gold, gliptins, spironolactone, amoxicillin, ciprofloxacin, potassium iodide
- Usually goes into remission once medication is stopped

Overall Work-Up for Pemphigoid

- Biopsy for H&E and DIF (see biopsy section)
  - BP/PG/MMP: linear C3, IgG4, and IgG1 at BMZ (be sure to also assess for IgA).
  - Start with DIF. If that is negative but high suspicion, repeat and do IIF on salt split skin and ELISA for BP 230/180.
  - DIF is most sensitive (90.8%) > IIF (76%), ELISA (BP 180 > BP 230).
    ELISA can be falsely negative in ~8% of patients with BP because the antigen maps to regions outside of the NC16A domain.

ELISA can sometimes correlate with disease activity.
- False-positive DIF can be seen in bullous scabies.

- Indirect immunofluorescence
  - BP/PG: 60–80% with detectable autoantibodies
  - Salt split skin
    BP and PG limited to epidermal side (roof)
    MMP antibodies to integrin and BP 180 limited to epidermal side
    MMP laminin 5 antibody limited to dermal (floor)

Overall Treatment Recommendations

- Bullous pemphigoid:
  - High-potency topical steroids for local disease
    Clobetasol may be superior to systemic steroids even in extensive disease, 30–40 g/day application.
  - Mild disease: tetracycline-type antibiotic and nicotinamide
    200 mg/day doxycycline + nicotinamide
  - Prednisone (0.5–1 mg/kg/day)
    Try to limit use/get down to physiologic dosing as soon as you can.
    If can get prednisone <10 mg/day, consider adjuvant.

- See prednisone in the dermatopharmacology section for bony, PCP ppx, and other guidelines for administration.
  - Rituximab
  - Nonsteroidal immunosuppressants with plan to taper over months
    Azathioprine (75–150 mg/day), mycophenolate (1–1.5 g BID), methotrexate (5–15 mg/week).
    See dermatopharmacology section for monitoring/screening before starting.
  - Other off-label treatments
    Dupilumab.
    Omalizumab.

- In patients with elevated IgE and/or eosinophilia
  Dapsone (50–100 mg/day).
  Combination of rituximab and/or IVIg for nonresponders may be helpful.

  - Pemphigoid gestationis

    Topical steroids/systemic antihistamine (diphenhydramine, chlorpheniramine, loratadine, cetirizine, levocetirizine [category B]) for prebullous stage
    Bullous stage: 0.5–1 mg/kg/day prednisone
    Potent immunosuppression postpartum if necessary

  - Mucous membrane pemphigoid

    Rituximab
    Prednisone
    Dapsone (50–150 mg/day)
    Cyclophosphamide (1–2 mg/kg/day) may be necessary + steroid for rapid ocular disease; oral steroid (usually insufficient alone)
    Work-up for malignancy in laminin 5+ patients

Linear IgA Bullous Disease

- Immune-mediated subepidermal vesiculobullous eruption that occurs in adults and children.
- In adults, LABD is frequently drug-induced.
- Antibodies
  - IgA1 ab to LABD 97 (a cleaved ectodomain of BP180)
- Associations
  - GI disease, autoimmune disease, malignancies, infections; gluten-sensitive enteropathy
- Important clinical features
  - Variable findings: can look like BP or dermatitis herpetiformis.
  - Frequently polycyclic or annular.
  - Perioral and genital involvement.

- Kids

  Annular erythema and blisters (crowns of jewels) predominantly in flexural areas esp. lower trunk, thighs, and groin

- May also present as a variant of mucous membrane (cicatricial pemphigoid with oral, nasal, pharyngeal, and esophageal lesions); the ocular form of LABD is indistinguishable from MMP.
- Natural course of disease: persistence for several years with eventual spontaneous remission in many patients; childhood LABD remits within 2–4 years.

• Drug-induced

- Can have more widespread bullous involvement with macular erythema
- Vancomycin (most common), beta-lactam abx (PCN), TMP-SMX, NSAIDs, furosemide, lithium, ACE inhibitor (captopril), amiodarone, phenytoin, diclofenac, cyclosporine, somatostatin, cefamandole, vigabatrin, rifampin, G-CSF, sodium hypochlorite (bleach)
- May be associated with IgA nephropathy

• Work-up
- Biopsy for H&E and DIF (see biopsy section)

  Band-like IgA at the DEJ
  Rule out dermatitis herpetiformis (DH)

- Indirect immunofluorescence

  Salt split skin limited to epidermal side, positive in 30% adults and 75% kids

• Treatment
- Stop culprit medication.
- Dapsone (usually 50–150 mg/day; kids 1–2 mg/kg/day), colchicine (1–1.5 g/day).
- Can add prednisone 40 mg to achieve complete control.

- Successful treatment in kids with oral antibiotics, dicloxacillin, erythromycin, tetracyclines, and TMS-SMZ, has been reported.

Dermatitis Herpetiformis (DH)

- Cutaneous manifestation of gluten sensitivity (~100%); however, only 20% of celiac patients have DH.
- Antibodies
  - IgA to transglutaminase 3 (TG3).
  - Antibodies to transglutaminase 2 seen in CD.
  - HLA-DQ2 strong association ≫ HLA-DQ8.
  - *Anti-endomysial antibodies are very specific for DH and CD*

    Found in 80% of DH and >95% of CD
  - *Levels indicate severity of gluten sensitivity enteropathy and reflect degree of compliance with dietary gluten restriction.*
- Common associations: *Hashimoto's, DM*, pernicious anemia, SLE, other autoimmune diseases; risk for possible enteropathy-related T cell lymphoma
- Important clinical features
  - Grouped papules and vesicles, excoriated papules, intensely pruritic.
  - Predominantly found over the elbow, knees, sacral back, buttocks, and occipital scalp.
  - Ingestion of iodide can worsen DH.
- Work-up
  - Biopsy for H&E and DIF (see biopsy section)
  - Granular pattern of IgA at the dermal papillae
  - Differentiates from linear IgA (linear band of IgA at basement membranse zone (BMZ))

- Serologic testing
  - Total serum IgA, anti-gliadin, anti-TG2 (anti-tissue transglutaminase), anti-TG3 (anti-epidermal transglutaminase), anti-endomysial IgA
- Treatment
  - Gluten-free diet.
  - Dapsone typically relieves pruritus within 24–48 hours; it recurs in 24–48 hours if dapsone is stopped.
  - Initial dose of dapsone 25–50 mg in adults maintenance of 0.5–1 mg/kg/day; 0.5 mg/kg in kids.
  - If cannot tolerate dapsone, sulfapyridine 500 mg TID up to 2 g TID; increase fluid intake and alkalinization of urine to avoid renal stones.

Epidermolysis Bullosa Acquisita (EBA)

- Rare, acquired, chronic, subepidermal bullous disease that is often recalcitrant to treatment
- Seen in both adults and kids
- Antibodies
  - Type VII collagen (major component of anchoring fibrils of DEJ)
- Important clinical features
  - Bullae + evidence of scarring/milia: Presents with either mechanobullous disorder mimicking dystrophic EB or clinical features indistinguishable from BP or more rarely mucous membrane pemphigoid

    Non-inflammatory bullae that heal with atrophic scar and milia.
    Acral blisters that heal with atrophic scarring and milia, PIH.
    Nail dystrophy/loss, scalp involvement in up to 20%.
    Mucous membrane: mouth, oropharynx, esophagus, and ocular involvement can be variable.
    Scalp involvement > scarring alopecia.

Childhood EBA have substantial overlap with childhood BP and LABD.

- Chronic and more refractory to treatment than BP

- Associations
  - IBD, myeloma, SLE, RA, diabetes, Crohn's (most frequent association)
- Work-up
  - Biopsy for H&E and DIF (see biopsy section)
  - Linear IgG and/or IgA, IgM, and C3 at basement membrane zone (BMZ)
  - Indirect immunofluorescence
  - Autoantibodies to type VII collagen
  - 50% with IgG > IgA
  - Salt split skin limited to floor side
- Treatment
  - Difficult: symptomatic – avoid trauma; treat wounds and secondary infections.
  - Prednisone (1 mg/kg and then taper) + nonsteroidal immunosuppressants (antineutrophilic in inflammatory subtype).
  - Dapsone (100–200/day).
  - Colchicine (1–2 mg/day).
  - Cyclosporine (higher doses may be required), azathioprine, methotrexate, mycophenolate mofetil.
  - IVIG, rituximab, extracorporeal photopheresis.

References

- Joost et al. *JAMA Derm.* 2019;155(2):158–165.
- Khalaf et al. *JAMA Derm.* 2019;155(2):166–171.
- Elston DM et al. *JAAD.* 2016;74(1):1–16.
- Meijer et al. *JAMA Derm.* 2019;155(2):158–65.
- Ahmed et al. *JAAD.* 2016;74(4):700–8.
- Kaye A et al. *JAMA Derm.* 2018;(10):1225–1226.
- Bolotin D et al. *JAAD.* 2011 64;(6):1017–24.
- Bolotin D et al. *JAAD.* 2011 64;(6):1027–33.
- Engineer L et al. *JAAD.* 2001 44;(5)818–28.
- Krindin K et al. *Dermatologic Clinics.* 2019;37(2):215–228.

Drug Reactions

All serious drug reactions require a drug timeline to be created to help decipher the culprit medication.

Steps When Evaluating a Possible Drug Reaction

1. Stop all unnecessary medications – just keep the bare essentials.
2. Ask about non-prescription medications (e.g., "what pills have you put in your mouth over the last 3 weeks?") and also eye drops, suppositories, injections, and recreational drugs, too.
3. No matter how atypical the patient's cutaneous reaction, always consider medication as a possible cause. Check the manufacturer reports.
4. <u>Make a drug-timing chart with dates across the top and all drugs taken within the last 2 weeks listed down the side.</u>
5. Assess likelihood of a drug to cause the patient's specific rash pattern.
   (a) Litt's Drug Eruption online (requires subscription)
   (b) literature review

Simple Drug Eruption

Occurs 7–10 days after first exposure, as early as 48 hours after subsequent exposure.

Typical features include:

- No facial involvement (unless HIV, then facial involvement may occur)
- No bulla
- No lymphadenopathy
- No mucous membrane involvement
- No systemic signs/symptoms
- Normal labs (some eos okay)
- Low-grade fever sometimes
- Usually pruritic (unlike viral, which is often non-pruritic and associated with conjunctivitis, URI symptoms, ± an enanthem)
- Rash typically polymorphous

- Simple drug eruption/"morbilliform drug eruption" is classically polymorphous with morbilliform or sometimes urticarial lesions on the limbs, confluent areas on the thorax, and purpuric lesions on the ankles and feet.
- Pruritus and low-grade fever are often present.
- On the trunk, the eruption may appear scarlatiniform.
- Annular plaques or atypical, irregularly shaped "target" lesions may be present, leading to the misdiagnosis, and thus overdiagnosis, of erythema multiforme.

- Typical medications to cause: aminopenicillins (penicillins, cephalosporins), sulfonamides, allopurinol, NSAIDs, anticonvulsants, but MANY drugs have been reported.
- Treatment is supportive: topical anti-pruritics, topical corticosteroids, PO antihistamines
- Typically resolves after 1–2 weeks without sequelae

Differential

- Viral (EBV, enteroviruses, adenoviruses, early HIV, HHV6/7, COVID-19) – should have viral prodrome, no meds, conjunctivitis/tongue findings, lymphadenopathy, and increased white count with lymphopenia. (Peripheral blood eosinophilia favors a drug reaction.)
- GVHD – >10 days after engraftment, folliculocentric to start, palmo-plantar and post-auricular involvement, diarrhea, LFTs (bili increased)
- Toxic shock syndrome, scarlet fever, Kawasaki disease, Still's disease also on DDx
- Early complex drug

Complex Drug Eruptions

Drug Reaction with Eosinophilia and System Symptoms/Drug-Induced Hypersensitivity Syndrome (DRESS/DIHS)

- Triad of morbilliform rash + fever + internal organ involvement

- Occurs >3 weeks after Rx started (mean = 22 days)
- Clinical features
  - Facial edema (can have facial pustules/facial crusting)
  - Rash (often urticarial/morbilliform; edematous, weeping at times)
  - Lymphadenopathy
  - Labs
    Eosinophilia >1500 absolute eos (no eos with dapsone)
- If eos > 4000, worry about cardiac infiltration.
  Atypical lymphocytes
  If doing poorly, HHV6/HHV7 serologies
- Early: multiorgan failure (hepatitis > nephritis > pneumonitis, encephalitis, myocarditis, pericarditis, pancreatitis, thyroiditis)
- Late
  - Autoimmune disease: thyroid disease, SIADH, dermatomyositis, SLE (due to decreased T-regs).
  - May have late relapse/recurrence
    4 months: can have myocarditis/STEMI.
  - 1 and 3 months after hospitalization: check thyroid function (TSH) and lytes.

Algorithms for Diagnosis

- RegiSCAR Criteria (European) – must have three of the four starred (*) for diagnosis:
  - Hospitalization
  - Reaction suspected to be drug-related
  - Acute rash*
  - Fever >38*
  - Lymphadenopathy in at least two sites*
  - Involvement of at least one internal organ*
  - Blood count abnormalities (lymphopenia or lymphocytosis*, eosinophilia*, thrombocytopenia*)

- RegiSCAR Criteria (Japanese) – must need seven of the nine:
  - Maculopapular rash developing 3 weeks after starting therapy of the suspected drug
  - Prolonged clinical symptoms 2 weeks after discontinuation of the suspected drug
  - Fever >38 °C
  - Liver abnormalities (ALT >100) or other organ involvement
  - Leukocyte abnormalities
  - Leukocytosis (>11 × 19^9/L)
  - Atypical lymphocytosis (>5%)
  - Lymphadenopathy
  - HHV6 reactivation

Summary of the Algorithms

- Common Medications to Cause
  - Anticonvulsants (phenobarbital, lamotrigine, carbamazepine, phenytoin)
  - Sulfonamides (especially sulfamethoxazole, sulfadiazine, and sulfasalazine)
  - Allopurinol
  - Nevirapine
  - Abacavir
  - Dapsone
  - Minocycline
  - Vancomycin
  - Gold
- Work-up
  - CBC w/ diff + ferritin; LFTs + GGT + PT/PTT; BMP; UA with protein/creatinine ratio and urinary eosinophil count; CK; LDH; triglycerides; TSH; parathyroid hormone; lipase; SPEP; CRP; HHV6/7, EBV, CMV; blood culture; ANA; EKG, echo; IgA level.
  - Evaluate CBC, LFTs, creatinine, and LDH at least twice per week.

- CXR if due to minocycline as commonly associated with interstitial PNA.
- LDH, methemoglobin level, albumin level if d/t dapsone (get hemolysis with resultant liver failure).
- There can be neurologic manifestations to DIHS that can look like CNS zoster but resolve quickly.
- Look for herpes viral reactivation in the setting of DIHS: HHV6, HHV7, CMV, HSV, and VZV.
- 1 and 3 months after hospitalization: check thyroid function (TSH) and lytes.

- Treatment
  - See chart below.
  - *Immediate withdrawal of offending drug.*
  - Prednisone or prednisolone 1–1.5 mg/kg/day gradually tapered over 3–6 months to avoid relapse (can take up to 9 months).

    If cases with no improvement, exacerbation of symptoms, and/or GI involvement: change to IV methylprednisolone.

    - Monitor CBC, LFT, lymph nodes, and organ tests.
  - Case reports of cyclosporine 5 mg/kg divided BID helping – can work quickly and be stopped without residual treatments required (Kirchhof M et al. *JAMA Derm* 2016;152:1254–7).

    Typically we consider these in cases of mild DRESS/DIHS.
  - Anti-herpes medications: valganciclovir.
  - N-Acetylcysteine may be added if hepatitis is present (most data with anticonvulsants).
    Can be associated with angioedema
  - Steroid-sparing strategies (do addition to steroids).
    High-dose IVIg (2 g/kg over 5 days)

    - Can help with viral reactivation.

- Add on if worsening on prednisone.
  Cyclosporine
  Cyclophosphamide
  Mycophenolate mofetil (for long-term steroid sparing treatment)

- Monitoring
  - Can get late relapse/recurrence of DRESS due to decreased T-regs

    Steroid therapy may promote reactivation of viruses (esp. herpes viruses) that can be associated with rare long-lasting steroid-dependent variant of DRESS.
  - 1 and 3 months after hospitalization: check thyroid function (TSH) and lytes.
  - If relapses/recurrence, increase prednisone, start IVIg, and consider mycophenolate mofetil for long-term steroid-sparing treatment.

    Ref: *JAAD*. 2012;66(6):e229–36
    Ref: *JAAD*. 2013;68(5):CME

- Mortality
  - Up to 10%: most from hepatic necrosis and also septic shock (bacteremia/fungemia)
  - Poor prognostic signs

    SIRS response: tachycardia/tachypnea
    High absolute eosinophil count (>6000/uL)
    Pancytopenia/thrombocytopenia/leukocytosis
    Coagulopathy
    GI bleeding
    H/o chronic renal insufficiency
    Multiple organ involvement
    Multiple underlying diseases

Specific findings with specific drugs in DRESS

- Anticonvulsant – as it evolves, it can get widespread pinpoint pustules (especially in darker Fitzpatrick skin types). Valproate is the safest alternative.
- Allopurinol – typically in patients with renal failure. HLA-B5801. Very slow to resolve. Requires months of steroids.
- Minocycline – often with interstitial pneumonia > ARDS.
- Dapsone – usually NO eosinophilia.

Can cautiously perform patch test or perform lymphocyte transformation test to establish culprit of DRESS /DIHS if needed. Lymphocyte transformation test should be performed 5–8 weeks after onset of DRESS/DIHS; patch testing should be performed 6+ months after recovery from symptoms. Positive findings are more informative than negative ones.

Ref: *JAAD*. 2012;66(6):e229–36 and *JAAD*. 2013;68(5):CME.
Ref: *JAAD*. 2013;68(5):CME.

Steven-Johnson Syndrome/Toxic Epidermal Necrolysis (SJS/TEN)

Nice quick overview available at DermNet NZ.

- Typically occurs 7–10 days after first exposure; 48 hours after subsequent exposures.
- Prodrome of fever and flu-like symptoms for a few days then.
- Skin lesions often start on the face and spread downward.
  - Macules > targets > bulla > slough
- Skin pain and sloughing (may begin with skin pruritus).
- Mucosal involvement (oral and conjunctival most frequent).
  - Ask regarding photophobia, difficulty swallowing, rectal erosions, painful urination, cough, and oral pain/erosions.
- SJS: can be caused by infection.
- TEN: never caused by infection (almost always due to drug).

A Note on Erythema Multiforme (EM)
Self-limited skin disease with abrupt onset of symmetric fixed papules, some of which are targetoid.

Often precipitated by infection.

Two forms: EM minor and EM major. Not thought to progress to TEN.

Typical targets have three zones: pink center surrounded by a white ring surrounded by red ring. Atypical targets are missing in one of these three zones.

- Erythema minor: Localized to extremities. No mucosal lesions or systemic symptoms.
- Erythema major: Lesions on extremities and face ± bullous lesions. Severe mucosal lesions may be present.
- Evaluation: HSV culture, skin biopsy. Consider mycoplasma titers and remove potential culprit drugs for EM major.
- Treatment: Acyclovir. Consider adding azithromycin for EM major.

SJS, TEN, and MIRM

- SJS and TEN on spectrum with each other. SJS sometimes due to infection; TEN almost always due to drug.
- MIRM (mycoplasma-induced rash and mucositis) with more mucosal than cutaneous findings and due to mycoplasma infection.
- See Table 3.14 for summary of findings in each and overview of treatment recommendations.

Common Drugs to Cause SJS/TEN

- Sulfonamides
- Anticonvulsants: lamotrigine, carbamazepine, phenytoin, phenobarbital
- Allopurinol
- NSAIDs (oxicam type most common)
- Lamotrigine
- Beta-lactam antibiotics: penicillin, cephalosporins
- Nevirapine
- Acetaminophen
- Note: NSAIDs and acetaminophen have been implicated as triggers and possibly exacerbants with other drugs and are best avoided during hospitalization for SJS/TEN

TABLE 3.14 Summary of findings, causes, and treatment recommendations for SJS/TEN and MIRM

	Mucosal and skin	% detach	Cause	Treatment
SJS	2+ mucosal (severe) Targets or morbilliform: Dusky macules with or without epidermal detachment *Macular* atypical targets Bullous lesions Trunk, face	<10%	HSV Mycoplasma Drug Rarely, immunizations	D/C drug Mycoplasma titers CXR HSV culture/PCR Biopsy IgA level BMP, mag, phos, uric acid, lipids, CBC HIV, hepatitis B Ab/Ag, hepatitis C Ab Ophtho consult Gyn consult (for females) Start: Azithromycin - until MIRM ruled out Acyclovir - until HSV/VZV ruled out Prednisone (IV methylpred 60 mg q6h [4 mg/kg/day for kids]) OR cyclosporine 4 mg/kg/day PO divided BID ± etanercept Rare progression to TEN

Mycoplasma-induced rash and mucositis[a]	Predominant mucosal	<10% usually	Mycoplasma	Biopsy CXR Mycoplasma IgM/PCR Oropharyngeal culture for mycoplasma Cold agglutinins[a] HSV culture/PCR Azithromycin IVIg may be beneficial for severe mucositis

(continued)

TABLE 3.14 (continued)

	Mucosal and skin	% detach	Cause	Treatment
SJS-TEN overlap	2+ mucosal	10–30%	Drug	D/C all non-essential drugs Mycoplasma titers CXR HSV culture/PCR Biopsy IgA level BMP, mag, phos, uric acid, lipids, CBC HIV, hepatitis B Ab/Ag, hepatitis C Ab Ophtho consult Gyn consult (for females) Worried that this may progress Start: Cyclosporine 3–5 mg/kg divided BID for 7–14 days ± etanercept 50 mg subQ injection × 1–2 OR High-dose steroids: dexamethasone 100 mg IV × 3 days or methylprednisolone 1000 mg IV × 3 days (if early in disease course) (IVIg 3–4 gm/kg/day divided over 4 days) Can start azithromycin and acyclovir, until infection (MIRM, HSV/VZV) is ruled out

TEN with spots	2+ mucosal Has targets and there is rash	>30%	Drug	D/C all non-essential drugs Mycoplasma titers CXR HSV culture/PCR Biopsy IgA level BMP, mag, phos, uric acid, lipids, CBC HIV, hepatitis B Ab/Ag, hepatitis C Ab Ophtho consult Gyn consult (for females) Start: Cyclosporine 3–5 mg/kg divided BID for 7–14 days ± etanercept 50 mg subQ injection × 1–2 OR High-dose steroids: dexamethasone 100 mg IV × 3 days or methylprednisolone 1000 mg IV × 3 days (if early in disease course) (IVIg 3–4 gm/kg/day divided over 4 days) Can start azithromycin and acyclovir, until infection (MIRM, HSV/VZV) is ruled out

(continued)

TABLE 3.14 (continued)

	Mucosal and skin	% detach	Cause	Treatment
TEN without spots	2+ mucosal Epidermal necrosis with erythema but not targets	>30%	Always drug	D/C all non-essential drugs Mycoplasma titers CXR HSV culture/PCR Biopsy IgA level BMP, mag, phos, uric acid, lipids, CBC HIV, hepatitis B Ab/Ag, hepatitis C Ab Ophtho consult Gyn consult (for females) Start: Cyclosporine 3–5 mg/kg divided BID for 7–14 days ± etanercept 50 mg subQ injection × 1–2 OR High-dose steroids: dexamethasone 100 mg IV × 3 days or methylprednisolone 1000 mg IV × 3 days (if early in disease course) Be sure to rule out *Staph*-scalded skin. Can do this via stat frozen biopsy to see if full epidermal necrosis versus split within granular layer Start on vancomycin/clindamycin if SSSS suspected Can start azithromycin and acyclovir, until infection (MIRM, HSV/VZV) is ruled out

[a]See below for MIRM

- But MANY drugs have been reported to cause SJS/TEN (look at DermNet NZ for longer list or look up individual drugs in Litt's Drug Eruption/PubMed).

Other Causes to Consider
- Vaccinations
- Contrast media
- Other chemical exposures
- Herbal medicines
- Radiotherapy
- Bone marrow transplantation (GVHD)

If having trouble determining which drug may be culprit, consider using ALDEN scoring system (Table 3.15).

Mycoplasma-Induced Rash and Mucositis (MIRM)

- Most common in children.
- Prodromal syndromes nearly universal (cough, malaise, fever) preceding eruption by about 1 week.
- The most common presentation is mucositis with sparse skin lesions; severe mucositis is the next most common presentation.
  - Mucosal surfaces: oral cavity/lips (94%), ocular involvement (82%), urogenital (63%)
  - Skin lesions can be absent, mild, or moderate and are polymorphous (vesiculobullous > targetoid lesions, papules, macules, morbilliform)
- Eighty-one percent make a full recovery.
- Treatment consists of antibiotics (although it is unclear if abx decrease the mucocutaneous eruption). Limited evidence that IVIg may be beneficial in patients with severe mucositis.

Table 3.15 ALDEN scoring system to help determine drug culprit for epidermal detachment

Criterion	Values	Rules to apply	Scoring
Delay from initial drug component intake to onset of reaction (index day)	Suggestive: +3	From 5 to 28 days	–3 to 3
	Compatible: +2	From 29 to 56 days	
	Likely: +1	From 1 to 4 days	
	Unlikely: –1	>56 days	
	Excluded: –3	Drug started on or after the index day. In case of previous reaction to the same drug, only changes for: Suggestive: +3 – from 1 to 4 days Likely: +1 – from 5 to 56 days	
Drug present in the body on index day	Definite: 0	Drug continued up to index day or stopped at a time point less than five times the elimination half-life[a] before the index day	–3 to 0
	Doubtful: –1	Drug stopped at a time point prior to the index day by more than five times the elimination half-life[a], but liver or kidney function alterations or suspected drug interactions[b] are present	
	Excluded: –3	Drug stopped at a time point prior to the index day by more than five times the elimination half-life[a], without liver or kidney function alterations or suspected drug interactions[b]	

Table 3.15 (continued)

Criterion	Values	Rules to apply	Scoring
Prechallenge/ rechallenge	Positive specific for disease and drug: 4	SJS/TEN after use of the same drug	–2 to 4
	Positive specific for disease or drug: 2	SJS/TEN after use of similar[c] drug or other reaction with the same drug	
	Positive unspecific: 1	Other reaction after use of similar[c] drug	
	Not done/ unknown: 0	No known previous exposure to this drug	
	Negative: –2	Exposure to this drug without any reaction (before or after reaction)	
Dechallenge	Neutral: 0	Drug stopped (or unknown)	–2 or 0
	Negative: –2	Drug continued without harm	
Type of drug (notoriety)	Strongly associated: 3	Drug of the "high-risk" list according to previous case-control studies	–1 to 3
	Associated: 2	Drug with definite but lower risk according to previous case-control studies	
	Suspected: 1	Several previous reports, ambiguous epidemiology results (drug "under surveillance")	
	Unknown: 0	All other drugs including newly released ones	
	Not suspected: –1	No evidence of association from previous epidemiology study with sufficient number of exposed controls[c] Intermediate score = total of all previous criteria	

(continued)

Table 3.15 (continued)

Criterion	Values	Rules to apply	Scoring
Other causes	Possible: –1	Rank all drugs from the highest to the lowest intermediate score If at least one has an intermediate score >3, subtract 1 point from the score of each of the other drugs taken by the patient (another cause is more likely)	–1
Final score: –12 to 10			

Clin Pharmacol Ther. 2010;88:60. www.nature.com/cpt

<0, very unlikely; 0 to 1, unlikely; 2 to 3, possible; 4 to 5, probable; ≥6, very probable

ATC anatomical therapeutic chemical, *SJS* Stevens-Johnson syndrome, *TEN* toxic epidermal necrolysis

[a]Drug (or active metabolite) elimination half-life from serum and/or tissues (according to pharmacology textbooks), taking into account kidney function for drugs predominantly cleared by kidney and liver function for those with high hepatic clearance

[b]Suspected interaction was considered when more than five drugs were present in a patient's body at the same time

[c]Similar drug = same ATC code up to the fourth level (chemical subgroups)

- See Table 3.16 for diagnostic criteria for MIRM.

Children with SJS/TEN

- Early in the disease process, children with TEN are at the greatest risk of airway compromise due to upper airway edema. Bronchoscope early if suspected airway involvement. Repeat bronchoscopy 24–48 hours later if normal.

  Reference: Rizzo JA et al. *Peds Derm.* 2015;32(5):704–9.

TABLE 3.16 Proposed diagnostic criteria for *Mycoplasma*-induced rash and mucositis (MIRM), including MIRM sine rash and severe MIRM

Classification	MIRM sine rash
Detachment	<10% BSA
No. of mucosal sites involved	≥2
Few and fleeting morbilliform lesions, or few vesicles	±
Evidence of atypical pneumonia	
1. Clinical	Fever, cough, positive auscultatory findings
2. Laboratory	Increase in MP IgM antibodies, MP in oropharyngeal or bullae cultures or PCR, and/or serial cold agglutinins
Classification	**Severe MIRM**
Detachment[a]	<10% BSA
No. of mucosal sites involved[b]	≥2
Extensive widespread blisters or flat atypical targets	Yes
Evidence of atypical pneumonia	
1. Clinical	Fever, cough, positive auscultatory findings
2. Laboratory	Increase in MP IgM antibodies, MP in oropharyngeal or bullae cultures or PCR, and/or serial cold agglutinins

BSA body surface area, *MIRM mycoplasma*-induced rash and mucositis, *MP mycoplasma pneumoniae*, *PCR* polymerase chain reaction

[a]Rare cases may have >10% BSA involvement

[b]Rare cases may have <2 mucosal sites involved

Work-Up for SJS/TEN

- Drug chart.
  - An algorithm for the assessment of drug causality in TEN (ALDEN) may be helpful.
- Calculate SCORTEN for prognosis (see below).
- CBC with diff, BMP, phosphorus, magnesium, LFTs, lipids, uric acid, hepatitis B and C, HIV.
- IgA level.
- Mycoplasma antibodies or PCR ± serial cold agglutinins.
  - Cold agglutinins: a quick bedside test can be performed by partially filling a purple top tube with blood and placing it in ice. A positive finding is one in which "grains of sand" appear on the glass portion of the tube.
- Aggressively culture at any sign of infection.
- Ophtho consultation.
- Gyn and vaginal dilator for women.
- Place Foley to prevent urinary strictures.
- CXR for pulmonary involvement.

Prognosis Scoring: SCORTEN

1 point for meeting each criterion. Predicts mortality risk at presentation

*S*ugar: blood glucose >252 mg/dL (14 mmol/L)
*C*ancer or hematologic malignancy
*O*ld: age >40 years
*R*ate: heart rate >120 beats per minute
*T*EN % BSA: involved body surface area >10% on day 1
*E*lectrolytes: serum bicarb <20 mEq/L (20 mmol/L)
*N*itrogen: BUN >28 mg/dL (>10 mmol/L or 10 mEq/L)

Mortality Rates

0–1 factor = 3%
2 = 12%
3 = 35%
4 = 58%
5+ = 90%

Note: Pulmonary/bronchial involvements are poor prognostic signs.

Dyspnea and hypoxia may be early signs of pulmonary decline and a CXR may be unreliable.

Treatment Considerations

- Pharmacotherapy
  - Lack of randomized control trials; no clear winning therapeutic treatment. Many studies show benefit, no benefit, and/or harm.
  - Corticosteroids – to be administered early (ideally when the skin is red and tender, before slough). NOT to be administered late.

    Dexamethasone 100 mg IV × 3 days
    Methylprednisolone 1000 mg IV × 3 days
    May be better for SJS rather than TEN

  - Cyclosporine 3–5 mg/kg orally (or IV equivalent) over 7 days – the only drug shown to have statistical significance in SJS/TEN
  - IVIg

    May not have a mortality benefit
    If going to administer, doses of at least 2 gm/kg (2–4 gm/kg) administered over 3–4 days recommended
    Pediatric IVIg dosing for TEN: 400 mg/kg/day as a continuous infusion × 5 days or until the lesions stopped progressing

  - TNF-alpha inhibitors

    Etanercept 50 mg subQ injection × 1–2
    Infliximab 5 mg/kg IV infusion

  - Others

    Plasmapheresis (one to four sessions)
    Dialysis

- Supportive care
  - Control fluid management, electrolyte disturbances, and temperature.
  - Nutrition enteral >>> parenteral
  - Infection surveillance

    Daily assessment of exudate.
    Skin cultures q48h.
    Regular cultures of blood, urine, and catheters.
    Discontinue any non-essential lines.
    Wood's lamp to assess for *Pseudomonas aeruginosa*

  - Pain control
- Skin/wound care
  - Strict contact precautions.
  - Aseptic handling and isolation.

    Droplet precautions when the skin is open

  - Minimize shear forces.
  - Cover intact skin with petroleum-based ointment.
  - In eroded skin, apply nonstick dressing.

    Vaseline gauze
    Silicone dressing
    Consider: 0.5% silver nitrate solution or dressings

  - Consider coverage with biologic dressing.
    Porcine xenograft

    Human allografts

  - Surgically debride slough.
- Pulmonary/airway
  - Dyspnea and hypoxia may be early signs of pulmonary decline, and a CXR may be unreliable.
  - Early in disease process, children with TEN are at risk of airway compromise d/t upper airway edema.

Bronchoscope early if suspected airway involvement. Repeat bronchoscopy 24–48 hours later if normal. Airway support may be required. **Ref**: Rissa JA et al. *Peds Derm*. 2015;(32):704–9

- Mucosal management
  - Oral

    Petrolatum TID-QID to lips
    Warm saline mouthwash
    Antiseptic mouth rinse

- Diluted chlorhexidine 0.2% mouthwash, swish/spit, or swab
  Clobetasol + Orabase for open erosions on lips/oral mucosa
  - Eyes/ocular

    Consult ophthalmology.
    Topical lubricant: non-preserved hyaluronate two drops in each eye QID
    Topical antibiotic prophylaxis: moxifloxacin
    Topical anti-inflammatory drops: non-preserved dexamethasone 0.1%/cyclosporine
    Daily mechanical separation of mucosal membranes to prevent scarring
    Amniotic membrane placement for slough of the cornea, conjunctiva, and lid margin
    Ref: John T. *Ophthalmology*. 2002:109;351–60
  - Nose/nares

    Nostrils cleaned daily with saline
    Petrolatum/antibiotic ointment application
  - Vulvovaginal

    Consult gynecology for a speculum exam
    Vaseline

Topical steroids: betamethasone or clobetasol ointment
Vaginal dilator/petrolatum-coated tampon placement

- Urethral

  Consult urology
  Vaseline
  Potent topical steroid if erosions
  Foley catheter placement if meatal involvement

- Pulmonary (respiratory tract involved in up to 25%)

  Supplemental O2
  Nebulized saline, bronchodilators
  Physical therapy
  CXR
  Bronchoscopy
  Intubation and mechanical ventilation

Expectations of Treatment

- Acute phase of SJS/TEN usually lasts 5–12 days.
- In studies, successful treatment often results in decreased detachment within 24–48 hours.
- Re-epithelialization usually starts within days and is completely within 3 weeks.

SJS/TEN Sequelae

- Cutaneous

  - Chronic xerosis/eczema
  - Persistent pigmentary changes (hyper-/hypopigmentation)
  - Eruptive melanocytic nevi
  - Hair loss

- Nail
  - Anonychia, dystrophic nails, longitudinal ridges, pterygium
- Ocular (most common, 43%)
  - Dry eye syndrome – most common
  - Corneal ulcers/opacities/scarring, ectropion/entropion, foreign body sensation, hyperemia, chronic conjunctivitis, trichiasis, corneal erosions, symblepharon, synechia, blindness
- Oral
  - Xerostomia, periodontal disease, synechia
- Genitourinary
  - Phimosis or vaginal adhesions
  - Urethral erosions/adhesions
- Gastrointestinal
  - Difficulty eating/speaking
  - Adhesions
- Joint contractures
- Lung disease
  - Bronchiolitis, bronchiectasis, obstructive disorders

References

- Worswick S and Cotliar J. Stevens-Johnson syndrome and toxic epidermal necrolysis: a review of treatment options. *Dermatologic Therapy.* 2011;24:207–18.
- Canavan TN, et al. Mycoplasma pneumonia-induced rash and mucositis as a syndrome distinct from Sevens-Johnson syndrome and erythema multiforme: a systemic review. *J Am Acad Dermatol.* 2015;72(2):239–45.

- American Burn Association protocol from 2008: https://evidencebasedpractice.osumc.edu/Documents/Guidelines/TEN_Guidelines.pdf.
- Yang Che-Wen et al. Long-term sequelae of Stevens-Johnson syndrome and toxic epidermal necrolysis. *Acta Derm Venerol.* 2016;96(4):525–9.
- DermNet NZ: https://dermnetnz.org/topics/stevens-johnson-syndrome-toxic-epidermal-necrolysis/.
- Downey A. *JAAD.* 2012;66:995–1003.
- Endorf F. *J Burn Care Research.* 2008;29:706–12.
- Rissa JA et al. *Peds Derm.* 2015;(32):704–9.
- Harris V. *J Int Mol Sci.* 2016;17:E2135.
- John T. *Ophthalmology.* 2002;109:351–60.
- Halebian PH. *Ann Surg.* 1986;204:503–12.
- Zimmerman et al. *JAMA Derm.* 2017.
- Schwartz RA. *JAAD.* 2013;69:187e1–16.
- Fischer M. *Br J Dermatol.* 2002;146:707–9.
- Yang CW. *Acta Derm Venereol.* 2016;96(4):525–9.
- Yang MS. *Plos One.* 2016;11(11):e0165933.

Acute Generalized Exanthematous Pustulosis (AGEP)

- Non-follicular pustules + fever + leukocytosis.
- *Scarlatiniform* erythema that begins as an edematous erythema in the body folds and face before generalizing to widespread non-follicular sterile pustules. It is associated with fever and neutrophilia. Usually pruritic.
- Develops suddenly within 24–48 hours of taking a medication (unless a cardiac med) – may be a viral reaction.
- Can have mucous membrane involvement but usually is confined to a single site (lips or buccal mucosa).
- Systemic involvement in 20%
  - Hepatic (hepatic pattern or cholestatic pattern)
  - Pulmonary involvement (b/l pleural effusions)

- Labs: neutrophilia in 90%, increased CRP.
- Mortality ~5%
  - Most often related to secondary infection.
  - Can be due to multiple organ dysfunction and DIC.
  - Diffuse mucous membrane involvement has worse outcomes.
- Upon discontinuation of the causative agent, resolution is usually within a few days. Can get wide spread desquamation as eruption clears.
- Nikolsky may be positive.
- Culprit medications
  - Ampicillin/amoxicillin.
  - Macrolides.
  - Quinolones.
  - Hydroxychloroquine – rxn may last longer than 2 weeks.
  - Sulfonamide antibiotics.
  - Fluconazole/ketoconazole.
  - Terbinafine.
  - Imatinib
  - Diltiazem
  - NSAIDs
  - Mercury
  - Radiocontrast
- Work-up
  - CBC, CMP (BMP and LFTs) + calcium
  - Skin bx
  - Abdominal ultrasound if abdominal pain
  - CXR if hypoxia, shortness of breath
  - Can do patch testing to confirm drug diagnosis 6+ weeks after resolution of eruption

- Treatment
  - Has a benign self-limiting course and resolves spontaneously in a few days
  - Removal of causative agent – usually leads to resolution in <15 days
  - Moist dressings and antiseptic solutions appropriate during the pustular phase to prevent infection
  - Topical steroids ± systemic steroids

    Tx with potent topical steroids correlated with decreased duration of hospitalization
  - Antihistamines for any associated pruritus

Reference: Szatkowski J, et al. Acute generalized exanthematous pustulosis (AGEP): A review and update. *JAAD*. 2015;73:843–8.

Other Drugs and Reactions Categorized by Pattern/Distribution

Symmetrical Drug-Related Intertriginous and Flexural Exanthema

A systemic contact dermatitis with patterned symmetrical erythema of the skinfolds due to a food/medication ingestion/systemic absorption to someone previously sensitized cutaneously (also known as baboon syndrome)

Requires four out of the five criteria (Tan et al. *Curr Opin Allergy Clin Immunol* 2011):

- Exposure to a systemically administered agent
- Distinct erythema of the gluteal, inguinal, or axillary area
- Involvement of at least one intertriginous site

- Symmetry
- Absence of internal organ dysfunction

Common meds: Beta-lactam antibiotics, mercury, heparin, IVIG, pseudoephedrine, aminophylline, terbutaline, codeine, allopurinol, cimetidine, nystatin

Other Medication Reactions (Table 3.17)

Drug-induced IgA deficiency: cyclosporine, NSAIDs, hydroxychloroquine, phenytoin, sulfasalazine

Drugs Interacting with OCPs

- Only proven significant with *rifampin and griseofulvin.*
- *ACOG*: tetracycline, doxycycline, ampicillin, and metronidazole do NOT affect OCP levels.
- Backup contraception is NOT necessary if reliable OCP user.

Oncodermatology

Common Terminology Criteria for Adverse Events

- Grade 1: mild; asymptomatic or mild symptoms; clinical or diagnostic observations only; intervention not needed
- Grade 2: moderate; minimal, local, or noninvasive intervention needed; limiting age-appropriate instrumental ADL*
- Grade 3: severe or medically significant but not immediately life-threatening; hospitalization or prolongation of hospitalization indicated; disabling; limiting self-care ADL**

TABLE 3.17 Cutaneous findings and potential causative drugs

Acanthosis nigricans	Nicotinic acid, insulin, pituitary extracts (somatotropin), glucocorticoids, diethylstilbestrol Rarely: OCPs, testosterone, triazinate, fusidic acid (topical), heroin, hydantoin, fibroblast growth factor receptor ligand (e.g., palifermin)
Acne and acneiform	Corticosteroids, androgenic steroids (danazol, stanozolol, nandrolone, testosterone), progesterone-only OCPs and hormonal (levonorgestrel-containing) IUDs, lithium, barbiturates, DHEA, halogens (bromines/iodides), cyclosporine, antiepileptics (carbamazepine, phenytoin, phenobarbital), anti-TB meds (ethionamide, isoniazid, rifampin), amoxapine, B vitamins (B6, B12), azathioprine, phenytoin, ACTH, psoralens, disulfiram EGFR inhibitors (acneiform pustular reaction – see below for details)
Acrodynia	aka pink disease. Due to mercury poisoning (usually in infancy); diagnose with mercury in urine. Painful swelling of hands/feet, hemorrhagic puncta
Acute generalized exanthematous pustulosis (AGEP)	Ampicillin/amoxicillin, macrolides, quinolones, hydroxychloroquine, sulfonamide antibiotics, fluconazole/ketoconazole, terbinafine, imatinib, diltiazem, NSAIDs, mercury, radiocontrast

TABLE 3.17 (continued)

Alopecia	Anagen effluvium: chemotherapy, gold, colchicine, poisoning with arsenic, bismuth, thallium, boric acid Telogen effluvium: Anticoagulants – heparin, warfarin Antihypertensives – beta-blockers, ACE inhibitors OCPs, hormone replacement therapy, androgens Anticonvulsants – valproic acid, carbamazepine Retinoids: acitretin > isotretinoin Others: cimetidine, allopurinol, lithium, etretinate, indomethacin, levodopa, just starting minoxidil (before it starts to work), methotrexate, cholesterol-lowering drugs, interferons, amphetamines, NSAIDs, bromocriptine, levodopa, tricyclic antidepressants
Angioedema	ACE inhibitors (d/t accumulation of bradykinin (lisinopril and enalapril are the more common cause than captopril)) > ARBs
DRESS (drug rash with eosinophilia and systemic symptoms)/ drug-induced hypersensitivity syndrome (DIHS)	See section "DRESS/DIHS"
Anticoagulant skin necrosis	Warfarin: onset 3–5 days, decreased in hepatic disease and with antithrombotic factors (protein C and S deficiency) Treat with vitamin K and protein C Heparin: onset 6–12 days. Causes antiplatelet Ab (anti-PF4) thrombosis and low platelets
Aplasia cutis congenita	Methimazole

(continued)

Table 3.17 (continued)

Symmetrical drug-related intertriginous and flexural exanthema (SDRIFE)	Beta-lactam antibiotics, mercury, heparin, IVIG, pseudoephedrine, aminophylline, terbutalinePCNs, pseudoephedrine, codeine, allopurinol, cimetidine, nystatin
Bactrim (TMP/SMX) rash in HIV	Rash in 45% of patients treated for PCP
Dermatomyositis	Penicillamine, HMG-COa reductase inhibitors (statins), NSAIDs, hydroxyurea
Eczematous	Calcium channel blockers
Eruptive xanthomas	Protease inhibitors, olanzapine, systemic retinoids (isotretinoin and bexarotene), estrogen, alcohol consumption
Erythroderma	Top suspects: allopurinol, antiepileptics (phenytoin, phenobarbital, carbamazepine), antihypertensives, antibiotics, calcium channel blockers See section "Erythroderma" for others
Erythema multiforme	Sulfonamides, NSAIDs, anticonvulsants, barbiturates, nitrofurantoin, phenothiazines <u>Radiation-induced EM:</u> phenytoin (at XRT port)/amifostine, EM-like reaction upon withdrawing steroids (can be at radiation ports as steroids are tapered); may appear like SJS/TEN and spread caudad
Erythema nodosum	OCPs, sulfonamides, halogens (bromides/iodine), tetracyclines, NSAIDs, gold, sulfonylureas
Exogenous ochronosis	Antimalarials (hydroxychloroquine, chloroquine), topical phenol, resorcinol, hydroquinone, Castellani's paint

TABLE 3.17 (continued)

Fixed drug reaction	Pigmented: aspirin, acetaminophen, tetracyclines (doxycycline, minocycline), barbiturates, benzodiazepine, chlordiazepoxide, dapsone, NSAIDs (naproxen, ibuprofen), sulfonamides (TMP-SMX, sulfasalazine), phenolphthalein (in laxatives), erythromycin, ACE inhibitors, OCPs, quinine Non-pigmented: pseudoephedrine
Flagellate	Bleomycin, shiitake mushrooms (toxin = lentinan), docetaxel (also Still's disease and dermatomyositis)
Flushing	Niacin, calcium channel blockers and other vasodilators, nitroglycerin, cholinergics, beta-blockers, ACE inhibitors, vancomycin, cyclosporine, methylprednisolone (high dose), IV contrast, sildenafil, muscle relaxants, thiopental, ciguatera Foods: capsaicin, nitrate, EtOH + topical calcineurin inhibitors, EtOH in patients with aldehyde dehydrogenase gene polymorphism, sulfites, scombroid fish poisoning (dark fish – releases histamine) MAOI + SSRI > serotonin syndrome + flushing Also: SSRIs, tricyclic antidepressants, monoamine oxidase inhibitors, or opiates + triptans, antibiotics, antiemetics, cough syrups, herbal remedies, or illicit drugs > serotonin syndrome as well

(continued)

TABLE 3.17 (continued)

Granulomatous drug eruptions	Drug-induced interstitial granulomatous: calcium channel blockers (most common), ACE inhibitors, lipid-lowering agents, brompheniramine, H2 receptor antagonists, furosemide, carbamazepine, bupropion and tricyclic antidepressants, TNFa inhibitors, lenalidomide, sennoside, herbal medications, beta-blockers, ganciclovir, sorafenib, strontium ranelate, febuxostat, anakinra, trastuzumab, darifenacin Drug-induced accelerated rheumatoid nodulosis: methotrexate (most common), TNFa inhibitors, aromatase inhibitors, azathioprine, leflunomide Drug-induced granuloma annulare: TNFa inhibitors (most common), amlodipine, gold, allopurinol, diclofenac, intranasal calcitonin, immunizations (hepatitis B and tetanus), paroxetine (photo-distributed GA, pegylated IFNa, desensitization injections, topiramate Drug-induced sarcoidosis: IFNa (most common), TNFa inhibitors, hyaluronic acid cosmetic fillers, zinc, desensitization injections, ipilimumab, ophthalmic drops containing sodium bisulfite, tattoos
G-CSF	Sweet's, small vessel vasculitis, psoriasis
Gingival hyperplasia	Cyclosporine (most common), tacrolimus, sirolimus Anticonvulsants: sodium valproate, phenobarbitone, vigabatrin, primidone, mephenytoin, and ethosuximide Calcium channel blockers: nifedipine, nitrendipine, felodipine, amlodipine, nisoldipine, verapamil, and diltiazem

Table 3.17 (continued)

Acral hyperpigmentation	Emtricitabine, zidovudine, B12 deficiency, tegafur, capecitabine, quinacrine (yellow acrally and sclera) Nails Brown/black – zidovudine, psoralens, hydroxyurea, chemo Yellow – tetracyclines, old nail polish Blue/gray – minocycline Brown – antimalarials (hydroxychloroquine, chloroquine)
Hyperpigmentation	Minocycline, tetracycline, antimalarials, amiodarone, clofazimine (violet brown in leprosy areas), zidovudine (nails), hydroxyurea (nails), imipramine, phenothiazines (chlorpromazine, promethazine, prochlorperazine), chemos (busulfan, cyclophosphamide, hydroxyurea, dactinomycin, methotrexate, 5-FU), heavy metals (silver, gold, bismuth (gums), arsenic (black trunk with white raindrops), diltiazem (follicular accentuation), quinacrine (yellow acrally and sclera)
Hypertrichosis	Oral minoxidil, diazoxide, phenytoin, cyclosporine, streptomycin, penicillamine, corticosteroids, danazol and anabolic steroids, psoralens, PUVA, androgens, streptomycin, acetazolamide Eyelashes: IFN, AZT, cyclosporine, bimatoprost Also remember: PCT, anorexia nervosa, malignancy
Small vessel vasculitis/LCV – leukocytoclastic vasculitis	Penicillins, sulfonamide, quinolones, allopurinol, propylthiouracil, valproic acid, phenytoin, anti-TNF alpha agents, and hydralazine

(continued)

Table 3.17 (continued)

Lichenoid drug eruption	Antihypertensives (ACE inhibitors [captopril]), beta-blockers, calcium channel blockers (nifedipine), methyldopa Diuretics: HCTZ, furosemide, spironolactone Sulfa-containing drugs: sulfonylureas, dapsone, mesalazine, sulfasalazine NSAIDs Phenothiazine derivatives Anticonvulsants (carbamazepine, phenytoin) Antimalarials (quinacrine and others) Anti-TB medications Others: ketoconazole, gold, NSAIDs, penicillamine, PPIs, HMG-COa inhibitors /statins, sildenafil, chlorpromazine, iodides, radiocontrast, IFNa, omeprazole, tetracyclines, TNFa inhibitors, misoprostol, vaccines (influenza, herpes zoster, hepatitis B) Mucosal: gold/mercury amalgams Mucous membrane rare in LDE (except with NSAIDs and diuretics (lower lip)) Photolichenoid: thiazides, NSAIDs, diltiazem, amiodarone, tetracyclines, antimalarials
Linear IgA	Vancomycin (most common), beta-lactam abx (PCN), TMP-SMX, NSAIDs, furosemide, lithium, ACE inhibitor (captopril), amiodarone, phenytoin, diclofenac, cyclosporine, somatostatin, cefamandole, vigabatrin, rifampin, G-CSF, sulfisoxazole, sodium hypochlorite (bleach)
Livedoid eruption	Amantadine (most common), quinidine, quinine, minocycline, catecholamines, NSAIDs

TABLE 3.17 (continued)

Lupus	Antihistone (serositis predominant): hydralazine, INH, procainamide, sulfonamides (sulfasalazine), penicillamine, anticonvulsants, minocycline, PTU, PUVA, quinidine, methyldopa, levamisole (cocaine contaminant), pembrolizumab True SLE lupus (anti ds-DNA): penicillamine, TNFa inhibitors SCLE (+ anti-Ro/SSA): hydrochlorothiazide > terbinafine, diltiazem, ACE inhibitors, NSAIDs (naproxen), griseofulvin, antihistamine, glyburide, anticonvulsants, piroxicam, spironolactone, sulfonylureas statins, IFN, PUVA, TNFa, PPIs, taxols (docetaxel)
Milia	Phenol, hydroquinone, 5-FU, topical steroids, tyrosine kinase inhibitors
Morbilliform drug eruption (simple drug eruption)	Aminopenicillins (penicillins, cephalosporins), sulfonamides, allopurinol, NSAIDs, anticonvulsants, but MANY drugs have been reported
Nicolau syndrome	Arterial thrombosis after IM injections "embolia cutis medicamentosa"
Onycholysis	Retinoids, captopril, quinolone, quinine, thiazide diuretics, phenothiazines, clofazimine, sodium valproate, capecitabine, paclitaxel/docetaxel, etoposide Photo-onycholysis: tetracyclines (doxycycline), OCPs, fluoroquinolones, psoralens, mercaptopurine, chloramphenicol, benoxaprofen
Paronychia	Retinoids, EGFR inhibitors (most common); methotrexate, cyclosporine, antiretrovirals
Orange-red urine	Rifampin
Pellagra-like rash	INH, azathioprine, 5-fluorouracil, ethionamide, prothionamide, pyrazinamide

(continued)

TABLE 3.17 (continued)

Pemphigus	Penicillamine, & captopril (most common two), pyritinol, penicillin, ampicillin, rifampin (may be drug-triggered; rash does not resolve with stopping medication), cephalosporins, ACE inhibitors (likely to cause vegetans), piroxicam, gold, phenylbutazone, propranolol, carbamazepine, thiopurine, thiamazole, 5-thiopyridine, pyrazolone derivatives (phenylbutazone, aminopyrine, azapropazone, oxyphenbutazone), levodopa, heroin, progesterone, phenobarbital, lysine, aspirin Usually PF > PV; DIF may or may not be positive Associated with malignancies of the larynx and esophagus
Pemphigoid	Beta-blockers, furosemide, NSAIDs (ibuprofen), sulfa-containing drugs (sulfasalazine), terbinafine, estrogen (OCPs), PCN, penicillamine, captopril, gold, gliptins, spironolactone, amoxicillin, ciprofloxacin, potassium iodide
Penicillamine	EPS, anetoderma
Pityriasis rosea-like rash	ACE inhibitors, arsenic, bismuth, barbiturates, beta-blockers, ergotamine, gold, imatinib, ketotifen, organic mercurials, metronidazole, NSAIDs, penicillamine, clonidine, isotretinoin, omeprazole, sulfasalazine
Photoallergic reactions	Sunscreens (benzophenones and cinnamates), fragrance (musk ambrette, sandalwood oil), chlorhexidine, fenticlor, hexachlorophene, NSAIDs(diclofenac, ketoprofen, celecoxib), phenothiazines (chlorpromazine, promethazine), quinidine, griseofulvin, quinine, quinolones, glipizide, sulfonamides, tricyclic antidepressants

TABLE 3.17 (continued)

Phototoxic reactions and photosensitivity	Antibiotics: tetracyclines (doxycycline), fluoroquinolones, sulfonamides NSAIDs (ibuprofen, naproxen, ketoprofen, celecoxib) Diuretics: furosemide, bumetanide, HCTZ Retinoids: isotretinoin, acitretin Sulfonylureas (glipizide, glyburide) Phenothiazines (chlorpromazine, fluphenazine) Voriconazole Others: chlorprothixene, vemurafenib, dabrafenib, vandetanib, psoralens, amiodarone, diltiazem, quinine, hydroxychloroquine, enalapril, dapsone, 5-aminolevulinic acid, methyl-5-aminolevulinic acid, 5-FU
Phytophotosensitivity	Lime, fig, carrot, parsley, celery, wild parsnip, bergamot, mango, perfumes, weeds
Pseudoporphyria	NSAIDs (naproxen, piroxicam) (most common), HCTZ, furosemide, HCTZ-triamterene, bumetanide, chlorthalidone, isotretinoin/acitretin/etretinate, OCPs, sulfonamides, dapsone, tetracyclines (doxycycline), furosemide, nalidixic acid, ciprofloxacin, sun itself/tanning bed/phototherapy, dialysis, excessive Coca-Cola consumption
Porphyria exacerbation	Barbiturates, estrogens/ethanol, griseofulvin, sulfa
Pseudolymphoma	<u>B cell (most common)</u> Adverse drug (sulfa, anticonvulsants, dapsone, imatinib, sulfa, ARBs, antipsychotics/antidepressants) (also: *Borrelia* bite, herpes zoster, acupuncture/gold jewelry, tattoo) Insect bite (persistent) <u>T cell</u> Antidepressants, antihistamines, calcium channel blockers, statins, anticonvulsants, (also: bites, contact)

(continued)

TABLE 3.17 (continued)

Psoriasis	Beta-blockers, lithium, terbinafine, prednisone, antimalarials (hydroxychloroquine, chloroquine, quinidine), amoxicillin (but it may be the infection that causes it), G-CSF, ACE inhibitors, cytokines (IL2, G-CSF, INF-gamma or INF-alpha), TNFa (palmo-plantar)
Pruritus	Opioids Chemotherapeutic agents Chloroquine (especially in patients of African ancestry) Antimicrobials: penicillin G, amoxicillin/clavulanate, ampicillin, cefotaxime, ceftazidime, erythromycin, ciprofloxacin, vancomycin, clindamycin, tetracyclines (minocycline), rifampin, trimethoprim/sulfamethoxazole Oral antifungals: terbinafine Antimalarials: chloroquine, amodiaquine ACE inhibitors: captopril, enalapril, lisinopril Calcium channel blockers: amlodipine, diltiazem, verapamil ARBs: candesartan, irbesartan Diabetic medications: metformin, gliclazide Neuropsychiatric medications: amitriptyline, citalopram, fluoxetine, paroxetine, sertraline, carbamazepine, phenytoin, topiramate, chlorpromazine, phenothiazine, risperidone Steroids and hormones: danazol, some oral contraceptive pills Chemotherapeutics and immunological agents: chlorambucil, gemcitabine, nilotinib, vemurafenib, temsirolimus, ipilimumab, cetuximab, rituximab, panitumumab, gefitinib Other medications: aspirin, clonidine, methyldopa, amiodarone, allopurinol, alcohol, dextran, enoxaparin, hydroxyethyl starch, radiopaque contrast agents, scopolamine

Table 3.17 (continued)

Pyogenic granuloma	EGFRs, indinavir, retinoids (isotretinoin, acitretin)
Pyoderma gangrenosum	Levamisole (cocaine), systemic retinoids (isotretinoin, alitretinoin), PTU, adalimumab, etanercept, infliximab, azacitidine, imatinib/sunitinib, ipilimumab, enoxaparin, EPO, G-CSF, IFN
Vancomycin flushing syndrome (VFS)	Vancomycin
Serum sickness	Antivenoms and anti-toxins
Serum sickness-like reaction	Cefaclor (kids): 1 week after treatment in kid with otitis media or URI Penicillins (including amoxicillin), other antibiotics, and NSAIDs, following immunizations for hepatitis B, tetanus toxoid, and rabies Bupropion (serum sickness + urticaria)
Sticky skin	Isotretinoin/acitretin/etretinate Ketoconazole + doxorubicin in prostate cancer
Sweet's-like syndrome	GM-CSF, OCP, TMP/SMX, minocycline, carbamazepine
SJS/TEN	Sulfonamides, especially TMP/SMX Anticonvulsants: lamotrigine, carbamazepine, phenytoin, phenobarbital Allopurinol NSAIDs (oxicam type most common) Beta-lactam antibiotics: penicillin, cephalosporins Nevirapine Acetaminophen (especially kids) Many other reports including acetaminophen. See SJS/TEN section.
Texier's disease	Pseudosclerodermatous changes after vitamin K injection (similar to L-tryptophan-induced EMS)

(continued)

Table 3.17 (continued)

Telangiectasias	Calcium channel blockers (photo-distributed) amlodipine, lithium, isotretinoin, IFNa, thiothixene
Urticaria	PCN (most common – even PCN in dairy products), NSAIDs (ibuprofen, naproxen, diclofenac), TMP-SMX, cephalosporins, tetracyclines, griseofulvin, opiates (morphine/codeine), radiocontrast agents, ACE inhibitors salicylates (aspirin, especially with nasal polyps, asthma, food-induced anaphylaxis) but MANY Others: macrolides, aminoglycosides, vancomycin, polymyxin B, tubocurarine, fluoroquinolones, anticoagulants, anticonvulsants, alkylating agents, taxanes, methotrexate, betadine/iodine, dextrans, dextromethorphan, trypsin, streptokinase, chymopapain, hydantoins, hydralazine, mannitol, atracurium, vecuronium, succinylcholine, curare, insulin, corticotropin, vasopressin, progesterone, quinidine, sorbitol, corticosteroids, alteplase, urokinase, vaccines, tubocurarine Bupropion (serum sickness + urticaria)
Ulceration/erosion	Lower extremity ulceration: hydroxyurea, sunitinib Penile erosions: foscarnet, lamivudine Scrotal erosions: all-trans-retinoic acid Methotrexate (at psoriatic sites) IFN-beta (at inoculation sites) Oral ulcers: imatinib Skin popping of illicit drugs
Urticarial vasculitis	ACE inhibitors, PCN, sulfonamides, fluoxetine, thiazides

TABLE 3.17 (continued)

Vasculitis	Small vessel/LCV: Common – NSAIDs, COX-2 inhibitors, leukotriene inhibitors, beta-lactam antibiotics (PCN), quinolones, TNFa inhibitors, G-CSF, hydralazine, anti-thyroid agents, cocaine with levamisole, sulfonamides, quinolones, valproic acid, phenytoin, anti-TNF alpha agents, and hydralazine Occasional: ACE inhibitors, allopurinol, furosemide, coumarin, quinine, macrolides, thiazides, sulfonylureas, vancomycin, IFN, beta-blockers, phenytoin, streptokinase, propylthiouracil (PTU), valproic acid, Radiocontrast ANCA-associated PTU + hydralazine Eosinophilic granulomatosis with polyangiitis: leukotriene inhibitors (Polyangiitis with granulomatosis-like with levamisole)

- Grade 4: life-threatening consequences; urgent intervention indicated
- Grade 5: death related to adverse effect

*Instrumental ADL refers to preparing meals, shopping for groceries or clothing, using the telephone, managing money, etc.

**Self-care ADL refers to bathing, dressing, undressing, feeding oneself, using the toilet, managing medications, and not being bedridden.

See link for specific criteria for grading of specific cutaneous adverse events: https://ctep.cancer.gov/protocolDevelopment/electronic_applications/docs/CTCAE_v5_Quick_Reference_8.5x11.pdf.

Summary of Targeted Therapy Pathways (Fig. 3.9)

Chemotherapy-Associated Cutaneous Reactions

Cutaneous reactions are the most common adverse effect with targeted therapies. See Table 3.18 for specifics.

Acral Toxic Erythema of Chemotherapy

Palmar-Plantar Erythrodysesthesia

Burning sensation on palms and soles + erythematous macules ± edema which can lead to bullae and desquamation

Implicated chemotherapeutics:

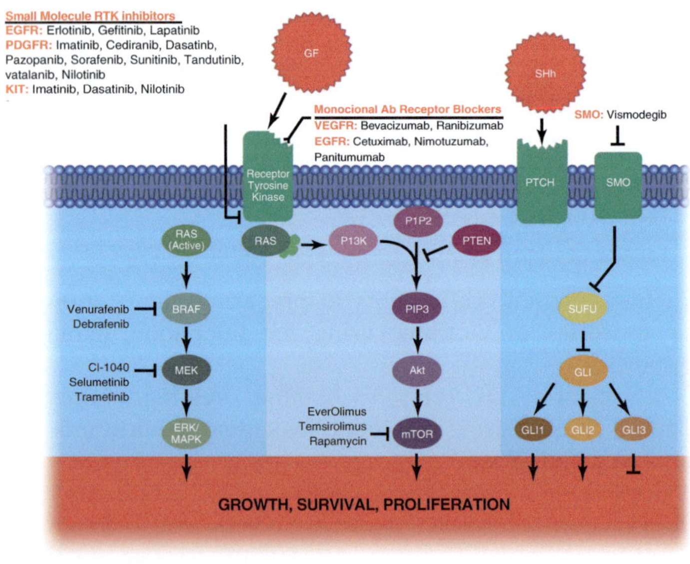

FIGURE 3.9 Molecular pathways important for targeted therapeutics. GF growth factor, RTK receptor tyrosine kinase, SHb sonic hedgehog, SMO smoothened. (Figure from Macdonald JB. *JAAD*. 2015;72:203–18)

Table 3.18 Dermatologic findings and typical culprit chemotherapeutic agents

Acneiform	Dactinomycin, fluoxymesterone, medroxyprogesterone, vinblastine, EGFR inhibitors (erlotinib, gefitinib, cetuximab, necitumumab)
Acral reactions	See below for Acral Toxic Erythema of Chemotherapy
Acral sclerosis	Bleomycin
Alopecia	Anthracyclines, bleomycin, busulfan, cyclophosphamide, chlorambucil, doxorubicin, hydroxyurea, methotrexate, mitomycin, mitoxantrone, platinum agents, procarbazine, taxanes, vinblastine, vincristine, vinca alkaloids
Contact dermatitis	L-Asparaginase, paclitaxel, mitomycin C, topical BCNU, squaric acid, DPCP
Eccrine squamous syringometaplasia	Liposomal doxorubicin (most common) and combination of cytostatic drugs administered in autologous hematopoietic stem cell transplant regimens; busulfan, bleomycin, carmustine, cisplatin, cyclophosphamide, cytarabine, dabrafenib, daunorubicin, doxorubicin, etoposide, 5-FU, imatinib, melphalan, methotrexate, mitoxantrone, pemetrexed, suramin, sunitinib, thiotepa, vemurafenib
Erythema multiforme	Busulfan, chlorambucil, cyclophosphamide, diethylstilbestrol (DES), etoposide, hydroxyurea, mechlorethamine methotrexate, mitomycin C, mitotane, paclitaxel, suramin
Erythema nodosum	Busulfan

(continued)

TABLE 3.18 (continued)

Extravasation injury	Irritant (phlebitis, cellulitis) or vesicant (blisters, bullae, ulcers) Anthracyclines (doxorubicin/daunorubicin), actinomycin D, docetaxel, paclitaxel, vinblastine, vincristine, etoposide, 5-FU Tx: elevate extremity, aspirate fluid, d/c line, cool compresses; warm compress for vinca alkaloids
Fixed drug	Dacarbazine, hydroxyurea, paclitaxel, procarbazine
Folliculitis	Actinomycin D, daunorubicin, 5-FU, methotrexate
Hair changes	INFa: increased eyelash growth Cyclosporine: hypertrichosis Cisplatin: platinum hair Methotrexate: flag sign Cyclophosphamide: hair color darkening
Hyperpigmentation	Bleomycin: flagellate pigmentation in areas of trauma, palm creases, striae 5-FU: serpentine supravenous pigmentation proximal to injection site Cyclophosphamide: patchy (palm, soles, nails, teeth) or generalized Doxorubicin/daunorubicin/dactinomycin: nail, tongue, skin Nitrogen mustard: localized to treatment areas Cisplatin: patchy pigmentation of dorsal extremities, nail, sites of trauma Carmustine (topical): occurs in occluded areas Methotrexate: diffuse brown pigmentation Thiotepa (alkylating agent): occurs in occluded areas Other hyperpigmentation under bandages: topical carmustine (BCNU), ifosfamide, docetaxel, cisplatin Imatinib: localized/generalized HYPOpigmentation Others: busulfan, ifosfamide, hydroxyurea (DM-like), doxorubicin, daunorubicin, cyclophosphamide, adriamycin, hydroxyurea

Table 3.18 (continued)

Inflammation of AKs	Systemic 5-FU, capecitabine, pentostatin, multikinase inhibitors (imatinib, dasatinib, nilotinib) (usually 1 week after chemotherapy)
Inflammation of SCC	Fludarabine
Inflammation of SKs	Cytarabine, docetaxel
Livedo	Hydroxyurea
Lichenoid	Hydroxyurea, tegafur
Lupus	Aminoglutethimide, hydroxyurea, leuprolide, tegafur
Neutrophilic eccrine hidradenitis	Cytarabine (most common), anthracyclines, bleomycin, cetuximab, dabrafenib, 5-FU, imatinib, methotrexate, mitoxantrone, vemurafenib, vinca alkaloids
Nail abnormalities/ shedding	Capecitabine, paclitaxel/docetaxel, etoposide, EGFR inhibitors, taxanes, vinca alkaloids
Melanonychia	Melphalan, hydroxyurea, bleomycin, capecitabine, doxorubicin (also, zidovudine, lamivudine, minocycline)
Mucositis	Many. Cyclophosphamide, chlorambucil, busulfan, procarbazine, EGFR inhibitors, tyrosine kinase inhibitors
Papular eruption resembling flat warts	Palifermin
Photo-onycholysis	>2 weeks after chemo (mercaptopurine)
Photosensitivity	Dacarbazine, 5-FU, tegafur, vinblastine, flutamide (photoallergic)
PR-like eruption	Imatinib
Pyogenic granulomas	EGFR (periungual)

(continued)

Table 3.18 (continued)

Radiation enhancement	Bleomycin, dactinomycin, doxorubicin, fluorouracil, hydroxyurea, mercaptopurine, methotrexate Chemo enhances toxicity of XRT if given within 7 days
Recall reaction: UV or XRT	Erythema, vesiculation, ulceration at XRT port >1 week after XRT XRT: cytoxan, 5-FU/capecitabine/gemcitabine, dactinomycin, actinomycin D, doxorubicin, daunorubicin, bleomycin, IFN, methotrexate, taxanes, vinca alkaloids UV: methotrexate
Raynaud's phenomenon	Bleomycin
Serum sickness	Antithymocyte globulin
Splinter hemorrhages (painful)	Bevacizumab
Scleroderma-like reaction	Taxanes (docetaxel, paclitaxel) Bleomycin (acral sclerosis)
Sticky skin	Doxorubicin + ketoconazole Also seen with etretinate
TEN	L-Asparaginase, bleomycin, chlorambucil, cytarabine, doxorubicin, 5-FU, methotrexate, cladribine, plicamycin, procarbazine, suramin
Ulceration	Leg ulcers: hydroxyurea Ulceration over pressure areas: bleomycin, methotrexate (see table above for other medications that can induce ulcerations/erosions)

Table 3.18 (continued)

Urticaria	Amsacrine, bleomycin, busulfan, carboplatin, chlorambucil, cisplatin, cyclophosphamide, cytarabine, daunorubicin, diaziquone, didemnin, DES <docetaxel, doxorubicin, epirubicin, etoposide, 5-FU, mechlorethamine, melphalan, methotrexate, mitomycin C, mitotane, mitoxantrone, paclitaxel, pentostatin, procarbazine, teniposide, thiotepa, trimetrexate, vincristine, zinostatin
Vasculitis	Busulfan, cyclophosphamide, cytarabine, hexamethylene bisacetamide (HMBA), hydroxyurea, levamisole, 6-mercaptopurine, methotrexate, mitoxantrone, tamoxifen

Liposomal doxorubicin, cytarabine (dose related and duration related), capecitabine, taxanes (docetaxel, can be dorsal hand instead of palm), 5-FU, epirubicin, gemcitabine,

– Bullous variant: methotrexate, cytarabine

Hand-Food Skin Reaction

Focal blistering and perilesional erythema on pressure points followed by a hyperkeratotic phase with tender keratoderma-like plaques

Usually is dose-dependent. Drug formulations that prolong serum drug levels or concentrate drug at affected sites have higher rates.

Implicated medications: multiple kinase inhibitors – sorafenib, sunitinib (can cause bullous reaction), axitinib, pazopanib, regorafenib, vemurafenib; liposomal doxorubicin +5-FU, bevacizumab + sorafenib combination, cabozantinib

Grading and Cares (Table 3.19)

Summary of Cutaneous Reactions with Targeted Therapies

Targeted therapy targets specific genes, proteins, or tissue environment that contributes to cancer growth and development. Cutaneous reactions are the most common with tar-

TABLE 3.19 Grading of acral toxic reactions and recommended managements based on grade

Grade	Management
Pretreatment	Evaluation with podiatry to treat preexisting hyperkeratotic plaques and prescribe orthopedic sole with wide, flexible shoes BID application of urea cream or other keratolytic agent to keratotic plaques/papules
Grade 1 – NIH/NCI criteria: minimal skin changes without pain WHO criteria: dysesthesia/paresthesia, tingling in hands and feet	Emollients, keratolytic creams, gel- or foam-based shoe inserts No dosage adjustment typically needed
Grade 2 – NIH/NCI criteria: skin changes with pain-limiting instrumental ADL WHO criteria: discomfort in holding objects and upon walking, painless swelling and erythema	Potent topical corticosteroid applied consecutively for 7–10 days in addition to treatment measures for grade 1 toxicity Targeted treatment dose reduction by 50% should be considered
Grade 3 – NIH/NCI criteria: severe skin changes with debilitating pain-limiting self-care ADL WHO criteria: painful erythema and swelling of palms and soles, periungual erythema and swelling	Local antiseptic bath of blisters and eruptions plus all recommendations below Treatment should be interrupted for at least 1 week and resumed at reduced dose after recovery of toxicity to grade 0 or 1

Table 3.19 (continued)

Grade	Management
Grade 4 – no NIH/NCI grade 4 WHO criteria: desquamation, ulceration, blistering, severe pain	Local antiseptic bath of blisters and eruptions plus all recommendations below Treatment should be interrupted for at least 1 week and resumed at reduced dose after recovery of toxicity to grade 0 or 1 Consider measures below
Other recommendations	Regional cooling using frozen gloves and socks just prior, during, and for 15 minutes after each chemotherapy session Topical application of antiperspirant prior to treatment Systemic agents Oral pyridoxine Dexamethasone Celecoxib – systemic review found only this effective to prevent hand-foot syndrome

geted therapies such as epidermal growth factor receptor, KIT, BCR-ABL, angiogenesis, and multikinase inhibitors.

Cutaneous Effects of EGFR Inhibitors (Table 3.20)
Drugs

- Small molecule tyrosine kinase inhibitors specific for EGFR
  - Erlotinib, gefitinib
- Dual kinase inhibitors of EGFR and HER2
  - Lapatinib, neratinib, afatinib
- Inhibitors of erbB receptors
  - Canertinib
- Multikinase inhibitors
  - Vandetanib

Table 3.20 Dermatologic effects of kinase inhibitors and recommended management

Dermatologic adverse effect	Management
Acneiform papulopustular eruption	Preventative: low-potency topical steroids, sunscreen, systemic antibiotics (tetracyclines) Treatment: low-potency topical steroids, clindamycin 1% topically, tetracycline antibiotics, isotretinoin (20–30 mg/day)
Xerosis/fissures	Bland emollients, keratolytics (urea, salicylic acid, lactic acid), zinc oxide, medium- to high-potency topical steroids; liquid glues
Hair changes (kinking, trichomegaly, hirsutism, alopecia [pattern or cicatricial], poliosis)	Non-scarring hair loss: topical minoxidil Scarring hair loss: topical steroids, topical/PO tetracycline antibiotics Hypertrichosis: eyelash trimming, eflornithine, laser hair reduction
Mucositis	Topical steroids, anesthetic rinses
Nail changes (paronychia, onycholysis, pyogenic granuloma-like lesions, brittle nails)	Antiseptic (dilute vinegar) soaks Topical steroids Biotin for brittle nails
Photosensitivity	Strict sun precautions, UVP clothing, broad-spectrum sunscreen
Pruritus	Can be managed with aprepitant

- Monoclonal antibodies that bind to a component of EGFR and prevent epidermal growth factor from binding
  - Cetuximab, necitumumab, panitumumab

References

- Macdonald JB. *JAAD*. 2015;72:203–18.
- Fabbrocini. *J Ex Clin Cancer Res*. 2012;31(1):50.

Cutaneous Effects of KIT and BCR-ABL Inhibitors (Table 3.21)

Inhibit the *bcr-abl* fusion protein, c-Kit, and platelet-derived growth factor receptors (PDGFRs).

Drugs

- Imatinib, nilotinib, dasatinib

Cutaneous Effects of Angiogenesis Agents (Table 3.22)

Inhibit vascular endothelial growth factor (VEGF) and activin receptor-like kinase-1 (ALK1).

Drugs

- Bevacizumab
- Ranibizumab

Table 3.21 Dermatologic effects of KIT/BCR-ABL inhibitors and recommended management

Dermatologic adverse effect	Management
Edema (facial typically)	Limited sodium diet (2 g/day); diuretics if severe
Morbilliform eruption – begins typically at week 9 of treatment initiation	Topical steroids or short course of oral steroids. Treatment interruption if grade 3/4
Pigmentary changes	Typically reversible with dose reduction/termination
Others: lichenoid reaction, psoriasis, PR-like eruptions, AGEP, DRESS/DIHS, SJS-TEN, urticaria, acute neutrophilic dermatosis, photosensitivity, pseudolymphoma, porphyria cutanea tarda, small vessel vasculitis, panniculitis, perforating folliculitis, erythroderma	

Cutaneous Effects of Multikinase Inhibitors (Table 3.23)
Affect many tyrosine kinase systems (e.g., PDGFR, EGFR, VEGF, KIT, RET, Flt3, RAF) and result in many skin-related adverse effects
Drugs

- Sorafenib

Table 3.22 Cutaneous effects of angiogenesis agents

Dermatologic adverse effect
Mucocutaneous hemorrhage
Disturbed wound healing

Table 3.23 Dermatologic effects of multikinase inhibitors

Dermatologic adverse effect	Management
Hyperkeratotic hand-foot syndrome	See above section related to acral reactions
Inflammatory eruptions (chloracne-like eruption, erythema multiforme-like eruption, SJS-TEN, DRESS/DIHS)	
Hair changes (alopecia, reversible hair depigmentation, yellowing of hair and skin)	
Skin pigmentation	
Localized eruptions of the scrotum/vulva (erythema, psoriasiform, lichenoid, desquamative)	
Facial edema	
Pyoderma gangrenosum-like ulceration	
Eruptive nevi	
Subungual hemorrhages	
Xerosis	
Photosensitivity	
Acute folliculitis	
Development of blue-gray macules (vandetanib)	

- Sunitinib
- Pazopanib
- Vandetanib

Adverse Effects of Hedgehog Signaling Inhibitors (Table 3.24)
Drugs
Smoothened inhibitors

- Vismodegib
- Sonidegib
- Erismodegib

Common side effects include muscle spasms (71%), alopecia (58%), dysgeusia (71%), and development of keratoacanthomas.
See prescribing information for more details.

Melanoma Therapeutics
See Fig. 3.10.

Cutaneous Effects of BRAF and MEK Inhibitors (Tables 3.25 and 3.26)
BRAF Inhibitors
Drugs

Table 3.24 Cutaneous adverse effects of hedgehog signaling inhibitors

Dermatologic adverse effect	Management
Keratoacanthomas	Surgical management or intralesional therapies (See keratoacanthoma section); regular skin examiantions
Hair loss	No treatment or minoxidil (Rogaine)
Mild folliculitis	Topical benzoyl peroxide wash, topical clindamycin
Dermal hypersensitivity reactions	Topical / oral steroids
Pruritus	Topical / oral steroids, anti-histamines, light therapy

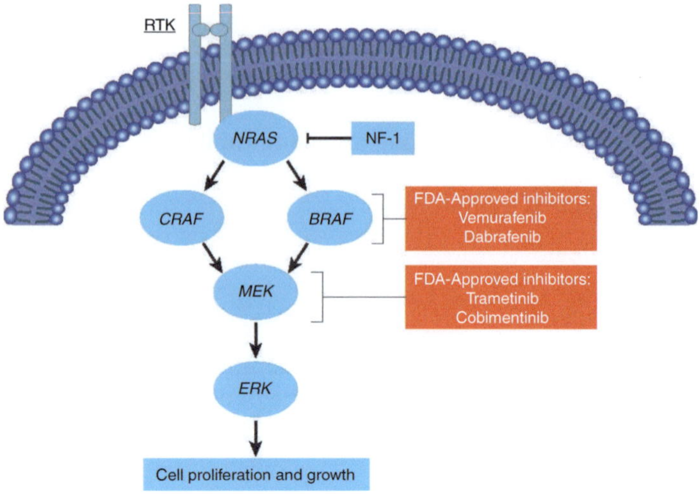

FIGURE 3.10 Molecular pathway and therapeutics targeted in melanoma

TABLE 3.25 Cutaneous adverse effects of BRAF inhibitors

Dermatologic adverse effect	Management
Maculopapular skin rash	Topical steroids, oral corticosteroids, emollients
Photosensitivity	Sun avoidance, protective clothing with UPF, broad-spectrum sunscreens
Palmoplantar hyperkeratosis	Urea cream; avoid friction
Verrucous keratosis	Cryotherapy – monitor for SCC
Alopecia	Minoxidil topically
Other hair changes: structural changes to hair (straight > curly), color changes (turning gray)	

(continued)

TABLE 3.25 (continued)

Dermatologic adverse effect	Management
SCC	Regular skin examinations and excision; consider acitretin
Panniculitis	Oral corticosteroids, NSAIDs
Melanocytic proliferations	Regular skin examinations, biopsy and excision as required; photoprotection
BCC	Excision or other therapy as required

TABLE 3.26 Cutaneous adverse effects of MEK inhibitors

Dermatologic adverse effect	Management
Acneiform papulopustular rash	Topical antibiotics, oral tetracyclines, oral steroids, oral isotretinoin

- Vemurafenib
- Dabrafenib

MEK Inhibitors
Drugs

- Trametinib
- Cobimetinib

Checkpoint Inhibitors (See Fig. 3.11)
Cutaneous Adverse Effects of Immune Checkpoint Inhibitors (Tables 3.27 and 3.28)
CTLA-4 Inhibitors
Drugs

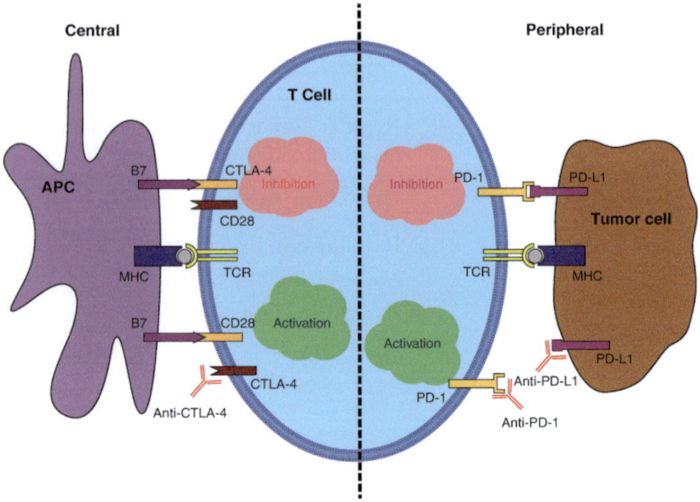

FIGURE 3.11 Molecular pathway and targets for immunotherapy/immune checkpoint inhibitors

TABLE 3.27 Cutaneous adverse effects of CTLA-4 inhibitors

Dermatologic adverse effect	Management
Morbilliform skin rash	Topical steroids, oral corticosteroids, emollients
Pruritus	Oral antihistamines, topical steroids
Lichenoid eruption	Topical steroids
Dermatitis	Topical steroids, emollients
Vitiligo – positive sign	Topical steroids, topical calcineurin inhibitors

Table 3.28 Cutaneous adverse effects of PD-1 inhibitors

Dermatologic adverse effect	Management
Morbilliform rash	Topical steroids, oral steroids
Pruritus	Topical steroids, oral antihistamines
Vitiligo – positive sign	Topical steroids, topical calcineurin inhibitors
Psoriasis	Topical steroids
Autoimmune blistering disorders	Oral steroids, topical steroids
Lichenoid eruption	Topical steroids
Dermatitis	Topical steroids, emollients, oral steroids

- Ipilimumab

  PD-1 Inhibitors
  Drugs

- Nivolumab
- Pembrolizumab
- Lambrolizumab

Less common reactions with melanoma immunotherapies include xerosis, photosensitivity, pyoderma gangrenosum-like ulcerations, Sweet's syndrome, cutaneous sarcoidosis, seborrheic keratoses, SJS-TEN, and DRESS/DIHS.

Reference: Russo I et al. *Scientifica*. 2018. PMID 30693134.

Other Drug Cutaneous Effects (Table 3.29)

TABLE 3.29 Select medications and their cutaneous side effects

G-CSF	Sweet's syndrome, psoriasis flare, LCV, localized pruritus and erythema
GM-CSF	Maculopapular exfoliative dermatitis, urticaria, pruritus, purpura, alopecia, flushing, exacerbation of vasculitis, localized wheals, localized erythema
Erythropoietin (Epo)	Abnormal hair growth, widespread eczema, palpebral edema, localized rash
Interleukins (IL)	IL-2: erythema, pruritus, urticaria, exacerbation of autoimmune skin disorders, telogen effluvium, ulcers, erythema nodosum, TEN, hypersensitivity to iodine contrast material IL-3: hemorrhagic rash, facial flushing, thrombophlebitis, urticaria IL-4: Grover's disease, papular rash, facial/peripheral edema IL-6: erythematous scaling macules and papules
Interferons (INF)	INFa: alopecia, pruritus, exacerbation of preexisting herpes labialis, cutaneous vascular lesions, psoriasis, eosinophilic fasciitis, anasarca, SLE, paraneoplastic pemphigus, and xerostomia INF-b: local reaction, fatal pemphigus vulgaris (when combined with IL-2) INF-g: relapses in melanoma, localized inflammation

Graft-Versus-Host Disease

Common complication of hematopoietic cell transplantation (HCT)

Acute GVHD

Usually occurs within days to weeks after HCT (typically within the first 100 days). Characterized by erythematous morbilliform eruption associated with fever, diarrhea, and elevated serum bilirubin. Erythematous macules and papules being on the face, *ears*, and palmar and plantar surfaces and may have perifollicular accentuation. Can become confluent progressing to erythroderma, bulla, and desquamation that can mimic TEN.

Acral erythema with violaceous discoloration of the pinna of the ear can be suggestive of acute GVHD.
Acute GVHD is a risk factor for developing viral coinfection (CMV, VZV, EBV, hepatitis viruses, parvovirus B19, respiratory viruses). Antimicrobial prophylaxis and monitoring of diagnostic infectious markers are recommended in suspected reactivation (viral DNA loads and cultures).

Infections and Acute GVHD

- CMV – reactivates in 20–40%. Presents as fever, malaise, myalgias, cervical LAD, and nonexudative pharyngitis with generalized petechial exanthem and can progress to LCV. Test via PCR. Prophylax/treat with ganciclovir/valganciclovir.
- VZV – disseminated VZV = presence of >10 nondermatomal lesions. Treatment: acyclovir/valacyclovir or famciclovir and foscarnet for acyclovir-resistant cases. (Note valacyclovir can cause nephrotoxicity.)
- EBV – presents with fever, cervical lymphadenopathy, and pharyngitis along with brawny morbilliform eruption on the extremities, although it can be urticarial or scarlatiniform. Periorbital edema and palatal petechiae can be seen. Can cause post-transplant lymphoproliferative disorder in certain patients. Most reactivations are subclinical. Treatment recommended if viral load >10,0000. Test via monospot, PCR, and EBV DNA.
- Parvovirus – often presents in transplant patients with pruritic, migratory erythema on the neck, upper extremities, and gluteal region. Lasts 1–2 weeks. Can have associated anemia, arthritis, and vasculitis. Mimics aGVHD. Dx: serum IgG and PCR. *Rule out parvovirus before starting treatment for aGVHD.*
- HHV6 – can be confused with aGVHD because both present with fever, diarrhea, and morbilliform rash. Characteristic presentation is 2–3 mm rose-pink blanchable macules and papules. Small vessel vasculitis (LCV)

can occur. Reactivation is usually 16 days post-transplant. Symptoms include cytopenia, pleurisy, encephalitis, seizures, and interstitial pneumonia. Dx: IgG or DNA-PCR. Tx: ganciclovir, foscarnet, cidofovir (HHV6 is less sensitive to acyclovir).

Chronic GVHD

Pleomorphic, multiorgan syndrome involving tissue inflammation and fibrosis that causes permanent organ dysfunction. Caused by replacement of host's immune system with donor cells.

Typically occurs within the first year after transplantation but 5–10% of patients develop it later. Thirty percent are de novo without any preceding aGVHD.

Can have lichenoid or sclerodermoid/fibrotic/poikiloderma-like presentations

Oral changes usually affect the buccal mucosa and tongue and include lichenoid changes, white patches, hyperkeratotic plaques, and ulcerations.

Can be triggered by UV light, trauma, and zoster or *Borrelia* infections.

2014 NIH Criteria for Diagnosis of cGVHD

(a) At least one diagnostic clinical sign of cGVHD
(b) At least one distinctive manifestation confirmed by biopsy or testing involved organs(s)

"Diagnostic" manifestations may be found in the skin, mouth, GI tract, lung, fascia, and genitalia (e.g., lichen planus, lichen sclerosus, poikiloderma, sclerosis, esophageal webs).

"Distinctive" features include papulosquamous lesions, oral ulcers, onycholysis, or dry gritty eyes.

Confirmatory tests are tissue biopsies (e.g., skin, mouth, lung, liver, GI, genitalia), organ-specific testing (PFTs, Schirmer tests), imaging (e.g., barium swallow showing an esophageal ring), or evaluation by a specialist (e.g., ophthalmologist or gynecologist) conforming GVHD.

Treatment: first line – systemic corticosteroids plus systemic calcineurin inhibitor, topical in mild/limited cases. Second line: thalidomide, mycophenolate mofetil, IL-2

Atypical Variants of GVHD

- Follicular/keratotic
- Thick-appearing white porcelain tongue
- Pityriasis rosea-like
- Keratosis pilaris-like cGVHD
- Overlap acute and chronic GVHD

Summary

Common manifestations of aGVHD: maculopapular rash, generalized erythroderma, bullae

Common manifestations of cGVHD: alopecia, angiomatous papules, bullae, erythema, hyper-/hypopigmentation, maculopapular eruption, poikiloderma, sweat impairment, ulceration.

And may resemble ichthyosis, LP, KP, lichen sclerosus, morphea, or scleroderma

Less common manifestations for acute or chronic GVHD: see references

References: *J Am Acad Dermatol.* 2015;72:690–5; *J Am Acad Dermatol.* 2015;72:696–702; Lee SJ. *Blood.* 2017;129(1):30–7.

Cutaneous Malignancies

Please refer to the NCCN Guidelines for the most updated management recommendations for conditions mentioned in this section.

Melanoma

ABCDs

ABCDE Adult

Asymmetry, border (irregular), color (irregular), diameter (>6 mm), evolution

ABCD Pediatric

Additional ABCD detection criteria (amelanotic; bleeding, bump; color uniformity; de novo, any diameter) used together with conventional ABCDE criteria may facilitate earlier recognition and treatment of melanoma in children.

ABCDEF for Nail Pigmentation

A: Age 50–70; African/Asian ancestry
B: Band – >3 mm; brown/black
C: Change – nail band/nail morphology
D: Digit involved – thumb, hallux, single nail involvement
E: Extension – Hutchinson's sign
F: Family and personal history – dysplastic nevus syndrome or previous melanoma

Work-Up of Primary Melanoma

- Biopsy primary site of concern.
  - Shave biopsy is preferred over punch biopsy if able to remove lesion in its entirety.
  - If punch biopsy is performed, punch out entire lesion.
  - Excisional biopsy can be used for larger lesions not able to be removed with shave biopsy.
- Palpate lymph nodes.

Sentinel Lymph Node Biopsy Recommendations

- According to NCCN Guidelines (2019)
  - Evidence supporting routine SLNB for patients with thin melanomas (<1 mm) is controversial.
  - NCCN does not recommend SLNB for patients with lesions of 0.75 mm or thinner (but should be discussed with lesions of 0.75 mm or greater depth).
  - The European Society for Medical Oncology (ESMO) recommends SLNB for lesions >1 mm and/or with ulceration.
- Gene expression profiling can aid in helping to predict if a patient is going to do poorly.

AJCC Scoring for Melanoma (Fig. 3.12)

Stage may change across care (clinical physical exam, imaging, biopsies, other diagnostics, surgical findings, after therapy, with recurrence). Pathology and radiology contribute staging information, but the clinician ultimately decides the stage across patient care continuum.

AJCC Melanoma of the Skin Staging
8th Edition

Definitions

Primary Tumor (T)

- **TX** Primery tumor cannot be assessed (for example, curettaged or severely regressed melanoma)
- **T0** No evidence of primary tumor
- **Tis** Melanoma in situ
- **T1** Melanomas 1.0 mm or less in thickness
- **T2** Melanomas 1.1 - 2.0 mm
- **T3** Melanomas 2.1 - 4.0 mm
- **T4** Melanomas more than 4.0 mm

NOTE: a and b subcatrgories of T are assigned based on ulceration and thickness as shown belowt:

T CLASSIFICATION	THICKNESS (mm)	ULCERATION STATUS
T1	≤ 1.0	a: Breslow < 0.8 mm w/o ulceration b: Breslow 0.8-1.0 mm w/o ulceration or ≤ 1.0 m wf ulceration.
T2	1.1-2.0	a: w/o ulceration b: w/ ulceration
T3	2.1-4.0	a: w/o ulceration b: w/ ulceration
T4	>4.0	a: w/o ulceration b: w/ ulceration

Regional Lymph Nodes (N)

- **NX** Patients in whom the regional nodes cannot be assessed (for example previously removed for another reason)
- **N0** No regional metastases detected
- **N1-3** Regional metastases based on the number of metastatic nodes, number of palpable metastatic nodes on clinical exam, and presence or absence of MSI[2]

NOTE: N1-3 and a-c subcategories assigned as shown below:

N CLASSIFICATION	# NODES	CLINICAL DETECTABILITY/MSI STATUS
N1	0-1 node	a: clinically occult[1], no MSI[2] b: clinically detected[1], no MSI[2] c: 0 nodes, MSI present[2]
N2	1-3 node	a: 2-3 nodes clinically occult[1], no MSI[2] b: 2-3 nodes clinically detected[1], no MSI[2] c: 1 node clinical or occult[1], MSI present[2]
N3	>1 node	a: >3 nodes, all clinically occult[1], no MSI[2] b: >3 nodes, ≥1 clinically detected[1]or matted, no MSI[2] c: >1 node clinical or occult[1], MSI present[2]

Distant Metastasis (M)

- **M0** No detectable evidence of distant metastases
- **M1a** Metastases to skin, sub cutaneous, or distant lymph nodes
- **M1b** Metastases to lung
- **M1c** Metastases to all other visceral sites
- **M1d** Metastases to brain

NOTE: Serum LDH is incorporated into the M Category as shown below:

M CLASSIFICATION	SITE	Serum LDH
M1a-d	Skin/subcutaneous/nodule (a), lung (b) other visceral (c), brain (d)	Not assessed
M1a-d(0)	Skin/subcutaneous/nodule (a), lung (b) other visceral (c), brain (d)	Normal
M1a-d(1)	Skin/subcutaneous/nodule (a), lung (b) other visceral (c), brain (d)	Elevated

ANATOMIC STAGE/PROGNOSTIC GROUPS

Clinical Staging[3]				Pathologic Staging[4]			
Stage 0	Tis	N0	M0	0	Tis	N0	M0
Stage IA	T1a	N0	M0	IA	T1a	N0	M0
Stage IB	T1b	..	..		T1b	..	..
	T2a	..	..	IB	T2a	..	..
Stage IIA	T2b	N0	M0	IIA	T2b	M0	M0
	T3a	..	..		T2a	..	..
Stage IIB	T3b	..	..	IIB	T3b	..	..
	T4a	..	..		T4a	..	..
Stage IIS	T4b	..	..	IIC	T4b	..	..
Stage III	Any T	≥N1	M0	IIIA	T1-2a	N1a	M0
	..	..	..		T1-2a	N2a	..
	..	..	..	IIIB	T0	N1b-c	M0
	..	..	..		T1-2a	N1b-c	..
	..	..	..		T1-2a	N2b	..
	..	..	..		T2b-3a	N1a-2b	..
	..	..	..	IIIC	T0	N2b-c	M0
	..	..	..		T0	N3b-c	..
	..	..	..		T1a-3a	N2c-3c	..
	..	..	..		T3b-4a	Any N	..
	..	..	..		T4b	N1a-2c	..
	..	..	..	IIID	T4b	N3a-c	M0
Stage IV	Any N	Any N	M1	IV	Any T	Any N	M1

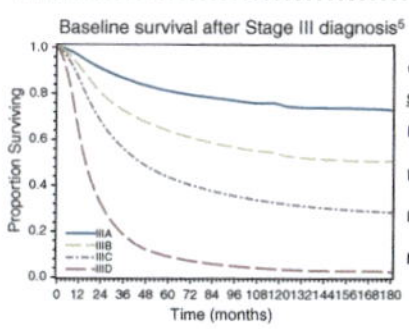

Conditional, 5-year survival (%)[5]

Stage	Baseline	3y survivors
IIIA	81.4	83.1
IIIB	64.0	76.0
IIIC	44.5	66.7
IIID	9.8	40.6

Notes

[1]Nodes are designated as 'clinically detectable' if they can be palpated on physical exam and are confirmed melanoma by pathology following excision/biopsy.
[2]MSI comprise any satellite, locally recurrent, or in transit lesions.
[3]Clinical staging includes microstaging of the primary melanoma and clinical/radiologic evaluation for metastases. By convention it should be used after complete excision of the primary melanoma with clinical assessment for regional and distant metastases
[4]Pathologic staging includes microstaging of the primary melanoma and pathologic information about the regional lymph nodes after partial or complete lymphadenectomy. Pathologic Stage 0 and 1 patients are the exceptions; they do not necessarily require pathologic evaluation of their lymph nodes. Physicians should "discuss and consider" SLNB for patients with T1b Stage IA disease; physicians should "discuss and offer" SLNB for patients with Stage IB disease.
[5]From Haydu et al., Journal of Clinical Oncology, 2017.

Produced following the 8th Ed. AJCC guidlines released January 1, 2017. Contact Dr. M. Gormally (mvgg07@gmail.com) for reprint.

FIGURE 3.12 AJCC scoring system for melanoma. (Gershenwald S et al. *CA Cancer J Clin.* 2017 [Epub ahead of print]. https://cancerstaging.org/references-tools/deskreferences/Pages/Supplemenatry-Material.aspx)

Clark Levels

I	Confined to epidermis and its appendages
II	Extends into papillary dermis
III	Extends throughout papillary dermis, impinging on reticular dermis
IV	Invades reticular dermis
V	Invades subcutaneous fat

Margins for Melanoma Excision

MIS or lentigo maligna = 5 mm margin
Melanoma 0–1 mm = 1 cm margin
Melanoma >1 cm = 2 cm margin

Types of Melanoma

- Non-chronically sun-exposed skin
  - Intermittently sun-exposed skin of trunk/ext
  - Superficial spreading melanoma, nodular melanoma, spitzoid melanoma
  - Superficial spreading: most common type
    60–70% of all MM.

    Trunk of men and legs on female are the most common sites.
  - Nodular: second most common type

    15–30%; can occur at any site; most commonly on trunk
    Arises without horizontal growth phase
- Chronically sun-exposed skin (head/neck)
  - Lentigo maligna (MIS on sun-damaged skin), lentigo maligna melanoma, desmoplastic melanoma

    Desmoplastic melanoma: dermoscopy shows atypical vascular structures, peppering, ± melanocytic structures
  - In contrast to trunk/extremities, focal changes can be very important for diagnosis and selection for biopsy – biopsy darkest/most popular area with broad shave
- Mucosal melanoma
  - Hard palate most common place.

- Don't forget to examine oral and genital mucosa during skin exams.

- Acral lentiginous melanoma
  - Most common presentation in Fitzpatrick skin types IV–VI
  - Dermoscopy patterns

  Need to biopsy

- Parallel ridge pattern
- Lesion >7 mm

Mutations in Melanoma

- BRAF mutation
  - Substitution of glutamic acid (E) for valine (V) at codon 600 (V600E) > activation of MAPK pathway; 80% of BRAF mutations
  - 40–60% of melanomas; seen in younger age onset

    Mutation also seen in 80% of acquired nevi

  - Most commonly arising in intermittently sun-exposed skin

- CDKN2A
  - Tumor suppressor gene.
  - Encodes *p16*INK4A and *p14*ARF
  - 20–40% of melanoma-prone families.
  - Associated with atypical mole – familial melanoma syndrome (BK mole)
  - Associated with pancreatic cancer.
  - Consider this gene mutation in patients with invasive melanoma AND ≥ 2 relatives affected by cutaneous melanoma and/or pancreatic cancer on one side of the family OR ≥ 3 primary melanomas in the individual.

- CDK4 mutation
  - Renders CDK4 resistant to p16

  Phenotype indistinguishable from CDKN2A phenotype

- KIT mutation
  - Mucosal (40%)
  - Acral (35%)
  - Chronically sun-damaged skin (25–30%)
- NRAS mutation
  - 10/15–20% of melanomas; nodular melanoma, acral and mucosal
  - Most often seen in later age onset
  - Also seen in congenital melanocytic nevi
- HRAS
  - Spitz nevus, rarely found in spitzoid melanoma
- GNAQ mutation
  - Uveal melanomas (45%)
  - Malignant blue nevi (i.e., melanoma arising from blue nevi)
- BAP1 (BRCA-associated protein)
  - Tumor suppressor; inactivated in 85% or uveal MM with mets
  - COMMON syndrome: cutaneous and ocular melanomas, characteristic melanocytic proliferation, and other internal neoplasms
  - *Uveal MM*, mesothelioma, MM, renal cell CA, lung CA, meningioma, *atypical spitz* or other *cutaneous to pink-colored intradermal tumors*
- TERC
- MITF/MITF p.E318K
  - Patients with MITF pancreatic or renal cancer > higher risk of melanoma
- BRCA1 or BCRA2
  - Increased risk of breast, ovarian, prostate, and pancreatic cancer and an up to twofold increase in risk of melanoma

- Melanoma and gene expression profile
  - Comparative genomic hybridization

    Compared to melanocytic nevi, 96% of melanoma had some form of chromosomal aberration compared to only 13% of nevi (all were spitz nevi with gain of 11p). Gain of 6p was seen in the thickest melanomas.
    6p and 1q gains had the lowest overall survival rates.
  - FISH

    Melanomas demonstrate changes in 11q and 6p (not seen in common nevi).
    Four-probe assay is currently available for testing:

    - 6p25, 6p23, 11q13, and centromere 6
    - Spitzoid melanoma: gain of 11q, loss of 9p

Ref: *JAAD CME.* June 2015.
Ref: Ransohoff et al. and Soura et al. *JAAD.* 2016;74(3):CMEs.

Genetic Testing

- *Send to genetics for genetic counseling and testing*
- Before undergoing genetic studies, ascertain a three-generation pedigree for all melanoma and non-melanoma cutaneous and visceral/heme malignancies. Discuss basic genetics, likelihood of hereditary melanoma, known melanoma loci, probability of detecting a CDKN2A (or other) mutation, availability and coverage of testing, possible results, clinical utility, and discrimination (Soura et al. *JAAD.* 2013;74(3):CME).
- Patients should be reassured that per the Genetic Information Nondiscrimination Act (GINA) of 2008 (http://www.ginahelp.org), familial genetic tests and genetic counseling cannot be used to deny health insurance or employment (in places with ≥15 employees). GINA does not protect against discrimination from life insurance, disability insurance, or long-term care insurance companies. GINA does not protect or apply to the US military or employees of the federal government who get care through the Federal Employees Health Benefits Plan (Table 3.30).

TABLE 3.30 Chromosomal aberrations in melanoma

Chromosome locus	Associated gene	Gain or loss	Others
6p25	RREB1	+	4-probe FISH, poor prognosis
6q23	MYB	±	4-probe FISH
11q13	CCND1	+	4-probe FISH
Centromere 6	CEP6	Gain or loss of chromosome 6	4-probe FISH
8q24	MYC	+	Aggressive melanoma, amelanotic MM
10q23	BRAF	–	
7	BRAF	+	
1q23	BRAF	+	
11q13	NRAS	–	Acral melanoma, poor prognosis
12q13	CDK4	–	
9p21	CDKN2A (p16)	–	
Chromosome 10	PTEN, BRAF	–	
11p		+	Spitz nevi, not melanoma

Melanoma Treatments

Please refer to NCCN Guidelines for the most up-to-date recommendations.

- Ninety percent of all recurrences occur during the first 5 years.
- Follow up dermatology visits:
  - Invasive melanoma

Q3-month skin checks for the first 2 years.
Q6-month skin checks for 3 years.
Then yearly skin exams for life.
If familial mole syndrome considered, Q3–6-month skin checks for life ± full-body photography ± referral to an internist for w/u of other visceral malignancies.
Dermoscopy to all nevi.
Education of ABCDEs.
Recommend monthly self-skin exams.
Counsel patients on standard eye and dental exams.

- Recommend that all first- and second-degree relatives have a dermatologic evaluation.

- Other therapies
  - Adjuvant therapy

    Goal: eliminate clinically inapparent micromets; resected high-risk stage II or III.
    INFa: sign of autoimmunity is associated with better prognosis.

  - Immunotherapy

    IL2 – used for distant mets usually.
    CTL4 blocker; autoimmunity is associated with better response.
    Vaccine.
    Targeted therapy.

  - Kinase inhibitors: BRAF and MEK

    Small molecules, orally taken.
    Specific mutations.
    Rapid tumor response.
    High response rate.
    Develop resistance.

  - BRAF inhibitors: vemurafenib, dabrafenib

    Specific V600E mutation
    Most common AE: photosensitivity, increase risk of new melanomas, SCCs/keratoacanthomas, rash

- MEK inhibitors: trametinib, cobimetinib

  Shown to increase median survival in patients with BRAF V6004/K mutation
  No increase in NMSC/SCC seen
  Most common AE: rash or acneiform eruption

- Immunostimulators

  Ipilimumab
  For advanced MM

- Programmed death 1 receptor blockers

  Nivolumab, lambrolizumab, pembrolizumab
  For advanced MM
  AE: pneumonitis, vitiligo, colitis, hepatitis, hypophysitis, thyroiditis

Keratinocyte Carcinomas

Keratinocyte carcinomas = basal cell carcinomas and squamous cell carcinomas

Risk factors

- Genetics
  - Fitzpatrick skin types I–III
- UVR
  - BCC: intermittent sun exposure also, medications that increase risk of sun sensitivity associated with more keratinocyte carcinomas (e.g. HCTZ, voriconazole)
- Tanning
  - 2.5 odds ratio for SCC; 1.5 for BCC
- UV therapy
  - PUVA: 8.6× increase for doses 100–337
- Ionizing radiation
  - >12015Gy; most appear ~20 years after initial exposure

- Occupational
  - Airline, farmers, sailors, outdoor occupations
- Chemical
  - Pesticides, asphalt, tar, polycyclic aromatic hydrocarbons, arsenic (acts as a tumor promoter by modulating signaling pathway for cell growth)
- HPV
  - SCC: HPV subtypes are thought to act as co-carcinogens in conjunction with UVR.
  - HPV DNA found in ~70–90% transplant-associated SCC
- Organ transplant
  - SCC: 40–250× increase
  - Cumulative sun exposure, age at transplantation, degree and length of immunosuppression
- Medications
  - Immunosuppressant medications

    SCC
    Risk related to length of immunosuppressive drug
  - BRAF inhibitors

    KAs/SCCs
- HIV infection
  - SCC – including perianal/HPV
- Other risk factors
  - Chronic ulcer, smoking, thermal burns, high attitudes
- Actinic keratosis
  - Risk of evolving into SCC: 0.065–0.096% per lesion per year

Management of Keratinocyte Carcinomas

- Excision is the most common therapy with Mohs for certain tumors (see Mohs Appropriate Use Criteria in Procedural Dermatology section).

- ED&C.
- Topical therapies, such a 5-FU/imiquimod /PDT, for certain superficial/in situ lesions.
- Cryotherapy can be used in certain cases.
- Localized radiotherapy.
- Watchful waiting/observation sometimes used in the extreme elderly or those with low-risk lesions and short life expectancy.

Management Pearls for BCCs

- Mohs surgery is the gold standard for most BCCs; if Mohs Appropriate Use Criteria are not met, then surgical excision preferred.
- Localized superficial BCC on low-risk sites (<trunk and extremities other than shin, hands, and feet, <2 cm,) in patients with low cosmetic concerns without hx of radiation or immunosuppression may consider ED&C.
- Field therapy with 5-FU (BID for 3–6 weeks) or imiquimod (5×/week for 6 weeks) or PDT.
- For people with mulitple BCCs, consider prevention with nicotinamide 500 mg BID
- If not a surgical candidate, may consider systemic treatment:

  – Vismodegib PO 150 mg daily or alternative therapeutic regimens:

    One week on and one week off for 1 months, then 1 week on and 2 weeks off for 2 months, and then 1 week on and 3 weeks off for 3 months.
    Monitor for side effects and titrate down or stop if loss of taste leads to weight loss or other effects which are not tolerable.

Management Pearls for SCCs

- Mohs surgery is the gold standard for most SCCs; if Mohs Appropriate Use Criteria are not met, then surgical excision preferred.

- Low-risk site/superficial SCC can consider ED&C, intralesional methotrexate 1 ml in 25 mg/ml every 2 weeks ×4, or intralesional 5-FU 50 mg/ml weekly ×4–8.
- In solid organ transplant patients, or other high-risk patients, consider chemoprevention with acitretin 10 mg daily and/or nicotinamide 500 mg BID and if many/severe SCCs, consider coordinating with transplant team to optimize/change immunosuppression.
- Metastasis is a concern for high-risk anatomical sites such as the lip and ear.
- Perform total body skin check and check lymph nodes on exam q3–6 months.
  - Monitor burn scars, chronic wounds, and any areas that underwent radiation closely for any primary/recurrent SCC.
- Survival benefit of sentinel lymph node bx with complete lymph node dissection unclear.
- If multiple high-risk features (see staging systems), consider adjunctive radiation with Mohs surgery/excision. Caveat: can usually only radiate effectively once. Survival benefit of radiation as an adjunct treatment unclear.
- If not a candidate for surgery, consider a systemic treatment (together with medical oncology).
  - Cetuximab, pembrolizumab, nivolumab, capecitabine

Staging Systems for Squamous Cell Carcinoma (Tables 3.31 and 3.32)

TABLE 3.31 Modified Brigham and Women's Hospital staging system: tied to prognosis (From: Jambursaria-Pulahani, et al. JAMA Dermatology. 2013;149(4):402–410.

T-staging	Definition	% of disease-specific death
T0	In situ SCC	
T1	0 risk factor	0%
T2a	1 risk factor	0%
T2b	2–3 risk factors	83%
T3	4 risk factors or bone invasion	17%

Table 3.32 Stage of tumor and associated risk factors

Stage	Risk factors
Clinical tumor stage	Low risk: tumor diameter ≤2 cm High risk: tumor diameter >2 cm
Pathological tumor stage	No risk: tumor thickness ≤2 mm Low risk: tumor thickness >2 mm and ≤6 mm High risk: tumor thickness >6 mm
Co-risk factors	Immunosuppression Desmoplastic type or poor differentiation Localization of ear

Breuginger et al. in Roscher et al. *JAMA Dermatol.* 2018;154(4):428–34

Risk factors include tumor diameter >2 cm, poorly differentiated histologic characteristics, perineural invasion (of any caliber, but esp. of nerves >0.1 mm that have increased risk of nodal involvement), and tumor invasion beyond subcutaneous fat (excluding bone as that automatically makes the staging T3) and also potentially tumors on the lip/ear and immunosuppressed patients.

Stages T2b and 3 must be considered for sentinel lymph node biopsy, further imaging, and/or radiation.

Ref: Jambursaria-Pulahani et al. *JAMA Derm.* April 2013.

Ref: Roscher et al. JAMA Dermatol. 2018;154(4):428–34.

Cutaneous Lymphoma

Good reading: http://www.bloodjournal.org/content/110/6/1713?sso-checked=true

Types of Cutaneous Lymphomas (Tables 3.33, 3.34, and 3.35)

3.9% of all non-Hodgkin lymphomas are cutaneous lymphomas.

T cell is the most common at 75–80% of all primary cutaneous lymphomas; 20–25% are B cell.

Refer to NCCN Guidelines for more information on staging and management.

Usually lymphoma work-up and treatment are done in a team approach together with medical oncology.

TABLE 3.33 Types of cutaneous T and NK lymphomas

Lymphoma	5-year survival
Mycosis fungoides (50%)	88%
MF variants and subtypes	
Folliculotropic MF	80%
Pagetoid reticulosis	100%
Granulomatous slack skin	100%
Sezary syndrome	24%
Adult T-cell leukemia/lymphoma	
Primary cutaneous CD30+ lymphoproliferative d/o (30%)	
Primary cutaneous anaplastic large cell lymphoma	95%
Lymphomatoid papulosis	100%
Subcutaneous panniculitis-like T-cell lymphoma (a/b type only)	82%
Extranodal NK/T-cell lymphoma, nasal type	NR[a]
Primary cutaneous peripheral T-cell lymphoma, unspecified	16%
Primary cutaneous aggressive epidermotropic CD8+ T-cell lymphoma[b]	18%
Cutaneous d/g T-cell lymphoma (including g/d type of SPTCL)[b]	NR[a]
Primary cutaneous CD4+ small-/medium-sized pleomorphic T-cell lymphoma[b]	75%

[a]NR = not reached (i.e., VERY poor prognosis); [b]provisional entities

Connective Tissue Diseases

Antibodies in Connective Tissue Diseases

- Antinuclear antibody (ANA) preferentially target cellular structures vital to cellular function (DNA, RNA-binding proteins), primarily IgG class.

TABLE 3.34 Cutaneous B-cell lymphomas

Lymphoma	5-year survival
Primary cutaneous marginal zone B-cell lymphoma	99%
Primary cutaneous follicle center lymphoma	95%
Primary cutaneous diffuse large B-cell lymphoma, leg type	55%
Primary cutaneous diffuse large cell B-cell lymphoma, others	50%
Intravascular large B-cell lymphoma	65%

TABLE 3.35 Precursor hematologic neoplasm

Lymphoma	5-year survival
CD4+/CD56+ hematodermic neoplasm (blastic NK-cell lymphoma)	?

  - ANA assay identifies autoantibodies present in serum that bind to autoantigen present in the nuclei (or cytoplasm) of mammalian cells.
- Assay *titer:* reflects the serial serum dilution necessary for fluorescence to disappear (depends upon subjective interpretation by lab technicians)
  - Usually >1:80 is reported as abnormal (but <1:160 often is true cutoff).
- Immunofluorescence patterns
  - See below.
  - Are usually of little specificity and value to disease except centromeric pattern: reflection of antibody binding to polypeptide components of chromosomal centromeres (CENP-B); primarily associated with limited form of systemic sclerosis (SSc).
- Normal vs abnormal ANA levels (Table 3.36)
  - ANA can be falsely elevated in normal population.
  - See below.

TABLE 3.36 ANA patterns

ANA	Predominant Ag	Disease
Peripheral	Native “n” DNA	SLE (esp. renal disease)
Homogenous	nDNA, histones	SLE
Nucleolar	Nucleolar RNA	SSc, SLE
Centromere	Kinetochore	CREST
Speckled	Various ribonucleoproteins (Ro, La, U1RNP)	Sjogren’s, SSc, SLE, MCTD
Particulate		SCLE

- Certain autoantibodies have significant disease specificity.
  - Anti-dsDNA, anti-Sm = systemic lupus
  - Anti-Mi-2 = classic dermatomyositis
  - Anti-Jo-1 = antisynthetase syndrome of dermatomyositis
  - Anti-topoisomerase 1 (Scl-70), anti-RNA polymerase (RNAP), anti-centromere for clinical forms of systemic sclerosis
  - Cytoplasmic antineutrophil cytoplasmic antibodies (C-ANCA) for granulomatosis with polyangiitis
- Absolute blood levels of few autoantibodies can correlate positively with underlying autoimmune disease activity.
  - Anti-dsDNA in SLE

    Rising level correlates positively with disease activity, especially when associated with falling complement values.
    High levels reflect increased risk of lupus nephritis.
  - C-ANCA in granulomatosis with polyangiitis
  - Presence of anti-RNP aAb: a risk factor for development of renal crisis in scleroderma; prognostic value; does not correlate with disease activity
- Extractable nuclear antigen (ENA).
  - Sm, RNP (U1 RNP), Ro/SSa, La/SSb, Scl-70, Jo-1

- Ro/La: human cytoplasmic RNP (hYRNP) – present in cytoplasm and nucleus
- Ro/La are linked; thus rare for them to be positive alone; anti-Ro aAb can occur alone; anti-La is very rare.

SLE: ANA+ in 95%; 60% dsDNA (specific and correlates with renal disease), 35% SSA, 20% histone, 20% Smith; sometimes +RF; SLE with negative ANA often + ssDNA.

Drug SLE: 95% have histone antibodies.
Discoid LE: 30–50% have +ANA.
SCLE: 70% with + Ro.
Sjogren's: 70% + SSA (Ro), 30% + SSB (La). Often + RF.
Scleroderma/Systemic Sclerosis (SSc): 35% SCL-70.
Dermatomyositis: 60–80% + ANA.
Normal: 10% + ANA.

Other Conditions with + ANA

- Elderly persons
- Pregnant women
- Relatives of patients with CTD
- Other autoimmune diseases (e.g., primary biliary cirrhosis, autoimmune thyroiditis)
- Drugs (e.g., procainamide, hydralazine)
- Chronic infections
- Neoplasms
- Healthy persons (up to 15% can have a positive ANA)

Lupus Erythematosus (LE)

Work-Up of Cutaneous LE

- History.
- Skin biopsy ± DIF.
- CBC with differential.
- UA, BUN, creatinine.
- Serologies: ANA, anti-dsDNA, Smith, Ro/SSA.
- Complement: total complement – if abnormal, get C2, C3, and C4.
- SPEP.
- ± antiphospholipid antibodies.

Cutaneous Lupus
Chronic Cutaneous Lupus

- Discoid lupus (localized, generalized)
- Hypertrophic lupus
- Lupus panniculitis
- Tumid lupus
- Chilblain lupus

Subacute Cutaneous Lupus

- Papulosquamous pattern
- Annular-polycyclic pattern

Acute Cutaneous Lupus

- Malar rash - High association with systemic disease (virtually 100%)
- Bullous lupus

Systemic Lupus Erythematosus
Diagnostic Criteria for SLE (Table 3.37)

Clinical Criteria: Further Information

1. Acute or Subacute Cutaneous Lupus (ALE, SCLE)
   Acute cutaneous lupus: malar rash (mixed, flat erythema, flat or raised over malar eminences, tending to spare the nasolabial folds – do not count if malar discoid), bullous lupus, TEN variant of SLE, maculopapular lupus rash, photosensitive lupus rash (in the absence of dermatomyositis)

   Subacute cutaneous lupus: non-indurated psoriasiform and/or annular polycyclic lesions that resolve without scarring, although occasionally with post-inflammatory pigmentary changes ± telangiectasia
2. Chronic Cutaneous Lupus (CLE)
   Classic discoid rash (raised red patches with adherent keratotic scale and follicular plugging; atrophic scarring in older lesions) localized (above the neck) or generalized (above and below the neck), hypertrophic (verrucous) lupus, lupus panniculitis (profundus), mucosal lupus, lupus erythematosus tumidus, chilblains lupus, discoid lupus/lichen planus overlap

TABLE 3.37 SLICC classification criteria for systemic lupus erythematosus

Clinical criteria	Immunologic criteria
1. Acute/subacute cutaneous lupus	1. ANA
2. Chronic cutaneous lupus	2. Anti-DNA
3. Oral or nasal ulcers	3. Anti-Sm
4. Non-scarring alopecia	4. Antiphospholipid Ab
5. Arthritis	5. Low complement (C3, C4, CH50)
6. Serositis	6. Direct Coombs test (do not count in the presence of hemolytic anemia)
7. Renal	
8. Neurologic	
9. Hemolytic anemia	
10. Leukopenia	
11. Thrombocytopenia (<100,000/mm^3)	

Requirements: ≥4 criteria serially OR simultaneously (at least 1 clinical and 1 laboratory criteria) OR biopsy-proven lupus nephritis with positive ANA or anti-dsDNA

3. Oral ulcers OR nasal ulcers
   Oral: palate, buccal, tongue
   Nasal ulcers
   Usually painless
   In the absence of other causes, such as vasculitis, Behcet's disease, infection (herpes), inflammatory bowel disease, reactive arthritis, and acidic foods
4. Non-scarring alopecia
   Diffuse thinning or hair fragility with visible broken hairs in absence of other causes, such as alopecia areata, telogen effluvium, iron deficiency, and androgenetic alopecia
5. Synovitis involving two or more joints

Characterized by swelling or effusion

OR tenderness in two or more joints and at least 30 minutes of morning stiffness

6. Serositis

   Typical pleurisy for more than 1 day OR pleural effusions OR pleural rub

   Typical pericardial pain (pain with recumbency improved by sitting forward) for more than 1 day OR pericardial effusion OR pericardial rub OR pericarditis by EKG

   In absence of other causes, such as infection, uremia, and Dressler's pericarditis
7. Renal

   Urine protein-to-creatinine ratio (or 24-hour urine protein) representing 500 mg protein/24 hours OR red blood cell casts
8. Neurologic

   Seizures, psychosis, mononeuritis multiplex (in absence of other known causes such as primary vasculitis), myelitis, peripheral or cranial neuropathy (in the absence of other known causes such as primary vasculitis, infection, and diabetes mellitus), acute confusional state (in absence of other causes including toxic/metabolic causes, uremia, drugs)
9. Hemolytic anemia
10. Leukopenia (<4000/mm^3) OR lymphopenia (<1000/mm^3)

    Leukopenia at least once in absence of other known causes like Felty's syndrome, drugs, and portal hypertension

    Lymphopenia at least once in absence of other known causes such as corticosteroids, drugs, and infection
11. Thrombocytopenia (<100,000/mm^3)

    At least once in the absence of other known causes such as drugs, portal hypertension, and thrombotic thrombocytopenic purpura

Immunologic Criteria

1. ANA level above reference range – an abnormal titer of antinuclear antibody by immunofluorescence or an equivalent assay at any point in time and in absence of drugs known to be associated with "drug-induced lupus" syndrome

2. Anti-dsDNA antibody above laboratory reference range (or two-fold of the reference range if tested by ELISA)
3. Anti-Sm
4. Antiphospholipid antibody positivity as determined by: Positive test for lupus anticoagulant

   False positive to RPR (syphilis test) – known to be positive for at least 6 months and confirmed by negative *Treponema pallidum* immobilization or fluorescent treponemal antibody absorption test

   Medium- or high-titer anticardiolipin antibody level (IgA, IgG, or IgM)

   Positive test result for anti-2-glycoprotein (IgA, IgG, or IgM)
5. Low complement (C3, C4, CH50)
6. Direct Coombs test (in absence of hemolytic anemia)

Progression to SLE

Overall: 10% of CLE progress to SLE; over the mean time of 8 years

DLE (localized) = 5% progression
DLE (generalized) = 20% progression
SCLE = 50%

Chronic Cutaneous Lupus

Discoid Lupus

Risk of progressing to SLE

- 5–10%; may be up to 28%.
- Generalized lesions, periungual telangiectasias, and arthralgias/arthritis.
- Lab factors: anemia, leukopenia, elevated ESR, and high ANA titer.
- Anti-RNP antibody titers may be associated with severe disease and systemic involvement.

Lupus Panniculitis

- Buttocks, chest, shoulder, and face.
- Heals with atrophy often.
- Some will have DLE lesions overlying panniculitis: "lupus profundus."

- Can present very similarly both clinically and pathologically to subcutaneous panniculitis-like T-cell lymphoma (!)
- 10–15% meet criteria for SLE.
- 30% have DLE.
- *Some patients with lupus panniculitis may have occasional subclinical PCT, and treating with hydroxychloroquine may lead to acute hepatic toxicity (abdominal pain, nausea/vomiting/diarrhea, transaminitis).*

Chilblain LE

- Acral dusky purple papules, plaques associated with acrocyanosis, minimal atrophy, scarring; acral sites, nose, ears.
- Brought on or exacerbated by moist cold climates.
- Most commonly will have +ANA, less likely +anti-Ro/Las, and cardiolipin antibodies.
- 18% of patients will develop systemic LE.

Monitoring Cutaneous LE

- Patients should be evaluated for systemic progression at each visit (e.g., fatigue, fever, arthritis, oral ulcers, nonscarring alopecia).
- ANA, CBC, and UA annually.
- Vitamin D level yearly if practicing strict photoprotection.
- Consider expanded annual labs (ESR, ENA, dsDNA, complement) for 1–2 years; thereafter do based on review of symptoms.

FYI

- Patients of African ancestry with +dsDNA, low C3/C4, even if no systemic symptoms, check serial UA; they are at higher risk of lupus nephritis.
- Low complement
  - C2, C4; many will have annular SCLE-like lesions and + Ro antibody.
  - C4 deficiency; often have hyperkeratosis of palms/soles.
  - May have nephritis and increase risk of infection.
- Anti-dsDNA, anti-C1q antibody: highly specific for active nephritis.

Subacute Cutaneous Lupus Erythematosus (SCLE)

- Photosensitivity; *midface usually spared*, while sides of the face, upper trunk, and upper extremities are commonly involved.
- Lesions will result in dyspigmentation but typically no scarring.
- 60–80% + ANA, 60–90% + anti-Ro.
- ~ 80% of patients with SCLE will have positive Ro/SSA Ab.
- More than 1/3 could be attributed to drugs.
- Fifty percent will eventually meet SLE criteria.
- 10–15% may develop internal disease (nephritis).
- With anti-Ro antibody association: some will also have Sjogren-like symptoms; patients with SCLE and Sjogren's have worse prognosis than without Sjogren's.

Neonatal Lupus

- Mother has anti-Ro autoantibodies.
- Subsequent risk of NLE in the next child is 25%.
- Systemic involvement
  - Congenital heart block (with or without cardiomyopathy); *almost always present at birth, rarely develops after birth.*
  - Hepatobiliary disease and TCP; many present within first few weeks of life.
  - Anti-U1RNP antibody not associated with congenital heart block.

Drug-Induced Lupus

Antihistone (serositis predominant): hydralazine, INH, procainamide, sulfonamides (sulfasalazine), penicillamine, anticonvulsants, minocycline, PTU, PUVA, quinidine, methyldopa, levamisole (cocaine contaminant), pembrolizumab

True SLE lupus (anti-ds-DNA): penicillamine, TNFa inhibitors

- Different than regular drug-induced SLE:
  - Prominent cutaneous findings

- Photosensitivity
- ANA+, *dsDNA antibody* +
- Less likely to have +antihistone antibody

SCLE (+ anti-Ro/SSA): *hydrochlorothiazide* > *terbinafine, diltiazem, ACE inhibitors*, NSAIDs (naproxen), griseofulvin, antihistamine, glyburide, anticonvulsants, piroxicam, spironolactone, sulfonylureas, statins, IFN, PUVA, TNFa, *PPIs*, taxols (docetaxel)

- Drugs may induce or exacerbate SCLE.
- ~20–30% of newly dx SCLE have drug as trigger, maybe higher in patients >50 years old.
- PPI-induced SCLE: younger than 40, lansoprazole >omeprazole, onset after 8 months of meds, resolution 3 months after stopping
  - 61% ANA+, 73% Ro+, 33% La+, 8% dsDNA+, 8% antihistone+

Prevention of CLE Flares

- Avoid sunlight and artificial sources of UV (tanning bed, fluorescent bulbs).
- Broad-spectrum physical block sunscreens (SPF 50+); adding in iron oxides to sunscreens help to protect against visitble light
- Heliocare supplements to reduce photosensitivity.
- Photoprotective clothing.

Treatment

Topical

- Topical corticosteroids
  - Face: low potency.
  - Trunk/extremities: mid potency.
  - Scalp, soles, palms: high potency.
  - Consider intralesional triamcinolone for DLE.
- Topical calcineurin inhibitors – can combine with top steroids to increase efficacy or be used alone

Systemic

Antimalarials

- Hydroxychloroquine
- Quinacrine (must get from compounding pharmacy)
- Chloroquine
  - Effects of antimalarials may take up to 2–3 months to work.
  - Smoking cessation required.
  - Aplastic anemia reported at doses of quinacrine >100 mg/day.
  - See dermatopharmacology section for more information

Immunosuppressives

- Corticosteroids – short bursts during flares helpful; response to DLE unreliable
- Methotrexate (PO or IM) – helpful for all CLE
- Mycophenolate mofetil – helpful for all CLE
  - If GI side effects, consider mycophenolate sodium, which is enteric coated.
- Azathioprine – helpful for DLE
- Cyclosporine – for resistant cases
- Rituximab – for refractory cases and bullous lupus

Immunomodulators

- Dapsone – for bullous lupus, lupus panniculitis, SCLE, and possible DLE
- Thalidomide – helpful for CCLE, SCLE, and tumid lupus
- Lenalidomide

Others

- IVIg
- Acitretin and isotretinoin

Therapeutic ladder

- Start hydroxychloroquine.
- Add quinacrine.
- If hydroxychloroquine-quinacrine combo fails, stop hydroxychloroquine, and start chloroquine in combination with quinacrine (to protect the retina).
- Add/change to an immunosuppressant.

References

- Chang YA and Werth VP. Treatment of cutaneous lupus. *Curr Rheumatol Rep.* 2011;13(4):300–7.
- Petri M et al. *Arthritis and Rheumatism.* 2012;64(8):2677–86.
- Eastham et al. *JAMA Derm.* 2014;150(3):344.
- Sandholdt et al. *Br J Derm.* 2014;170(2):342–51.

Dermatomyositis

Dermatomyositis (DM) vs polymyositis (PM) (Table 3.38)

Diagnostic criteria for dermatomyositis (Table 3.39)

Antibodies in dermatomyositis and their clinical significance (Table 3.40)

Tender palmar papules (inverse Gottron's papules) have been recently described in DM patients; presence of these lesions is often associated with anti-MDA5 (CADM140) phenotype. Neopterin and factor VII-related antigen (von Willebrand Factor) reported to correlate with juvenile DM.

Systemic Disease

- Proximal muscles weakness, especially extensor muscles (triceps, quadriceps).
- Most commonly overlaps with other CTD (CREST)
  - Raynaud's
  - Dysphagia (should evaluation for possible scleroderma overlap)
  - GERD (esophageal dysfunction)

Table 3.38 Dermatomyositis vs polymyositis

Dermatomyositis	**Polymyositis**
Without muscle weakness (amyopathic DM or dermatomyositis sine myositis) - amyopathic have increased risk of malignancy	Adult Pediatric Inclusion body myositis Overlap (myositis associated with a connective tissue disease)
With muscle weakness	
Adult	
Malignancy associated	
Not malignancy associated	
Pediatric	

TABLE 3.39 Diagnostic criteria for dermatomyositis

1.	Skin lesions: (1) Heliotrope, red-purple edematous erythema on the upper palpebra; (2) Gottron's sign, red-purple keratotic atrophic erythema or macules on the extensor surface of finger joins; (3) Erythema on the extensor surface of extremity joints, slightly raised red-purple erythema over elbows or knees
2	Proximal muscle weakness (upper or lower extremity and trunk)
3.	Elevated serum creatinine kinase or aldolase level
4.	Muscle pain on grasping or spontaneous pain
5.	Myogenic changes on electromyography (short-duration, polyphasic motor unit potentials with spontaneous fibrillation potentials)
6.	Positive anti-Jo-1 antibody test (histidyl-tRNA synthetase)
7.	Non-destructive arthritis or arthralgias
8.	Systemic inflammatory signs (temperature: >37 °C at axilla, elevated CRP, or ESR >20 mm per hour by Westergren)
9.	Pathologic findings compatible with inflammatory myositis (inflammatory infiltration or skeletal evidence of active regeneration may be seen)

Criteria no. 1 + four other criteria from no. 2–9 = DM; four criteria from no. 2–9 = polymyositis

- Pulmonary disease: 15–30% of patients – diffuse interstitial fibrosis similar to RA and scleroderma patients can lead to ARDS.
- Cardiac disease: usually asymptomatic – usually presents as arrhythmias or conduction defects (poor prognostic indicator, major indicator of death!).
- Other organs: renal, joint, neuropathy, Raynaud's, pulmonary, etc. can suggest overlapping systemic autoimmune connective tissue disease.

TABLE 3.40 Antibodies in dermatomyositis

Target	Median prevalence	Molecular specificity	Clinical association
High specificity for DM/PM			
P155	80% amyopathic, 20–30% classic	c (TIF1-G)	Clinically amyopathic DM; in adult-classic DM, increased risk of *malignancy* *Low risk of ILD*
Mi-2	15–20%	Helicase nuclear proteins	Gottron's papules/ sign, shawl sign, periungual telangiectasia, cuticular overgrowth/ dystrophy, good prognosis
Jo-1	20%	Histidyl-tRNA synthetase	Most common anti-synthetase antibody: Antisynthetase syndrome: arthritis, Raynaud's interstitial lung disease, mechanical hands; poorer prognosis
PL-7	5%	Threonyl-tRNA synthetase	Antisynthetase syndrome (see above)
PL-12	3%	Alanyl-rTNA synthetase	Antisynthetase syndrome (see above)
OJ	Rare	Isoleucyl-tRNA synthetase	Antisynthetase syndrome (see above)
EJ	Rare	Glycyl-tRNA synthetase	Antisynthetase syndrome (see above), possibly increased frequency of skin changes

(continued)

Table 3.40 (continued)

Target	Median prevalence	Molecular specificity	Clinical association
SRP	5%	Signal recognition particle (intracytoplasmic protein translocation	Associated with polymyositis; fulminant/acute DM/PM, cardiac involvement
Fer	Rare	Elongation factor 1-alpha	
Mas	Rare	Small RNA	
MDA5/ CADM-140	–15%	IFN induced with helicase C domain protein/ melanoma differentiation-associated gene 5	*Asian patients* Clinically amyopathic DM, rapidly progressive interstitial lung disease, palmar papules, painful ulcers with associate vasculopathy, gum pain, alopecia, calcinosis
Low specificity for DM/PM			
ANA	40%		Clinically amyopathic DM (65%), most common IF patterns: speckled, nucleolar
ssDNA	40%	ssDNA	SLE, SSc, morphea
PM-Scl (PM-1)	10%	Ribosomal RNA processing enzyme	Overlap with SSc

TABLE 3.40 (continued)

Target	Median prevalence	Molecular specificity	Clinical association
SSA/Ro (esp. 52 kDa Ro)	15%	hYRNP	Overlap with SjS, SCLE neonatal LE/CHB, SLE
U1RNP	10%	Spliceosome RNP	Overlap with other CTDs
Ku	3%	DNA end-binding repair protein complex	Overlap with SSc and SLE
U2RNP	1%	Spliceosome RNP	Overlap with SSc RF: elevated in 20% – most often in overlap syndromes

Paraneoplastic Dermatomyositis

- Reported frequency of <10%–50%.
- Patients with amyopathic DM appear to be at increased risk of associated malignancy.
- Antibodies: TIF1G (p155), NXP2
  - Patients with TIF-1γ have more extensive skin disease.
  - Characteristic palmoplantar hyperkeratotic papules.
  - Psoriasis-like lesions.
  - Hypopigmented and telangiectatic patches.
  - Less likely: Raynaud's, arthritis, ILD
- GU malignancies; ovarian and colon cancer are overrepresented.
- Others: breast, lung, gastric, pancreatic, lymphomas.
- Risk of malignancy returns to normal after 2–5 years.

Laboratory Manifestations of Dermatomyositis

- Muscle enzyme evaluation
  - Proximal extensor inflammatory myopathy: deltoid muscle biopsy or MRI
- Serum aldolase, ALT, LDH, CK, AST, carbonic anhydrase isoenzyme II

Work-Up

- Skin biopsy, muscle biopsy/EM
- ANA, Jo-1, Mi-2, and other antibodies as needed (see Table 3.40)
- Serum aldolase, ALT, LDH, CK, AST, carbonic anhydrase isoenzyme II
- CXR
- Pulmonary function test (even if CXR is normal and there are no symptoms)
- EKG
- CBC, CMP, UA, CK, and aldolase
- ESR: elevated in 50%; does not correlate with disease
- RF: elevated in 20% – most often in overlap syndromes
- EMG: myopathic pattern, 10% false negative
- Physical examination – including rectal, breast, and pelvic exam ± pelvic ultrasound (for females).
- CBC, CMP, UA, TFTs.
- CXR.
- PFTs (even if CXR is normal and there are no symptoms).
- Consider esophageal studies (barium swallow).
- CT of the chest/abdomen/pelvis (may substitute ultrasound of pelvis in women).
- Repeat CXR, stool guaiac, pelvic and pap, breast, and mammogram yearly for 3 years.
- If normal at 3 years, can revert to age-appropriate screening.

Treatment

- Oral corticosteroids: 1 mg/kg/day tapered to 50% over 6 months and to zero over 2–3 years.
- Elevated CK >1000 U/L suggests disease that is more difficult to control and may need higher doses or longer course of corticosteroids + nonsteroidal agent.
- Methotrexate (5–20 mg/week); azathioprine (2–3 mg/kg/day), IVIg, rituximab.
- Need regular examinations q4–6 months for at least 2–3 years with surveillance for malignancy.
- Patients with DM sine myositis usually do not require long-term oral corticosteroids control often gained with

alternative treatment (hydroxychloroquine, methotrexate+ topical steroids, sunscreen, Heliocare).

- Anti-interferon: alpha and beta.
- Jak inhibitors

- Calcinosis cutis: can be treated with diltiazem or surgical excision
  - Treatment of DM does not necessarily lead to resolution of calcinosis, which may be difficult to treat.

References
- Waldman et al. *JAAD*. 2020;82(2):283–296.
- DeWane et al. *JAAD*. 2020;82(2):267–281.

Cutaneous Sarcoidosis

Reading: Wanat KA and Rosenbach M. Clinics in chest medicine. 2015;36(4):685–702

Noncaseating granulomas of unknown cause

Skin disease typically present at disease onset and can correlate with systemic inflammation.

Clinical manifestations can be variable:

- Macules/papules – may be red/violaceous, skin colored to brown, hypopigmented. Can be disseminated or concentrated in a certain area such as the face, extremities, and areas of trauma.
- Plaque – typically found on the face, back, buttocks, and extensor surfaces of arms. Annular is a variant of plaque.
- Lupus pernio – specific presentation of red-to-violaceous indurated plaques of the nose, central face, and cheeks. Most common in patients of African ancestry. Can be disfiguring.
- Subcutaneous (Darier-Roussy) – affects deep dermis and subQ tissue. Firm, nontender, mobile subcutaneous nodules; often do not have associated redness. Most common on arms.
- Scar/tattoo – may be the sole cutaneous manifestation of sarcoidosis or can be seen in association with other morphologies.

- Less common: psoriasiform sarcoid, lichenoid sarcoidosis, verrucous sarcoidosis, ichthyosiform sarcoidosis, lymphedema, atrophic and ulcerative sarcoidosis, hypopigmented, angiolupoid (characterized by prominent telangiectasias within a plaque or nodule), erythroderma, pigmented purpuric-like sarcoidosis, photoinduced sarcoidosis with seasonal variation

Nonspecific lesions

- Erythema nodosum
- Digital clubbing (may be related to underlying pulmonary disease)
- Calcinosis
- Neutrophilic dermatoses (Sweet's syndrome and pyoderma gangrenosum)
- Sarcoidosis-lymphoma syndrome

Systemic sequelae or other findings can include:

- Bony cysts
- Pulmonary fibrosis
- Uveitis
- Involvement of the mucosa/sinuses/oropharynx (any portion of oral cavity can be affected)
- Nasal ulceration and septal perforation
- Severe, recalcitrant arthritis
- Erythema nodosum

Drug-induced:

IFNa (most common), tattoos, TNFa inhibitors, hyaluronic acid cosmetic fillers, zinc, desensitization injections, ipilimumab, ophthalmic drops containing sodium bisulfite,

Work-up

- Diascopy for apple-jelly or yellow-brown discoloration
- Biopsy of lesion
- CXR
- Pulmonary function tests (including diffusion capacity for carbon monoxide)
- Ophthalmologic examination
- CBC

- BMP
- LFTs
- UA (if history of stone, then 24-hour urine calcium)
- ECG, transthoracic echocardiogram, Holter monitor (consider additional testing if symptomatic)
- PPD or interferon-gamma release assay (T-SPOT/quant gold)
- Vitamin D_{25} and vitamin $D_{1,25}$
- TSH (thyroid dysfunction reported in association with cutaneous disease)

Treatment Options (from Wanat KA and Rosenbach M. *Clinics in Chest Medicine*. 2015;36(4):685–702):

Topical: mid- to high-potency corticosteroids, tretinoin, tazarotene

ILK every 4–8 weeks as needed

UVA, PDL, CO_2, KTP, ruby laser

Immunomodulatory: hydroxychloroquine 200–400 mg daily, chloroquine 250–500 mg daily, tetracyclines 100 mg daily, pentoxifylline 400 mg TID, apremilast 20 mg BID, isotretinoin 20–60 mg daily, acitretin 25 mg daily

Immunosuppressants: prednisone 10–60 mg daily, methotrexate 7.5–25 mg weekly, azathioprine 50–200 mg daily, mycophenolate mofetil 500–1500 mg BID

TNF inhibitors: adalimumab 40 mg weekly (or every other week), infliximab 3–5 mg IV week 0, 2, and 6 and then every 4–8 weeks

Behcet's Disease

Diagnostic Criteria

A. Recurrent oral ulceration at least three times during a period of 12 months

B. Plus two of the following:

  - Recurrent genital ulceration
  - Eye lesions
    Anterior/posterior uveitis, cells in vitreous, retinal vasculitis
  - Skin lesions

    Erythema nodosum, pseudofolliculitis, papulopustular lesions, or acneiform nodules
  - Positive pathergy = pustule at site of needle prick after 24–48 hours

Common Clinical Features

- Oral ulcers (99%)
- Genital ulcers (83%)
- Uveitis (39%)
- Retinal vasculitis (19%)
- Positive pathergy test (33%)
- Pathergy equivalent (9%)
- Arthritis (28%)
- Meningoencephalitis (17%)
- Vascular lesions (20%

Common Cutaneous Features

- Papulopustular (44%)
- Erythema nodosum (37%)
- Pseudofolliculitis (7%)
- Acneiform nodules (7%)
- Pyoderma gangrenosum-like (3%)
- Nondescript (1%)

Treatment: colchicine, dapsone, thalidomide, TNFa inhibitors

Reference

- Criteria for diagnosis of Behcet's disease. *Lancet.* 1990;335(8697):1078–80.

Various Fibrosing Disorders (Table 3.41)

Vasculitis

Vasculitis is an inflammatory process affecting the vessel wall that can be limited to the skin. It can also be a presenting sign of a systemic process (polyarteritis nodosa, granulomatosis with polyangiitis, eosinophilic granulomatosis with polyangiitis) or a secondary process (infection, malignancy, drug).

It is categorized based on the size of the vessel involved. Skin is affected in small vessel vasculitis and medium vessel vasculitis but usually not in large vessel vasculitis.

Small vessel vasculitis findings: palpable purpura, urticaria, vesiculobullous lesions, targetoid lesions

Medium vessel vasculitis findings: subcutaneous nodules, livedo reticularis, ulcers, infarcts, digital pitted scars, gangrene

Most common causes of cutaneous vasculitis:

- Infections (22%)
- Drugs (20%)
- Connective tissue disease (12%)
- Henoch-Schonlein purpura (10%)
- <5% for malignancy, primary systemic vasculitis, and systemic inflammatory disease such as sarcoidosis and cryoglobulinemia

ACR Classification Criteria for Vasculitis
Large Vessel Vasculitis

- *Giant-cell (temporal) arteritis (GCA)*
  - Three criteria classify GCA with sensitivity = 93.5% and specificity = 91.2%.
  - Age > 50 years at onset.
  - New type of headache.
  - Early: erythematous or cyanotic skin alopecia, purpura, tender nodules on frontotemporal scalp, abnormal tem-

TABLE 3.41 Summary of fibrosing disorders of the skin

Disorder	Clinical manifestations	Pathologic features
Nephrogenic fibrosing dermopathy (NFD) / Nephrogenic Systemic Fibrosis (NSF)	Firm, thickened skin; papules and subcutaneous nodules on extremities and trunk; usually spares face History of MRI with gadolinium in setting of renal disease	Early lesions: thickened collagen bundles with clefts, *CD34+*, spindle cells, mucin Late lesions: less clefting and mucin, fewer CD34+ cells, elongated elastic fibers
Scleromyxedema	Waxy, linear distributed papules on the face and neck, furrowing of glabella, sclerodactyly, paraproteinemia	Thickened collagen bundles, stellate fibroblasts, mucin poor, lymphoplasmacytic infiltrate
Morphea	Ivory-colored plaque with violaceous borders (if active) or depressed areas of the skin with thickening/fibrotic feeling	Thickened, homogenized collagen bundles, lymphoplasmacytic infiltrate, atrophy of adnexae, mucin in early stages
Systemic sclerosis	Diffuse, local, or widespread sclerosis; sclerodactylyl; subcutaneous calcification, telangiectasias, facial constriction; pulmonary, cardiac, renal involvement; small ulcerations of fingertips (early sign)	Thickened, homogenized collagen bundles, vascular fibrosis, calcification, less inflammation than seen in morphea *DDx*: GVHD, PCT, PKU, progeria, Werner, EF, NSF

TABLE 3.41 (continued)

Disorder	Clinical manifestations	Pathologic features
Porphyria cutanea tarda	Bullae, scarring, and milia in photosensitive areas, hypertrichosis, skin thickening	Non-inflammatory subepidermal bulla with festooning base; caterpillar bodies; IgG/C3 deposition at DEJ and in vessel walls in linear fashion
Eosinophilic fasciitis	Swelling, induration of extremities, "groove sign"	Hyalinization and thickening of collagen of deep fascia and subcutis; focal collections of eos
Eosinophilia-myalgia syndrome	Diffuse skin thickening, papules on trunk and face – spares hands and feet – peripheral eosinophilia, severe myalgias	Thickened collagen bundles, variable inflammatory infiltrate, mucin deposition

poral artery on clinical examination (tenderness on palpation or decreased pulsation).
- Late – ulceration and/or gangrene of the frontotemporal scalp/tongue.
- Elevated erythrocyte sedimentation rate.
- Temporal artery biopsy showing vasculitis.

- *Takayasu's arteritis (TA)*
  - Three criteria classify TA with sensitivity = 90.5% and specificity = 97.8%.
  - Age less than 40 years at onset.
  - Limb claudication.
  - Decreased brachial artery pulses BP > 10 mm Hg difference between two arms.
  - Bruits.
  - Arteriogram abnormality.

Medium Vessel Vasculitis

Larger/deeper vessel involvement with livedo reticularis and tender subQ nodules. Usually no signs of small vessel vasculitis

- *Classic systemic polyarteritis nodosa (PAN)*
  - Palpable purpura, livedo racemosa, retiform purpura, "punched-out" ulcers
  - Weight loss
  - Livedo reticularis
  - Testicular pain/tenderness
  - Myalgias, myopathy, or tenderness
  - Neuropathy
  - Hypertension (diastolic >90 mm Hg)
  - Renal impairment (elevated BUN or creatinine)
  - Hepatitis B virus
  - Angiography showing microaneurysms
  - Biopsy of artery showing PAN
- *Cutaneous PAN*
  - Painful or tender subQ nodules
  - Livedo racemosa
  - Cutaneous necrosis/ulcers
  - P-ANCA more commonly positive in cPAN than systemic PAN

Small-Medium (Mixed) Vessel Vasculitis

Palpable purpura with associated livedo racemosa, retiform purpura, ulcers, subcutaneous nodules, and digital necrosis

- *Cryoglobulinemia*
- *ANCA-associated*
  - *Microscopic polyangiitis*
  - *Granulomatosis with polyangiitis*
  - *Eosinophilic granulomatosis with polyangiitis*
- *Secondary Causes*
  - *Infections*
  - *Inflammatory disorders (AI-CTD)*

Small Vessel Vasculitis

Skin lesions appear 7–10 days after an inciting event. Palpable or macular purpura often in dependent areas. Systemic symptoms may occur along with arthralgias, arthritis, and GI/GU/renal involvement. Leukocytoclastic vasculitis (LCV) is seen on pathology.

- *Henoch-Schonlein purpura (IgA vasculitis)* – see pediatrics section for more information.
- *Acute hemorrhagic edema of infancy*
- *Urticarial vasculitis*
- *Erythema elevatum diutinum*
- Secondary causes
  - Drug exposure
  - Infections
  - Malignancies (often hematologic)

Systemic Diseases that Mimic Vasculitis

- <u>Hemorrhage</u> (trauma, actinic purpura, thrombocytopenia, coagulopathies, viral exanthems, scurvy, primary systemic amyloidosis)
- <u>Thromboses</u> (hypercoagulable state, livedoid vasculopathy, purpura fulminans, heparin necrosis, coumadin necrosis, thrombotic thrombocytopenic purpura, hemolytic uremic syndrome, paroxysmal nocturnal hemoglobinuria, DIC)
- <u>Emboli</u> (cholesterol, cardiac-originated [endocarditis], fat, air)
- <u>Inflammation</u> (pigmented purpura, hypergammaglobulinemic purpura of Waldenstrom)
- <u>Infectious</u> (Lucio's phenomenon, strongyloidiasis)
- <u>Functional</u> (fibromuscular dysplasia, vessel spasm, drug-induced vasospasm, atherosclerosis, drugs: ergots, cocaine)
- <u>Malignancy</u> (intravascular lymphoma)

Labs for Vasculitis

- *Biopsy* for H&E, DIF, and sterile/tissue culture.
- *CBC, BUN/creatinine, LFT, UA* – evaluate for hematologic, renal, and other organ involvement.
- *Blood cultures* – rule out infection.

- *ESR/CRP* – high value suggests inflammatory disease and, in the setting of IgA vasculitis in adults, a higher likelihood of renal insufficiency.
- *Rheumatoid factor* – very high titers in RA, Sjogren's, and cryoglobulinemia-associated vasculitis.
- *Antinuclear antibody* – screen for SLE and Sjogren's syndrome.
- *Complements (C3, C4, CH50)* – low levels suggest consumption by immune complexes (SLE and cryoglobulinemia). In urticarial vasculitis, normal complements suggest cutaneous only disease, in which hypocomplementemia in this setting is associated with systemic disease.
- *Cryoglobulins* – seen in mixed essential or secondary cryoglobulinemia.
- *ANCAs (C-ANCA and PR3, P-ANCA and MPO)* – C-ANCA pattern specific for granulomatosis with polyangiitis; P-ANCA pattern occurs with other vasculitides.
- *Creatinine phosphokinase (CPK)* – elevation suggests myositis, which can occur in many vasculitis syndromes.
- *RPR/VDRL* – rule out syphilis.
- *SPEP* – evaluate for plasma cell dyscrasias.
- *Hepatitis B and C serology* – rule out hepatitis.
- *HIV.*
- *Anti-glomerular basement membrane* – rule out Goodpasture's syndrome, which can mimic vasculitis and cause pulmonary hemorrhage.

Approach to Small Vessel Vasculitis/LCV

<u>Four-step process:</u>

- *Confirm the diagnosis of LCV with biopsy (H&E, tissue culture/sterile biopsy, and also DIF on an early lesion).*
- *Establish etiology if possible.*
  - *Infection* – consider HCV, HBV, Strep, deep fungus, TB, meningococcal disease, HIV, and endocarditis (can look like LCV, so work up for these).
  - *Meds* – sulfa, penicillin, phenytoin, NSAIDs, allopurinol, thiazides.

  - *Autoimmune* – (get ROS ± tests for) SLE < Sjogren, RA, IBD, Behcet's cryoglobulinemia.
  - *Malignancy* – ensure that patients are up to date on routine screening. Hematologic malignancy is the most likely type to be associated with LCV (esp. IgA vasculitis), so palpate nodes, liver, and spleen, and check CBC and SPEP. Consider CT C/A/P.
  - *Dysproteinemia.*
  - Note: 50% of cutaneous LCV cases are idiopathic (the above w/u is unrevealing)

- *Look for systemic involvement.*
  - Inquire about fever, weight loss, joint aches/pains, GI/GU upset, pleuritis, and oral symptoms.
  - Check UA, creatinine, and fecal occult blood tests (GI bleeds are a major source of mortality in children with vasculitis).
  - If suspecting systemic disease, a complete head/neck, cardiopulmonary, abdominal, musculoskeletal, and neurologic examination should be performed.

- *Employ a therapeutic ladder.*
  - *General measures*

    Most cases are self-limited and short-lived (few weeks to several months).
    Exclude systemic disease per above.

  - *Mild skin-limited disease*

    Leg elevation, avoid tight clothing, symptomatic therapy (antihistamines, NSAIDs) as needed

  - *Chronic (>4 weeks) or moderate skin disease*

    Colchicine 0.5 mg BID-TID, dapsone 50–200 mg/day (alone or in combination)

  - *Severe, ulcerating, progressive skin disease*

    Oral prednisone (up to 1 mg/kg/day) tapered over 4–6 weeks
    Low-dose methotrexate
    Dapsone

– *Systemic involvement*

Systemic steroids ± additional immunosuppressive medication (azathioprine, cyclophosphamide, methotrexate)

– *Mixed vessel, medium vessel, large vessel*
Get rheum involved due to risk for serious sequelae.

Monitoring
For relapsing disease, start a steroid-sparing agent, such as methotrexate.

Adults with IgA vasculitis are more likely to have renal involvement and develop chronic renal insufficiency.

Clinical Clues of Different Vasculitides
Cutaneous

- Palpable purpura = post-capillary venules – any type of vasculitis except giant cell arteritis and Takayasu's arteritis
- Skin ulcers or gangrene in an extremity = arterioles and small arteries – polyarteritis, eosinophilic granulomatosis with polyangiitis
- Granulomatosis with polyangiitis and hypersensitivity vasculitis also with cutaneous manifestations

GI Tract

- Abdominal pain or mesenteric ischemia – small- to medium-sized arteries = Henoch-Schonlein purpura, polyarteritis, eosinophilic granulomatosis with polyangiitis
- Gastrointestinal bleeding – capillaries to medium-sized arteries = Henoch-Schonlein purpura, polyarteritis, eosinophilic granulomatosis with polyangiitis
- Mesenteric ischemia – PAN

Renal

- Glomerulonephritis – capillaries = microscopic polyangiitis, granulomatosis with polyangiitis, cryoglobulinemia, eosinophilic granulomatosis with polyangiitis, Henoch-Schonlein purpura. Rare in PAN
- Renovascular hypertension – seen in PAN
- Ischemic renal failure – small- to medium-sized arteries = polyarteritis, Takayasu's arteries; less commonly

eosinophilic granulomatosis with polyangiitis and granulomatosis with polyangiitis

Pulmonary

- Pulmonary hemorrhage – capillaries = less commonly small- to medium-sized arteries: microscopic polyangiitis, granulomatosis with polyangiitis
- Pulmonary infiltrates or cavities – small- to medium-sized arteries = eosinophilic granulomatosis with polyangiitis vasculitis, microscopic polyangiitis

Neurologic

- Peripheral neuropathy – small arteries = polyarteritis, eosinophilic granulomatosis with polyangiitis, granulomatosis with polyangiitis, cryoglobulinemia
- Stroke – small, medium-sized, or large arteries – giant cell arteritis, SLE-associated vasculitis
- Mononeuritis multiplex – PAN

Retiform Purpura

Reticulate eruptions due to cutaneous blood vessel compromises > skin ischemia, purpura, and necrosis. Non-blanchable lesions often with necrotic centers. Can be bullous.

Due to:

- Vessel wall damage (vasculitis/depositional disease/angioinvasion by an organism)
- Vessel lumen occlusion (thrombosis or embolic disease)

Biopsy required
Differential and etiologies are vast – the key is to identify early for proper management and avoidance of long-term complications.

Five-step approach to work-up (based on *JAAD*. 2020:82(4):783–796).

1. Confirm morphology and assess patient status: Perform biopsy (required) and start labs to determine if vessel lumen vs vessel wall damage is occurring (see Fig. 3.13). For acute presentation of retiform purpura/if patient is severely ill, consider rapidly progressive fatal causes (Fig. 3.13).
   - Biopsy for H&E, DIF, & Tissue cultures - collect tissue from peripheral purpuric rim of a lesion. When hemorrhagic bullae are present, fluid can be obtained for culture; blister roof can be scraped for KOH.
   - Labs can be tailored to the individual, but in all patients, obtain CBC, UA, BUN, creatinine, LFTs, coagulopathy work-up (see below), and if acutely ill also a blood culture.
2. Consider medications?
   - Assess for medication causes (e.g., warfarin/heparin).

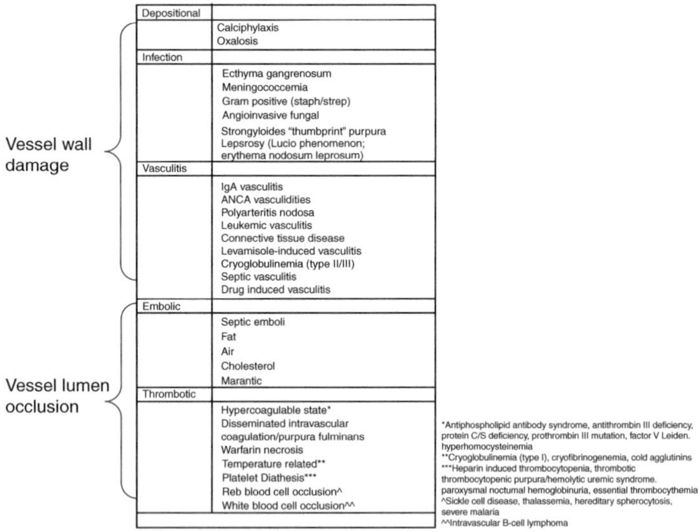

FIGURE 3.13 Diagnostic considerations for retiform purpura based on clinical/pathological findings. ANCA = antineutrophil cytoplasmic autoantibody

Start broad-spectrum antibiotics and antifungals (anti-helminth in right setting) while cultures are pending.

3. Where is/are the lesion(s)?

   – All patients should receive a full skin examination (including nails). Some etiologies have classic locations:

   Ear – levamisole (in cocaine)
   Periumbilical (thumbprint purpura) – strongyloides
   Acral – embolic, cold-associated disease (e.g., cryoglobulinemia), endocarditis

- Acral lower extremities – vasculitis
  Fatty areas – warfarin-/heparin-induced skin necrosis; calciphylaxis

   – If disseminated, can be infectious or noninfectious in etiology.
   – See Fig. 3.14 for summary of etiologies based on location.

4. Past medical history/family history - including history of illicit drug use (Table 3.42)

5. Perform a comprehensive review of systems.

   – Travel history
   – Pulmonary/GI symptoms
   – Abdominal pain, joint pain, change in urine color, blood in stool, neurologic complaints

See Fig. 3.14.

Coagulopathy Work-Up

- CBC with diff
- PT/INR, PTT
- Cryoglobulins, cryofibrinogen
- Homocysteine level
- ANA

Table 3.42 Historical components and etiologies to consider for vasculitis (based on JAAD. 2020:82(4)):783–796)

History	Etiologies to consider
End-stage renal disease	Calciphylaxis
Stroke, miscarriage, lupus/ connective tissue disease	Antiphospholipid syndrome, cryoglobulinemia
Ear/nose/airways: asthma, nasal polyposis	ANCA-associated vasculitis: Eosinophilic granulomatosis with polyangiitis, polyangiitis with granulomatosis
Hepatitis	Cryoglobulinemia types II and II, polyarteritis nodosa
Malignancy	Vasculitis
Hemoglobinopathy	
Recent cardiac procedure	
Recent/active infections	DIC and purpura fulminans: encapsulated Gram-positive bacteria Ecthyma gangrenosum: Gram-negative sepsis HUS: Shiga toxin-producing *E.coli*, pneumococcus, influenza Cold agglutinins: *Mycoplasma pneumoniae* Cutaneous polyarteritis nodosa: streptococcal infections IgA vasculitis (Henoch-Schonlein purpura): *Streptococcus* infection
New medications? Warfarin, heparin, TNF inhibitor, propylthiouracil, hydralazine, minocycline, rituximab, statin, cocaine (levamisole)	

- Anticardiolipin antibody
- Antithrombin III
- Lupus anticoagulant
- Protein C and S
- Factor V Leiden mutation
- Prothrombin gene mutation
- B2 glycoprotein 1 antibody
- Heparin/PF4 complex immunoassay (if concern for HIT)
- Peripheral smear

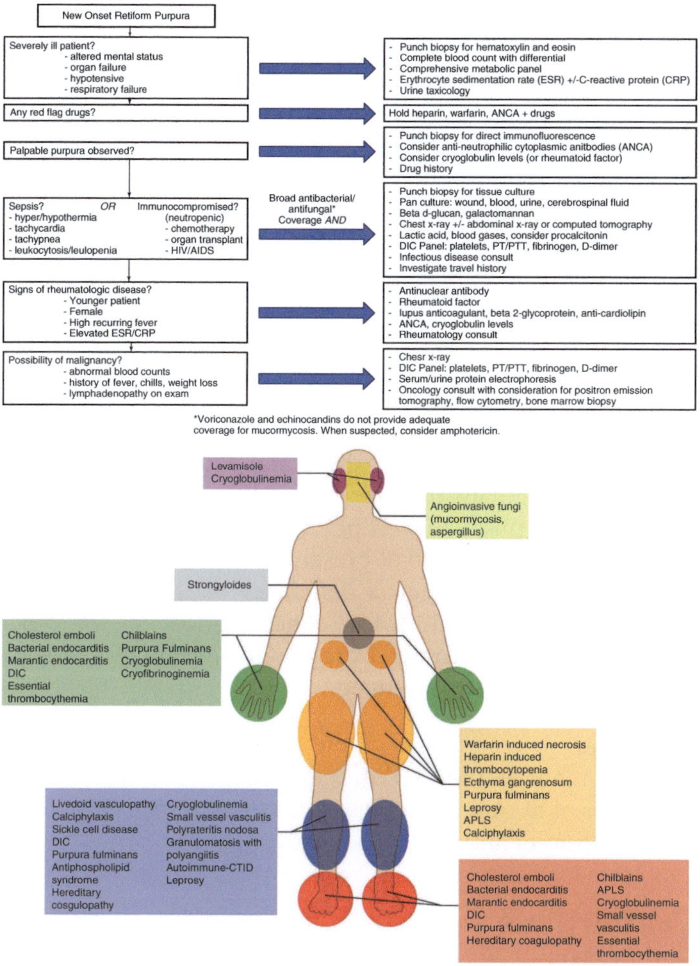

FIGURE 3.14 (**a**) Work-up for new onset retiform purpura. DIC disseminated intravascular coagulation, PT prothrombin time, PTT partial thromboplastin time. (**b**) Anatomic disrtibution of common causes of retiform purpura. APLS antiphospholipid antibody syndrome, CTD connective tissue disease, DIC disseminated intravascular coagulation

Pitfalls

- Genetic tests are essentially unaffected by heparin or warfarin therapy.
- Acute DVT/PTE by itself can transiently reduce the plasma concentration of antithrombin and occasionally protein C and protein S.
- Heparin: can produce up to a 30% decline in the plasma antithrombin concentration over several days.
- Warfarin: produces a marked reduction in the functional activity of protein C and protein S and a lesser decline in immunologic levels. Warfarin rarely elevates antithrombin concentrations in patients with antithrombin deficiency, sometimes into the normal range.
- Recommend testing for these deficiency states at least 2 weeks after completing the initial 3–6-month course of oral anticoagulant therapy following a thrombotic event. If, however, plasma levels of antithrombin, protein C, and protein S are obtained at presentation and are well within the normal range, then a deficiency of these proteins is essentially excluded. A low concentration, on the other hand, must be confirmed by repeat testing after anticoagulation has been discontinued.

References

- Khetan P et al. *Indian J Med Res.* 2012;135(1):107–33.
- Goeser et al. *Am J Clin Dermatol.* 2014;15(4):299–306.
- Fiorentino et al. *JAAD.* 2003;48(3):311–40.

Calciphylaxis

Multifactorial etiology with unknown trigger/cause. Can be uremic or non-uremic.

Lesion morphology

- Progress from livedo reticularis to livedo racemosa to retiform purpura to black eschars to necrotic, ulcerate, malodorous plaques that can appear gangrenous.
- Pain is severe and typically unaffected by opiates.

Characteristics of uremic

- Most common on legs, abdomen, and buttocks.
- Proximal, adipose-rich sites have a worse prognosis.

Work-up

- Diagnosis can be clinical or confirmed with:
  - Biopsy
    Can be non-diagnostic
    May cause localized progression and ulceration
    Contraindicated in penile calciphylaxis
    Histology: medial calcification and proliferation of the intima of small- to medium-sized arteries ± lobular and septal panniculitis and extravascular soft tissue calcification/stippled calcification of eccrine sweat glands
  - Imaging

    X-ray: Tram-Track calcifications
    Also, MRI, CT, ultrasound, nuclear bone scintigraphy, spectroscopy, mammography

- Labs: LFTs, BMP (including calcium), PTH, serum albumin, blood cultures, hypercoagulability work-up ([see above] antiphospholipid Ab, protein C and S, factor V Leiden, antithrombin III, homocysteine, methylenetetrahydrofolate reductase mutation, cryoglobulins), rheumatoid factor, ANA, ANCA.
- Medication assessment: stop warfarin.

Management

- Multifactorial management (dermatology, nephrology, pain management, wound care, plastic surgery, nutrition, hyperbaric oxygen specialists).
- No tried and true treatment algorithms are available.
- Medical treatments
  - STOP warfarin.
  - Anticoagulation (excluding warfarin).
  - Becaplermin (recombinant plate-derived growth factor).
  - Bisphosphonates (pamidronate, aldenodrate).

  - Cinacalcet (in the setting of elevated PTH).
  - Discontinue medications that may contribute to calciphylaxis (warfarin, steroids).
  - Sodium thiosulfate (chelates calcium and thought to have antioxidant and vasodilatory properties) – can be given intralesional and/or intravenous.
  - Non-calcium-containing phosphate binders (sevelamer).
  - Pentoxifylline.
  - Prostaglandins.
  - Vitamin K Supplementation.

- Surgical treatments
  - Debridement (in appropriate candidates, could worsen so proceed with caution)
  - Dermal regenerative template
  - Parathyroidectomy
  - Renal transplantation

- Miscellaneous
  - Hyperbaric oxygen therapy
  - Local wound care

    Including maggot therapy to debride the tissues

  - Pain management

Prognosis: 60–80% mortality rate

- 30% at 6 months, 50% at 12 months, 80% at 2 years.
- Sepsis secondary to the ulcers is the leading cause of death.

Reference: Khanna U et al. *Cutis*. 2018;102(6):395–400.

Cryoglobulins

Note that drawing cryoglobulins is a tricky task and should be done after reviewing with the attending physician. Must be delivered to the lab immediately by physician after drawing to ensure that the cryoglobulins do not precipitate out of solution en route.

Summary of Cryoglobulinemia in Tables 3.43 and 3.44

TABLE 3.43 Cryoglobulinemia summary

	Type I	Type II	Type III
Essential (72%)	30%	70%	57%
Secondary (28%)	70%	30%	43%
Associated diseases	LPD >>> essential > CTD, CLD	Essential ≫ LPD > CLD > CTD	Essential ≫ CLD ≫ CTD
Signs and symptoms			
Purpura	+	+++	+++
Gangrene/ acrocyanosis	+++	+ to ++	±
Arthralgias, arthritis	+	++	+++
Renal disease	+	++	+
Neurologic	+	+	++
Liver disease	±	++	+++

CLD chronic liver disease, *CTD* connective tissue disease, *LPD* lymphoproliferative or plasmaproliferative disorder

TABLE 3.44 Cryoglobulinemias

Type	Monoclonal Igs	Polyclonal
I	IgM, IgG, and IgA or light chains	None
II	IgM usually or IgG	IgG/IgM
III	None	IgG or IgM

Rheumatoid factor is a “poor-person's” cryoglobulin that can screen for type II and III cryoglobulins.

- Type I: monoclonal immunoglobulin (Ig) typically IgG or IgM, typically associated with multiple myeloma or Waldenstrom's macroglobulinemia, respectively. Often associated hyperviscosity syndromes (Raynaud's phenomenon, digital ischemia, livedo reticularis, or purpura) present
- Type II: mixture of polyclonal Ig in association with a monoclonal Ig, typically IgM or IgA, with rheumatoid factor (“poor man's cryo), often due to persistent viral infections (particularly HCV and HIV). Most often produce constitutional and nonspecific symptoms, such as arthralgias, fatigue, and myalgias; also palpable purpura due to cutaneous vasculitis and sensory changes or weakness due to peripheral neuropathy Melzer's triad: purpura, arthralgias, and weakness
- Type III: mixed polyclonal Ig, often secondary to connective tissue diseases. The same presentation as type II

Cutaneous manifestations: inflammatory macules/papules, pigmentary changes/petechiae, ulcers, leg edema, livedo reticularis, hemorrhagic crusts, infarction, urticaria, NXG

Treatment Options
- Prednisone
- Cyclophosphamide
- Plasmapheresis/plasma exchange (will get rid of the cryos but then will make more)
- IVIg
- Rituximab
- INF, ribavirin if hepatitis C related

Neutrophilic Dermatoses

Pyoderma Gangrenosum

- *History*
  - Painful ulcer preceded by papules, pustule, or vesicle
  - Rapid progression – starts quite suddenly usually at the site of minor injury as a small pustules and then rapidly progresses
  - Pathergy
  - Associated disease – inflammatory bowel disease (ulcerative colitis/Crohn's diseases), rheumatoid arthritis, IgA paraproteinemia/monoclonal gammopathy, myeloma/leukemia (AML), hypogammaglobulinemia, PAPA syndrome, sarcoidosis, chronic active hepatitis, CVD, levamisole-adulterated cocaine
  - Drug history – levamisole (cocaine), systemic retinoids (isotretinoin, alitretinoin), PTU, adalimumab, etanercept, infliximab, azacitidine, imatinib/sunitinib/gaffinitib, ipilimumab, enoxaparin, EPO, G-CSF, IFN
- *Physical exam*
  - Ulcer with an irregular, violaceous border and undermined, rolled edges. May have a cribriform appearance. May be bullous
- *Skin biopsy*
  - Specimen from inflamed border – routine H&E and for tissue culture (sterile biopsy) for bacteria, fungus, and AFB
- *Laboratory*
  - CBC, ESR, LFTs, BUN/Cr, SPEP (for IgA gammopathy), CXR, Pt/PTT, colonoscopy, Antiphospholipis Antibodies, ANCAs, cryoglobulins, venous and arterial function studies

- *Diagnostic criteria*
  - Need the major criterion +4+ minor criteria (sensitivity 86%, specificity 90%)
  - Major criterion

Histopathology of ulcer edge must show a neutrophilic infiltrate.

  - Minor criteria

Exclusion of infection
Pathergy
History of inflammatory bowel disease or inflammatory arthritis
History of papule, vesicle, or pustule ulcerating within 4 days
Peripheral erythema, undermining border, tenderness at the ulcer site
Multiple ulcers, at least one on the anterior lower leg
Cribriform or wrinkled paper scars at the site of the healed ulcer
Decreased size of the ulcer within 1 month of initiating immunosuppressive medication

- *Treatment*
  - *Debridement contraindicated (2/2/ pathergy phenomenon)*
  - Local wound care.
  - Topical, intralesional, oral steroids.
  - Topical immunomodulators (e.g., tacrolimus).
  - Minocycline/doxycycline.
  - Steroid-sparing agents: dapsone, sulfapyridine, sulfasalazine, colchicine
  - Immunosuppressants: azathioprine, cyclosporine, mycophenolate, methotrexate.
  - TNFa inhibitors, ustekinumab.
  - Others: thalidomide, SSKI.
  - Control for wound infection.
  - Skin grafting can be tried when active stage is over.

- *Follow-up*
  - Monitor response to therapy.
  - If no response, reconsider diagnosis and repeat biopsy.

Sweet's Syndrome (Acute Febrile Neutrophilic Dermatosis)

Diagnostic criteria: requires two major and two minor criteria

Major criteria

1. Abrupt onset of tender or painful red or purplish plaques or nodules.
2. Biopsy shows inflammation that is composed mainly of neutrophils without vasculitis.

Minor criteria

1. Preceding fever or infection
2. Accompanying fever, painful joints, conjunctivitis, or underlying cancer
3. Raised white cell count on blood testing
4. Improvement with systemic antibiotics and not with antibiotics
5. Increased erythrocyte sedimentation rate (ESR)

Variants

- Bullous Sweet's syndrome
- Histiocytoid variant – hard to differentiate from leukemia cutis; strong association with hematologic malignancies
- Neutrophilic dermatosis of the dorsal hands – localized variant
- Necrolytic or resemble necrotizing fasciitis – often with more SIRS symptoms/even mimicking sepsis

Treatment

- Systemic corticosteroids
- Potassium iodide (SSKI)
- Colchicine

- Dapsone, sulfapyridine, sulfasalazine
- Indomethacin/NSAIDs
- Clofazimine
- Doxycycline, minocycline

Nutritional Deficiencies (Table 3.45)

Infectious Dermatology

Bacterial Disease

Normal skin flora

- Aerobic cocci: *Staphylococcus aureus* (35% nares, 20% perineum, 5–10% toewebs), *S. saprophyticus*, *S. epidermidis*, *Micrococcus luteus*, *M. roseus*, *M. varians*
  - All body sites, especially intertriginous areas
- Aerobic coryneform bacteria: *Corynebacterium minutissimum*, *C. lipophilicus*, *C. xerosis*, *C. jeilelium*, *Brevibacterium epidermidis*
  - Intertriginous areas
- Anaerobic coryneform bacteria: *Propionibacterium acne*, *P. granulosum*, *P. avidum*
  - Sebaceous glands and hair follicles
- Gram-negative bacteria: acinetobacter
  - Axillae, perineum, antecubital fossa
- Yeast: *Malassezia furfur (Pityrosporum)*
  - Skin rich in sebaceous glands (scalp/face)

Gram-Positive Bacteria

Impetigo

- *Staphylococcus aureus* > *Streptococcus pyogenes*
- Common infection in kids
- Nasal carriers of staph are at a particular risk.

TABLE 3.45 Summary of nutritional dermatoses

Nutrient	Clinical manifestations
Vitamin A	Phrynoderma "toad" skin, keratosis-like papules on extremities, night blindness, conjunctival white Bitot spots, keratomalacia
Vitamin B1 (thiamine) (beriberi)	Red burning tongue (glossodynia), edema, cardiac enlargement, peripheral neuropathy
Vitamin B2 (riboflavin)	Oro-oculo-genital syndrome: atrophic tongue, cheilitis, photophobia, scrotal/ groin dermatitis
Vitamin B3 (niacin) (pellagra)	Diarrhea, dermatitis (Casal's necklace; scrotal and perineal erythema; fissured, atrophic mucous membranes; seborrheic dermatitis; photosensitivity with erythema), dementia, death (similar to tryptophan deficiency). DDx: INH, 5-FU, azathioprine
Vitamin B6 (pyridoxine)	Atrophic glossitis with ulceration, seborrheic dermatitis, cheilitis, intertrigo, neurologic abnormalities (similar to pellagra)
Vitamin B12/folate	Glossitis, hyperpigmentation, canities, weakness, paresthesias, ataxia, megaloblastic anemia
Vitamin C	Perifollicular petechial hemorrhages, hyperkeratotic plugs, corkscrew hairs
Vitamin D	Alopecia, osteopenia, rickets
Vitamin K	Purpura, hemorrhage, ecchymoses
Iron	Koilonychia, glossitis, cheilitis, telogen effluvium, dysphagia (Plummer-Vinson syndrome)
Biotin	Alopecia, lethargy, hypotonia, periorificial dermatitis, brittle nails (similar to zinc deficiency)

(continued)

TABLE 3.45 (continued)

Nutrient	Clinical manifestations
Essential fatty acid	Periorificial dermatitis, alopecia, fair hair (similar to zinc deficiency)
Zinc	Acrodermatitis enteropathica, alopecia, nail dystrophy, diarrhea, poor wound healing, lethargy
Selenium	Hypopigmentation, leukonychia, cardiomyopathy, muscle pain, weakness
Copper	Pale, twisted hair
Protein-energy	Marasmus = prolonged calorie deficiencies, <50% ideal body weight, no edema; loss of buccal fat pad causes "monkey facies" and dry, loose, wrinkled skin Kwashiorkor = protein deficiency, closer-to-normal caloric intake, 60–70% ideal body weight, edema, potbelly "red" children, hypopigmented dry hair, "flaky paint" skin, "flag" sign in hair

- Can be non-bullous or bullous
  - Non-bullous: staph and strep – usually at sites of trauma
  - Bullous: localized production of exfoliant toxins (ETA, ETB) by phage II *Staphylococcus aureus* at sites of cutaneous infection > Dsg 1 cleavage; more likely to develop on clinically intact skin
- Treatment: mupirocin, oral b-lactamase-resistant penicillin or first-generation cephalosporin

Folliculitis

- *Staphylococcus aureus* is the most common.
- Gram-negative folliculitis develops in acne with long course of oral antibiotics, isotretinoin.
- *Pseudomonas* cause hot tub folliculitis.

Abscess, furuncles, carbuncles

- Abscess and furuncles are collection of pus that are walled off from surrounding tissue.
  - Furuncle – involves hair follicle

  Carbuncle = collection of furuncles (can extend deep with sinus tracts)
  - Abscess can be anywhere.
- *Staph* is the usual cause.
  - Furuncles most frequent manifestation of community-acquired MRSA
- Treatment
  - Simple furuncles: warm compresses, incision, and drainage
  - Antibiotics: doxycycline, TMP-SMX, clindamycin

Staphylococcal scalded skin syndrome (SSSS)

- Exfoliative toxin (ET) cleaves Dsg1.
- Systemic symptoms with prodrome of malaise, fever, irritability, and severe tenderness of the skin.
- Erythema of the head and edema within 48-h generalization > skin becomes wrinkled with flaccid bullae > intertriginous sites are first to exfoliate > desquamation.
- Periorificial crusting is characteristic, with radial fissures.
- Treatment: oral antibiotics (cephalexin, dicloxacillin).

Scarlet fever

- Group A strep: exotoxins A, B, and C
- Sore throat, headache malaise, n/v, fever
- 12–48 hours later: blanchable erythema on the neck, chest, and axilla > sand paper texture, Pastia's lines in the folds; beefy red tongue; desquamation 7–10 days later
- Treatment: amoxicillin 10–14 days (drug of choice)

Erysipelas and cellulitis

- Cellulitis – infection of cutaneous lymphatics in subcutis. Well-defined erythema.
- Erysipelas – infection of superficial lymphatics in the upper dermis. Sharply demarcated borders.

- Most frequently caused by *Strep. pyogenes* and less often *Staph. aureus*, *Enterobacteriaceae*, and anaerobes.
- Early treatment necessary to prevent sepsis, skin necrosis, and permanent tissue damage.
- Treat with oral antibiotics; if no improvement after 24 hours, consider changing to IV.

Corynebacteria

- Gram-positive rods
- Likes warm moist environments
- Three main types in the skin:
  - Erythrasma: *C. minutissimum*

    Produces protoporphyrin IX – Woods lamp it

  - Treatment: topical clindamycin, erythromycin, oral erythromycin
  - Pitted keratolysis: *Kytococcus sedentarius* (aka micrococcus); corynebacteria and actinomyces
  - *Trichomycosis axillaris*: *Corynebacterium tenuis* – shave affected hair

Gram-Negative Bacteria
Pseudomonas

- Gram-negative aerobic bacillus
- Produces colors
  - Greenish blue: pyocyanin
  - Yellow green: fluorescein
  - Brown black: pyomelanin
- Cutaneous infections are varied:
  - Green nail
  - Pyoderma and blastomycosis-like pyoderma
  - Otitis externa
  - Hot tub folliculitis
  - *Pseudomonas* hot-foot syndrome
  - Ecthyma gangrenosum
  - Gram-negative toeweb infection

Mycoplasma

Mycoplasma-Induced Rash and Mucositis (MIRM) (see section on MIRM above)

- Most common in children.
- Prodromal syndromes nearly universal (cough, malaise, fever) preceding eruption by about 1 week.
- The most common presentation is mucositis with sparse skin lesions; severe mucositis is the next most common presentation.
  - Mucosal surfaces: oral cavity/lips (94%), ocular involvement (82%), urogenital (63%).
  - Skin lesions can be absent, mild, or moderate and are polymorphous (vesiculobullous > targetoid lesions, papules, macules, morbilliform).
- Eighty-one percent make a full recovery.
- Treatment consists of antibiotics (although it is unclear if abx decrease the mucocutaneous eruption). Limited evidence that IVIg may be beneficial in patients with severe mucositis.

Bacterial Decolonization

Staph Eradication Steps

To eradicate staph (a type of skin bacteria that can cause problems) from your skin, you have to target both your skin and the environment you live in. These are the recommended steps:

- Soak in a bleach bath at least every other day for 2–4 weeks for 10 minutes (see below for details). Once done with the daily baths, continue with a weekly bleach bath, or switch to using a benzoyl peroxide wash in the shower at least weekly.
- Apply the mupirocin in the nose for 5 days in a row and then for the first 5 days of every month.
- Wipe down all common surfaces with Lysol (or a similar) disinfecting wipes or a similar wipe. This includes things like *cellphone/house phones, door knobs, light switches, refrigerator/microwave/stove handles, sink handles, toilet*

seat and toilet flusher handle, remote control, toys, and any other common surfaces.

- Wash all clothes, towels, and bedding in warm/hot water.
- Stop smoking (MRSA exposed to cigarette smoke was harder to kill and had increased keratinocyte adherence than MRSA not exposed to smoke).
- Continue to be gentle with your skin; otherwise use gentle skin cleansers.

Bleach Baths

Note: must use only pure bleach (sodium hypochlorite). Other "cleansers" are NOT a substitute.

1/4–1/2 cup of bleach in a whole tub of warm water. (1–2 cap fulls in a baby-sized tub).

Can add 1 tbsp. of salt if the bleach leads to stinging.

Soak for up to 10–20 minutes.

Viral Diseases

Herpes

Antiviral Therapy for HSV

Genital Herpes

- Initial therapy
  - Acyclovir 400 mg PO TID for 7–10 days or 200 mg PO five times a day for 7–10 days
  - Valacyclovir 1 gram BID for 7–10 days
- Recurrent
  - Immunocompetent

    Acyclovir: 400 mg TID for 5 days or 800 mg BID for 5 days – initiate at earliest signs of symptoms.

    Famciclovir 125 mg BID for 5 days or 1 gram BID for 1 day.

    Valacyclovir 500 mg BID for 3 days.
  - Immunocompromised (e.g., HIV+)

Acyclovir 400 mg q4h while awake (5×/day) for 7 days
Famciclovir 500 mg BID for 5–10 days
Valacyclovir 1 gram BID for 5–10 days

- Suppressive doses (recommended by ACOG if only 1 partner has HSV-2)
  - Immunocompetent

    Acyclovir 400 mg BID for up to 12 months or 200 mg 3–5×/day
    Valacyclovir 500 mg or 1 gram daily
    Famciclovir 250 mg BID

  - Immunocompromised (e.g., HIV+)

    Acyclovir 400–800 mg BID to TID
    Famciclovir 500 mg BID
    Valacyclovir 500 mg BID

- Herpes simplex/orolabial herpes
  - Initial therapy – no guidelines.
  - Recurrent

    Valacyclovir 2 gram BID for 1 day if given during prodrome/within 24 hours of symptom onset

  - For prophylaxis for dental work or laser resurfacing, famciclovir 250 mg BID or valacyclovir 500 mg BID started the day before and continued 10–14 days afterward.
  - For suppression, acyclovir 400 mg BID.
  - Therapies outlined above for genital herpes may prove helpful as well.

<u>Herpes Zoster</u>

- Ideally started within 24 hours of the rash/symptom onset.
- There is no evidence for treatment beyond 72 hours of rash onset.
- Adult dosing
  - Acyclovir 800 mg PO five times per day × 7–10 days
  - Valacyclovir 1 gram TID for 7 days

- Famciclovir 500–750 mg TID
- Famciclovir 500 mg TID for 7 days

Varicella

- Children: >2 years and >40 kg. Ideally started within 24 hours of rash: acyclovir 20 mg/kg up to 800 mg QID × 5 days. Check baseline creatinine in kids if concern for dehydration.
- Adults/people >13 years old: there is a risk of severe fulminant disease with visceral complications – treat aggressively.
  - Immunocompetent: 800 mg PO QID for 5 days
  - 10 mg/kg IV every 8 hours adjusted for creatinine clearance for 7–10 days

Post-herpetic Neuralgia

- Gabapentin, pregabalin, and tricyclic antidepressants are generally the drugs of first choice.
- Gabapentin 300 mg PO on day 1, 300 mg BID on day 2, and 300 mg TID on day 3. May increase dose up to 1800 mg/day (divided TID). Adjust for renal failure.
- Pregabalin
  - For normal renal function (>60 mL/min creatinine clearance)
  - Regular-release capsules

    Initial: 150–300 mg/day PO divided q8–12h
    Maintenance: may increase to 300 mg/day divided q8–12h after 1 week, as needed

  - Extended-release tablets

    Initial: 165 mg PO qDay
    Maintenance: may increase to 330 mg PO qDay within 1 week based on response and tolerability; not to exceed 330 mg PO qDay
    Patients who experience insufficient pain relief following 2–4 weeks of treatment with 330 mg PO qDay and tolerate the ER tablets may be treated with up to 660 mg PO qDay.

- Amitriptyline
  - Start at 10 or 12.5 mg PO qhs titrating up to effect/side effect, typically to 25 mg PO qhs.
  - Max dose of 150 mg PO qhs.
- Others
  - Steroids

    Prednisolone 50 mg/day tapered in 2 weeks (started with acute zoster to reduce pain, but no acute on post-herpetic neuralgia)

    Lidocaine patches: 5% patch 1–3 patches on for 12 hours and then off for 12 hours

    - Topical lidocaine may provide short-term relief

    Capsaicin 0.025–0.075% cream applied 3–5 times daily

    - Can take up to 4 weeks to work but generally poorly tolerated

Warts and Molluscum

Topical therapeutics are many. Be cautious on the face to only perform the mildest of therapies so that the scar/mark risk is minimized.

- *Cryotherapy*
  - *Do not perform in higher Fitzpatrick skin types or patients with a tan due to risk of permanent hypopigmentation.*
  - Try to limit surrounding skin that is treated with the cryo.

    Pulse the spray to minimize surrounding tissue damage.

  - Be extremely cautious around the eye.

    For the face/sensitive areas, either spray into an otoscope tip (not favored as the lesion cannot be seen well) or use a cotton swab or forceps to dip into the liquid nitrogen, and then touch lightly/repeatedly for cryotherapy.

- On average, treat each lesion with 10 seconds of cryotherapy; let the area rewarm, and then retreat with another 10 seconds of cryotherapy.
- Post-cryo expectation: the areas will get pink and may form a shallow blister. That blister should crust and fall off in about 7 days. The goal is that the lesion will fall off with the crust.
- If bothersome, patient can apply Vaseline ± Band-Aid to the area(s).
- Set up appointment for 3–4 weeks to assess need for retreatment.

• *Salicylic acid liquid or plasters*

- Good to pair with cryotherapy. Should start using about 4–6 days after cryo on the wart itself. Replace daily until next appointment (ideally in 3–4 weeks).

• *Pulsed dye laser*

- Pare down, ~ 3 pulses per lesion, 7 mm spot, cryo off (or on), 8 J, 0.45 ms
- Make sure to wear N95 mask and have smoke evacuator running so that the wart virus is not vaporized and then inhaled.

• *Cantharidin*

- Use plain cantharidin rather than the bottle that has the salicylic acid mixed in since the salicylic acid adds irritation (that preparation should only be used for very thick, hyperkeratotic warts).
- Apply the cantharidin with a thin tipped Qtip right on the wart itself with as little as possible placed on the normal skin.
- Don't use on the face/neck and be very careful in intertriginous areas.
- For thick warts, can place tape over the wart after application to enhance potency (let the cantharidin dry first so it isn't wicked into the tape, though).
- Wash off with soap and water, not just water, after about 4 hours for molluscum and until bedtime for warts (if treating a second time, leave on 1–2 hours lon-

ger for molluscum and until morning for warts). Can wash off sooner if there is pain.
- For molluscum, may only want to treat 20 or so in patient with innumerable lesions; can get more of them at next visit.
- Flat warts tend to form "ring warts," so consider not treating these.
- Tip: end visit by asking "So, what time are you going to wash these off?"

- *Curettage*
  - Wart: anesthetize, cauterize, and then curette: cure rate okay with one treatment
  - Mollusca: try EMLA under occlusion for 15–20 minutes; easy to flick off with curette; high cure rate.

- *Imiquimod* (Aldara)
  - Tiny packets make for difficult application, but the tip is to use a pin to poke a tiny hole into the packet and then squeeze the cream out of that. Only need a little to be placed on the wart.
  - Wart: once a night, soak in warm water, pare or use a fresh emery board to file down the wart, and then apply a thin amount of imiquimod.
  - Genital warts: apply 3–5 times per week.
  - Avoid in patients with immunodeficiency and autoimmune conditions.

- *Podofilox*
  - Used in anogenital warts
  - Apply with cotton-tipped applicator (solution) or finger (gel) q12h for 3 days and then no treatment for 4 days.
  - May repeat in 1 week, cycle up to 4 times.

- *Squaric acid (SADBE)*
  - Can sensitize with 1–2% on the upper arm or hip.
  - Can also apply directly to warts for sensitization.
  - Give patient rescue clobetasol script for rash.
  - The goal is to create an allergic contact dermatitis.

- Penn State Protocol helpful to follow: https://www.pennstatehershey.org/c/document_library/get_file?uuid=b0f83ec7-ba9f-484d-b9c7-2c2e3dc56e66&groupId=102184.

- *Topical 5-FU* (Efudex)
  - For warts: soak warts in warm water for 15 minutes to soften, then pare with a razor blade, or file with a fresh emery board until pinpoint bleeding.
  - Add a thin layer of topical 5-FU to warts nightly for up to 3 months.
  - Avoid scrotal contact, and keep away from pets (can kill them).
  - Rarely patients with dihydropyrimidine dehydrogenase deficiency can have systemic side effects including mucositis, fatigue, fever, and extreme lethargy with topical 5-FU.

- *Intralesional Candida antigen*
  - Inject 0.15 to 0.3 mL total – repeat monthly. If no change after 3 months, cease treatment. If getting some improvement, can go up to six treatments.
  - Avoid in the immunosuppressed.

- *Bleomycin*
  - Cure rate between 50 and 100% depending on the type of wart (76–94% for periungual wart)
  - Consent should include ESCHAR × 4 weeks, PAIN × 72 hours, erythema, and hematoma. Rare reports of: hypopigmentation, scarring, restricted joint movement, narrowing of fingertips, gangrene, nail atrophy, nail ridging, onychodystrophy, nail loss, and Raynaud's. Contraindicated in pregnancy.
  - Concentration of reconstituted bleomycin should be 1%. Activity is enhanced by addition of local anesthetic.
  - Consider paring wart prior to injection.
  - Blanching on injection indicates infiltration is at the appropriate depth.
  - Maximum dose of bleomycin per wart is 4 mg/session. Generally need two to three sessions scheduled 4 weeks apart.

- *Cimetidine*
  - 30–40 mg/kg/day (*Eur J Dermatol.* 2003)
  - Adjuvant treatment. Helps to increase Th1 profile (IL-2, IFN-gamma)
- *Topical cidofovir*
  - Topical: 1% or 3% cidofovir cream with or without occlusion once or twice a day.

    Most common side effect: irritation
  - Consider intralesional therapy.
  - Can work in immunocompromised patients.

COVID-19 Skin Manifestations

The AAD maintains a resource center for updated clinical guidance, teledermatology, legal and practice management, as well as a library section that includes checklists and other guidelines (https://www.aad.org/member/practice/coronavirus).

It is unclear at this time if skin manifestations are directly virally mediated or an indirect response by the immune system to the infection.

Skin manifestations can include:

- Urticaria
- Pernio-like presentation "COVID toes" (not just in acral locations)
- Livedoid eruption
- Petechiae

Occupational hazards for the skin:

- Hand washing-induced dry skin and dermatitis with increased hand hygiene
- Skin damage from N95 respirator mask, surgical masks, or other protective equipment

Pediatric concerns

- While most children are more likely to present with a milder disease course, some children show a risk for more significant illness.

- Multisystem inflammatory syndrome in children (MIS-C) involves persistent fever, inflammation, and multiorgan dysfunction in the context of exposure to SARS-CoV-2:
  - May mimic Kawasaki disease
  - Have a low threshold of suspicion for hospitalization

Testing

- If suspecting COVID-19, rapid testing (<24 hours turnaround time) and standard PCR testing (approx. 72 hours turnaround time) are available.
  - Nasopharyngeal or oropharyngeal swabs
- Antibody testing (for cases that may have recovered from COVID-19 >14 days ago) has mixed evidence in terms of reliability and validity at the time of this publication.

Treatment (at this time) – dexamethasone, tocilizumab (monoclonal antibody) remdesivir +/- baricitinib, molnupiravir (awaiting FDA approval) More up-to-date information available at: https://www.health.harvard.edu/diseases-and-conditions/treatments-for-covid-19

Vaccines have been shown to be safe and effective in the prevention of severe COVID

Social distancing and wearing a surgical mask in daily activities (especially if social distancing cannot be maintained) are recommended.

Special contact precautions by healthcare personnel in the care of patients include mask and goggles or face shield.

Check your local state/government recommendations in elective procedures, patient care, and other required and recommended precautions.

Antifungals

Topical Mycotic Treatment

Azoles: good for yeast and fungus (and some, like ketoconazole, have mild antibacterial properties as well)

Nystatin: yeast only

Terbinafine (Lamisil): fungus only

For oral pharmacotherapy (griseofulvin, terbinafine, fluconazole, itraconazole), see dermatopharmacology section

Note: Oral ketoconazole is no longer used for cutaneous indications.

Parasitic Infestations

Scabies

- *Permethrin 5%* (Elimite)
  - Infants >2 years old and adults
  - Bathe *before* applying. Apply thin layer from neck to toes, including all body folds, under the nails, in the gluteal crease, in the umbilicus, and between the fingers/toes. Infants and children need to treat their scalp, temples, and forehead. *Do NOT* apply to the nose, lips, or eyelids or around the eyes or mouth. If wash hands after applying, reapply.
  - Apply before bed. (Must stay in place for 8–14 hours before washing it off.) In the morning, wash off and place all clothes, towels, and sheets/blankets in the wash and clean with hot water. Repeat ALL STEPS in 1 week. (Similarly treat all people with whom the patient has skin-to-skin contact with; however, no need to repeat in 1 week).

    Scabies don't like mature sebaceous glands or maybe they have territorial fights with the demodex mites, but in any case, they generally don't go above the neck in adults/postpubertals/kids over 2 years old.
  - For children <2 years old or immunocompromised, treat from scalp down (avoid eyes and mouth).
- *Ivermectin* (not FDA approved, but widely used)
  - 200 mcg/kg PO × 1; may repeat in 1 week
  - Ideal for treating multiple patients in a nursing home setting

Scabies Adjunctive Therapies
Mites can survive for days without human skin.

- Wash your clothes, bedding, towels, sheets, comforters, blankets, and other items.
  - Wash all items in a washing machine. Use the *hottest* water possible.
  - After washing, dry everything in a dryer, using the *hot* setting.
- For things that cannot be washed in a washing machine, dry it in the dryer and/or seal it in a plastic bag for a least 1 week.
- Vacuum the entire home on the day the treatment is started. Vacuum the carpet, area rugs, and all upholstered furniture. Upon completing vacuuming, throw away the bag. If your vacuum does not have a bag, empty the canister. You should wash a removable canister with hot, soapy water. If you cannot remove the canister, wipe it clean with a damp paper towel.
- No need to treat pets.

Head Lice
Can either treat the whole household (like scabies) or just those with head-to-head contact in the past 4–6 weeks

All treatments should be given twice, 7 days apart. Must also treat linens, fomites, headgear, sheets, clothes, and towels on hot cycle. All products should avoid the eyes.

- *Permethrin 1% cream rinse* (Nix) – apply overnight (8–12 hours), and then wash off.
- *Pyrethrin cream rinse* (Rid) – apply for 10 minutes, and then wash off.
- *Malathion 0.5% lotion* (Ovide) – flammable! – apply 20 minutes and then wash off.
- *Lindane 1% shampoo* (Kwell) – unsafe in children d/t neurotoxic issues – leave on for 4 minutes, and then wash off.
- *Ivermectin* (not FDA approved) – 200 mcg/kg × 1

Additionally, professional lice/nit removal clinics are widely available.

Chapter 4
Pediatric Dermatology

Infantile Hemangiomas

- Fastest growth is between 5 and 7 weeks of life. Deep hemangiomas often present later than superficial hemangiomas.
- Propranolol is the treatment of choice for high-risk hemangiomas.
- Propranolol initiation is ideally around 4–8 weeks of life and continued until 9–12 months of age. Earlier discontinuation is associated with a higher rate of rebound growth.
- There is not a universally accepted dosing or medication initiation protocol, but gradual dose increases with monitoring are recommended.

Example Protocols

Inpatient Start Protocol
- Initiation phase (oral)
  - 0.17 mg/kg q8h × 2 doses then.
  - 0.33 mg/kg q8h × 2 doses then.
  - 0.67 mg/kg q8h × 2 doses.
- Maintenance phase: 0.67 mg/kg/dose TID
  - Treatment is continued for 6–12 months (sometimes longer).

S. Hylwa et al., *Pocket Dermatology*,
https://doi.org/10.1007/978-3-030-83602-3_4

- Doses are adjusted for weight gain on a monthly basis.
- At the conclusion of treatment, can be tapered off with 50% reduction in dose for 1–2 weeks prior to d/c.

- *Vitals and blood glucose taken 1 h after each dose until dose stabilized*

Outpatient Start Protocol

- Week 1: 0.5–1 mg/kg/day *divided TID*
- Week 2: 1–1.5 mg/kg/day *divided TID*
- Week 3: 2 mg/kg/day *divided TID*
- Maintenance therapy
  - Clinic visits every 4–8 weeks (younger infants every 4 weeks) for vital signs and weight-based dose adjustments
  - Treat until 9–12 months of age
- Safety concerns
  - *Hold propranolol if <50% of normal intake or GI illness.*
  - Doses should be at least 6 h apart.
  - Infant must feed every 6–8 h when on propranolol including overnight.
  - Doses that are spit-up/vomited should not be redosed.

Side Effects of Propranolol

- Well tolerated in most cases
- Common side effects: reflux, cool extremities, sleep disturbance, diarrhea, fatigue, coughing
- Less common and worrisome: sweating, pallor, agitation/irritation, dyspnea/wheezing, hypoglycemia (jitteriness, lethargy)
  - Somnolence, hypotension, bradycardia, bronchospasm, and hypoglycemia are emergencies. These are very rare but more common in younger/smaller infants. Dose reduction with inpatient monitoring is suggested if propranolol is needed.

Infants with five or more infantile hemangiomas should receive a hepatic ultrasound. If diffuse hepatic hemangiomas are present, lab studies including TSH, T4, reverse T3, and LFTs should be performed and ECHO should be considered to evaluate for evidence of high-output cardiac failure. Propranolol should be initiated pending cardiac evaluation.

Propranolol Alternatives

- Topical timolol: 0.25% or 0.5% gel-forming solution. Dosing should be limited to a total of 2–3 drops/day in small infants.
- Limited safety data is available for oral nadolol and atenolol.

Management of Ulcerated Hemangioma

- *Wound cares*: cleanse wound daily with mild cleanser. Keep the wound covered with a petrolatum-based emollient and a wound dressing.
- Infection prevention: topical antibiotic ointment. Mupirocin ointment or wound culture and treat accordingly.
- *Pain management*: topical lidocaine (limit quantity based on weight due to cardiac toxicity), scheduled acetaminophen.
- *Healing*: Pulsed dye laser, topical timolol (limit quantity based on weight, especially if used in conjunction with oral propranolol). Topical becaplermin.

Ongoing use of systemic propranolol: rapid dose escalation or high dose may result in worsened ulceration (CB author opinion, not yet published).

Questionnaire for Propranolol Follow-up:

Has your child experienced any of the following?:

Yes	No	
☐	☐	Sleep disturbance
☐	☐	Nausea/vomiting
☐	☐	Coughing or breathing difficulties

☐	☐	Sweating
☐	☐	Changes in appetite
☐	☐	Fainting or decreased consciousness
☐	☐	Agitation/irritation/changes in activity
☐	☐	Seizures
☐	☐	Other

PHACE Syndrome

Posterior fossa malformations–hemangiomas–arterial anomalies–cardiac defects–eye abnormalities–(sternal cleft and supraumbilical raphe) syndrome.

Striking female predominance (88% females with PHACE).

PHACE syndrome should be considered in infants with large plaque-type facial hemangiomas (Fig. 4.1).

- One-third of patients with large facial hemangiomas have extracutaneous manifestations, most commonly cerebrovascular (72%) and cardiovascular anomalies (50%).

PHACE is associated with large segmental hemangiomas (>5 cm) and >1 facial segment involved.

- S2 has significantly lower likelihood of PHACE if it is the only segment involved.
- S1 (S4) involvement has higher risk of CNS anomalies
- S3 involvement has higher risk of cardiac anomalies.

Workup for PHACE

- Head and neck MRI/MRA (including the aortic arch)
- Echocardiogram
- Dilated eye exam
- Consultation with cardiology and/or neurology if abnormal imaging studies *prior* to initiation of propranolol

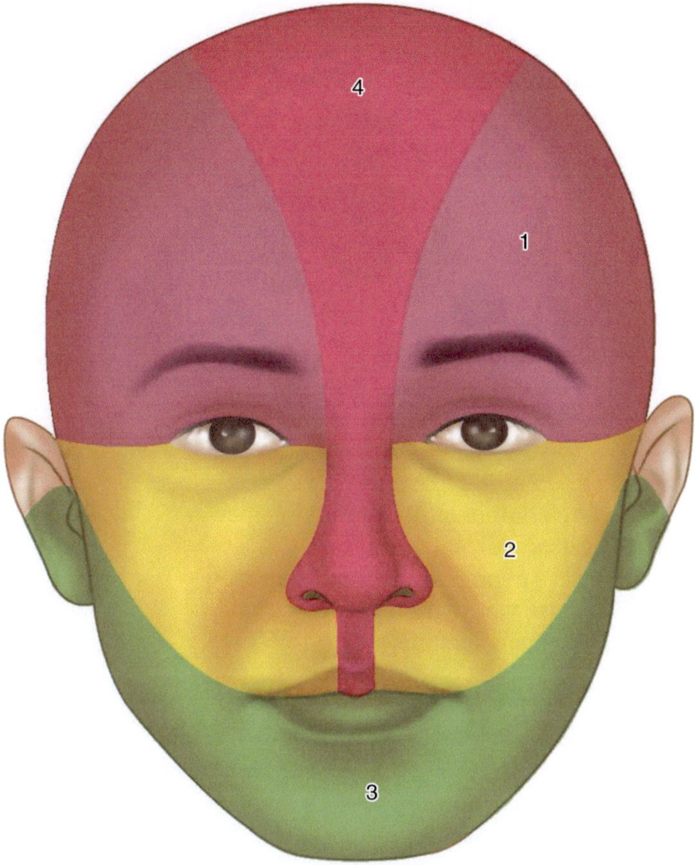

FIGURE 4.1 Segmental hemangioma patterns. (1) Frontotemporal; (2) Maxillary; (3) Mandibular; (4) Frontonasal

Erythroderma in the Newborn

Differential Diagnosis

- Infectious diseases
  - Staphylococcal scalded skin syndrome
  - Candida/other fungal infections
  - Rare: HSV, syphilis
- Inflammatory
  - Atopic dermatitis
  - Seborrheic dermatitis
  - Psoriasis
  - Rare: Diffuse mastocytosis
- Immunologic
  - Severe combined immunodeficiency
  - Omenn syndrome
  - Bruton's hypogammaglobulinemia
  - Common variable immunodeficiency
  - Graft-versus-host disease (GVHD)
- Ichthyosiform
  - Nonbullous ichthyosiform erythroderma
  - Bullous ichthyosis (epidermolytic hyperkeratosis)
  - Netherton syndrome
  - Sjögren-Larsson syndrome
  - Keratosis-ichthyosis-deafness (KID) syndrome
  - Trichothiodystrophy
  - Neutral lipid storage disease
- Metabolic
  - Zinc deficiency
  - Biotinidase deficiency
  - Holocarboxylase deficiency
  - Essential fatty acid deficiency
  - Cystic fibrosis (due to nutritional deficiency)
  - Rare

Cobalamin deficiency
Maple syrup urine disease
Carbamoyl phosphate synthetase deficiency
Argininosuccinic aciduria
Methylmalonic aciduria
Propionic acidemia

- Others
  - Chondrodysplasia punctata
  - Ectodermal dysplasias

Workup for Erythroderma in a Newborn (Fig. 4.2)

- CBC with differential
- BMP with electrolytes (mag, phos, calcium)
- Liver function tests
- Blood cultures
- Skin cultures for bacteria, herpes simplex virus, and yeast from lesional sites and orifices
- KOH preparation of skin scraping (if candidiasis is suspected)
- Skin biopsy
- Consider: chest X-ray (evaluates thymic shadow), rapid plasma regain (RPR), peripheral smear, zinc level, immunologic testing, metabolic testing, hair mount

Bullous Diseases in the Newborn

Differential Diagnosis

- Infectious:
  - Bullous impetigo
  - Staphylococcus scalded skin syndrome
  - Group B strep
  - Pseudomonas
  - Congenital syphilis
  - Neonatal VZV/HSV

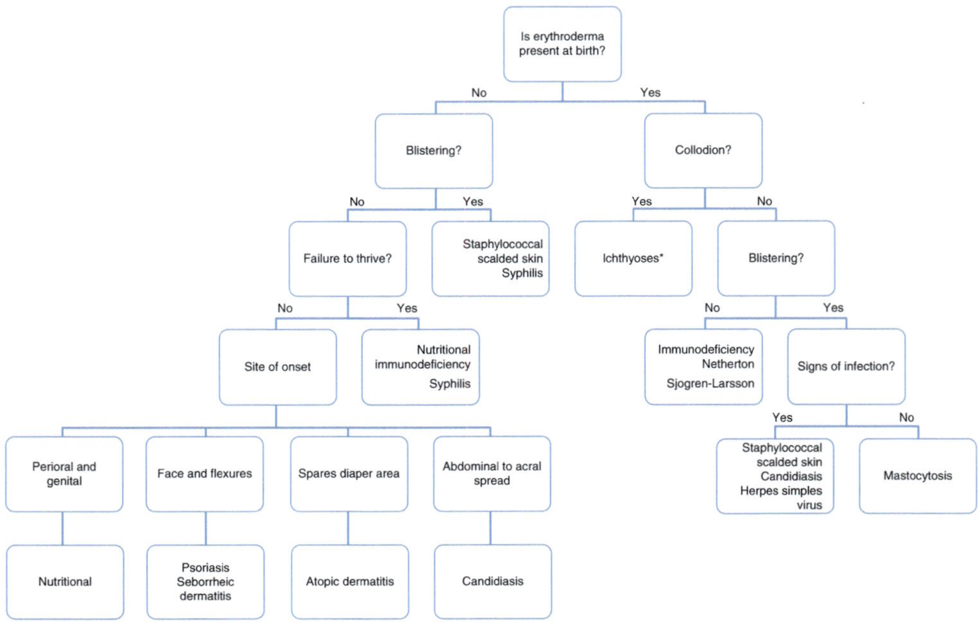

FIGURE 4.2 Stepwise approach to erythroderma present at birth. (From: Boull and Hook. 2017)

- Inherited
  - Epidermolysis bullosa
  - Epidermolytic hyperkeratosis
  - Porphyria (CEP)
  - Absent dermal ridges and congenital milia syndrome
- Inflammatory
  - Bullous mastocytosis
  - Maternal bullous disease: pemphigus foliaceus, pemphigus vulgaris, pemphigoid gestationis
  - Neonatal lupus
  - Primary immunobullous diseases: Congenital bullous dermatosis of childhood, bullous pemphigoid
  - Congenital GVHD (from a primary immunodeficiency syndrome)
- Other
  - Acrodermatitis enteropathica
  - Sucking blister
  - Aplasia cutis congenita
  - Transient porphyrinemia (secondary to hemolysis)
  - Trauma, burns

Workup
- Maternal and neonatal history
- Skin biopsy of infant (and mother if applicable) +/– DIF +/– EM
- Touch prep of biopsy for gram stain and KOH
- Rapid plasma reagin (RPR)
- Gram stain and bacterial culture; Tzanck; DFA, viral culture
- Serum zinc level and alk phos
- Serum, urine, and fecal porphyrins

Pustular Disease in the Newborn

Differential Diagnosis

- Infectious: Group A strep, neonatal or congenital candidiasis, HSV, scabies, impetigo, listeria, *Haemophilus influenzae*, *Pseudomonas*, VZV, CMV, *Aspergillus*
  - Congenital candidiasis often begins at the umbilicus and spreads acrally. Scraping the umbilical cord can help with diagnosis. The prognosis is poor in small preterm infants and presents as "burn-like" erythema. Prognosis is correlated with birth weight (neonates <1000 g have mortality rate of 40%; neonates >1000 g 8%). Treatment most commonly is amphotericin B.
- Inflammatory:
  - Common: erythema toxicum neonatorum (eosinophils on scraping), neonatal pustular melanosis (neutrophils on scraping), miliaria, neonatal acne
  - Less common: eosinophilic folliculitis, acropustulosis of infancy
  - Rare: congenital self-healing reticulohistiocytosis (Langerhans cell histiocytosis), neonatal Behcet's, neonatal psoriasis, Down syndrome-associated vesiculopustular eruptions
- Inherited: Incontinentia pigmenti, hyper IgE syndrome (eosinophilic folliculitis)

Workup

- Maternal and neonatal history
- Skin biopsy
- Rapid plasma regain (RPR)
- Gram stain and bacterial culture; Tzanck smear, DFA, viral culture
- KOH prep and fungal culture
- Scabies prep

Henoch-Schonlein Purpura

Tetrad: Palpable purpura, arthritis, abdominal pain, hematuria.

American College of Rheumatology Criteria (2+ of the following):
- Patient age younger than 20 years
- Palpable purpura
- Abdominal pain/GI bleeding
- Extravascular or perivascular granulocytes on biopsy

Other Manifestations
- Recent URI or febrile illness (Group-A beta-hemolytic strep, *Yersinia*, *Campylobacter*, *Mycoplasma*)
- Arthritis or arthralgias (knees, ankles)
- Testicular pain/swelling
- Microscopic hematuria, proteinuria
- Leukocytoclastic vasculitis on biopsy, often, but not always, with IgA staining
- Skin lesions may blister and ulcerate

Workup
- CBC with diff, CMP, UA
- PT/PTT, DIC panel
- ESR/CRP
- C3, C4, CH50
- ASO/Anti-DNAse B titers and pharyngeal culture
- Stool culture and guaiac
- Blood culture
- Skin biopsy for H&E and DIF

Treatment
- Corticosteroids are controversial; many will initiate if nephrotic/nephritis syndrome or severe GI symptoms. Current consensus is that corticosteroids do not prevent renal disease but could be used to treat severe nephritis.

- Renal consult is recommended.
- Follow serial UA monthly × at least 6 months (nephritis may present late and predicts outcome); adults are more likely to have kidney disease.

Atopic Dermatitis

General Treatment Considerations for Children

- Ointments are preferred to cream vehicles due to less stinging and better moisturizing
- Topical calcineurin inhibitors (TCIs) (tacrolimus and pimecrolimus) and crisaborole may sting/burn when applied. Use topical steroids first to improve the dermatitis and then transition to one of these agents.
- Pimecrolimus is less effective than tacrolimus.
- TCIs can safely be used "off label" in infants and children <2 years.
- Thick creams or ointments are preferred moisturizers as lotions do not provide adequate skin hydration. Lotions may also contain irritants and cause stinging and burning of inflamed skin.
- Moisturizers should be applied within several minutes after bathing.
- Systemic antihistamines mainly aid with sleep as opposed to providing itch relief.
- Topical antihistamines and topical antibiotics should be avoided due to contact sensitization and lack of benefit in atopic dermatitis.
- Systemic steroids should be avoided in atopic dermatitis due to rebound flares and short- and long-term side effects including osteoporosis.
- Food allergy testing, especially by RAST, should be reserved for children with moderate to severe atopic dermatitis who do not respond to standard treatments. Testing should be limited to only the most common allergens. RAST testing has a high false-positive rate, so it should be

TABLE 4.1 Example of an eczema action plan

Green: Eczema under control	Daily moisturizer +/– prophylactic, intermittent use of topical steroids or topical calcineurin inhibitor
Yellow: Eczema worsening	Face: Tapering twice daily use of mild topical steroid or topical calcineurin inhibitor Body: Tapering twice daily use of mid-strength topical steroid
Red: Eczema out of control	Seek an appointment with a physician Face: Limited use of a mid-strength topical steroid then revert back to yellow Body: Limited time use of super-potent topical steroid then revert back to yellow

followed with prick testing and a food challenge test (gold standard).

- Development of an eczema action plan can be very helpful for patients and parents to understand when to ramp up and when to taper treatment (Table 4.1).

Treatment Instructions: Based on Treatment Guidelines Unless Noted to be Expert Opinion (E)

1. Take a 10 min tub bath daily (E). Consider the addition of ¼–½ cup bleach (not splashless) to ½ filled bathtub of water.
2. Cleansers should be soap-free, fragrance-free, and hypoallergenic.
3. After bathing, pat skin dry and immediately apply topical medications and emollient.
4. Use the lowest-strength topical steroid that is effective for body site, patient age, and disease severity.
5. Twice daily application of topical steroids every day until the skin lesions are clear is recommended over intermittent dosing.
6. When the skin is clear, prophylactic intermittent application of topical steroids or TCIs to problem areas can help to decrease the frequency of flares.

7. Topical steroids may be safely applied over open excoriations in atopic dermatitis.
8. Use of wet wraps (see instructions below) is more effective than use of topical steroids alone.
9. Steroid phobia is common among parents and should be addressed to maximize compliance.
10. TCIs can be used as steroid sparing agents and are especially useful for treating the face and skin folds.
11. Safety studies have shown no increased malignancy rates in children on TCI compared to the general pediatric population.

Home Wet Wrap Instructions

1. Bathe and apply topical medications and emollient.
2. Soak snug cotton pajamas in warm water, and wring out well.
3. Dress the child in the damp pajamas.
4. Cover the child in warm blanket/towel or a second dry pair of pajamas.
5. Wet wraps can be worn overnight but should be left in place for at least an hour.
6. Reapply an emollient after removing the wet wrap.

Calls that Need Urgent Attention and Notification of an Attending Physician

- Blistering from a laser procedure
- Blistering in the newborn
- Urticaria in the newborn (risk of autoinflammatory and immunodeficiency syndromes)
- Collodion baby
- Ulcerating hemangioma
- Propranolol overdose (have family contact EMS)

- Concern for:
  - Eczema herpeticum
  - Staphylococcal scalded skin syndrome
  - SJS/TEN
  - Drug-induced hypersensitivity syndrome (DIHS)
  - Reactive infectious mucocutaneous eruption (RIME)

Less Likely Pediatric Diagnoses and Potential Alternatives (Table 4.2)

Rule of thumb:

Consider imaging prior to any biopsy of a midline lesion in a child.

Table 4.2 Less likely pediatric diagnoses and potential alternatives

Less likely diagnosis	Alternate diagnoses to consider
Cherry angioma	Spider telangiectasia, pyogenic granuloma, small infantile hemangioma (infant), Spitz nevus
Lipoma	Deep infantile hemangioma (infant), deep granuloma annulare (child/teen)
Skin tag	Molluscum contagiosum, Spitz nevus, angiofibroma (rarely), basal cell carcinoma in basal cell nevus syndrome (rare)
Hemangioma in teen	Pyogenic granuloma, congenital hemangioma, vascular malformation (AVM, venous malformation, etc.)
Electrode marks of the scalp of an infant	Aplasia cutis congenita
Epidermal inclusion cyst	Abscess/furuncle, midline anomalies in infants, preauricular sinus, pilomatricoma
Cellulitis	Consider exuberant arthropod bite reaction

Unique Pediatric Diagnoses (Table 4.3)

Table 4.3 Unique pediatric diagnoses

Diagnosis	Clinical features
Idiopathic facial aseptic granuloma	Pink-red nodule(s) on the midface and eyelids of young children. Self-limited
Pedal papules of infancy	Flesh colored papules on the medial heels of infants. Benign, self-resolving
Calcinosis cutis due to heel sticks	Firm white subcutaneous papules on the lateral aspects of the plantar heel. Often history of multiple heel sticks. Self-resolving
Acropustulosis of infancy (rule out scabies)	Recurrent crops of monomorphic pustules on the palms and soles of infants. Topical steroids if pruritic, spontaneous resolution
Lichen striatus	Blaschkoid linear flesh-colored or pink plaques. Nails may be affected. Spontaneous resolution
Papular urticaria (more common in children)	Hypersensitivity reaction to arthropod bites presenting as pruritic pink/brown papules on exposed sites. Reactions may last into the late fall. Treat with topical steroids and scheduled antihistamines. Avoid bites
Slime dermatitis (irritant or allergic contact)	Contact dermatitis that can be induced by all types of slime. If ACD, allergen is usually methylisothiazolinone from the glue
Pseudomonas "hot foot"	Painful pink nodules on the soles. Contracted in pools or hot tubs. Variant of neutrophilic eccrine hidradenitis. Spontaneous resolution
Autoeczematization reaction "id"	Flesh-colored papules on the extensor surfaces, cheeks, ears. More common in children. Triggers include tinea capitis, molluscum, allergic contact dermatitis

Pediatric Skin Findings that Require Additional Workup (Table 4.4)

Table 4.4 Pediatric skin findings that require additional workup

>/= 5 infantile hemangiomas	Hepatic US
Segmental hemangioma on the face	See PHACE workup
Segmental hemangioma on the sacrum, perineum	LUMBAR workup: pelvic ultrasound, spinal imaging
Acne in age 2–6 years	Endocrine evaluation for hyperandrogenic state
Juvenile xanthogranuloma (two or more)	Eye exam for ocular JXG
Angiomas on the lips, palms, ears	Consider hereditary hemorrhagic telangiectasia evaluation
Angiofibroma	Genetics evaluation for tuberous sclerosis
Six or more cafe au lait macules >5 mm (prepubertal)	Genetics evaluation for NF1
Three or more hypopigmented macules	Consider TS workup
V1 capillary malformation	Eye exam
Large congenital melanocytic nevus Multiple congenital melanocytic nevi	Consider MRI of the brain and spine prior to age 4–6 months. Highest risk if axial location, extensive satellite nevi
COVID-related rashes	Please refer to infectious dermatology section

Diaper Dermatoses (Table 4.5)

TABLE 4.5 Diaper dermatoses

Diagnosis	Features	Treatment
Irritant diaper dermatitis variants: Erosive (Jacquet's) Granuloma gluteale infantum	Ill-defined erythema favoring the convexities where skin is most in contact with the diaper Spares the folds Circular erosions or pink/flesh colored papules on the scrotum, labia, perirectal area Multifactorial due to: High pH Frequent stooling Chronic moisture Candida Skin barrier dysfunction	Gentle skin cares Frequent diaper changes Wash area daily Avoid wiping (pat the skin) High-absorbent disposable diapers Thick barrier (zinc, petrolatum) with each change Topical nystatin Topical steroid (mid to high potency may be needed for granulomatous dermatitis)
Candidal diaper dermatitis	Pink papules in on the buttocks, lower abdomen, medial thighs	Gentle skin cares (see above) Topical nystatin
Perianal strep infection	Sharply marginated red perianal patch or plaque, often pruritic	PO penicillin or alternative
Psoriasis	Well-marginated confluent red scaling plaques Includes the folds	Gentle skin cares (see above) Topical steroids or TCI

TABLE 4.5 (continued)

Diagnosis	Features	Treatment
Acrodermatitis enteropathica	Red symmetrical erosive plaques with peripheral "chipped paint" scaling May have similar lesions in the periorificial distribution	Zinc replacement
Langerhans cell histiocytosis	Classically pink-brown papules in the inguinal creases, other flexures, scalp Many other morphologies have been described	Biopsy if suspicion

Pediatric Pharmacology

1 teaspoon = 5 mL or 5 cc.

Approximate Weight and Surface Area by Age (Table 4.6)
Body surface area (m^2) = $(\text{Height (cm)} \times \text{weight (kg)}/3600)^{0.5}$

Common Pediatric Medications and Dosages (Table 4.7)

Medications to Avoid in Pediatrics

- Tetracyclines in children younger than 8 years due to dental staining
- Quinolones in children whenever possible due to risk of cartilage concerns
- Aspirin due to (low) risk of Reye syndrome

Table 4.6 Approximate weight and surface area by age

Age	kg	m²
Newborn	3–4	0.2–0.25
6 months	7	0.3
1 year	10	0.5
3 years	15	0.7
5 years	20	0.8
8 years	25	0.95
10 years	30	1–1.1
15 years	50	1.5

Table 4.7 Common pediatric medications and dosages

Ensure that weight-based dosing does not exceed maximum dose in larger/older children

Drug	Dose	Interval	Taste	Other considerations
Analgesics				
Acetaminophen	10–15 mg/kg/dose	Div Q6h	Good	Alternate with ibuprofen to maximize anti-pyretic effect
Ibuprofen	10 mg/kg/dose	Div Q8h	Good	
Antibiotics				
Amoxicillin	40 mg/kg/day	Div Q8h	Good	80 mg/kg/d for otitis
Amoxicillin/ Clavulanate	40–80 mg/kg/day	Div Q8–12h	OK	Diarrhea common
Azithromycin	10–12 mg/kg	Div Q24h × 5d	Good	

TABLE 4.7 (continued)

Ensure that weight-based dosing does not exceed maximum dose in larger/older children

Drug	Dose	Interval	Taste	Other considerations
Cefdinir	14 mg/kg/day	Div Q12 or 24 h	OK	PO version of ceftriaxone
Cephalexin	25–50 mg/kg/day	Div Q6h	OK	
Clindamycin	30 mg/kg/day	Div Q6–8h	Bad	Risk of C. diff low in children
Dicloxacillin	30–40 mg/kg/day	Div Q6h	Bad	
Erythromycin	20–40 mg/kg/day	Div Q6h	Bad	Difficult to obtain, may need to compound
Trimethoprim-sulfamethoxazole	8–12 mg/kg/day (based on trimethoprim)	Div Q12h	OK	
Antifungals				
Griseofulvin microsize	*Microsized* 11 mg/kg/day as single dose or divided q12h (<2 years old efficacy not established) *Ultramicrosized* 7.3 mg/kg/day (<2 years old efficacy not established) Can be crushed and given with ice cream	Div Q12h or daily Treat for 8 weeks for tinea capitis		Ultramicrosized can be crushed and given with ice cream There is an oral suspension available but it is less readily absorbed than the tablets

(continued)

Table 4.7 (continued)

Ensure that weight-based dosing does not exceed maximum dose in larger/older children

Drug	**Dose**	**Interval**	**Taste**	**Other considerations**
Terbinafine	<25 kg: 125 mg 25–35 kg: 187.5 mg >35 kg: 250 mg	Daily × 6–8 weeks for capitis		Tabs only, can be hidden in "crunchy" foods
Antihistamines				
Non-sedating				
Cetirizine	2–5 years: 2.5–5 mg/day ≥6 years: 5–10 mg/day	Daily or Q12h	Good	
Loratadine	2–5 years: 5 mg ≥6 years: 10 mg	Daily	Good	
Fexofenadine	≥6 months to <2 years: 15 mg BID 2–11 years: 30 mg BID ≥12 years: 60 mg BID	BID	Good	
Sedating				
Diphenhydramine and hydroxyzine	0.5 mg/kg qhs	May dose 0.25 mg/kg Q6–8h	Good	Hydroxyzine 10 mg/tsp; diphenhydramine 5 mg/tsp

Table 4.7 (continued)

Ensure that weight-based dosing does not exceed maximum dose in larger/older children				
Drug	**Dose**	**Interval**	**Taste**	**Other considerations**
Anti-inflammatory				
Prednisolone	Doses vary; not to exceed 80 mg/day Common taper is: 2 mg/kg × 4d, then 1 mg/kg × 4d, then 0.5 mg/kg × 4d, then stop	Daily in am		15 mg/5 mL, liquid version of prednisone, dose-equivalent

Bibliography

Boull CL, Hook KP. Neonatal erythroderma–clinical perspectives. Res Rep Neonatol. 2017;7:1.

Eichenfield LF. Consensus guidelines in diagnosis and treatment of atopic dermatitis. Allergy. 2004;59:86–92.

Haggstrom AN, et al. Risk for PHACE syndrome in infants with large facial hemangiomas. Pediatrics. 2010;126(2):e418–26.

Harter N, Mancini AJ. Diagnosis and management of infantile hemangiomas in the neonate. Pediatr Clin. 2019;66(2):437–59.

Krowchuk DP, Frieden IJ, Mancini AJ, Darrow DH, Blei F, Greene AK, Annam A, Baker CN, Frommelt PC, Hodak A, Pate BM. Clinical practice guideline for the management of infantile hemangiomas. Pediatrics. 2019;143(1):e20183475.

Mathes E, Howard RM, Edwards MS. Vesicular, pustular, and bullous lesions in the newborn and infant. UpTo Date. Available. 2018 Dec 3.

Oni L, Sampath S. Childhood IgA vasculitis (Henoch Schonlein Purpura)—advances and knowledge gaps. Frontiers in pediatrics. 2019;27(7):257.

Paller AS, Fölster-Holst R, Chen SC, Diepgen TL, Elmets C, Margolis DJ, Pollock BH. No evidence of increased cancer incidence in children using topical tacrolimus for atopic dermatitis. Journal of the American Academy of Dermatology. 2020;83(2):375–81.

Chapter 5
Surgery in Dermatology

Surgical Danger Zones (Figs. 5.1, 5.2, and 5.3)

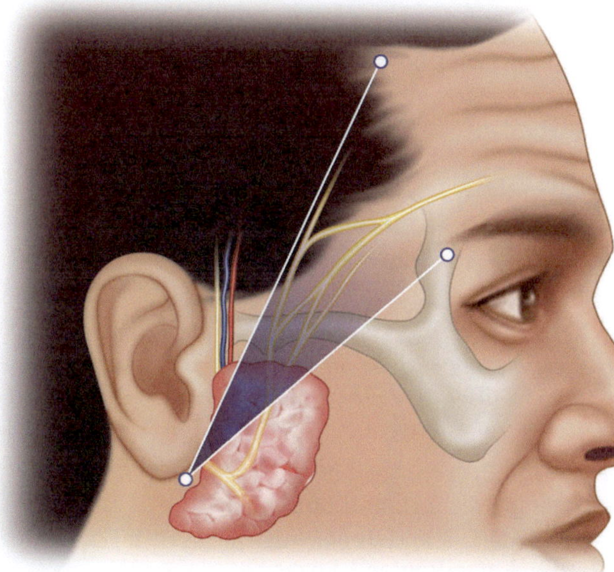

FIGURE 5.1 Temporal artery as it exits the parotid gland and crosses the zygomatic arch

S. Hylwa et al., *Pocket Dermatology*,
https://doi.org/10.1007/978-3-030-83602-3_5

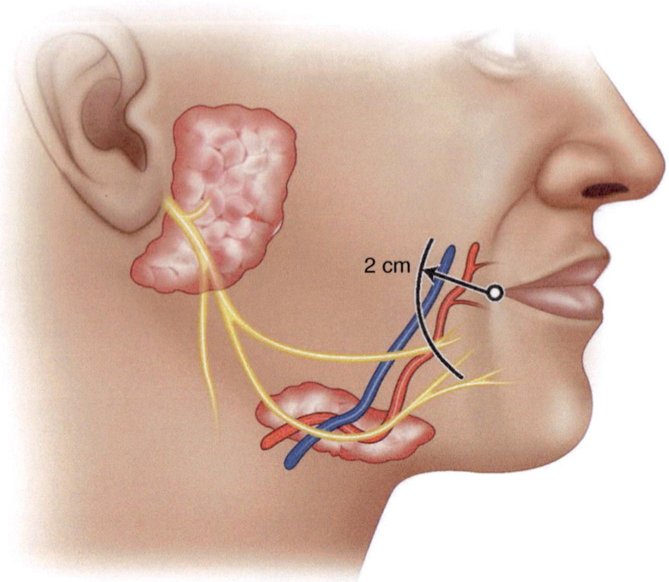

FIGURE 5.2 Marginal mandibular branch as it courses around the jaw

Other

- *Consider branches of facial nerve for surgery on face (to Zanzibar by motor car) motor nerve so paralysis can occur with branch damage.*
  - Temporal branch – forehead
  - Zygomatic – cheek and upper lip
  - Buccal – cheek and upper lip
  - Marginal mandibular – lower lip
- *Superior and inferior orbital rim are good landmarks* for supraorbital and supratrochlear as well as infraorbital nerves; these are sensory, so can create numbness and should include risk for damage in informed consent.

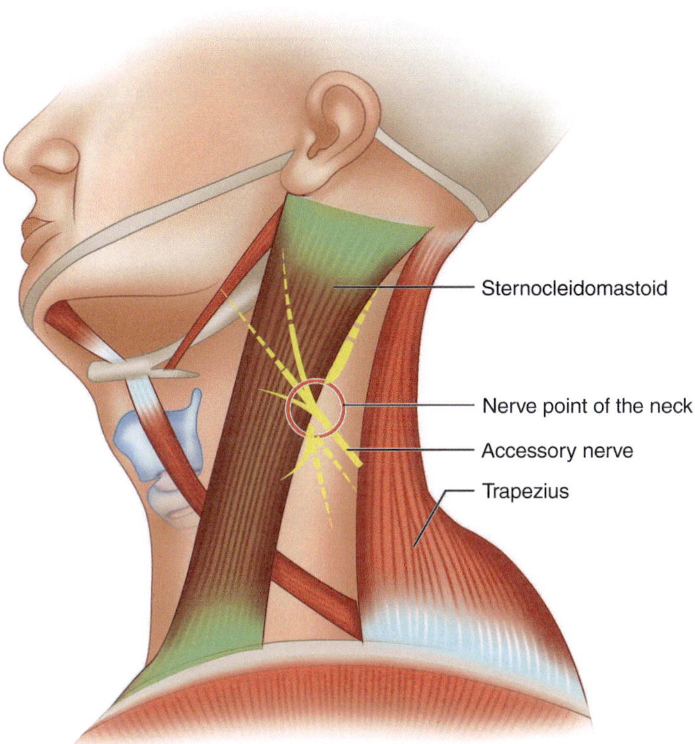

FIGURE 5.3 Erb's point: risks damage to the spinal accessory (CN XI), greater auricular, lesser occipital nerves
Erb's point is located on the posterior portion of the sternocleidomastoid muscle, midway on a line drawn from the mastoid to the clavicle

Mohs Appropriate Use Criteria (Table 5.1)

For the "mask areas" of the face (central face, eyelids [including inner/outer canthi], eyebrows, nose, cheeks, forehead, lips [cutaneous/mucosal/vermillion], scalp, chin, jawline, neck, ear and periauricular skin/sulci, temple), genitalia (including

TABLE 5.1 Mohs appropriate use criteria for BCC, SCC, lentigo maligna, and melanoma in situ

Area H	Appropriate	Uncertain	Inappropriate
BCC	Primary or recurrent: Aggressive Nodular Superficial		
SCC	Primary or recurrent: Aggressive Nonaggressive[a] Verrucous KA-type SCC[b] In situ SCC/Bowen		Primary or recurrent: AK with focal SCC in situ
LM and MIS	Primary or recurrent: LM MIS		
Area M	Appropriate	Uncertain	Inappropriate
BCC	Recurrent or primary: Aggressive Nodular Superficial (IC) Primary: Superficial > 0.6 cm	Primary: Superficial < 0.5 cm	
SCC	Primary or recurrent: Aggressive Nonaggressive[a] KA-type SCC[b] In situ SCC/Bowen		Primary or recurrent: AK with focal SCC in situ
LM and MIS	Primary or recurrent: LM MIS		

Table 5.1 (continued)

Area I	Appropriate	Uncertain	Inappropriate
BCC	Recurrent: Aggressive Nodular Primary: Aggressive ≥ 0.6 cm Nodular > 2 cm Nodular (IC) ≥ 1.1 cm	Primary: Aggressive ≤ 0.5 cm Nodular 1.1–2 cm Nodular (IC) 0.6–1 cm Superficial (IC) ≥ 1.1 cm	Recurrent: Superficial Primary: Nodular ≤ 1 cm Nodular (IC) ≤ 0.5 cm Superficial Superficial (IC) < 1 cm
SCC	Primary or recurrent: Aggressive Recurrent: KA-type SCC[b] Nonaggressive[a] Primary > 2 cm Nonaggressive[a] In situ SLC/Bowen Primary > 1.1 cm Nonaggressive (IC)[a] KA-type SCC[b] In situ SCC/Bowen (IC) KA-type SCC (IC) > 0.6 cm[b]	Recurrent: SCC in situ/Bowen Primary 1.1–2 cm Nonaggressive[a] SCC in situ/Bowen Primary ≤ 1 cm Nonaggressive (IC)[a] Primary 0.6–1 cm SCC: in situ/Bowen (IC) Primary ≤ 0.5 cm KA-type SCC (IC)[b]	Primary or recurrent: AK with final SCC in situ Primary < 1 cm Nonaggressive[a] KA-type. SCC[b] SCC in situ/ Bowen Primary < 0.5 cm SCC in situ/ Bowen (IC)
LM and MIS	Recurrent: LM MIS	Primary: LM MIS	

Listed indications are for both healthy and IC patients, and tumors of any size unless otherwise specified

Area H: 'Mask areas' of face (central face, eyelids [including inner/outer canthi], eyebrows, nose, lips [cutaneous/mucosal/vermillion], chin, ear, and periauricular skin/sulci, temple), genitalia (including perineal and perianal), hands, feet, nail units, ankles, and nipples/areola

Area M: Cheeks, forehead, scalp, neck, jawline, pretibial surface

Area I: Trunk and extremities (excluding pretibial surface, hands, feel, nail units, and ankles)

AK actinic keratosis, *BCC* basal cell carcinoma, *KA* keratoacanthoma, *IC* immunocompromised, *LM* lentigo maligna, *MIS* melanoma in situ, *SCC* squamous cell carcinoma

[a]SCC without aggressive features, <2 mm depth without other defining features, Clark level < III

[b]Not central facial

TABLE 5.2 Aggressive BCC and SCC morphologies

Aggressive BCC histology includes	Aggressive SCC histology includes
Morpheaform/ fibrosing/sclerosing	Sclerosing
Infiltrating	Basosquamous (excluding keratotic BCC)
Perineural	Small cell
Micronodular	Poorly or undifferentiated (Characterized by a high degree of nuclear pleomorphism, high mitotic rate, or low degree of keratinization)
	Perineural/perivascular
	Spindle cell
	Pagetoid
	Infiltrating
	KA-type (Central face)
	Single cell
	Clear cell
	Lymphoepithelial
	Sarcomatoid
	Breslow depth 2 mm or greater
	Clark level IV or greater

perineal and perianal), hands, feet, pretibial areas, nail units, ankles, and nipples/areola, Mohs is indicated for: Aggressive features of BCC and SCC found in Table 5.2.

Mohs Appropriate Use Criteria App

Available from the American Academy of Dermatology as a Free App)
Can be used for both healthy and immunocompromised patients and tumors of any size unless specified.

Excisional Margins of Lesions

- Benign – can be to edge to 1 mm
- Melanoma

  - In situ: 5 mm
  - <1 mm deep: 1 cm
  - 1–4 mm: 2 cm
  - >4 mm: 2–3 cm

- BCC low risk
  - If <2 cm in diameter: 4 mm (95% cure rate)

- SCC low risk
  - If <2 cm in diameter: 5 mm (95% cure rate)

Antibiotic Prophylaxis

Decision Tree

From the recommendations from Wright et al. Antibiotic Prophylaxis in Dermatologic Surgery JAAD. 2008;59(3):464–73.

1. Is the dermatologic procedure over a high risk site?
   (a) If yes, then offer ppx
2. If no, ask if there is a high risk of infective endocarditis or hematogenous total joint infection
   (a) If no, then no ppx
3. If yes, then ask if procedure includes oral mucosa or infected skin
   (a) If no, then no ppx
   (b) If oral mucosa involved, offer ppx
   (c) If infected skin, offer ppx and also tx infection

   For more considerations, see Table 5.3.

Locations/Techniques at a Higher Risk of Surgical Site Infection

- Lower extremity
- Groin

TABLE 5.3 Considerations for preoperative antibiotic prophylaxis for infective endocarditis or total prosthetic joint infection

Infective endocarditis high risk	Joint replacement high risk
Prosthetic cardiac valve Previous endocarditis Congenital heart disease Unrepaired cyanotic heart disease Completely repaired defects with prosthetic material/device Repaired congenital heart disease, but with residual impairment Cardiac transplant patients who develop valve disease	First 2 years after replacement Previous prosthetic joint infections Immunocompromised/suppressed Inflammatory arthropathies Insulin-dependent diabetes HIV infection Malignancy Malnourishment Hemophilia

- Wedge excision of lip or ear
- Skin flaps on nose
- Skin grafting
- Extensive inflammatory skin disease

Administer Antibiotics (Table 5.4) **30–60 min Prior to Procedure**

Consider postoperative antibiotics if
- >1 surgical site
- Ear, lip, nose, groin, hand, arm locations
- History of surgical site infection
- History of poorly controlled diabetes

Anesthetics

Topical Anesthetics

- Mucosal/conjunctiva: tetracaine 0.5% eye drops and proparacaine eye drops.

Table 5.4 Antibiotic indications based on site and penicillin (PCN) allergy status

	Non-PCN-allergic	**PCN-allergic**
Wedge excisions of ear/lip	Cephalexin 2 g po	Clindamycin 600 mg po or Azithromycin 500 mg po or Clarithromycin 500 mg po
Oral surgical site	Amoxicillin 2 g po	Clindamycin 600 mg po or Azithromycin 500 mg po or Clarithromycin 500 mg po
Lesions in groin and lower extremity	Cephalexin 2 g po	Bactrim DS one tab po or Levofloxacin 500 mg po

- Nasal: 4–10% cocaine solution (also is hemostatic).
- Oral: 2% viscous lidocaine, 2–4% lidocaine jelly, benzocaine, and anbesol.
- Skin
  - EMLA (Eutectic Mixture of Local Anaesthetics): 2.5% lidocaine + 2.5% prilocaine. Skin blanches; avoid eyes. Occlude it for 30–60 min before procedure.

    Do not use in children as prilocaine can increase risk of methemoglobinemia.

    Local reactions: erythema, pallor, and edema.
  - Topicaine: 4% lidocaine in lecithin gel provides rapid onset of anesthesia, associated with allergic contact dermatitis.
  - LMX: 4% for skin (OTC), 5% for mucosa (Rx). No occlusion required. Apply 15–40 min before procedure.
  - BLT (benzocaine 20%, lidocaine 6%, tetracaine 4%) – onset is 15–30 min. Since it contains and ester anesthetic, beware in those with para-amino contact allergy (e.g., allergic to PPD/hair dye, sulfonamides, thiazides, and azo dyes – see contact dermatitis section for more details).

Injectable Anesthetics (Tables 5.5 and 5.6)

- *Esters*: 1 "I" in name
  - All vasodilate except cocaine, which vasoconstricts
  - Hydrolysis by pseudocholinesterase in plasma to PABA
  - *Renal* excretion
  - Infrequent but possible allergy
  - Cross-reacts with PABA, PPD, PAS, sulfonamides, sulfonylureas, thiazides, and azo dyes so if patient is allergic to these, he/she can be allergic to esters (see contact dermatitis section for more details)
- *Amides*: 2 "I"s in name
  - N-dealkylated/hydrolyzed in *liver* P450
  - No allergic cross-reactivity with esters, rare allergy (usually related to additives)

Tumescent Anesthesia

- Must have ACLS certification.
- Subcutis lidocaine (0.05–0.1%) combined with sodium bicarbonate (generally 10 mEq/L) and epinephrine (0.65–1 mg/L).

TABLE 5.5 Pharmacokinetics of select anesthetics

Name	**Class**	**Speed**	**Duration (w/o epi)**	**Duration (2/epi)**
Procaine	Ester	Slow	15–30 min	30–90 min
Tetracaine	Ester	Slow	120–140	240–480
Lidocaine	Amide	Fast	30–120	90–200
Prilocaine[a]	Amide	Fast	30–120	60–240
Bupivacaine[b]	Amide	Moderate	120–240	240–600

[a]Prilocaine – methemoglobinemia that is dose dependent (if use <500 mg), peds cases; metabolized to ortho-toluidine

[b]Bupivacaine side effects: Greater cardiac toxicity than lidocaine, ventricular arrhythmia, cardiovascular collapse

Table 5.6 Maximum doses of cutaneous injectable anesthetics

Med	Dose	Max volume for 70 kg patient
1% lidocaine, NO epi	5 mg/kg	35 mL
1% lido with epi 1:100,000	7 mg/kg	50 mL
1% lido with epi 1:1,000,000	35–50 mg/kg	2500 mL
Tumescent anesthesia (1% lido with epi 1:1,000,000)	MAX: 55 mg/kg	

1% solution is 10 mg/mL (1 g/100 mL)

- Maximum dose is 35 mg/kg although doses of 55 mg/kg have been reported as safe.

Lidocaine

- Pregnancy category B
- Signs of lidocaine toxicity
  - 1–5 μg: tinnitus, lightheadedness, circumoral numbness, metallic taste, double vision
  - 5–8 μg: nystagmus, speech slurring, muscle twitching, fine tremors
  - 8–12 μg: seizures
  - 20–25 μg: respiratory depression and coma

Epinephrine

- Less anesthetic required because local vasoconstriction keeps medication local and reduces anesthetic clearance, thus lasts longer (prolonged anesthetic duration by 100–150%), and decreases systemic absorption. Also provides hemostasis
- *Contraindication (absolute): hyperthyroidism, pheochromocytoma*

- Relative contraindications: hypertension, coronary artery disease, pregnancy (can induce premature labor), beta-blocker use, narrow angle glaucoma (not to use around the eye), phenothiazine, MAO inhibitors, tricyclic antidepressants (e.g., amitriptyline, nortriptyline), acral sites (may be safe if do not perform a full ring block but proceed with caution), peripheral vascular disease, patients on beta-blockers
- Side effects: tachycardia, hypertension, skin necrosis, palpitations, arrhythmias

Adverse Events

- Vasovagal: Due to low BP and decreased pulse
  - Treatment: Cold compresses on head, stimulation, Trendelenburg positions, IVF if prolonged
- Anaphylaxis: Due to decreased BP and increased pulse
  - SubQ epinephrine, IVF, prednisone, Benadryl, airway if needed
- Epinephrine: Causes increased BP and increased pulse, sense of anxiety
  - Reassurance, will pass [8]

Allergy to Anesthetics

Options include injecting *diphenhydramine 1%* or *bacteriostatic saline +/– 0.9% benzyl alcohol.* BE SURE TO CREATE A WHEAL as the wheal is anesthetic in itself.

Refrigerant sprays, ethyl chloride, and dichlorotetrafluoroethane sprays can be used in preparation for other anesthetic administration. The duration of anesthesia is 4–6 s.

Sutures (Figs. 5.4 and 5.5; Tables 5.7 and 5.8)

Suture packets contain information such as the type of suture, its size (e.g., how many 0s (5-0, 4-0, 3-0)), and the type and size of the needle.

Postsurgical Infectious Assessment (Fig. 5.6)

Electrosurgery

Always ask before starting electrosurgery if patient has an implanted device.

Before starting electrosurgery, wipe off any flammable materials, such as aluminum chloride or alcohol.

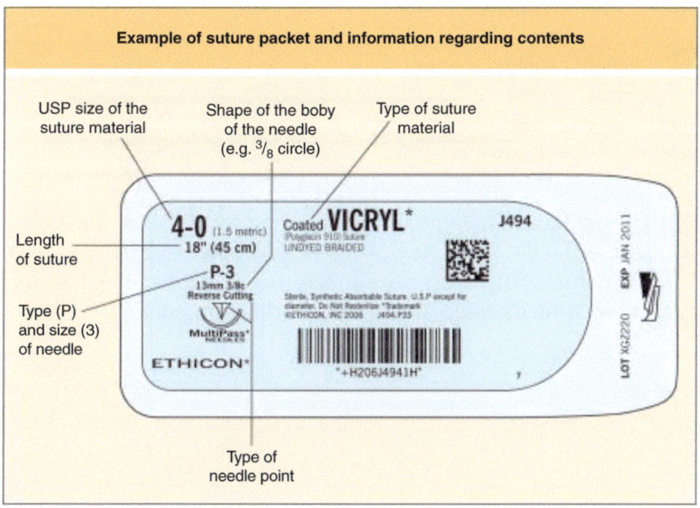

FIGURE 5.4 Example of suture packet and relevant information

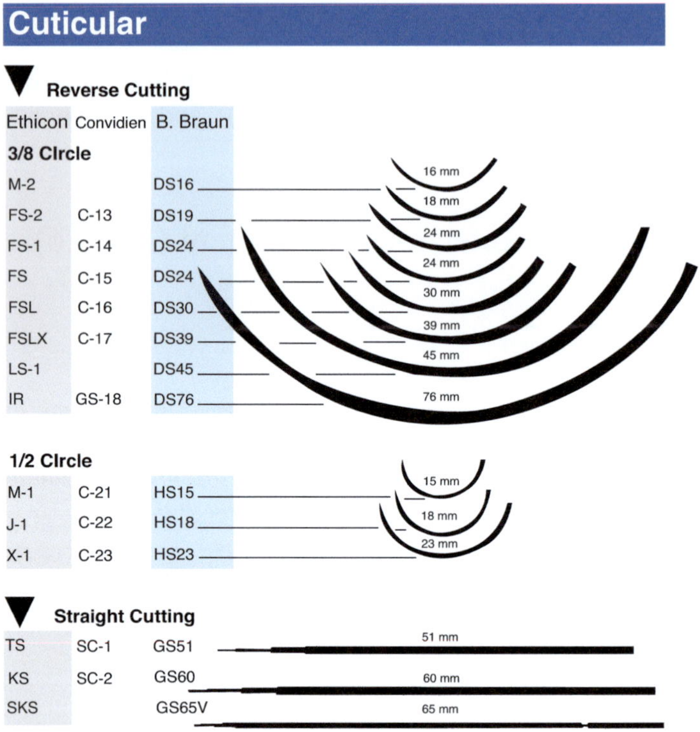

FIGURE 5.5 Suture needle shapes. (https://www.aesculapusa.com/assets/base/doc/DOC571RevC-AesculapNeedleComparisonChart-3-foldBrochure.pdf; https://woundclosure.ethicon.com/sites/com.wcrc_v2_rest/files/needle_true_to_scale_diagram.pdf)

Plastic / Cosmetic

Premium Reverse Cutting with Micropoint

Ethicon	Covidien	B. Braun
3/8 Circle		
P-6	P-16	DSMP7
P-1	P-10	DSMP11
P-3	P-13	DSMP13
PS-3	P-11	DSMP16
PS-2	P-12	DSMP19
PS-1	P-14	DSMP24
PS	P-15	DSMP24
PSL	C-16	DSMP30
PSLX	C-17	DSM39

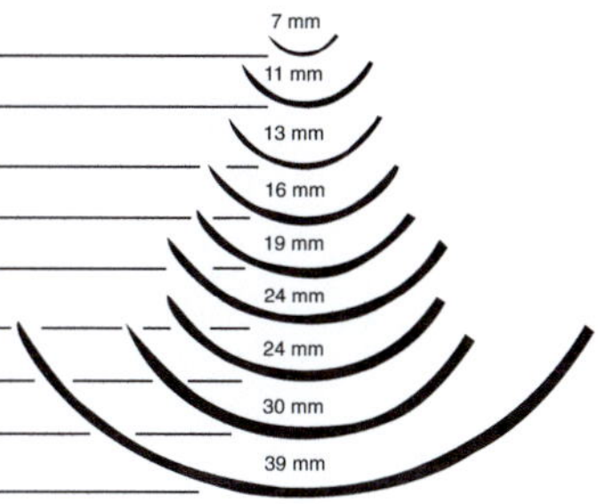

Premium Cutting with Micropoint

3/8 Circle

PC-1	PC-13	DSMP13
PC-3	PC-11	DSMP16
PC-5	PC-12	DSMP19

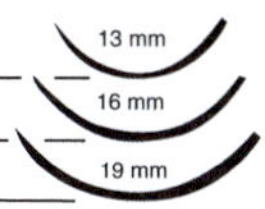

1/2 Circle

P-2	P-21	HSMP9
PS-5	P-22	HSMP12
PS-4	P-24	HSMP15
PC-12	DXH-16	HSMP15

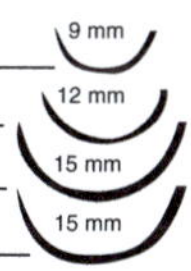

FIGURE 5.5 (continued)

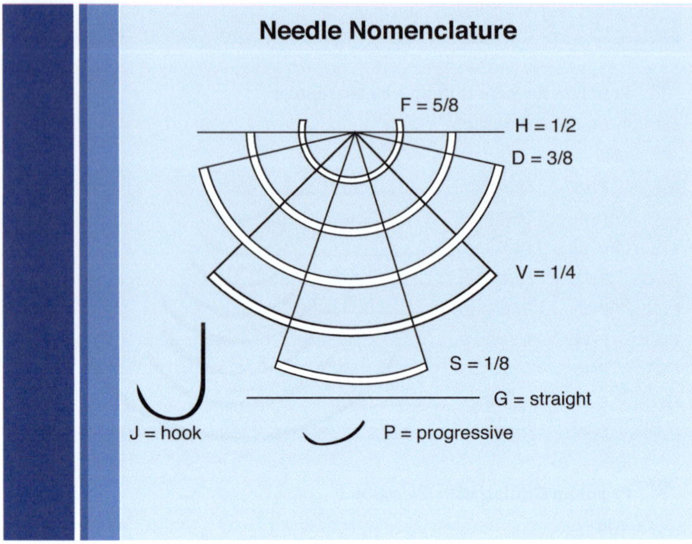

Aesculap Closure Technologies

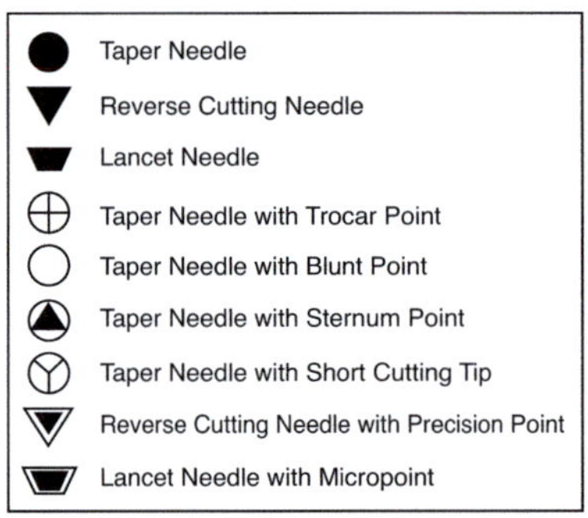

Figure 5.5 (continued)

Table 5.7 Physical properties of absorbable sutures

Name	Configuration	Raw material	Tensile strength	Complete absorption	Tissue reaction
Plain gut	Polished and spun ribbons	Collagen from the submucosal layer of sheep intestine or serosa layer of beef intestine	7–10 days	70 days	Moderate
Fast absorbing gut	Polished and spun fibers	Heat-treated surgical gut	5–7 days	*Weakest*	Moderate
Chromic gut	Polished and spun fibers	Chromium salts added to surgical gut to decrease. inflammation	10–14 days	90 days	< plain gut
Coated polyglactin 910 (Vicryl)	Coated, braided	Co-polymer of lactide and glycolide	75% at 14 days, 50% at 21 days	Complete in 56–70 days	Mild
Coated Vicryl Rapide	Coated, braided	Partially hydrolyzed, gamma irradiated co-polymer of lactide and glycolide	50% at 5 days, 0% by 10–14 days	42 days	Mild
Poliglecaprone 25 (Monocryl)	Monofilament	Co-polymer of glycolide and epsilon-caprolactone	Undyed 50–60% at 7 days; 20–30% at 14 days	91–119 days	Minimal
Poly-dioxanone (PDS II)	Monofilament	Polyester poly (p-dioxanone)	70% at 14 days, 50% at 28 days, 25% at 42 days	6 months STRONGEST	Minimal

TABLE 5.8 Physical properties of non-absorbable sutures

Name	Type	Advantages	Disadvantages
Silk (Sofsilk, Perma-Hand)	Non-absorbable, but will absorb over many months Dyed black for visibility	Does not tear tissue Useful for *mucosal surfaces* and areas of thin skin (*eyelids*)	WEAKEST: Low tensile strength High reactivity Braiding increases the risk of infection
Nylon (Ethilon, Monosof, Dermalon)	Monofilament Hydrolyzes very slowly (over many months)	High tensile strength Minimal tissue reactivity Inexpensive Very slowly absorbed	
Polypropylene (Prolene)	Monofilament Polymer of propylene	Smooth surface makes ideal for running intradermal closure HIGH TENSILE STRENGTH LEAST tissue reaction	Poor knot security (slippery) High memory (stiff)

Avoid electrosurgery/electrocautery in hair-bearing areas, especially if wearing hair spray or hair products.

Do not use electrosurgery/electrocautery if patient is on oxygen.

Types of Electrosurgery (Table 5.9)

Guidelines for Surgery for a Patient with an Implanted Device

Types of implanted electronic devices (IED):
- Pacemaker
- Defibrillator

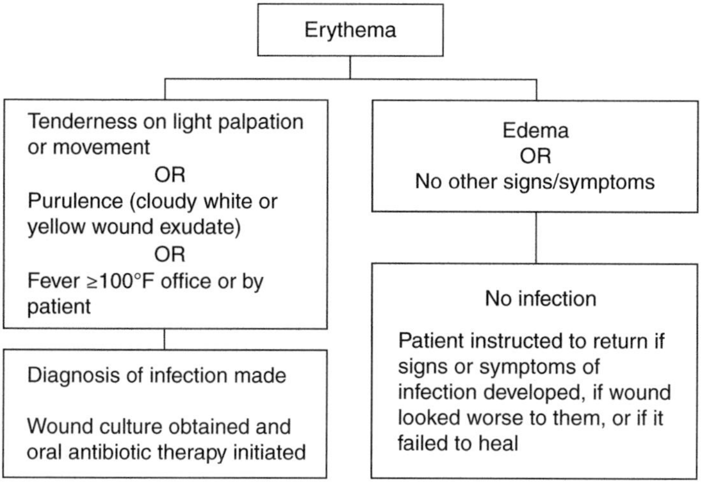

FIGURE 5.6 Stepwise approach to an erythematous surgical wound

- Deep brain stimulator
- Spinal cord stimulator
- Vagal and phrenic nerve stimulator
- Gastric stimulator
- Bone stimulators
- Cochlear implants

Electromagnetic interference adverse effect of performing electrosurgery due to the electromagnetic waves themselves that interfere with or damage the device's functionality. Each type of electrosurgery carries a different risk (Fig. 5.7).

Types of Hemostasis

1. *Electrocautery* – no use of electric current. Heat generated which when in direct contact with tissue provides hemostasis.

TABLE 5.9 Types and characteristics of differing forms of electrosurgery

Method	Tip	Current	Terminal	Damage	Uses
Electrocautery	Hot	*Direct* Low voltage	None	+++	Burn tissue
Electrodessication	Cold	Alternating; High voltage, low amps	Mono	+	Superficial ablation (SK, skin tags) Low penetration
Electrofulguration	Cold	Alternating; High voltage, low amps	Mono	+	Very superficial ablation: Electrode at a slight distance from skin and creates a *spark*
Electro-coagulation	Cold	Alternating; Moderate voltage, high amps. Greatest amount of tissue char/destruction	Bi	+++	Hemostasis Deeper ablation than electrodessication or electrofulguration. Current may move along vessels and beyond site and cause pain/bleeding later
Electrocutting/ electrosection	Cold	Alternating; Low voltage, high amps	Bi	+++	Excision/incision For example, rhinophyma

Destruction or removal of tissues by conversion of electric energy into heat through tissue resistance to the passage of high-frequency alternating current (electrocautery is DIFFERENT because it is direct current)

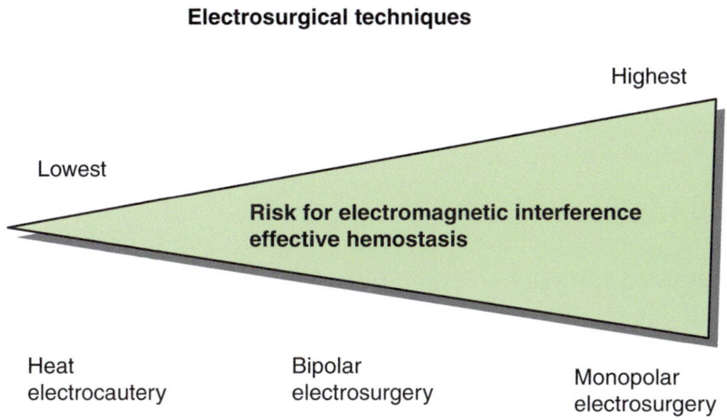

FIGURE 5.7 Risk for electromagnetic interference by type of electrosurgical technique

2. *Electrosurgery*

- *Monopolar* – current delivered to surgical site through one electrode
  - Hospital/OR – high-powered electrical units generate high currents that travel from the electrode to the surgical site, through the patient's body, to a grounding pad (return electrode) and back to the electrosurgical unit to complete a circuit.
  - Office-based (hyfrecator) – low-powered monopolar device. Given low power, grounding pad is optional, and when absent, the current disperses throughout the body. Because the current flows beyond the surgical side, the use of this low-powered unit without a grounding pad has the potential to cause interference with IEDs.
- *Bipolar* – current travels through a two-electrode instrument from one electrode, through tissue, to a second adjacent electrode, completing an electrical circuit. Current is concentrated across the tips, so a grounding pad is not required. Less capable of interfering with an IED than monopolar device.

Monopolar and electrocuting devices carry the most risk.

Electromagnetic interference is more likely to occur within 15 cm of the device or its lead or when monopolar cautery is used in long (>5 s) or frequent (<5 s) bursts.

Guidelines

Stepwise approach to evaluating electrical devices in Figs. 5.8 and 5.9

- Inquire on every patient before using electrosurgery if they have an IED.
- For unplanned procedures, verbal confirmation of the presence or absence of an IED is sufficient.
- For planned procedures, if pt does have an IED, ask about the type of device, its medical indication, and which physician he/she sees to evaluate it.
  - Type and location of IED, date of implantation and last interrogation, programmability, symptoms when device is turned off, and need for postoperative interrogation are important.

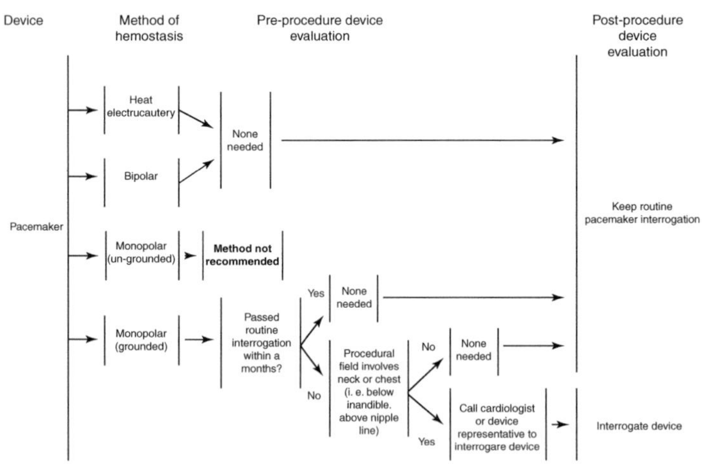

FIGURE 5.8 Stepwise approach to evaluating pacemakers

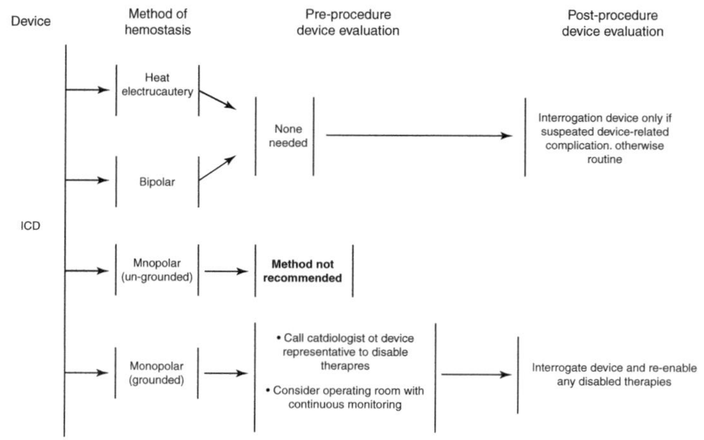

FIGURE 5.9 Stepwise approach to evaluating ICDs. (Adapted from: Howe and Cherpelis [3]; Voutsalath et al. [9])

Overall: Attempt to avoid electrosurgery in patients with implantable devices.

Safest: Thermal/heat electrocautery is the safest as it delivers no current to the patient. Avoid using directly over IED as this can damage the device itself.

For neuronal devices:

Unlike cardiac implanted devices, neuronal implanted devices often can be turned off with a remote control and should be turned off for a procedure if possible.

Turn off device before procedure.

Heat cautery or bipolar forceps favored over monopolar with a grounding pad directed away from the device. If monopolar use, select low voltage at the lowest possible setting.

Monopolar cautery without a grounding pad should be avoided.

For cochlear implants:

Attempt to reduce the voltage to zero and turn the device off. Remove the external sound processor before surgery.

Monopolar use is strictly prohibited.

Bipolar is considered safe if used no closer than 3 cm from the implant device and its electrodes.

Damage to the cochlear implant can be permanent and make reimplantation not possible.

For cardiac devices:

Ok to use heat cautery.

If electrosurgery is required, see below for details, but it should not be performed within 6 inches (15 cm) of a cardiac device or lead system without prior consultation.

Minimum power and shower, intermittent, irregular bursts (<1 s duration) should be used.

- *Pacemakers*
  - Heat cautery is safe to use.
  - Bipolar forceps are considered safe in patients with pacemakers.
  - Do not use within 6 inches of device or leads.
  - Magnet application – magnets are applied by a pacemaker to change the program to an asynchronous or fixed-rate mode.
- ICDs
  - Heat cautery is safe to use.
  - Preoperative cardiology consultation recommended if anything greater than heat cautery is expected.
  - Bipolar cautery is most likely safe to use as well. Do not attempt to use within 15 cm of the device or its leads.
  - Magnet application – Applying a magnet to an ICD prevents tachyarrhythmia detection and treatment while ensuring proper pacing in the pacemaker-dependent patient. The magnet should be left in place only during the delivery of the electrosurgical current and then should be removed. It should be noted, however, that some magnets may permanently disable an ICD, temporarily disable it, or have no effect at all, so preoperative cardiology recommendations and postoperative device interrogation are recommended.

Blood Thinners

Summary of Anticoagulants (Table 5.10) *and Antiplatelet Agents* (Table 5.11).

Drug Interactions with Oral Anticoagulants

Check Medscape Drug Interactions before starting on any of these medications.

Warfarin

- Potentiation: fluconazole, ciprofloxacin, cotrimoxazole, isoniazid, metronidazole, erythromycin, amiodarone, sertraline, fish oil, cimetidine, omeprazole, levofloxacin, tetracycline, aspirin, grapefruit
- Inhibition: nafcillin, rifampin, griseofulvin, methylprednisolone, dicloxacillin, azathioprine

Dabigatran

- Pantoprazole, clopidogrel, ketoconazole, verapamil, amiodarone, quinidine, rifampin; P-glycoprotein inhibitors/inducers

Rivaroxaban and Apixaban

- P-glycoprotein and CYP3A4 inhibitors: ketoconazole, itraconazole, erythromycin, fluconazole
- P-glycoprotein and CYP3A4 inducers: rifampin, carbamazepine, phenytoin, St. John's wort

Supplements with increased bleeding risk: garlic, ginseng, gingko, vitamin E, fish oil, ethanol.

Current recommendation is to continue antiplatelet and anticoagulation for dermatologic surgery as the "magnitude of potential harm to patients with perioperative discontinuation is demonstrably greater than the potential risks of bleeding complications incurred when anticoagulation is continued during cutaneous surgery" [1].

Table 5.10 Summary of anticoagulants from Brown et al. [1]

Agent	FDA approval	MOA	Onset of action	Half-life	Metabolism/ excretion	Monitoring	Reversal	Notes
Warfarin	Ppx and tx of DVT, PE, VTE complications with AF, cardiac valve replacement, risk reduction for embolic events after MI	Vit K epoxide reductase inhibitor	90 min	36–42 h	CYP2C9 Renal excretion	INR	Vit K; fresh frozen plasma	May induce a short-term hypercoagulable state as protein C&S inhibited earlier than the other compliments of the coagulation cascade Numerous meds and supplements have significant interactions with warfarin because of CYP2C9 Bleeding is a major risk; risk of hemorrhage increases significantly with INR > 4.5 See drug interactions below.
Dabigatran	Reduce the risk of CVA and VTE in patients with nonvalvular AF	Direct thrombin inhibitor (inhibits conversion of fibrinogen to fibrin)	2–3 h	8–17 h	Renal excretion	Thrombin or ecarin clotting time	Hemodialysis; PCC	Common SE includes bleeding and GI symptoms. Patients >75 y/o with increased bleeding compared to warfarin

Agent	FDA approval	MOA	Onset of action	Half-life	Metabolism/ excretion	Monitoring	Reversal	Notes
Rivaroxaban	Reduce the risk of CVA and VTE in patients with nonvalvular AF; treatment of DVT/PE; prophylaxis of DVT after hip or knee replacement	Factor Xa inhibitor Inhibits free and clot-associated factor Xa.	2–4 h	5–12 h	65% renal excretion; 35% CYP3A4 metabolism then fecal/biliary excretion	Prothrombin time No routine monitoring assays are available	PCC, recombinant factor VIIa	Pharmacokinetics and pharmacodynamics are predictable; thus, can be given at a fixed dose without routine monitoring Significant interactions with Rx metabolized by the CYP3A4 system (inducers or inhibitors) P-glycoprotein Patients on this have lower fatal/serious bleeding but higher GI bleeding than patients on warfarin
Apixaban	Reduce the risk of CVA and VTE in patients with nonvalvular AF	Factor Xa inhibitor	1 h	12 h	O-demethylation, sulfation, and hydroxylation. 50% fecal, 25% renal, 25% biliary excretion	Prothrombin time No routine monitoring assays are available	PCC, recombinant factor VIIa	Only severe renal disease results in prolonged effects. Ok for patients with moderate liver disease Interactions similar to rivaroxaban Incidence is lower than patients on warfarin

TABLE 5.11 Summary of antiplatelet agents from Brown et al. [1]

Agent	FDA approval	MOA	Onset of action	Half-life	Metabolism/ excretion	Monitoring	Reversal	Notes
Aspirin (acetylsalicylic acid)	Secondary prevention of ACS/CVA; pain relief; antipyretic	Irreversible COX-1 inhibitor	30–40 min	3 h	Deacetylation in the liver; Renal excretion	Platelet function assay; serum drug levels	ddAVP – off label	
Clopidogrel (Plavix)	ACD (reduce risk of death); secondary prevention of CVA, MI, and vascular death in patients with recent MI, CVA, or PAD	P2Y12 ADP receptor antagonist Inhibition of ADP signaling lasts for the life of the platelet (~1 week)	2 h	6 h (single 75 mg dose)	Inactivation via esterase hydrolysis 50% renal/50% fecal excretion	Platelet function assay	ddAVP – off label	Drugs metabolized by the CYP450 pathway can reduce metabolism of clopidogrel (e.g., PPIs) More bleeding complications than with aspirin
Prasugrel (effient)	Reduce thrombotic cardiovascular events in patients with ACS, including stent thrombosis	P2Y12 ADP receptor inhibitor	15–30 min	2–15 h	Activated by CYP3A4/2B6 Renal (68%) and fecal excretion	Platelet function assay	ddAVP – off label	More rapid and thorough platelet inhibition and less interindividual variability than clopidogrel

Agent	FDA approval	MOA	Onset of action	Half-life	Metabolism/ excretion	Monitoring	Reversal	Notes
Ticagrelor (Brilinta)	Reduce thrombotic cardiovascular events in patients with ACS, including stent thrombosis	P2Y12 ADP receptor inhibitor	15–30 min	6–8 h	CYP3A4 metabolism Biliary excretion	Platelet function assay	ddAVP – off label	Faster platelet recovery when medication stopped than clopidogrel (more rapid reversal, though takes 72 h) Increased risk of intracranial and GI bleeds when compared to clopidogrel
Dipyridamole/ aspirin (Aggrenox)	Reduce risk of stroke in patients with TIA or CVA Primarily used as a vasodilator for coronary artery and peripheral arterial disease. Has antiplatelet effects	PDE 3/5 inhibitor > increased camp > decreased platelet aggregation and vasodilation	2–2.5 h	19 h	Glucuronidation Enterohepatic recirculation with biliary excretion	None	ddAVP – off label	Dipyridamole itself does not increase the risk of bleeding

Suggested guidelines for perioperative management of PO anticoagulant and antiplatelet regimen [1]

- Continue if patient has + PMHx or physician recommendation; just manage intraoperative hemostasis thoroughly as well as postop pressure dressing for at least 24–48 h.
- ASA: if taking for ppx or pain, may d/c 3d preop and resume 3d postop.
- Warfarin: obtain recent INR within 1 month before surgery to make sure it is within therapeutic range (2–3.5). IF > 3.5, postpone surgery if possible.
- No specific recs for other RX.
- Supplement: if taking for ppx, d/c 7d preop, and restart 7d postop.
- Alcohol: avoid 3d preop to 3d postop.

Postop Pearls for Patients with Bleeding Risk

- Pressure dressings with added dental rolls can be helpful, as well as wrapping extremities, or scalp for 1 week postop (Kerlix, ACE).
- If patient has held pressure for 15 min × 2 and still oozes through dressing, they should be seen.

Postop Pain Management Tips

Based on and adapted from recommendations published in JAAD [4].

Decision Tree

1. Are there risk factors for increased opioid pain (surgical sites on lower extremity, scalp, lip, ear, or genitals; anxiety about pain, current opioid user, current smoker, female, multiple same day procedures, age younger than 64 years old)?
    (a) If no, then use nonopioid analgesia (alternate acetaminophen/NSAIDs, rest, ice, elevate).
    (b) If yes, and second intention wound healing

Still use non-opioid analgesia.

(c) If yes and advanced reconstruction (flap, graft), prescribe for 6 tabs opioids maximum.

2. Only consider opioids for limited time (<36 h) in addition to nonopioid recs first.
3. Do not provide refills. The patient should schedule return visit if still in need of opioids after 36 h/6 tabs for evaluation of postop complications.
4. For primary closures, consider extent of tissue rearrangement and size of defect.

Protocol Recommendations

Treatment of Actinic Keratoses

- Imiquimod: Apply thin layer once a day 3 times a week for 16 weeks – complete clearance in 45–57%.
  - Alternative: 3 times a week for 4 weeks, then a break for 4 weeks, then 3 times a week for 4 weeks if needed.
- 5-FU (Efudex 5% cream): Use BID for 4 weeks. Check-in with them 2 weeks into treatment and 4 weeks post-treatment. 47% clear (see below for care instructions).
  - Efudex chemo wraps are another option that can work well for legs/arms
  - Protocol: wipe down affected area with washcloths and dry. Apply 10 g 5% 5-FU to affected extremity (20 g total each visit), followed by an Unna boot: Viscopaste zinc wrap, then a thin layer of Kerlix, and then Coban. Keep dry, and sponge baths only/tub for rest of body. Keep on for up to one week. Take off and shower on the day of the appointment prior to replacing the wraps. Do for 4–20 weeks according to the response. Maintenance therapy can be considered, such as appling Efudex cream at night (no wrap) weekly (up to forever).

  - Some risk for systemic absorption, so consider CBC for neutropenia Possible hair loss or mucositis. Beware of patients with dihydropyrimidine dehydrogenase deficiency as they can manifest systemic symptoms of from 5-FU from even topical use.

- 5-FU (Carac 0.5% cream): Use daily for 4 weeks (47–58% clear)
- Photodynamic therapy

  - Scrub face with acetone wash to remove oils and debris.
  - Break Levulan Kerastick as directed.
  - Paint entire treatment area.
  - Incubate for 60–120 min in dark room with lights off/minimal light.
  - Blu-Lite for 16 min, 40 s (1000 s).
  - Apply sunscreen and have patients avoid any sun for 24–48 h following treatment.

- 5-FU + calcipotriene

  - Apply 5-FU 5% cream + Calcipotriene BID × 4 days [2]

- Cryosurgery: Freeze quickly with border of 1–2 mm; maintain freeze with border for 10 s with intermittent spray technique. Thaw time is thus 30–60 s – do not hasten thaw time by warming/touching. Hypertrophic AK may require more prolonged freeze; thin AKs may require less.

5-fluorouracil (Efudex/Carac) Patient Instructions
Topical 5-FU (brand names Efudex, Carac, and Fluoroplex) is a cream that is used to treat sun-damaged skin, precancerous skin lesions (actinic keratoses) and certain skin cancers. (Actinic keratoses are precancerous growths that have the capacity to develop into squamous cell carcinoma, a type of skin cancer.) Also called "5-FU," this topical medication has been used for over 30 years to treat pre-skin cancers as well as superficial skin cancers.

- *Topical 5-FU cream is generally used once or twice daily.* Use this medication sparingly; you do not need to use a lot of it.

- *You can apply the medication with your bare hands, but wash your hands after using it.* Try to keep the medication away from your eyes.
- *Generally, after a week or two of application, your skin will start to look red;* ***this is expected***. When applied to the areas of sun-damaged skin, the 5-FU will "find" damaged skin cells and destroy them. As the cream destroys the precancers or skin cancers, they will become red, inflamed, irritated, and slightly sore. Sometimes, itching may also develop. This is the expected, normal response and is not an allergic reaction! Some patients using 5-FU show minimal redness and scaling while others have a very "vigorous" response where the skin scabs and peels. The important thing to realize is that 5-FU is treating sun-damaged skin that carries skin cancer risk. If your symptoms are severe, call and let us know.
- *The medication is used from 2 to 6 weeks depending on what is being treated.* For treatment of precancers (actinic keratoses), if your skin is very irritated and the symptoms are really bothering you, then you can stop after 2 weeks, but let the doctor know. However, if it is not bothering you too much, you should try to treat for a full 4 weeks. For treatment of skin cancers, the medication is generally used for the full 6 weeks.
- *If you have never used the medication before, it is preferable to schedule an appointment about 3 weeks into your treatment, so we can see if you are responding as expected.*
- *If you have any questions during the treatment, call us or make an appointment to come in.*
- *Avoid prolonged sun exposure* while you are using this cream. If you do go out in the sun, use a broad-spectrum sunscreen.
- *Side effects of this medication include* redness, inflammation, erosions, formation of ulcers, and sometimes inflammation of the eyes if it gets near the eyes.
- Very rarely the medication can cause systemic symptoms such as mucositis, nausea or fatigue. Please let us know if this occurs.

- Once you finish the medication, the area of skin treated will be red and raw. It generally takes about 3–4 weeks for all of the inflammation to resolve. You may use Vaseline (petroleum jelly) or another bland cream, such as Vanicream, Vaniply, or Aquaphor, to soothe the skin. Alternatively, you may apply some 1% hydrocortisone ointment to the affected areas. This is available over-the-counter via several name brands. If you get an area that is really open/sore/scabbed, then apply some antibiotic ointment such as bacitracin. If the irritation is quite bad, please call the office as we can give you a prescription cream to help soothe things and heal a little faster.
- Once your skin completely heals from the treatment, your skin should be smoother, and many of the red spots should be gone.
- Keep in mind that the reason you are going through all of this is to destroy precancers and early skin cancers to hopefully reduce your risk of larger and more serious skin cancers that may require surgery.
- *This medicine is extremely toxic to dogs and cats. Less than a gram can kill a small dog. DO NOT leave the tube where your dog or cat could get it.*
- Do not confuse where to put this cream with other creams you may have at home or that were prescribed for you today.
- If you have questions or concerns, please call us!

Keratoacanthomas

Intralesional Methotrexate

- Exclude patients who might be pregnant, breast-feeding, with significant renal or hepatic disease, or with any blood dyscrasia.
- Can apply topical anesthetic agent before injecting if needed (e.g., EMLA).
- Infiltrate with 0.4–0.5 mL of 12.5 mg/mL methotrexate divided into five injection sites – each quadrant at a shoul-

der and again in the center of the lesion (small lesions you can just aim for the center). Aim for depth of 2–8 mm (lesion should blanche).

- Less painful than intralesional 5-FU.

- Reported adverse effects with intralesional methotrexate:
  - Pain at time of injection (moderate), nausea, malaise, oral aphthae, leukopenia/thrombocytopenia/pancytopenia, erythema, inflammation, dermatitis, photosensitivity, pigment ulceration, urticaria, reversible alopecia, and radiation recall.
- Follow-up every 2 weeks and re-inject until resolved.
  - There is no consensus when to stop injections.

Intralesional 5-FU

- Exclude patients who might be pregnant, breast-feeding, with significant renal or hepatic disease, or with any blood dyscrasia.
- 5-FU 15 mg (50 mg/mL) infiltrated to each quadrant at shoulder and again in center of lesion weekly for 3–4 weeks. Most effective in stages of active growth or large lesions such as KCM.
- Reported adverse effects with intralesional 5-FU:
  - Discomfort at time of injection, focal irritation and necrosis, temporary hypopigmenation, purulent exudate, erythema, swelling, lymphedema, irregular scar formation, leukopenia, and thrombocytopenia.

Intralesional Bleomycin

- Exclude patients who might be pregnant, breast-feeding, with significant renal or hepatic disease, or with any blood dyscrasia.
- Bleomycin 0.2–0.4 mg injected weekly for 2–6 weeks.
  - Can apply topical anesthetic before injection (which can increase efficacy).

- Adverse effects:
  - Pain with injection, pigmentary changes, and erythema [5].

Light-Based Therapy

Photodynamic Therapy Protocol

Photodynamic Therapy Questionnaire

□ No history of photosensitive diseases (lupus, porphyria)
□ Not currently pregnant/breastfeeding
□ Not taking deferoxamine
□ Not currently undergoing chemotherapy or radiation therapy
□ Not taking any cytostatic drug (these patients will have increased healing time after procedure)
□ Prescribed tretinoin 0.025% cream as pre-treatment (tell patient to start using pea-sized amount on the face 2 weeks before procedure)
□ Prescribed physical block sunscreen for post-treatment
□ Review that the patient must bring protective clothing, sunglasses, or hat to appointment
□ History of herpes labialis? If yes, acyclovir 400 mg po BID for 4 days to be given
□ Any evidence of scaling disorder of the face (e.g., seb derm)? If yes, treat this first before undergoing PDT
□ Review post-care instructions and make sure they understand/are willing to comply

Levulan Sticks

- 6 come in a pack.
- Do not have to be refrigerated.
- Has a shelf-life of 2.5 years.
- One stick is usually enough to cover a whole face twice.

Physician Mandated Procedures

- Applying the ALA
- Positioning the patient and turning on the light

PDT Protocol

Pre-PDT

1. Go through questionnaire per above:
   (a) If herpes, give acyclovir 400 mg bid for 5 days.
   (b) For everyone if tolerated: tretinoin 0.025% cream 2 weeks prior to PDT. Can also consider pre-treatment with efudex for 1-2 weeks if many AKs.
   (c) For everyone: Sunscreen with physical block to have available post PDT, and patient brings protective clothing/sunglasses/hats.
2. Consider d/c NSAIDS or antioxidants (VIT C or E) 2 days prior to PDT.
3. DO NOT d/c photosensitizing meds if they are medically required.
4. Skin conditions that promote parakeratotic scale, such as seborrheic dermatitis, should be treated and controlled before PDT.

Day of PDT

1. Check vitals
2. Counseling/informed consent
   (a) Most likely will experience stinging/burning/discomfort while light is on; however, most people tolerate it without difficulty.
   (b) If on photosensitizing meds (see list below), may have more brisk response.
   (c) If on cytostatic drugs (chemo, AZA, hydroxyurea), may have prolonged healing.
   (d) There is a theoretical risk of hyper or hypopigmentation (rare).
   (e) The patient MUST avoid sun completely for 3 days following treatment by use of opaque clothing, hat, or mineral-based or physical sunblocks applied thickly.
3. Steps
   (a) Cleanse – this allows for a more uniform penetration and subsequent photoactivation.

(i) Chlorhexidine gluconate 2%.
(ii) Followed by acetone (for degreasing), but if this is not tolerated, isopropyl alcohol or alpha-hydroxy/salicylic acid cleansers may suffice.
(iii) Avoid periorbital, ocular, mucosal regions.

(b) Prep skin for penetration of ALA.

(i) Curette any HAKs.
(ii) Gauze abrasion rubbed on the skin, oscillating brushes, microneedling rollers, and/or fractional non-ablative and ablative fractional lasers to enhance delivery.

(c) Apply ALA (Levulan Kerastick – break the stick according to the directions and apply to the areas to be treated – the goal is to crush it so that it breaks both the vials. Use the crusher applicator (line up A with A and B with B and then crush it; then, shake the stick to mix the ingredients)).

(i) Place the patient in a slightly reclined position.
(ii) Kerastick cotton-tipped applicator facilitates placement.
(iii) Application to full face is best accomplished by expressing the solution onto the treatment area and with a gloved hand evenly wiping it over the face *in 2 coats* – put it on once and then let it dry and then put it on again.
(iv) Take care not to drip the solution.
(v) Can put gauze pads over the eyes.

(d) For nonfacial areas (e.g., extremities), occlusion with plastic wrap can be used to increase penetration and then cover with longer sleeves or a warming area. Also, applying a warming blanket can enhance penetration.
(e) Incubation times – vary on type of treatment (cosmetic/medical). Must incubate in a dark room, devoid of as much ambient light as possible. Discomfort during light treatment will increase with longer incubation times.

(i) See table below for treatment protocols and different indications.

1. In general, for actinic damage, face: 1–2 h; scalp, 2 h; and arms/hands, 3 h
2. Maximum clearance of AKs with 3 h incubation

(f) After incubation, the targeted area may be gently washed with water and a cleanser.

(g) Irradiation.

(i) Put a warning on the door that the light is being used.

(ii) Perform in a room without windows and low ambient light. Room should have adequate cooling and ventilation.

(iii) *Everyone in the room is to wear eye protection before the light is turned on (!!!)* (prolonged exposure to blue and UV light is damaging to the retina and increases risk of cataracts (red light does not seem to result in the same retinal toxicity) *Patients and clinicians both have goggles.*

(iv) See table below for specific treatment protocols for different indications.

1. General: Light treatment with Blu_U light PDT illuminator model 4170 (peak emittance at 417) for 16 min and 40 s.

(v) No skin surface closer than 2 inches to device and no further than 4 inches.

(vi) Stay in the room with the patient for the first 6 min, and then after that, if they are doing well, they can be in there themselves with a buzzer.

(vii) If the treatment is overly painful:

1. Cool air blown on face may help.
2. Injectable anesthetics (without vasoconstrictor) may help.

3. Interruption of treatment (3 min break with cold spray [cold packs reduce efficacy]).
4. Consider instead trying daylight PDT (protocols vary based on weather).

4. Post-irradiation
   (a) Cleanse with tepid water and pat dry.
   (b) Apply mineral based sunscreen and protective clothing.

5. Post-care
   (a) Pain tends to subside quickly after light source is terminated
   (b) Immediately after erythema can occur to varying degrees but can be profound; edema may be present

6. Side effects
   (a) Erythema – peaks at 1–2 h and resolves within 1–2 weeks (rarely lasts >3 months).
   (b) Edema.
   (c) Urticaria – consider ppx antihistamines.
   (d) Infection – risk small. Development of sterile pustules may be seen when treating acne.
   (e) Scarring.
   (f) Pigmentary changes – both hyper and hypopigmentation.
   (g) If you get it in the eye, it does burn and is more due to the alcohol in it than the ALA. Do a very good eyewash if this occurs.

Ideal treatment regimen is a 2-treatment process with treatments 8 weeks apart. If you wait more than 12 weeks before treatments, then you essentially would need to restart.

Note that treatment responses can vary between patients and between times patients receive the treatment (e.g., varying amounts of erythema, crusting, etc.).

Sample Care Instructions for Patients Following Photodynamic Therapy

After your treatment, you may experience these most common side effects:

- Burning/stinging, which could be severe, may last up to 24 h after your treatment.
- Redness and swelling and scaling/crusting which may last up to 4 weeks after your treatment.

Day of Treatment

- Remain indoors and avoid direct sunlight for 36 h (3 days). *THIS IS VERY IMPORTANT!!!* Do NOT sit by a window (must be at least 6 feet away from windows).
- Cover all treated areas like by wearing a broad hat or opaque clothing.
- Sunscreens do not block all rays of light and are less helpful than clothing or staying inside and away from windows. If you are to wear a sunscreen, wear a mineral or physical block sunscreen (zinc oxide and titanium dioxide) ideally with iron oxide as well to block visible light (e.g., Vanicream sunscreen, baby sunscreens, Elta MD SPF 41) and apply thickly.
- Try to limit exposure to screens (TV/computers) as well as fluorescent lights.
- Wash your face twice daily with a gentle cleanser (like Cetaphil or CeraVe liquid cleanser).
- Apply a bland moisturizing cream four times per day (like Vanicream, Cetaphil, or CeraVe).
- Take analgesics, such as ibuprofen, if there is any pain.
- If you have any discomfort, apply ice packs to the treated area for 5–10 min every few hours. This will help to keep the area cool and alleviate any discomfort as well as keep down any swelling. Swelling will be the most evident around the eyes and is usually prominent in the morning.
- Redness of the face may be very intense for the first day or two.

Day 2–7
- Wash the face twice a day with a gentle cleanser.
- The skin will feel dry and tightened; a bland moisturizing cream should be used twice a day.
- You may begin applying makeup once crusting has healed. The area may be red for 3–5 days. If makeup is important to you, please use mineral makeup, which is all natural, inert, and less inflammatory and acts as a concealer with sunscreen. It is especially effective to mask redness.
- When outdoors, use a "physical block" sunscreen with zinc oxide and titanium dioxide and a minimum SPF 30, such as Vanicream, Neutrogena Pure Baby, and Elta MD 41 tinted, Cotz sensitive skin.

If you feel pain, this most likely is because you are being exposed to a light source, such as a window or an indoor light (particularly fluorescent light). You are encouraged to stay 6 feet away from windows for the 3 days after treatment.

If you have any questions, please do not hesitate to call the office.

7. Follow-up:

   (a) Acne: 4–5 monthly tx
   (b) AKs one to two tx
   (c) Follow-up in 6 weeks to see if repeat treatment is required (for AKs)

Photodynamic Therapy-Specific Treatment Protocols for Different Indications (Table 5.12)

Photosensitizing Medications (Table 5.13)

Storage of the Light
- Put the locks in place on the wheels.
- Put the light down over the base.
- Keep it plugged in.
- Make a copy of a key so that we have more than one.

TABLE 5.12 Photodynamic therapy specific treatment protocols for different indications

Indication	Topical photosensitizer	Incubation period	Light source	Dose	Comments
Actinic keratosis	ALA MAL	1–4 h 1–4 h 0.5 h 1–3 h	Blue light Red light Daylight Red light	10 J/cm^2 750–150 J/cm^2 35–75 J/cm^2	Requires 1–2 sessions of PDT for optimal results Sunscreen applied after incubation for daylight PDT; patients are then instructed to walk/sit outside for 2 h. Studies done between June and October
Bowen disease/ SCCIS	ALA MAL	4 h 3 h	Red light Red light	>100 J/cm^2 75–100 J/cm^2	Requires 2–3 sessions of PDT for optimal results
Superficial BCC	ALA MAL	3–6 h 3 h	Red light Red light	>60 J/cm^2 37–75 J/cm^2	Requires 2–3 sessions of PDT for optimal results
Acne vulgaris	ALA MAL	3 h 3 h	Blue light Red light Red light	10 J/cm^2 37 J/cm^2 37 J/cm^2	2–3 treatments, repeated biweekly
Photorejuvenation	ALA MAL	30 min–3 h 30 min–1 h	Blue light Red light Red light	10 J/cm^2 37 J/cm^2 37 J/cm^2	2–3 treatments, repeated monthly

From Ozog et al. [7]

Lasers

Chromophores (Fig. 5.10)

- Melanin: absorption peaks at 418 nm then slowly decreases as wavelength increases.
- Hemoglobin: separate peaks at 418, 542, and 577 nm.

TABLE 5.13 Photosensitizing medications

Acitretin	Chlorothiazide	Dacarbazine	Flutamide (photoallergic)	Gemifloxacin	Methotrexate	Ofloxacin	Tazarotene
Alitretinoin	Chlortetracycline	Dapsone	Furosemide	Grepafloxacin	Minocycline	Psoralens	Tetracycline
Aminolevulinic acid	Ciprofloxacin	Demeclocycline	HCTZ/hydrochlorothiazide	Griseofulvin	Moxifloxacin	St. John's wort	Thorazine or phenothiazine
Bexarotene	Coal tar	Doxycycline	Hydroxychloroquine	Isotretinoin	Norfloxacin	Sparfloxacin	TMP-SMX
Capecitabine	Clotrimazole	Fluorouracil	Gatifloxacin	Levofloxacin	NSAIDS	Sulfa drugs	Tretinoin

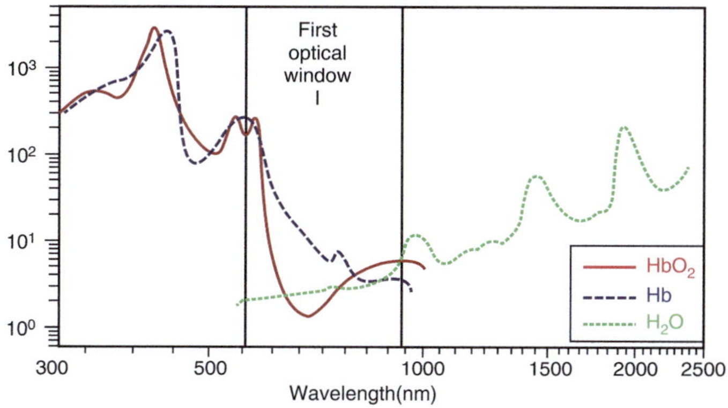

FIGURE 5.10 Hemoglobin and water absorption spectrum curves

Laser Safety

- Before starting laser treatment, everyone in the room must be equipped with eye protection and the door must be closed with the laser sign visible.
- Goggles must have an OD (optical density) of at least >/= to 4 for the wavelength of the laser being used.
- Fire hazard:
  - Drapes, clothing, dry hair, and plastic material can be ignited, especially when oxygen is IN use.
  - Greatest risk with CO2 and erbium: YAG lasers used for skin resurfacing and ablative fractional treatments.
  - Remember to place the laser in STANDBY mode when not using the laser.
  - Alcohol, acetone, and other flammable skin-cleaning solutions must dry completely before laser use.
  - Moisten any hair-bearing areas near the treatment field; remove mascara and eye makeup when working around the eyelids.
  - A fire extinguisher and water should be readily available.
- Prevention of laser "plume" biohazards:
  - Smoke evacuator and good ventilation are most effective measures.

- Sub-micrometer surgical filter masks provide some protection when worn properly.
- Q-switched lasers capture particulate material in plastic cones.
- Wearing an N95 mask or PAPR can be considered.

Various Lasers and Their Typical Uses (Table 5.14)

PDL 595 nm Suggested Settings

Refer to Your User Manual for Specifics as not all may be Best for Your Device

- Warts: 0.45 s, cryo off, 8 J. Suggested 3 pulses per lesion, may be more or less depending on size, previous response,

Table 5.14 Various lasers and their typical uses

Laser	Wavelength (nm)	Mode	Typical uses
Excimer	308	Pulsed	Psoriasis, vitiligo
Argon	488, 514	CW	Vascular lesions
Argon dye	630	CW	PDT
Copper vapor	512	Quasi-CW	Vascular lesions
KTP	532	Quasi-CW	Vascular lesions
Pulsed dye	585–600	Pulsed	Vascular lesions
Ruby, Q-switched	694	Pulsed	Hair removal, tattoos, pigmented lesions, nevus of Ota
Alexandrite, Q-switched	720–850	Pulsed	Hair removal, tattoos, pigmented lesions
Diode	800–810	CW/pulsed	Type I–V hair removal, leg veins
Q-switched Nd:YAG	1065	Ns pulsed	Tattoos (black)
Nd:YAG	1064	Pulsed	Hair removal, leg veins, Type IV–VI hair removal
Erbium	2940	Pulsed	Rhytides, scars, photodamage
CO2	10,600	CW/pulsed	Vaporizing/coagulation

depth, etc. IN GENERAL, though, avoid lasers on a wart due to smoke plume or take necessary precautions.

- Port wine stain: 1.5 ms, cryo 30, 10 J/cm^2 and increased as tolerated.
- Hemangiomas: 3–6 ms, 8–10 J, slowly increase fluence.
- Cherry or spider angiomas: 11.5 J at 3 ms, 30 ms cryo; single pulse.
- Telangiectasias: Pulse width depends on vessel size – 10 J, 30/20 cryo; single pulse, small vessels, 6 ms; large vessels, 20–30 ms; purpuric doses.
- Venous lakes: 13 mJ at 10 ms, 30/20 cryo; low risk of bruising; pulse width 30% overlap if needed (approx).
  - Expect two to three treatments with 50% improvement on first. Total improvement about 80%.
  - Try topical benzocaine for a few minutes first.
  - Can increase duration of pulse after first treatment depending on results.
- Granuloma faciale: 8 J at 0.4 ms, 7 mm spot
- Poikiloderma: 10 ms, 8–9 J, 30 ms cryo. Risk of scarring!
- Scars and striae: 5–6 J at 0.45–3 ms, 30/20 cryo, 7 mm spot with 10% overlap. Repeat q4 weeks as needed.
- SLE active lesions: 7 mm at 5.5 J, 0.45 ms, overlap 10–20% with cryo.

Intense Pulsed Light (IPL)

- Wavelength of filter: powered using a xenon flash lamp (also used for camera flashes). Produces a spectrum of light form 400–1200 nm.
- Different filters can remove the lower wavelengths.
  - For vascular/rosacea treatments, a 515 or 540 nm filter is used.
  - Photodamage: a 540 or 590 nm filter is used.
  - Example: a 590 nm filter would reduce the wavelength from 400–120 nm to 590–120 nm – the longer wavelength is still present!!
- Risks:
  - For men, if the area of facial hair growth is treated, this could result in temporary shunted hair with possible

hair loss (especially if longer wavelengths are not filtered).
- If patient has dark skin, tan, or a sunburn, then this will reduce the effectiveness of the treatment.
- The operator presses too hard with the handpiece; the effectiveness of the treatment will be reduced because the pressure will cause blanching of the skin and therefore less blood, and blood is the most common target of the IPL.
- If the energy levels are too high, this can result in purpura or blistering.

Excimer
- 308 nm.
- Approved indications: psoriasis, vitiligo, leukoderma, eczema.
- Treatment algorithm is based on Fitzpatrick skin type and thickness of lesion to be treated.
- Goal is to be pink but not tender at treatment site with each treatment – percentage adjustment made up or down if no response or too much response if treating psoriasis. (For vitiligo, standard dose increase or decrease is based on response – not percentage).

Phototherapy

Reading:
Zanolli and Feldman [10]; Olsen et al. [6].

UV Light
- UVC 200–280 nm
- UVB 280–320 nm
- UVA 320–400 nm
  - UVA II 320–240 nm
  - UVA 1 340–400 nm

Types of Therapeutic Ultraviolet Therapy
- UVA
- UVA1

- Broadband UVB
- Narrowband UVB – most common
- Hand/foot UVA/UVB

Remember:
Narrowband uses far more Joules than broadband; do not switch them!

Before Starting Therapy

Patient screening
- Patients must be reliable/committed and able to stand.
- Contraindications to phototherapy
  - History of photosensitive disorders (SLE, porphyria, XP, dermatomyositis)
  - History of melanoma
  - History of organ transplantation/on immunosuppression (GVHD an exception)
  - On any photosensitizing medications (see below)
- Contraindications to PUVA specifically
  - Renal disease
  - Liver disease
  - Pregnancy
- Relative contraindications
  - History of multiple nonmelanoma skin cancers
  - History of eye disease (cataracts)
  - Arsenic exposure
  - Radiation in the past
- If patient is pregnant, avoid PUVA, and remember to increase folic acid daily dosing.

If the patient has a history of HSV, consider premedication with acyclovir/valacyclovir.

Before starting a patient on phototherapy, be sure to perform a medication reconciliation and check if the patient is on any photosensitizing medications (Table 5.15).

TABLE 5.15 Photosensitizing medications

Acitretin	Chlorothiazide	Dacarbazine	Flutamide (photoallergic)	Gemifloxacin	Methotrexate	Ofloxacin	Tazarotene	Trioxsalen
Alitretinoin	Chlortetracycline	Dapsone	Furosemide	Grepafloxacin	Minocycline	Psoralens	Tetracycline	Vinblastine
Aminolevulinic acid	Ciprofloxacin	Demeclocycline	HCTZ/ hydrochlorothiazide	Griseofulvin	Moxifloxacin	St. John's wort	Thorazine or phenothiazine	Zalcitabine
Bexarotene	Coal tar	Doxycycline	Hydroxychloroquine	Isotretinoin	Norfloxacin	Sparfloxacin	TMP-SMX	
Capecitabine	Clotrimazole	Fluorouracil	Gatifloxacin	Levofloxacin	NSAIDS	Sulfa drugs	Tretinoin	

Setting Patient Expectations and Informed Consent

- Light therapy is not a cure.
- Onset of action typically 6–12 weeks.
- Duration of treatment is often 4–6 months but may be longer (maintenance phase).
- Side effects: pinkness/redness of the skin, sunburn reaction, corneal burn or cataracts if eye protection is not worn during treatment, photoallergic dermatitis, freckling, premature aging, and increased risk of skin cancer (although it is generally believed that nbUVB therapy results in fewer skin cancers than other forms of UV-therapy such as UVA).
- Do not apply sunscreen, calcipotriene, or calcitriol before treatment; patients should use SPF 15+ for remainder of treatment day, however.
- Cover sensitive areas during treatment (genitals, nipples, eyes, and potentially face).
- Apply a thin layer of petroleum jelly/Vaseline or mineral oil immediately before treatment (except for itch and vitiligo patients) as this helps the light to penetrate.
- For PUVA, also need to wear *sun protective sunglasses* from moment of 8-MOP ingestion for 24 h after PUVA treatment.
- PUVA in Caucasian patients with >250 treatments does increase risk of skin cancer in the future.
- It is important to adhere to the treatment regimen; missing treatments can produce less reliable results and possibly treatment failure.

Photograph patients before starting to determine whether they are improving as clearance is sometimes slow and not immediately noticeable.

Definitions

- *Minimal erythema dose* – the minimal amount a particular type of UVR that leads to erythema of the exposed skin
- *Irradiance/power (watts)* – the intensity of UVR to which the patient is exposed

- *Exposure time (seconds)* – the length of time a patient undergoes UVR treatment
- *Dose (J/cm2)* – amount of light energy a patient to which a patient is exposed. Dose = irradiance ($J/s.cm^2$) × exposure time (s)

Proposed Skin Type Classification and Questions to Help Determine Skin Type (From Eilers et al. JAMA Dermatol. 2013;149(11):1289–1294)

- Question 1: If after several months of not being in the sun, you stayed outdoors for about 1 h at noon for the first time in the summer without sunscreen, what would happen to your skin?
  - Always burn
  - Usually sunburns
  - Minimally sunburns
  - Rarely sunburns
  - Never sunburns
- Question 2: Over the next 7 days, would you develop a tan or notice your skin becoming darker?
  - Never tan
  - Minimally tan
  - Moderately tan
  - Deeply tan
  - No noticeable change in color of skin

  Categorization of these answers into Fitzpatrick skin type:

  I. Always burns and never develops a tan (painful burn at 24 h and no tan at 7d)
  II. Easily burns and then develops a light tan (painful burn at 24 h and a light tan at 7d)
  III. Mild or moderate burning, skin irritation, tenderness, or itching in sun-exposed skin, then develops a medium tan or skin becomes slightly darker in sun-exposed sites (slightly tender, itching at 24 h, moderate tan or slightly darker at 7d)

IV. Minimal skin irritation, tenderness, or itching in sun-exposed skin, then develops a deep tan or skin becomes darker in sun-exposed sites (no skin irritation, tenderness, or itching at 24 h and a tan or darker skin at 7d)
V. Occasional/rare skin irritation, tenderness, or itching in sun-exposed skin, then always develops darker skin in sun-exposed sites in temperate climates
VI. Never burns: No skin irritation, tenderness, or itching in sun-exposed skin, no noticeable change in skin in sun-exposed sites in temperate climates

nbUVB

Steps before starting

☐ Skin type graded and documented in chart
☐ Patient information sheet given to patient and consent signed
☐ Patient has appropriate history (see above)
☐ Is body surface examined for moles or other abnormal skin chart and documented in chart?
☐ For male patients: has patient obtained an athletic supporter and cup?

Contraindications and Cautions

- Patients must be reliable/committed and able to stand.
- Contraindications to phototherapy
  - History of photosensitive disorders (SLE, porphyria, XP, dermatomyositis)
  - History of melanoma
  - History of organ transplantation/on immunosuppression (GVHD an exception)
  - On any photosensitizing medications (see below)
- Relative contraindications
  - History of multiple nonmelanoma skin cancers
  - History of eye disease (cataracts)
  - Arsenic exposure

- Radiation in the past

- *If patient is pregnant, avoid PUVA, and remember to increase folic acid daily dosing.*

Before every treatment, optimize UV absorption into the skin by descaling/removing crusts, and applying emollients prior to therapy as hydrated skin transmits UVR more easily.

- Petrolatum/Vaseline or mineral oil should be applied to affected areas prior to treatment (can skip in itch patients and vitiligo).

Dosing for nbUVB (Tables 5.16, 5.17, 5.18, and 5.19)

Maintenance
- Hold dose and incrementally decrease frequency of treatment/per chart below.
- Maintain at minimum frequency necessary to control skin disease and not increase risk of burn due to loss of tolerance.
- All patients should follow-up in 6–8 weeks after the start of phototherapy.
- Erythema/Burn Guidelines (Table 5.19)

TABLE 5.16 nbUVB dosing based on Fitzpatrick skin type

According to skin type:

Skin type	Initial UVB dose (mJ/cm²)	UVB Increase after each treatment (mJ/cm²)	Maximum dose (mJ/cm²)
I	130	15	2000
II	220	25	2000
III	260	40	3000
IV	330	45	3000
V	350	60	5000
VI	400	65	5000

Initial dosing 3×/week

[a]For vitiligo, use Fitzpatrick I skin type as dose regimen

Table 5.17 nbUVB dosing based on MED

According to MED:	
Initial UVB	50% of MED
Treatments 1–20	Increase by 10% of initial MED
Treatments ≥21	Increase as ordered by physician
If subsequent treatments are missed for:	
4–7 days	Keep dose same
1–2 weeks	Decrease dose by 25%
2–3 weeks	Decrease dose by 50% or start over
3–4 weeks	Start over

Table 5.18 Maintenance schedule for nbUVB phototherapy

Maintenance therapy for NB-UVB after >95% clearance:		
1×/week	NB-UVB for 4 weeks	Keep dose same
1×/2 weeks	NB-UVB for 4 weeks	Decrease dose by 25%
1×/4 weeks	NB-UVB	50% of highest dose

Table 5.19 Protocols for erythema for phototherapy

Skin response	**Adjustment**
No erythema	Increase as prescribed
Barely perceptible erythema or asymptomatic erythema that has resolved	Decrease by 10%, resume previous schedule of dose increases on subsequent treatments
Marked erythema with or without edema, with or without symptoms	Hold until resolved and then give 80% of last dose. MD to determine subsequent schedule
Severe erythema (blisters and edema), painful	Hold until resolved and then given 50% of last dose. MD to determine subsequent schedule

PUVA

Steps before starting

- ☐ Patient history taken and contraindications to therapy reviewed
- ☐ Patient information sheet given to patient and consent signed

Unique to oral PUVA: UV protective eye wear should be worn when outdoors for 24 h post-ingestion

- ☐ Is body surface examined for moles or other abnormal skin chart and documented in chart?
- ☐ Baseline eye examination ordered
- ☐ Baseline BMP, LFTs, and ANA, Ro/La (if indicated)
- ☐ Follow-up labs: every 6 months to 1 year – skin exam and ophtho exam
- ☐ For male patients: has patient obtained an athletic supporter and cup?

Contraindications to PUVA

- Females who are pregnant or nursing
- History of photosensitive disorders (e.g., SLE, porphyria, XP, dermatomyositis)

- History of organ transplantation/on immunosuppression (GVHD an exception)
- History of arsenic intake
- Previous treatment with ionizing radiation therapy
- History of melanoma or multiple nonmelanoma skin cancers
- Any medical condition that is severe enough that patient cannot tolerate heat or prolonged standing in light box
- Severe liver disease that could lead to toxic levels of psoralens
- Allergy to psoralens

Caution should be exercised in patients with the following conditions:

- Skin types I and II who tend to burn easily
- Females who are pregnant or nursing (contraindicated)
- *Patients with potential drug interactions*
  - Caution when patient is taking other photosensitizing medications (see list above)
  - Patients on other medications which can be toxic to the liver (e.g., methotrexate, cyclosporine)
  - Should decrease UVA dose by one-third if oral retinoids are started while patient is receiving PUVA

Psoralens

Topical

Topical Dosing

- Use 0.1% 8-methoxypsoralen in emollient and treat two to three times/week
- Apply 30 min before UVA
- Start at 0.25–0.5 J/cm^2, increase by 0.25–0.5 J/cm^2

Bath Dosing

- 20–30 min pre-exposure; mix psoralen in water
  - 50 mg of 8-methoxypsoralen (Oxsoralen Ultra) in 100 L of water (whole body) or 1% methoxsalen solution 0.4 mL/L of warm water (dilute 0.5 mL of 8-MOP 10 mg/mL per 1 L warm water); can use 2 L approximately for hands and feet
- Soak skin for 15 min. Pat dry the skin.
- Start UVA at 0.5 J/cm^2 for all skin types.
- Post-treatment, thoroughly wash skin.
- Increase treatments by 0.5 J/cm^2 every treatment as tolerated to a max of 2.5 J/cm^2 or more.
- Treat two to three times per week.
- Maintenance can be once weekly or every other week.

Duration of Treatment

- May take 30 treatments to have noticeable response.
- Single course usually is 30–40 treatments.
- May be repeated as indicated.

Oral

Dosing

- 8-Methoxypsoralen (Oxsoralen Ultra), 0.4–0.6 mg/kg
- Taken 1–2 h before exposure to UVA
- Other available forms of psoralen include 5-methoxypsoralen and trimethylpsoralen

Psoralen Dosing (Table 5.20)

PUVA Dosing (Table 5.21)

Lifetime Maximum of PUVA Treatments of 250 in Fitzpatrick I–II Skin Type

Duration of Treatment

- Initial improvement frequently seen within 1 month of therapy.
- Single course is typically 20–25 treatments.
- May be repeated as indicated.

Table 5.20 Dosing of 8-methoxypsoralen for oral psoralen with UVA phototherapy

Dosing of 8-methoxypsaralen for oral psoralen plus ultraviolet A		
Patient weight		
Pounds	**Kilograms**	**Drug dose, mg**
<66	<30	10
66–143	30–65	20
144–200	66–91	30
>200	>91	40

TABLE 5.21 Dosing of UVA with oral psoralens based on Fitzpatrick skin type

Dosing of ultraviolet A radiation for oral psoralen plus ultraviolet A			
Skin type	**Initial dose (J/cm^2)**	**Increments (J/cm^2)**	**Maximum dose (J/cm^2)**
I	0.5	0.5	8
II	1.0	0.5	8
III	1.5	1.0	12
IV	2.0	1.0	12
V	2.5	1.5	20
VI	3.0	1.5	20

Initial treatments 3×/week

Regular skin cancer screenings and eye examinations are required for patients on PUVA (Table 5.22).

Side Effects Associated with PUVA (Table 5.23)

Other Treatment Regimens

Goeckerman

For psoriasis:

5 times/week, patient gets UVB per guidelines above. Then, patient is coated in 2% tar (or 5% tar for experienced patients), wrapped in saran wrap, and put into a surgical scrub suit to be left on for 4–6 h. They relax and then shower the tar off 4–6 h later. After shower, apply heavy emollient (Aquaphor). UVB doses are increased per above.

Ingram

5 times/week, patient gets UVB per above. Then, patient is coated with anthralin 0.1% paste to psoriatic areas except the

TABLE 5.22 American Academy of Dermatology monitoring recommendations for patients on PUVA

Monitoring	
Baseline	**Ongoing**
Skin cancer screening	Regular full skin examination because of potential increased risk of photocarcinogenesis in Caucasians
Eye examination; however, recent evidence demonstrates no increased risk of cataract in patients who receive PUVA	In patients who are noncompliant with eye protection, yearly eye examination
If indicated by history: ANA panels (anti-Ro/La antibodies) Liver enzymes	

TABLE 5.23 Side effects possible with PUVA

Toxicities	
Acute	**Chronic**
Nausea and vomiting are common	Photocarcinogenesis (SCC, BCC, and possible melanoma)
Dizziness and headache are rare	Increased risk of photocarcinogenesis in Caucasians with skin types I–III after 200 treatments; this risk is less present for non-Caucasians
Erythema: peaks at 48–95 h	Photoaging and lentigines are common, especially in patients of skin types I–III and are cumulative UVA dose dependent
Pruritus	
Tanning: starts at 1 week after PUVA	
Blisters, photo-onycholysis, melanonychia	

face and body folds. Protect normal skin around plaques with Vaseline. Cover with saran wrap and a surgical scrub body suit. Keep in place for 2 h and then shower off. Use Aquaphor or equivalent at night. Increase UVB per above. Anthralin concentration can be increased every third treatment or so: 0.25%, 0.5%, 1%, 2%, 3%, and 4% (max).

Home phototherapy units

Are available for prescription by:

- Daavlin
- National Biologic Corporation
- UVBioTek, LLC
- Solarc Systems, Inc.

Reading for how best to prescribe a phototherapy unit for home: Anderson and Feldman. J Am Acad Dermatol. 2015;72(5):868–78.

Patients should be counseled to measure out distance from the device exactly and place a piece of tape on the floor to avoid burns from standing too close.

References

1. Brown DG, Wilkerson EC, Love WE. A review of traditional and novel oral anticoagulant and antiplatelet therapy for dermatologists and dermatologic surgeons. J Am Acad Dermatol. 2015;72:524–34.
2. Cunningham TJ, et al. Randomized trial of calcipotriol combined with 5-fluorouracil for skin cancer precursor immunotherapy. J Clin Invest. 2017;127:106–16.
3. Howe N, Cherpelis B. Obtaining rapid and effective hemostasis: Part II. Electrosurgery in patients with implantable cardiac devices. J Am Acad Dermatol. 2013;69(5):677.e1–9.
4. J Am Acad Dermatol. 2019;80(3):746.
5. Kiss N, et al. Intralesional therapy for the treatment of keratoacanthoma. Dermatol Ther. 2019;32(3):e12872.
6. Olsen EA, et al. J Am Acad Dermatol. 2016;72(1):27–58.

7. Ozog DM, et al. Photodynamic therapy: a clinical consensus guide. Dermatol Surg. 2016;42:804–27.
8. Park K, Sharon V. A review of local anesthetics: minimizing risk and side effects in cutaneous surgery. Dermatol Surg. 2017;43(2):173–87.
9. Voutsalath MA, et al. Electrosurgery and implantable electronic devices: review and implications for office-based procedures. Dermatol Surg. 2011;37(7):889–99.
10. Zanolli MD, Feldman SR. Phototherapy treatment protocols. 3rd ed. Boca Raton: CRC Press; 2016.

Chapter 6
Cosmetic Dermatology

Cosmetic Consultation

- Ask before all cosmetic procedures (45 minutes).
  - What are the top three things that you would like addressed?
- Take pictures before you start any injections.
- Take patients off ASA, fish oil, and vitamin E for 1 week before the procedure (if used for ppx).
- Assess a face.
  - Look for symmetry from the nose, through the eyes, and then down.
  - Assess the face vertically in thirds (hairline to the bottom of the eye, eye to mouth, mouth to jowl). All these thirds should be equal.
  - Assess the face horizontally in fifths (nose, mid cheek, lateral cheek – all of these should be equal).
  - Looking at the chin, have patients say "January, February, March" and assess for dimpling in those areas – will want to fill those areas.
  - Look for jowling.
  - Look for asymmetry in the brows (the goal is for lateral brow to be at the same height as the medial brow).

S. Hylwa et al., *Pocket Dermatology*,
https://doi.org/10.1007/978-3-030-83602-3_6

Botulinum Toxin

Toxins are FDA approved primarily for the glabellar region but can treat multiple areas including muscle-mediated dynamic horizontal forehead lines, periorbital smile lines (i.e., "crow's feet"), upper and lower lip vertical rhytids, and cobblestoned mental creases. They can reshape the face by selective muscle relaxation including an upturning of the upper lip, rounding of a square mandibular contour, and widening of the eye aperture to an almond shape. They can reshape a smile, lowering the lip to prevent the show of gums. Injections reduce scar formation in healing surgical or traumatic sounds. Off the face treatments include platysmal banding upon tooth clenching and chest rhytids. Hyperhidrosis on the palms, axillae, and to some degree on the soles of the feet can also be treated.

Common areas of the face that can be injected (Fig. 6.1) and facial musculature anatomy to know for botulinum toxin injections (Fig. 6.2)

Types of Toxins

Type A Toxins

- OnabotulinumtoxinA (Botox)
- AbobotulinumtoxinA (Dysport)
- IncobotulinumtoxinA (Xeomin)

1 unit of ona- or inco-toxin is equivalent to 2.5 units of abo-toxin.

Type B Toxin

- RimabotulinumtoxinB (Myobloc) – used less frequently because of shorter duration of action

Diluting Toxins

Typical dilutions are 1–10 mL per standard vial (100 units of ona- or inco-toxins; 300 units of abo-toxin).

Concentrated solutions offer more precision because of minimal diffusion and minimal induration of intracutaneous blebs, although more toxin can be lost through drops during reconstitution and preparation.

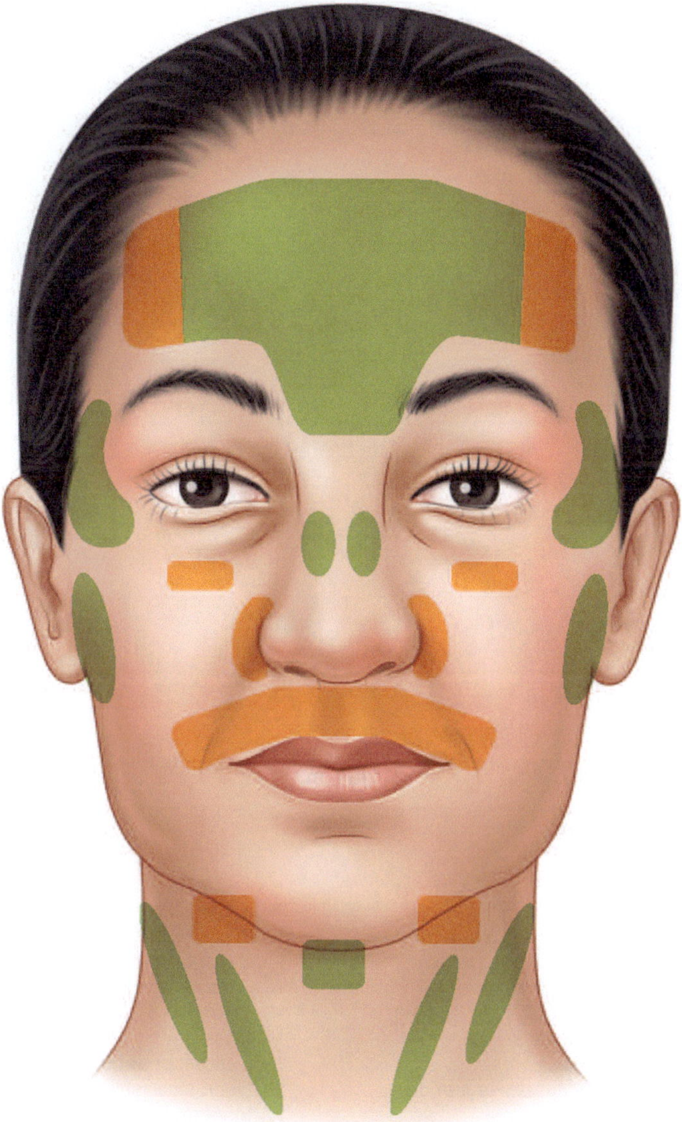

FIGURE 6.1 Areas of the face that can be safely injected with botulinum toxin (green areas) and those that can be injected with caution (yellow areas). (Adapted from Alam and Tung [1])

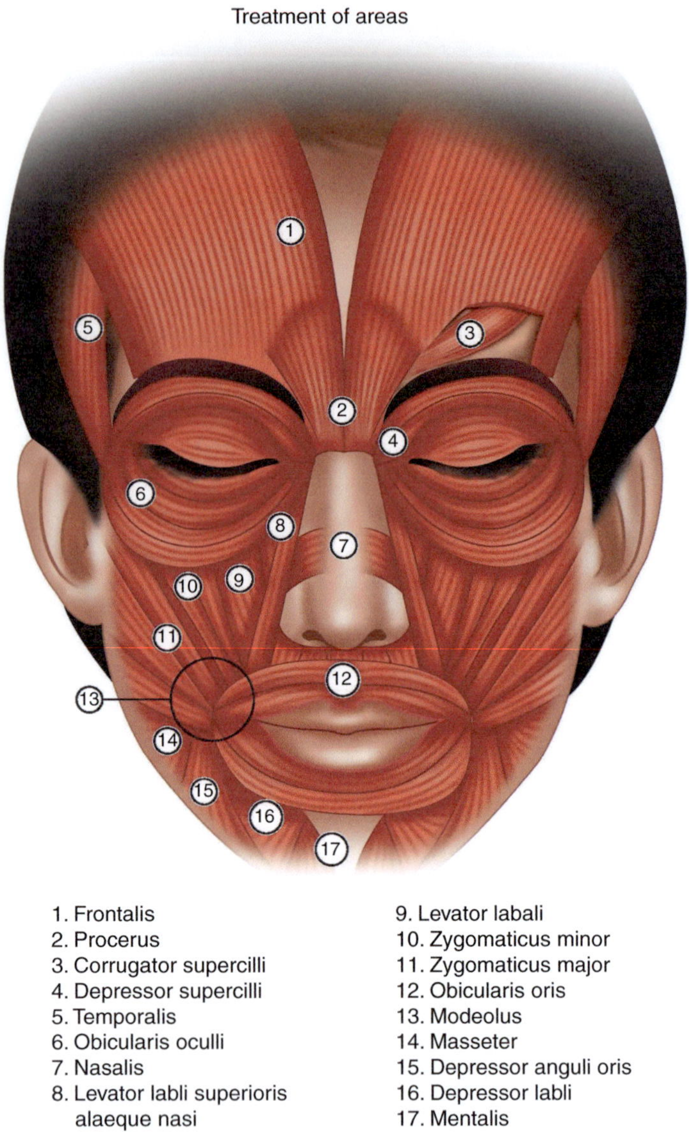

FIGURE 6.2 Muscles of the face pertinent for botulinum toxin injections

Dilute solutions can treat a wider area with a smaller dosage but can leave visible blebs after injection and be less precise.

Steps to administering Botox

- Questions to ask:
  - Known allergy to Botox?
  - Pregnant or nursing?
  - History of myasthenia gravis, Eaton-Lambert syndrome, ALS, or other musculoskeletal syndrome?
  - History of adverse reactions to Botox in the past?
  - Other allergies?
  - On any medications (particularly aminoglycosides)?
- *Sign informed consent*: see below.
- Discuss price.
- *Take photo of the face both at rest and in action.*
- Apply BLT or other topical anesthetic if you wish.
- Plan sites to administer.
- Draw up Botox.
- Prep and administer.
- Review after care.
- Offer 2-week follow-up.
- Schedule 3 months' follow-up.

Adverse Events

- Small erythematous macules at the site of injection – resolve spontaneously.
- Brow ptosis and eyelid ptosis – avoid by not injecting low and close to the midbrow.
- Ectropion – avoid by not injecting in older individuals with skin and muscle laxity.
- Unilateral lip droops if injecting midface.
- Headaches.

Eyelid Ptosis Management

Apraclonidine (Iopidine) – an alpha-2 adrenergic agonist

Contraindications

- Hypersensitivity to neurotoxins
- Infection at site of planned injection

Avoid if

- Botulism history
- Neurologic disease (ALS, peripheral motor neuropathy, myasthenia gravis, other muscle disease)
- Double vision, blurred vision, retrobulbar hemorrhage or compromised retinal circulation, corneal ulcer
- Upper lid ptosis at baseline
- Decreased lung function
- Trouble breathing or swallowing
- Pregnancy: may cause fetal harm
- Breastfeeding
- Coagulopathy
- Safety and efficacy not established in patients under 18 yo

Filler

Temporary injectable fillers can correct aging-related volume loss, depressed scars (most commonly rolling scars with acne), and fat atrophy (including coup de sabre, HIV lipoatrophy, progressive hemifacial atrophy). Body indications include horizontal creases of the neck, fine rhytids of the upper chest and décolletage, and dorsal hand atrophy with a veiny appearance.

Types of Filler

- Hyaluronic acid derivatives
- Calcium hydroxylapatite (CaHA)
- Poly-L-lactic acid

All are biocompatible, biodegradable, and unlikely to migrate from the point of injection.

Filler Properties

Five parameters can characterize fillers:

- G* – measures hardness
- G′ – measures elastic properties
- G″ – measures viscous properties
- tan∂ – the ratio of viscous to elastic
- Cohesivity – measure of internal adhesion forces (resistance to vertical compression or spreading)

The ideal filler is viscoelastic – sufficiently viscous to be injected and sufficiently elastic to retain some shape when placed in the skin.

Harder fillers are typically injected deeper and are used in areas such as the upper cheekbones, deeply creased nasolabial folds, nasal dorsum depressions, and chin notches.

Less cohesive fillers that spread to create a soft, diffuse correction used on lower cheeks and fine lines.

Hyaluronic acid filler characteristics:

- Hyaluronic acid is a naturally occurring linear glycosaminoglycan with a disaccharide unit, which repeats several thousand times. It is found in the extracellular matrix of the dermis. Its hygroscopic end absorbs water extensively, thus creating volume. Hyaluronic acids are biocompatible and have low potential for allergic reactions. They are reversible with hyaluronidase.
- Each HA filler differs from the others in polymer chain length, degree of HA concentration, particle size, gel consistency, gel hardness, gel viscosity, degree of water solubility, and degree of cross-linking.
- Cross-linking – essential to avoid enzymatic degradation by endogenous hyaluronidase (prolongs half-life). More cross-linking is associated with higher risk of inflammation and nodule formation, however. Cross-linkers used are 1,4-butanediol diglycidyl ether and divinyl sulfone.
- G′ (G-prime) – measures the firmness/stiffness of the filler and its resistance to deformation. High G′ is stiffer and is meant for deeper injection.
- Biphasic fillers – range of microsphere sizes (e.g., Restylane, Perlane).

- Monophasic fillers – homogenous microspheres (e.g., Juvederm, Belotero). Monophasic fillers are more cohesive and may not migrate as much following injections.

  Properties of common fillers: Table 6.1.

Calcium Hydroxylapatite

Tiny spherules of synthetic calcium hydroxyapatite are combined with a neutral gel matrix that dissipates after injection. Biodegradation occurs over a year. Is radio-opaque.

Injected deeper into the subcutis. Use 27- to 28-gauge needles.

Excess injection is corrected by a stab incision followed by extrusion via manual compression.

Poly-L-lactic Acid

Synthetic polymer powder reconstituted with sterile water before injection. Injected particles settle into the subcutis, and water is resorbed; the particles then stimulate neocollagenesis. Most appropriate for deeper injections. Does not induce an immediate correction and the post-injection contour can change/worsen as water is absorbed. Patients massage the area immediately after injection and then for 5 minutes, 5 times/day for 5 days to prevent nodules.

Tip to avoid clotting the needles: reconstitute with a larger volume of water than specified in the package and store for 48–72 hours before injecting.

Adverse Events

- Most common reactions: erythema, swelling, bruising, nodules, asymmetry
- Inadvertent intravascular injection
  - Usually results in pain and delayed reticulated erythema – usually resolves without sequelae but can scar.

TABLE 6.1 Physical properties of select hyaluronic acid fillers

Product	Material	Formulation	Cross-linker	Indication	Notes
Restylane	HA produced by fermentation of equine streptococci Passed through sizing screens and sieves to quantify the size	20 mg/mL	BDDE cross-link at 1%	Correction of moderate to severe facial wrinkle and folds (e.g., nasolabial folds)	Longevity = 6 months
Restylane-L	HA with lidocaine Passed through sizing screens and sieves to quantify the size	100,000 particles/mL; 20 mg/mL HA	BDDE	Correction of moderate to severe facial wrinkle and folds (e.g., nasolabial folds and perioral rhytids); lip augmentation	Addition of lidocaine does not affect the longevity of the filler SE: contusion, lip swelling, lip pain, unspecified lip disorder, headache
Restylane Silk	HA with lidocaine Passed through sizing screens and sieves to quantify the size	10,000 particles/mL; 20 mg/mL HA	BDDE	Specifically designed for lip augmentation; correction of perioral rhytids	Less viscous than restylane and requires less pressure to inject. To avoid swelling, recommend that this be injected slowly. A short course of oral prednisone may be administered after the procedure to treat any edema. Longevity = 6–9 months

(continued)

Table 6.1 (continued)

Product	Material	Formulation	Cross-linker	Indication	Notes
Restylane Lyft	HA with lidocaine	20 mg/mL	–	Correction of facial rhytids (nasolabial fold), cheek augmentation, midface contouring	SE: Injection site hematoma, pain, swelling, headache, hemorrhage Injection can be serial puncture (most common), linear antegrade threading, linear retrograde threading
Restylane Refyne	Uses XpresHAn Technology			Correction of moderate to severe facial wrinkles and folds	Lasts for ~ 12 months
Restylane Defyne	Uses XpresHAn Technology			Correction of moderate to severe deep facial wrinkles and folds	Lasts for ~ 12 months

Juvederm	NASHA (bacterium-derived) Monophasic gel	24 mg/mL	9% cross-linked Hylacross technology: cohesive molecules of cross-linked HA. Does not break up cross-linked HA by passing through a sizing screen	Correction of moderate to severe facial wrinkles and folds	High concentration of cross-linked HAs, which accounts for the longevity of the product Remains in the area where injected due to cohesive nature and high viscosity; therefore it fills more precisely and efficiently
Juvederm Ultra	Hyaluronic acid produced by *Streptococcus equi*	24 mg/mL of HA	9% cross-linked Hylacross technology: cohesive molecules of cross-linked HA. Does not break up cross-linked HA by passing through a sizing screen.	Correction of moderate to severe facial wrinkles and folds. Best for contouring and volumizing medium depth facial wrinkles and lip augmentation	Soft and easy to use Implanted mid-dermis with a 30-gauge needle

(continued)

Table 6.1 (continued)

Product	Material	Formulation	Cross-linker	Indication	Notes
Juvederm Ultra Plus		24 mg/mL of HA	11% cross-linked Hylacross technology: cohesive molecules of cross-linked HA. Does not break up cross-linked HA by passing through a sizing screen	Correction of moderate to severe facial wrinkles and folds Used for volumizing and correcting deeper folds	Soft and easy to use Longevity: about 12 months Implanted deeper than Ultra via a 27-gauge needle
Juvederm Voluma	HA with lidocaine, smooth, highly cohesive, viscous HA gel	20 mg/mL HA and 0.3% lidocaine	BDDE Vycross technology – combines low and high molecular weight HA	Deep injection for cheek augmentation	Higher G′ creates lift; low swelling capacity Longevity: 2 years Injection techniques: serial puncture, fanning, tunneling, cross-hatching SE: resolving in 2 weeks or less: tenderness, swelling, firmness, lumps/bumps. Lasting 30 days or more: injection site mass, induration, swelling, pain.

Belotero	HA with cohesive polydensified matrix technology, low elasticity, low viscosity	22.5 mg/mL HA	BDDE	Correction of moderate to severe facial wrinkles and folds (e.g., nasolabial folds)	Lowest G′ makes ideal for superficial injections (forehead lines, vermillion border, tear trough, atrophic scars, neck lines [off-label]) Longevity = 6–8 months Injection technique: threading or multiple puncture SE: injection site swelling, nodule formation, bruising, induration, erythema, pain, discoloration, pruritus

BDDE = 1,4-butanediol diglycidyl ether

Fillers can be injected using several techniques: serial puncture, linear threading, cross-hatching, fanning, and depot placement. Fillers are layered to correct areas where fine superficial lines overlie deeper volume loss. See below under administration for filler to read more on these techniques

  - Rarely retrograde movement to the retinal artery and can cause blindness. *Abundant superficial vasculature in the glabella and perinasal regions renders these locations particularly susceptible to vaso-occlusion.*

- Less frequent: contour irregularities, product migration, bluish discoloration (more likely to occur with superficial injections), nodules, infection, scarring, vascular occlusion leading to skin necrosis or blindness

Pain Management

- Many fillers have lidocaine built in.
- Topical ice.
- Topical anesthetics (lidocaine 2.5% and prilocaine 2.5%) applied under occlusion for 30–60 minutes before treatment.
- Infraorbital and mental nerve blocks.
- Avoid intralesional anesthetics because they distort the anatomy.

Prepping the Patient for Injection

- If going to do any injections in the tear trough region, ask an ocular history: history of contact lenses and glasses and history of visual abnormalities, and note any differences in pupil size – this area is quite tricky to get corrected.
- Consent and note the batch or lot number sticker (place with patient consent form).
- Point out baseline asymmetries and make sure to photodocument these.
- Take pretreatment photographs both head on and from a 45-degree angle.
- Apply mixture of Betacaine/lidocaine/tetracaine (BLT) - or other topical anesthetic - 30 minutes prior to treatment and use pretreatment ice to minimize pain associated with injections.

- Sterile technique is important in order to prevent infections, but there is no universal consensus on how to prep the face.

  One option: Have the patient wash the face with soap and water and then chlorhexidine, then wipe the areas with alcohol before injecting.

Filler Danger Zones – AVOID

- Glabella
- Periorbital area
- Tip of the nose

Drawing Out Where to Fill

- Have the patient seated upright (not laying back as this can mask the jowls).
- Draw straight lines from the tragus to the lateral eye canthus to the oral commissure and then back to the tragus. Draw a line straight down from the lateral canthus to the base of the triangle. Then, draw a line parallel with the base of the triangle 1/3 of the way from the top of the triangle (lateral canthus).
- The goal is to inject laterally on the 1/3 lines (this helps to soften the eye and helps with shadowing under the cheek fat pad and helps to correct a jowl).
- Another method is to draw from the tragus to the nasal ala and then from the lateral canthus to the commissure (Fig. 6.3).

Injection Techniques

- Almost all fillers are injected into the subcutis, usually in the high subcutis just below the dermis. Deeper injections can be wasteful as the space is deep and large quantities of

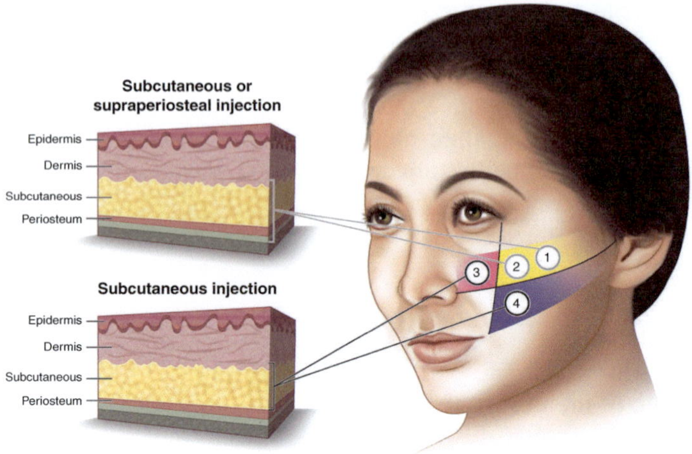

FIGURE 6.3 Outlining the face for zygomatic cheek filler injections

fillers can be placed that do not result in contour change. More superficially placed fillers in the dermis can lead to nodules, a bluish hue, or skin toned nodules for white fillers.

- Two main injection techniques include linear threading and serial puncture.
  - In linear threading, the needle is inserted at an acute angle (<90°) and then advanced laterally. Injection can be anterograde (commenced at the point of insertion and continued while the needle is advanced) or retrograde (initiated as the needle is withdrawn from the most distant point). Anterograde injections allow hydrodissection of the tissue which can facilitate needle insertion and thus cleave tissue planes naturally and deposit filler where it is required without the needle or cannula creating an artificial tunnel that transects planes or vessel lumina, and because a stream of soft extruded filler precedes the sharper tip of the needle/cannula, tissue trauma may be minimized. Retrograde injections provide security of preplanning and course of filler delivery as they offer more control over filler placement;

also, because the tunnel for injection already exists, less injection pressure may be needed to expel the filler from the syringe. Linear threading allows for less puncture marks to be made in the skin and a more uniform delivery of filler and less risk of dermal deposition of filler.
  - Serial puncture consists of numerous small injections. Each injection perforates the dermis followed by extrusion of a droplet of filler into the high subcutis. The needle is then withdrawn, repositioned a small distance away, and the process is repeated. Benefits of this are less risk of needle trauma to vessels, precise delivery to each location, and suitability for small defects.

- Other injection methods include cross-hatching and depot injections – these are generally used for large areas and deep soft tissue defects like atrophied cheeks.
  - Cross-hatching – placement of a row of linear threads followed by another row at right angles. To minimize trauma/multiple pokes, some injectors use a fanning pattern instead. Fans can be propagated from several entry points to create a cross-hatch pattern. These are placed in the superficial subcutis.
  - Depots – create a nodule of filler deep at the center of the defect, and then manual compression is used to spread this evenly. Spreading of the depot can be painful, though, so multiple smaller depot injections may be preferred.
  - More advanced techniques include cannulas.

- *Always aspirate before injecting.*
- Administer low volumes.
- Tent the skin prior to injecting more superficially to reduce risk of skin necrosis.
- Juvederm, Restylane, and Puragen are not fully hydrated with water in the syringe, and HA is known to be able to avidly bind water. Therefore, these products that absorb water after injections often slightly expand within 24 hours. It is important to note this as you may want to underfill, particularly the lips, to allow for expansion. Captique and Hylaform are completely hydrated.

Tips for Commonly Injected Areas

- Along the 1/3 triangle line: Inject 0.1cc, 0.2cc, 0.3cc, 0.2cc, and 0.1cc along that line. Always start laterally and move proximally along the zygomatic cheek so that you don't cannulate the artery.
- Nasolabial fold: Stay 1 cm from alar insertion.
- Marionette lines: place small amounts, into a K line to create scaffolding at the angle of lip.
- Lip proper: Ideal ratio of the lip is 1:1.6 (upper:lower). Want the larger/fuller part of the lip centrally below the nose. Conservative treatment is to take the cupid's bow and then inject in the lower lip about 1 mm below the line with a soft filler like Belotero.
- Using a cannula: Ideal in the lip and for the mesolabial folds. To do this, inject the area with a 25- or 27-gauge needle and then put in the cannula to do the feathering.
- Charting: Name of filler, quantity injected, and area injected should be noted in the chart.
- Avoid injecting into the dermis reduces the likelihood of nodule creating – persistent lumps may require hyaluronidase injections.

Post-care Wound Instructions

- Patient should refrain from massaging the area for 2 weeks unless otherwise directed.
- Avoid extreme temperatures (e.g., skiing, sauna).
- Swelling is to be expected and will minimize over the next few days.

Complications

- Early complications (up to 1 week after treatment)

- Lumping (somewhat expected) – molding performed immediately on recognizing it until the lump is flattened and any lumping reversed. Continue to have the patient mold the filler for up to 2 weeks postinjection.
- Bruising – immediate ice, observe, and then can use arnica gel, vitamin K cream, PDL, or IPL laser.
- Swelling – prednisone 30 mg daily for 3 days.
- Nodules – see below.
- Hypersensitivity.
- Tissue necrosis - see below.
- Blindness if injected in the periocular/glabellar area - see below.

Pathomechanism for blindness (Fig. 6.4)

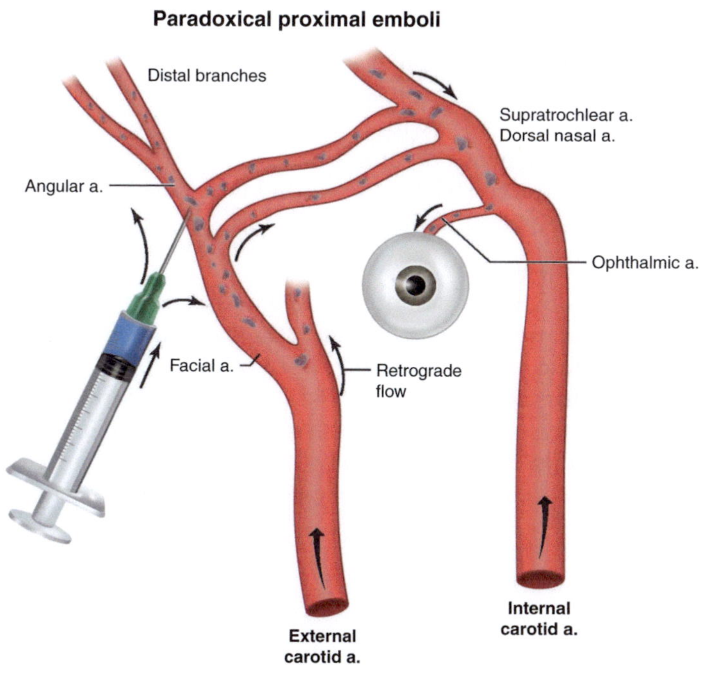

FIGURE 6.4 Mechanism for ocular blindness from periocular/glabellar filler injections

- Late complications (>1 week)
  - Infection
  - Biofilm formation
  - Granuloma formation

Algorithm for Treatment of Inflammatory Nodules
- I&D as much of the substance as possible.
- Send for culture.
- Oral antibiotics for at least 2–5 weeks. May need multiple agents if no response or IV antibiotics if severe.
- Avoid initial use of intralesional corticosteroids. Use only if the patient is already on an antibiotic regimen.
- Inject hyaluronidase if caused by hyaluronic acid filler.
- Excision or debridement of the nodule if no response and long-term persistence.

Algorithm for Treatment of Necrosis
- Impending necrosis presents in one of three patterns: immediate, early (within 24–48 hours), or delayed. Treatment depends on onset.
- If immediate, you will see white and then purple in area of injection. Acute treatment protocol is:
  - Stop injecting.
  - Applying warm compresses and massage.
  - Application of 2% nitroglycerin paste in the area to facilitate vasodilation and blood flow.
  - Skin testing with hyaluronidase could be performed, and if no hypersensitivity to this agent is seen, then 10–30 units diluted in a 1:1 ratio with saline should be injected per $2 \times 2\ cm^2$ area into the region of impending necrosis.

Bruising Management

- Fewer passes with a needle or cannula can help prevent microvascular injury.

- Vitamin K cream, arnica gel, and/or bromelain may prevent or treat injection-related bruising.
- Pulse dye laser promptly treating an ecchymosis on non-purpuric settings can speed resolution.

Emergency Use of Hyaluronidase Hyaluronidase Cosmetic Dermatology Hyaluronidase: Triaging Vascular Accident After Filler Injection

Sources: Vitrase (Bausch & Lomb Inc.), Amphadase (Amphastar Pharmaceuticals), and Hylenex (Halozyme Therapeutics).

In general: it typically takes several dozen to 100 units of hyaluronidase to dissolve a full syringe of HA. Delayed onset nodules may take repeat injections of several hundred units. As little as 3 units, though, may be required to dissolve small aliquots of filler in thin skin areas like the infraorbital areas.

- Administer aspirin.
- Apply warm compresses.
- Administer hyaluronidase: recommendations are 200 units of hyaluronidase at 3–4 cm intervals throughout the area of vascular compromise manifested by ischemic, mottled skin discoloration and tenderness.
  - This can be repeated at 60-minute intervals until reperfusion becomes evident and daily if needed.
  - Reading: Jones DH. JAMA Dermatology. 2018;154(7):763–764.

Retinal Artery Occlusion with Filler: Steps

Have your retinal specialist on speed dial, but also be prepared to intervene yourself – time is vision! Get a game plan in place before you treat your first filler patient and mentally walk through what would be needed. If you are not comfortable doing any of these steps, experts recommend to not offer filler for your patients.

- First sign is pain near or away from the site of injection.
- Ask the patient what is going on with the vision and try to get a quick visual acuity test (have them try to read something with the eye) and check pupil size.
- Have an ophthalmic emergency "crash cart" ready: 10 mL syringes, ample hyaluronidase (more than 2000 units at any one time), retrobulbar needles (also called Atkinson needle – 23- to 25-guage and 1.5 inches in length), and topical anesthetic eye drops.
- Perform retrobulbar injection of hyaluronidase – injection upwards of 10 mL into the area. Instructions on how to perform this type of injection (along with a video) can be found at: https://emedicine.medscape.com/article/2000744-overview?pa=m8P4lV7NFyK8VyJGgkpTqO%2Bdz6jYPNQ909MKWtS5sroM6yWKrzfhfYnRR2zJZj0fcFrqow%2Bf2%2F37XuRaZT6JAA%3D%3D#a3
- Reading: Fagien S. Dermatol Surg. 2018;44(3):437–42.

Nonemergency Use of Filler: Treatment of Granulomas, Other HA Reactions, and HA Misplacement

- Note that highly cross-linked fillers may require more hyaluronidase than lower cross-linked fillers.
- Start with 10 units of hyaluronidase (Vitrase) for each 0.1cc of Juvederm, 5 units for each 0.1cc of Restylane, and 30 units for each 0.1cc of Voluma (which is highly cross-linked).
- When attempting to remove smaller or partial amounts of filler, can dilute the hyaluronidase with normal saline to go from 20 units/0.1cc to 10 units/0.1cc or less.

Kybella (Deoxycholic Acid)

Injectable treatment is used for midline submental fat reduction. Full effect is visible at 3 months. Typically requires > 1 injection session for maximal improvement.

Need to assess facial functioning pretreatment.

Evaluate anatomy: thyroid gland palpation/swallow, larynx palpation, and location of sternocleidomastoid in the neck, and these areas should be marked on the surface with a cosmetic marker and avoided

Contraindications:
- Surgery on the face/neck/chin
- Medical conditions on the face/neck/chin
- Bleeding problems
- Trouble swallowing
- Pregnant/breastfeeding

Treatment Pearls: Main Treatment Areas and Botox Units
Frontalis: ~ 2 units per site (typically double for men)

- Caution: eyebrow ptosis – stay at least 2 cm above brows.
- Caution: Spock effect (compensatory lateral frontalis activity) – palpate lateral frontalis. To correct, use ~1 unit.

Glabellar complex: ~2–5 units per injection point (more medially, less laterally)

Lateral canthal lines/orbicularis oculi

- Target is orbital part of the muscle.
- ~2 units per injection site.

Perioral lines/orbicularis oris

- ~0.5 units per site, four sites upper cutaneous lip, two sites lower cutaneous lip

Gummy smile/hyperactive superior levator labii

- ~1 unit per injection site

Pebbly chin/peau d'Orange/Mentalis

- ~2 units per injection site

Adverse Effects
Most common are:

- Temporary swelling, pain, numbness, redness, and hardness in the treatment area

  Less common are:

- *Nerve injury* to the jaw with resultant uneven smile or facial muscle weakness 2/2 marginal mandibular nerve injury
- Trouble swallowing
- Bruising
- Hair loss in treatment area
- Open sores/ulcers/necrosis
- Intravascular injection

If suspect intravascular injection
Reading and based on McKay et al. [5].

Hypothesized mechanism:
Inadvertent injection into a blood vessel > direct cytolysis of endothelial cells of the vascular lumen. Irritation of the vessel wall then causes vasospasm.

Both can potentially result in ischemia and necrosis outside the treatment area.

Vascular occlusion is an unlikely result of intravascular deoxycholic acid injection, given that the product is a solution free of particulate matter.

Clues:
If the patient experiences significant pain and there is dusky discoloration

Treatment:
1. Warm compresses, nitropaste, and massage immediately applied to promote vasodilation.
2. Sublingual aspirin 325 mg and then baby aspirin PO (81 mg) for 7 days.

3. Topical desonide (or other steroid) ointment BID.
4. If significant swelling, start oral prednisone 20–40 mg for 3–5 days.
5. If significant pain/immediate duskiness, flood affected area with saline to dilute the product.
6. Advise patient to massage area with warm compresses 3×/daily until follow-up next day.
7. Patient follow-up next day, and continue daily follow-up until improvement. If improved, follow up in 7 days.

Latisse (Bimatoprost Ophthalmic Solution) 0.03%

- FDA approved for growing eyelashes for people with sparse or thin lashes.
- As lashes grow gradually over time; patients will see initial results at 4 weeks and full results at 16 weeks.
- Each kit comes with detailed instructions on how to use, daily use for 16 weeks, single use applicator, patient will apply to upper lash line only.
- Counsel patients that this product may:
  - Cause brown darkening of colored part of eye (can be permanent).
  - Cause eyelid skin darkening (may be reversible).
  - Hair may grow outside treatment area.
  - Common side effect is itchiness.
- If the treatment is discontinued, lashes gradually return to previous appearance.
- Important safety information:
  - Do not use in patients who are allergic to one of its ingredients or who use/have used prescription eye pressure products.

Vaginal Rejuvenation

- Laser device to address women's intimate wellness
- 15–20 minute in office laser procedure
- Can be based on CO_2 lasers or radiofrequency

For the internal treatment, the laser device is introduced into the vagina and slowly rotated out during the treatment.

For the external treatment, the laser touches and treats the labia majora and/or minora.

Can treat externally for:

- Pigment
- Tightening
- Lichen sclerosus et atrophicus

Off-label small clinical studies show that it may be beneficial for:

- Vaginal dryness/itchiness
- Stress urinary incontinence

Conservative treatment protocols are needed for internal use, and internal tightening of the vaginal canal is controversial.

Close collaboration with OB/GYN is needed, and referral to an experienced cosmetic dermatologist who has the device needed and can go over indications and contraindications with the patient in detail.

Skin Tightening

This usually requires referral to an experienced cosmetic dermatologist who has the devices available to offer. Below is an overview of what can be discussed during counseling with the patient.

Monopolar Radiofrequency Devices (MRF)

- Thermage Comfort Pulse Technology System

- Exilis
- Pelleve
- ThermiTight system
- TruSculpt System

Ultrasound

Ultrasound uses high-frequency sound waves to cause cellular membrane disruption through the transformation of acoustic (mechanical) energy into thermal energy. U/S can precisely target tissue, with minimal damage to surrounding structures. Two main types of ultrasound: microfocused ultrasound (MFU) and high-intensity focused ultrasound (HIFU). MFU is used in skin tightening; HIFU is used for noninvasive body contouring and the reduction of the appearance of cellulite.

Microfocused Ultrasound with Visualization (MFU-V)

Used for skin tightening. MFU delivers lower-energy pulses to the deep reticular dermis and subdermis, disrupting the underlying architecture of the skin and allowing for a significant increase in skin properties such as distensibility, elasticity, and viscoelasticity. Does this by delivering ultrasound energy that selectively heats dermal and subdermal tissues to greater than 60 °C in a linear array of tightly focused thermal coagulation points, stimulating long-term collagen remodeling through activation of the wound healing cascade and then collage contraction creating short and thick fibrils as well as the production of new viscoelastic collagen. This ultimately leads to tissue tightening and lifting without damage to the epidermal surface [4].

- FDA-approved technology for noninvasive brow lift and submental neck lift as well as improvement of rhytids of the décolletage

- Routinely used off-label to treat skin laxity of the submental areas, nasolabial folds, neck, knees, posterior arms, elbows, medial thighs, abdomen, and buttocks
- Can be used in a wide range of skin types as melanin does not absorb ultrasound energy

Body Contouring

Current techniques include invasive procedures (surgical correction, liposuction) and noninvasive procedures (mechanical suction, radiofrequency, cryotherapy, low-level laser, and ultrasound).

High-Intensity Focused Ultrasound

This HIFU targets subcutaneous adipose tissue and aims to destroy it without collateral damage. Does this by using acoustic energy to disrupt cell membranes which leads to cell death and leaving cavitation bubbles within the tissue architecture. At 47 °C acoustic energy is transferred into heat; 57 °C, proteins denature; at 70 °C, coagulative necrosis is induced, and adipose cells are destroyed. Two types of HIFU are available: (1) non-focused acoustic (disrupts cell membranes of adipocytes creating cavitary lesions) or (2) focused ultrasound (initiates coagulative necrosis of adipocytes). Also used in cellulite reduction (when fat strands become tethered to subcutaneous tissues resulting in skin dimpling).

Microneedling

Microneedling (collagen induction therapy) is a minimally invasive skin rejuvenation procedure that involves the use of a device with fine needles that puncture the skin at various depths to create a controlled injury. The punctures stimulate neovascularization and neocollagenesis which then fill the microscopic wounds leading to skin rejuvination. Outcomes of microneedling vary based on the device, depth of needle penetration, and number of passes.

It can be used in skin types I–VI

Needle sizes: 0.1–2.5 mm

Uses:
- Rhytids
- Surgical scars
- Acne scars – rolling and boxcar acne scars with better effect than ice pick scars
- Striae
- Burn scar contractures
- Pore reduction
- Possibly: hair loss, vitiligo

Contraindications:
- Scleroderma
- Collagen vascular disease/autoimmune diseases (e.g., lupus)
- Clotting disorders
- Active infection of the skin including active herpes labialis
- Immunosuppression/on chemo
- Isotretinoin within the last 6 months
- Pregnancy

Should Be Avoided in:
- Keloids/hypertrophic scars
- Inflammatory dermatoses
- H/o herpes simplex in perioral area (pre-treat with Valtrex)
- Any growth in the target area
- Diseases with koebnerization: psoriasis, lichen planus
- Areas of permanent makeup
- Laser procedure within the last month
- Botox within the last week
- Dermal filler administration within the last week
- Active infection
- Active sunburn/recent tanning

- *Caution is advised with concomitant use of topical products of any type during a microneedling procedure due to the risk of granuloma formation.*

Pretreatment Considerations:

- Liberal approach outlined by Alster and Graham [2]: All patients may continue the use of any home skin care regimen (including retinoids, antioxidants, and growth factors) up until the time of the procedure.
- Others recommend:
  - No retinoids for 1 week before (and 1 week after)
  - No anti-inflammatories (NSAIDs) 3 days before (and 1 week after)
  - No waxing, epilating creams, or electrolysis 1 week prior
- Anticoagulants do not have to be discontinued.
- The use of topical antioxidants has actually been shown to enhance the regenerative process of microneedling-induced wound healing (vitamin A and C).
- Although best to perform these on separate dates, if performing other cosmetic procedures on the day of microneedling, perform these deep to superficial (e.g., injectables before microneedling and/or laser irradiation) to maintain visual landmarks and prevent diffusion of injectables caused by tissue edema or bleeding.
- Photograph the treatment areas before each session.
- Go through informed consent including the contraindications: have the patient sign the informed consent.

General Steps for Performing:

- Lay all instruments on a cleaned tray with a clean sheet. Spray all with isopropyl alcohol and wipe down all instruments and bottles of creams thoroughly.
- Cover the cord of the microneedling device with the sheath and cover the body of the instrument with the adherent plastic wrap.
- Open a sterile tip and insert into the instrument.
- Have the patient clean off all makeup with a gentle soap and wash cloth

- Position the patient comfortable and then cleanse the skin aggressively with isopropyl alcohol and/or chlorhexidine. Rinse well if using chlorhexidine and be sure to avoid the ocular area.
- Optional: EMLA/BLT/ or other topical anesthetic applied to target area and allowed to sit for 20–30 minutes. Rinse off completely and wipe with acetone before microneedling.
- Microneedling pen depth is set based on anatomic location with an endpoint of pinpoint bleeding. Sebaceous skin typically requires deeper measurements than thin periorbital skin. General references:
  - Forehead: 0.5–1.5 mm depth
  - Nose and upper lip: 0.5–1 mm depth
  - Chin and cheeks: 1–2 mm depth
  - Neck: <1 mm generally, 1.5 mm max
  - Scars, abdomen striae: 2.5 mm goal
- Apply hyaluronic acid mixed with an emollient to the forehead (or area of treatment).
- Start on forehead with depth of 0.2 for two passes to get your patient used to it, and then dial into the starting point for 0.5 mm for the forehead.
- Overlap by 50%.
- 1–4 passes are the options (3 passes standard: vertical, horizontal, diagonal).
  - Look for light pinkness
  - For scars, additional passes at increased depths, such as 2.5 mm, may be useful using either a stamping method or figure of 8. Pinpoint bleeding to be expected.
- Depending on the specific location to be treated, it is often helpful to divide the area into quadrants so that they can be treated more individually and uniformly with the microneedling (e.g., the perioral area into upper left, upper right, lower left, lower right). Gentle traction of the skin with one hand while simultaneously lowering the microneedling device perpendicular to the skin with the other assists the smooth delivery of microneedles into the skin. It is important to apply sufficient hyaluronic acid gel on the treatment

area surface to facilitate the gliding action of the microneedling device. Combine horizontal, vertical, and diagonal passes over the treatment areas, repeating three to six times until pinpoint bleeding is observed. When treating deep rhytids or scars, a "rocking" or "stamping" technique can be used to increase the density of microneedling channels created. As needle lengths > 1.0 mm may not penetrate to the corresponding dermal depth, it is useful to use pinpoint bleeding as a clinical endpoint to treatment.

- General areas of treatment: Forehead, periocular area (only perform on bony ridge, do NOT perform over the globe), cheeks/nose, chin
- Can add PRP to the face before/after microneedling.
- At the end, ice water-soaked sterile gauze can be applied to remove excess blood and hyaluronic acid gel. A thin layer of hyaluronic acid gel can then be applied to the treatment area and allowed to dry.

Series of four to six treatment sessions recommended for maximum benefit

Sessions spaced 2–6 weeks apart. Scarring will take 5–6 months of treatments.

Post-procedure Recommendations

- For the first 4 hours after the procedure, the patient should apply a provided sample of hyaluronic acid gel to the skin.
- After 4 hours, 1% hydrocortisone cream or a nonallergic moisturizing cream can be applied to the treatment area two to four times daily for 2–3 days.
- The use of physical block sunscreens (nonchemical sunscreens) is advocated (on top of the moisturizer) during the first posttreatment week starting at 48-hour posttreatment
- Application of makeup may resume 2 days after the procedure, and any active skin care products that the patient used pretreatment can resume in 5–7 days (when all traces of erythema have resolved).
- Use growth factor serums after use.

- Wash only with water or a gentle cleanser like Vanicream, Cetaphil, and CeraVe for 3 days after the treatment.
- After 3 days, okay to resume normal skin care regimen.
- Do not resume retinoids for 1 week posttreatment.
- No NSAIDs or anti-inflammatories 3 days before and 1 week after.
- No swimming in a lake pool for 1-week posttreatment.
- Avoid exercise for 24–48 hours (sweat which irritates the skin).
- Avoid sun exposure until healed; do not use sunscreen for 3 days after treatment.

Side Effects and Complications

- Irritation of the face with a sunburn type of reaction that will last for 24–48 hours: mild erythema, localized edema, and skin flaking.
- Pain with washing.
- Increase skin sensitivity (transient).
- Acne breakouts.
- Pinpoint bleeding is expected and self-limited and typically resolved within minutes of the procedure with gentle manual pressure and ice water-soaked gauze.
- Dyspigmentation in darker skin types but is rarely seen in the absence of UV light exposure on microneedled treatment surfaces.
- Granuloma formation.

General Tips

- Microneedling can be performed over hair but *not* over permanent makeup.
- Do *not* combine with hydroquinone.
- Forehead is the most painful area generally as well as any areas over bony processes.
- Go up to the vermillion border but do not do the lips. Similarly, do not perform over the globe of the eye!
- For rhytids there is a lag time of at least 6–8 weeks from the time of initiation of treatment to clinically apparent results from dermal collagen production.

Sclerotherapy (Endovenous Chemical Ablation)

Reading:

Duffy DM. Sclerotherapy. Clin Dermatol. 1992;10(3):373–80.

Emedicine: http://emedicine.medscape.com/article/1271091-treatment.

Types of sclerosants (Table 6.2)

Detergents – disrupt vein cellular membrane

- *Sodium tetradecyl sulfate (Sotradecol)*
- *Polidocanol (Asclera, Aethoxysklerol)*
- Sodium morrhuate (Scleromate)

Osmotic Agents – damage cell membrane through shifting water balance and osmotic dehydration

- *Hypertonic sodium chloride solution*
- Sodium chloride solution with dextrose (Sclerodex)

Chemical irritants – caustic destruction of the endothelium

- *Chromated glycerin (Scleromo)*
- Polyiodinated iodine

Pretreatment assessment:

- On any blood thinners? Herbal medications?
- Any signs of arterial or venous insufficiency? If so, correct underlying pathology before pursuing sclerotherapy.
- Take pretreatment photographs.

Side effects: Pain, urticaria at sites of injections, bruising, telangiectatic matting and neovascularization, ischemic ulceration, lower extremity edema, extravasation, superficial thrombophlebitis (usually occurs in larger vessels), and postinjection hyperpigmentation (due to hemosiderin or postinflammatory change). Rarely: anaphylaxis (incidence 0.3% – can occur with any sclerosant), PE/DVT due to uncontrolled thrombosis, and death

Informed consent:

TABLE 6.2 Comparison of different sclerosants

Sclerosant	Clinical application	Dosage	Advantages	Disadvantages	Complications
Sodium tetradecyl sulfate (detergent)	Varicose and spider veins Esophageal varices	1% or 3% standard concentrations *Suggested concentrations*: 0.25–0.4% for reticular veins (2–4 mm) and venulectasias (1–2 mm) and 0.1–0.2% for telangiectasias (<1 mm) Maximum single treatment not to exceed 10 mL	FDA approved in 1946 for varicose veins Useful in large veins in higher concentrations Good for smaller vessels in lower concentrations	Mild discomfort on injection No more effective than saline for small vessels	Tendency to cause post-sclerotherapy hyperpigmentation in up to 30% of patients High likelihood of tissue necrosis upon extravasation (esp. when injected in high concentrations) PE/DVT Anaphylaxis *Death reported with therapeutic volumes and concentrations*

(continued)

Table 6.2 (continued)

Sclerosant	Clinical application	Dosage	Advantages	Disadvantages	Complications
Polidocanol: Hydroxypoly-ethoxy-decan polidocanol (non-ester local anesthetic)	Varicose and spider veins Esophageal varices and gastric varices Hemorrhoids 0.5–5%)	Not to exceed 2 mg/kg (maximum daily dose) *Suggested concentrations*: 0.5–1% for reticular veins (2–4 mm) and venulectasias (1–2 mm) and 0.25–0.75% for telangiectasias (<1 mm)	°CFDA approved 2010. Virtually painless to inject Does not produce tissue necrosis if extravasated Low incidence of allergic reactions No deaths reported in therapeutic doses or concentrations Low risk of allergies No cutaneous tissue necrosis at 3%	Transient urticaria and pruritus May produce hyperpigmentation	PE Anaphylaxis (few case reports) Death after overdose (600 mg) caused by pulmonary failure Noncontact cutaneous tissue necrosis

Sodium morrhuate	Varicose and spider veins Esophageal varices (5%)	Medium veins 50–10 mg (1–2 mL of 5% injection) Large veins 150–250 (3–5 mL of injection)	FDA approved in 1930 for varicose veins	Painful on injection	PE Antigenic *Death in therapeutic concentration volumes* Cutaneous tissue necrosis in full strength
Hypertonic Saline	Abortifacient Spider, small varicose veins (10–30%)	*Suggested concentrations*: 23.4% for reticular veins (2–3 mm), venulectasias (1–2 mm) 11.7% (half strength) for telangiectasias (<1 mm) Restrict volume in patients with salt-restricted diets	Absolute absence of allergens Off-label use Good for people who want "all natural"	Moderate discomfort during injection Muscle cramps High likelihood of post-sclerotherapy hemosiderin staining Generally ineffective for large varicose veins FDA approved as abortifacient only	PE Deaths not reported *Likely cutaneous tissue necrosis in concentrations > 10% and if extravasated (leading cause of malpractice)*

(continued)

TABLE 6.2 (continued)

Sclerosant	Clinical application	Dosage	Advantages	Disadvantages	Complications
Chromated glycerin	Varicose and spider veins (1.11% chromated glycerin)	Maximum at single session is 10 mL pure solution	Low incidence of side effects No cutaneous tissue necrosis in full strength Rarely causes posttreatment hyperpigmentation, telangiectatic matting, or tissue necrosis if extravasated	Not FDA approved Fairly weak and only good for superficial vessels Highly allergenic Painful to inject	Highly allergic Can lead to ureteral colic and hematuria
Polyiodide Iodine	Varicose veins (2–12%)	Maximum at single session is 3 mL of 6% solution	Allergies not reported	Not FDA approved *Iodine may cause anaphylaxis*	Cutaneous tissue necrosis with paravenous injections Contact allergies Varicophlebitis

Adapted from Duffy [3]

- Sclerotherapy is the use of a sclerosing agent to occlude the visible vessels in the skin so that they are made non-functional and absorbed slowly by the body.
- Minor complications include as follows: pain, hives at the site of injection, bruising, swelling of legs, formation of new veins around the area of injection (neovascularization), thromboses, pigmentation changes in the skin, brown spots due to hemosiderin (which should disappear with time), and/or post-inflammatory hyperpigmentation
- Major complications that have been reported include uncontrolled thrombosis (pulmonary emboli, deep venous thrombosis), anaphylaxis, unintended tissue necrosis, and even death.
- Often patients require multiple treatment sessions

Cutaneous ulceration/tissue necrosis can be broadly categorized into three types:

- Certain concentrations and volumes of specific agents produce necrosis when in direct contact with the skin (e.g., sodium morrhuate, 1% Sotradecol, 15% hypertonic saline).
- Vasospasm, local clotting leading to cutaneous skin breakdown.
- Ulceration in patients with very delicate veins, especially elderly with varicosities. These patients tend to have exaggerated vascular and perivenular destruction that occurs (usually in correlation with the concentration of sclerosant).

Tools needed/recommended:

- 30 or 31 # ½ inch long disposable needles
- 1cc syringes (can progress to 3cc syringes with experience)
- Magnifiers 2–4×, binocular or stereoscopic if possible
- 3/8 inch washers and tiny rubber bands to create three-ring syringe to allow one-handed injections
- Sclerosant of choice

- Injections of sodium chloride solution (to dilute any extravasated sclerosant)
- Cotton balls in cup of isopropyl alcohol or alcohol pads
- Cotton balls and tape for hemostasis
- 4 × 4 as sponges
- Strong light source
- ACE wrap or compression hose
- Disposable gloves
- Have on hand: nitroglycerin 2% paste, hyaluronidase (75 units in 3 mL syringe)

Principles of treatment

- Larger veins should be treated before smaller veins.
- Proximal sites should be treated before distal sites.

How to enter a delicate vessel sometimes smaller than the needle?

- Bend the needle about 30° with bevel up.
- Vessel is the runway, and needle is the plane trying to land.
- Gently glide the needle into the vessel; injection should be precise and slow.
- Stabilize the skin around the vessel with left hand for counter traction.
- Stay superficial – number 1 error is to go through and under vessel.
- Severe pain or burning is often a sign of extravasation.
  - If this occurs, inject the site with normal sodium chloride solution or lidocaine to dilute the sclerosant.
- Each injection is usually 0.1–0.4 mL; injections are carried out in 2–3 cm intervals until the entire vessel is clear

How to tell if needle is in vessel?

- Will see bevel in vessel
- Feel pop
- Feel give when plunger advanced
- See lightening as the blood is replaced by clear sclerosant

What to do if you extravasate?

- Don't panic – unlikely anything bad will happen.
- If pt has severe burning, inject liberally with bacteriostatic 0.9% saline – will dilute out the irritancy of the 24% hypertonic saline.
- Hyaluronidase 75 units decreases the rate of ulceration after extravasation.
- Porcelain white blanching is an early sign of arteriolar injection or spasm: recommend topical nitroglycerin 2% paste that can be used for prolonged blanching and immediate treatment with hyaluronidase (75 units in 3 mL). Injections of normal sodium chloride solution, lidocaine, or both are advised.
- A large extravasation means you are not paying attention – PAY ATTENTION

A few other tips:

- As you enter the skin, put slight pressure on the plunger, slowly advance – when the vessel is entered, you should feel it give. If you think you've gone through the vessel and note extravasation, pull back while gently advancing the plunger – you'll again feel the "give as a vessel lumen is entered."
- Maintain a comfortable position for yourself by having the patient move toward you – have him/her contort/twist, no you.
- If your needle catches or grabs as you try to penetrate the skin, replace the needle.
- Let patients know that popliteal and ankles areas are touchier and tend to hurt more.
- If the syringe is "dribbling," there are tiny bubbles within that expand with your finger head; express them.
- The pretibial area and ankle have the highest propensity for ulceration. Treatment in these areas should be limited in each session.
- Telangiectatic matting is due to injections that are administered too rapidly or in which the sclerosant concentration is too high. It usually resolves spontaneously but can be permanent.

- For superficial thrombophlebitis, treatment is with compression and NSAIDs. Evacuation of the liquefied thrombus is helpful.

Posttreatment patient reminders:

- As you inject, tell the patient that it is normal to see bright spots or hives on treated areas.
- Remind them that the legs will be tender and look like they have been brushed up in prickly bushes for a few days.
- Remind them that the brown spots may appear.
- Remind that symptomatic improvement usually occurs quickly after sclerotherapy, whereas cosmetic improvement may be more gradual.
- New vessels may develop over time, and repeat treatments may be required.
- If patient complains of painful sore, reassure and give Bactroban and Band-Aid and DuoDerm hydrogel dressing.

Posttreatment care:

- Once the needle is removed, compression with cotton balls and tape used.
- Once the entire treatment session is completed, wrap the leg in an ACE wrap or Jobst/Ted stocking at 20–30 mmHg minimum to be worn for 24 hours and then daily for 1–3 weeks.
  - Compression garments decrease the risk of pigmentation, edema, and DVT.
- Ask patients to perform lower extremity exercises immediately following sclerotherapy and then on a daily basis.
- Avoid aggressive exercise for 4 weeks.

Follow-up:

- In 2–8 weeks for repeat treatment (often of the same anatomic location)

Therapies for Hyperpigmentation

First line:

- Topical: hydroquinone, retinoids (tretinoin, tazarotene, adapalene), and azelaic acid
- Oral: tranexamic acid

Nonprescription medications (cosmeceuticals): aloesin; arbutin-deoxyarbutin; coffeeberry products; ellagic acid; emblica officinalis extract; glutathione; kojic acid; licorice extract; lignin peroxidase; mulberry; N-acetylglucosamine; niacinamide; oligopeptides (decapeptide-12); polypodium; procyanidin; resorcinol; retinol; soy; and vitamins A, C, and E

Photoprotection with sunscreens that bloack UVA, UVB, and visible light

Adjunctive therapies: microdermabrasion, chemical peels, lasers, energy-based devices, and microneedling

References

1. Alam M, Tung R. Injection technique in neurotoxins and fillers: indications, products, and outcomes. J Am Acad Dermatol. 2018;79(3):423–35.
2. Alster T, Graham P. Microneedling: a review and practical guide. Dermatol Surg. 2018;44(3):397–404.
3. Duffy DM. Sclerotherapy. Clin Dermatol. 1992;10(3):373–80.
4. Juhasz M, et al. A review of the use of ultrasound for skin tightening, body contouring, and cellulite reduction in dermatology. Dermatol Surg. 2018;44:949–63.
5. McKay C, et al. Vascular injury after deoxycholic acid injection. Dermatol Surg. 2019;45(2):306–9.

Chapter 7
Contact Dermatology

Patch Testing

Patch Testing: The method of applying small quantities of haptens onto the skin in order to diagnose allergic contact dermatitis.

Allergic Contact Dermatitis: Type IV hypersensitivity reaction mediated largely by Langerhans cells in the epidermis of the skin and T lymphocytes. Likelihood of allergens to cause sensitization. In general, allergens can be classified as low-molecular-weight (chemical) allergens and high-molecular-weight (protein) allergens.

Ref: Dermatitis Jan/Feb 2014

- Category 1: Extensive evidence of contact allergy (MCI/MI, DNCB, PPD)
- Category 2: A frequent cause of contact allergy but of less clinical significance than category 1 (formaldehyde, isoeugenol, methyldibromoglutaronitrile)
- Category 3: A common cause of contact allergy, perhaps requiring higher exposure compared with category 2 (abietic acid, eugenol, imidazolidinyl urea)

S. Hylwa et al., *Pocket Dermatology*,
https://doi.org/10.1007/978-3-030-83602-3_7

- Category 4: Infrequent cause of contact allergy in relation to level of exposure (benzocaine, hydroxycitronellal, resorcinol)
- Category 5: A rare cause of contact allergy in special circumstances (hexylcinnammal, isopropanol, parabens)
- Category 6: Non-sensitizing (xylene, glycerol, sodium lauryl sulfate)

Patch Testing Process (General)

- Day 1: History obtained, physical exam performed, allergens ordered and placed / taped onto the skin.
  - Patches are left in place for 48 hours.
- Day 3: Patches removed. First day reads performed.
  - Solid allergens (e.g. chunkies) may be reapplied on this day if no reaction has occurred at this read.
  - Many reactions on this day may be pure irritation of the skin and not a true Type IV reaction c/w ACD.
- Day 5: Final interpretive read done.
  - It can take up to 5 days for ACD reactions to form, so this is the more definitive read.
  - Irritant reactions that may have been visible on Day 3 should have diminished or disappeared.

Common modes of patch testing:

NEVER TEST TO A PRODUCT THAT YOU DO NOT KNOW WHAT IT IS / OR ITS INGREDIENTS.

- 'Closed' = Antigen placed on aluminum disc, covered with Scanpor tape. Antigens are typically diluted in petrolatum or aqueous solutions. Can apply personal care products that are meant to leave on the skin (e.g. moisturizers) in a closed fashion.
- 'Semi-open' = Used for 'wash-off' (e.g. shampoos, cleansers) or irritating (e.g. deodorants) products. Antigens/products are painted directly on skin, dabbed, left to dry some, and covered with Scanpor tape.

- 'Chunky' = Pieces of suspect materials are cut into 1" x 1" squares and applied directly to skin using Scanpor tape. Wet the chunkies with water prior to applying. These are often late reactors, if they react at all. Chunkies are typically reapplied at the 48-hour reading until the completion of testing if there is no reaction at the 48-hour read.
- Testing for fixed drug eruption = Paint suspect allergens directly to lesional skin.

Patch testing interpretation (performed on Day 3 and 5)

1. Mild – non-vesicular, non-infiltrated, pink barely palpable papule(s)
2. Strong – edematous or vesicular reaction
3. Very strong – bullae, spreading of the reaction beyond the patch test site, ulcerations
4. Borderline/doubtful – macular erythema
5. Irritant
6. Negative: normal appearing skin

Late development of positive tests (after day 5–7) can occur with:

- Metals (nickel, palladium, gold)
- Topical antibiotics (neomycin)
- Surfactants
- Methyl methacrylate
- Paraphenylenediamine
- Corticosteroids

Causes of long-lasting patch reaction: Gold and metal salts (nickel, chromate)

Determining Relevance

This is the hardest part – interpreting whether the patch tests are actually relevant to the patient's eruption. You can use the NACDG relevance coding criteria as a resource for understanding this or COADEX below.

NACDG Relevance Coding Criteria:

- Relevance will be considered definite if a use test with the putative item containing the suspected allergen is positive or positive patch to object/product.
- Relevance will be considered probable if the substance identified by patch testing can be verified as present in the known skin contactants of the patient.
- Relevance will be considered as possible if the patient is exposed to circumstances in which skin contact with materials known to contain the putative allergen will likely occur.

Recommended Dose Limits of Immunosuppressants for Patch Testing (Table 7.1)

- Tolerated medications
  - Methotrexate <0.25 mg/kg/week
  - Prednisone <10 mg/day or off for at least 1 (ideally 2) week(s)
  - Biologics (TNFa and IL12/23 inhibitors are okay)
- Contraindicated given high probability of impacting test results
  - Prednisone >10 mg/day
  - Cyclosporine >2 mg/kg/day
  - Dupilumab (Dupixent)
  - IM triamcinolone within the last 4 weeks
  - Topical steroids used on the testing site
  - Phototherapy or sunburn/tanning within the last 2 weeks.

Common Allergens (Tables 7.2 and 7.3)

Basics of Some Allergen Categories

Surfactants
- Decyl glucoside

TABLE 7.1 Recommended dose limits of immunosuppressants for patch testing: adapted from a consensus of the North American Contact Dermatitis Group (NACDG) members

Agent	General Recommnedations	NACDG consensus opinion
Topical corticoids on test site	Avoid for 3–7 days in test area(s)	Evenly split between 3 and 7 days
UV exposure at test site	Avoid for 2 weeks post exposure	Avoid for 1 week
Oral prednisone	OK to test on as long as <10 mg/day (best to DC_ for 1–14 days)	10 mg OK, but best if able to DC for 3–5 days
IM triamcinolone	Wait between 3 and 4 weeks post injection	Wait until 4 weeks after injection
Methotrexate	Unknown to little/no effect (Methotrexate <0.25 mg/kg/week may be okay)	Little to no effect
TNF-ct inhibitors	Unknown to little/no effect	Little to no effect
Ustekinumab	Unknown to little/no effect	Little to no effect
Azathioprine	Dose-dependent inhibition	Dose-dependent inhibition
Cyclosporine	Dose-dependent inhibition	Dose-dependent inhibition
Mycophenolate mofetil	Dose-dependent inhibition	Dose-dependent inhibition
Tacrolimus (systemic)	Dose-dependent inhibition	Dose-dependent inhibition

Adapted from: Fowler Jr JF, Maibach HI, Zirwas M, et al. Effects of immunomodulatory agents on patch testing. Dermatitis. 2012;23(6):301–2

DC indicates discontinue, *IM* intramuscular, *UV* ultraviolet

Table 7.2 Information on the NACDG standard series screening allergens

1	*Benzocaine* – Topical anesthetic. Cross-reacts with PABA (sunscreen), sulfa, aminobenzene, azo dyes (disperse blue 106 and 124 and orange #3), PPD
2	*2-mercaptobenzothiazole* – Rubber accelerator. Used in natural and synthetic rubber products and is commonly found in athletic shoes. #1 cause of ACD from shoes
3	*Rosin (colophony)* – Colophony, also known as rosin, comes from the sap of coniferous trees, such as pine. Its main allergen is abietic acid/abitol. It is found in personal care products (mascaras, diapers, and feminine napkins), adhesives (Band-Aids, ostomy appliances, DuoDERM), glues, dental materials, beauty products (wax depilatories), topical medications, glues, and waxes. It is used as a grip aid for certain sports (bowling, gymnastics, baseball, rock climbing) and as rosin for string instruments. Some individuals with this allergy have difficulty with pine trees and pine decorations
4	*Paraphenylenediamine* – Used in permanent and semi-permanent hair dyes, black henna, and black rubber products (black rubber hoses, tires, tool grips). Can cause purpuric ACD and acute swelling reactions. People can be allergic to other para-amino compounds, such as benzocaine PABA, sulfa, aminobenzene, IPPD, azo dyes (disperse blue 106 and 124 and orange #3), sulfa medications (thiazide diuretics, sulfonylurea antidiabetics, sulfa containing antibiotics), and 4,4-diaminodiphenylmethane (plastic eyeglass frames)
5	*Dimethylaminopropylamine (DMAPA)* – Surfactant impurity forms when cocamidopropyl betaine and oleamidopropyl dimethylamine are made by reacting fatty acids extracted from coconut oil with DMAPA
6	*Fragrance mix II* – Combo of six fragrance materials: amyl cinnamal, cinnamic aldehyde, cinnamyl alcohol, hydroxycitronellal, eugenol, isoeugenol, geraniol, oakmoss (evernia prunastri). Mix is emulsified in sorbitan sesquioleate

Table 7.2 (continued)

7	*Lanolin (Americhol)* – Aka lanolin alcohol. Vehicle. Wool fat obtained from the fleece of sheep. Commonly used in skin care products, cosmetics, topical medicines, and barrier creams. May cross-react with Eucerin/Aquaphor (has lanolin in it). Most common cause of allergic cheilitis. Lanolin paradox: lanolin-containing topical meds tend to be more sensitizing than lanolin-containing cosmetics (probably because meds are applied to damaged skin while cosmetics are applied to normal skin)
8	*Carba mix* – Rubber accelerator: the combination of three chemicals (diphenylguanidine, zinc dibutyldithiocarbamate, and zinc diethyldithiocarbamate) used in the manufacture of many rubber products, such as gloves and shoes. Can also be found in pesticides/herbicides. "Bleached rubber/elastic" releases carbamates but patch testing will be negative - need to clinically suspect. Cross-reacts with thiurams
9	*Neomycin* – Topical antibiotics, especially triple antibiotic ointments. Most frequent antibiotic causing contact sensitivity. Co-reactivity with bacitracin. Cross-reacts with gentamicin
10	*Thiuram mix* – Rubber accelerator: contains four chemicals (tetramethylthiuram monosulfide, tetramethylthiuram disulfide, tetraethylthiuram disulfide, dipentamethylenethiuram disulfide) used in the manufacture of many rubber products, such as gloves and shoes. Can also be found in pesticides/herbicides. #1 cause of glove dermatitis. Cross-reacts with carbamates. Cross-reacts with disulfiram (Antabuse)
11	*Polyhexamethylene biguanide/Polyaminopropyl biguanide* – Commonly used as antiseptic: used in a variety of products (wound care dressings, contact lens cleaning solutions, perioperative cleansing products, swimming pool cleaners)
12	*Ethylenediamine dihydrochloride* – substance used to manufacture various drugs and industrial compounds. Can be found in topical medications. Structurally related to hydroxyzine. Aminophylline = theophylline + ethylenediamine, promethazine, tripelennamine, piperazines (eg, cyclizine, cetirizine, meclizine)

(continued)

Table 7.2 (continued)

13	*Bisphenol A (epoxy resin)* – Epoxy resin: reactive in the "uncured" state but technically inert once cured. Found in plastics, paints, 2-part glues and adhesives, and flooring and composite materials with a curing agent. Must protect self with vinyl gloves since it will penetrate rubber gloves (although vinyl gloves may have bisphenol A as a component). Cured epoxy is not sensitizing.
14	*Quaternium-15* – Formaldehyde releaser. Most frequent preservative to cause ACD in the USA. Commonly found in clothing, personal products, personal care products/makeup/cosmetics
15	*4-tert-butylphenol formaldehyde resin* – Adhesive/glue. Used in shoes, upholstery, leather, carbonless copy paper, cardiac electrodes, and hearing aids. Leading cause of shoe dermatitis worldwide. Used in neoprene wet suits, shin guards, swim goggles, and sports equipment. Co-sensitivity with epoxy resin
16	*Ethylhexylglycerin* – Dual antimicrobial and emollient. Found in cosmetics and sunscreen. As formaldehyde and parabens fall out of popularity, EHG is increasingly being used in "formaldehyde-free," "paraben-free" baby and "hypoallergenic" products. Infrequent allergen
17	*Black rubber mix* – Rubber. Contains three chemicals used to manufacture black rubber products (PPD-derivatives: N-isopropyl-N-phenyl-4PPD, N-cyclohexyl-N-phenyl-4-PPD, and N-N′-diphenyl-PPD). Used in shoes, sports equipment, and tires. Also found in pesticides/herbicides. Can cross-react with paraphenylenediamine (PPD)
18	*Potassium dichromate* – Metal salt derived from chromium. Commonly found in metal objects, *wet* cement, tanned leather products, green felt/fabric, yellow-green pigment (tattoos, cosmetics), crude oil (engine, aircraft workers), chromic gut suture, and matches. May have cobalt and chromate co-reactivity in cement workers

Table 7.2 (continued)

19	*Myroxylon pereirae (balsam of Peru)* – Fragrance/flavoring. Resinous liquid with cinnamon vanilla odor harvested from trees grown in El Salvador. Allergens include cinnamon oils (cinnamates, eugenol, vanillin), eugenol/isoeugenol, ferulic acid, benzoic acid derivatives, and coniferin derivatives. Found in cosmetics, fragrances, medical supplies, and foods (citrus, sweets, tomatoes, spices, condiments, liquors). Cross-reacts with colophony, turpentine, and propolis
20	*Nickel sulfate* – Metal. Commonly found in metal/jewelry (white gold, 14-carat gold, chrome, bronze, brass, silvery metals), coins, keys, tools, clothing fasteners (buttons/snaps/zippers/underwires), personal care products (clippers, eyelash curlers, razors), eyeshadows, musical instruments, and medical implants. Dimethylglyoxime test determines release of nickel from metal objects.
21	*Diazolidinyl urea (Germall II)* – Formaldehyde-releasing preservative. Used in personal care products
22	*DMDM hydantoin (Glydant)* – Formaldehyde-releasing preservative with broad spectrum of activity. Used in personal care products
23	*Imidazolidinyl urea (Germall 115)* – Formaldehyde-releasing preservative. Used in personal care products
24	*Bacitracin* – Antibiotic. Topical antibiotic used alone and in triple-antibiotic ointments used to treat skin, eye, and ear infections. Common co-sensitization with neomycin
25	*Mixed dialkyl thioureas* – Antioxidants used in the manufacture of synthetic rubber: neoprene/spandex. Can also be found in pesticides/herbicides
26	*Methylchloroisothiazolinone/methylisothiazolinone (Kathon CG, Euxyl K 100)* – Preservative. Used in personal care products (cosmetics, wet wipes, personal hygiene products, bath and baby products, hair coloring agents, hair care products, nail polish), toiletries, household cleaning products (dish soap, stain removers, detergents, fabric softeners, cleansers), paint, and glues including school glue. Sodium bisulfite can inactivate MCI/MI in paint for occupational problems

(continued)

TABLE 7.2 (continued)

27	*Paraben mix* – Preservative. Widely used in cosmetics and foods in over-the-counter medications, cosmetics, personal care, and hygiene products. Least common sensitizer of all the preservatives
28	*Cinnamic aldehyde* – Perfume/flavor: chemical compound that gives cinnamon its flavor and odor
29	*Fragrance mix I* – Fragrance: combination of eight fragrance materials: citral, farnesol, coumarin, citronellol, a-hexyl cinnamaldehyde, hydroxyisohexyl 3-cyclohexene carboxaldehyde (lyrral). The mix is emulsified with sorbitol sesquioleate
30	*Amidoamine* – Surfactant. Intermediate contaminant in the process of making cocamidopropyl betaine. Commonly found in soaps, shampoos, conditioners, and hair products. Will not be on label; look for cocamidopropyl betaine.
31	*2-Bromo-2-nitropropane-1,3-diol (Bronopol)* – Formaldehyde-releasing preservative. Widely used in personal care and household products
32	*Sesquiterpene lactone (SL) mix* – Plant allergen from the Compositae family. Allergy can be from direct contact with the plant or from toiletry products or related foods that use the plant extracts. Most common plants: chrysanthemum, ragweed, feverfew, artichokes, and endives. Cross-reacts with permethrin *Bisabolol* is a sesquiterpene derivative in Aquaphor Healing Ointment
33	*2-Hydroxyethyl methacrylate* – Acrylates (salts polymerized to solid plastics – fully formed plastics are inert, but building block acrylates are strong irritants and allergens). Monomers found in UV inks, adhesives, lacquers, dental materials, and artificial nails (gel nails, dip nails, acrylic/sculpted nails). Can easily penetrate gloves, especially vinyl, nitrile, and latex
34	*Hydroperoxides of linalool* – Fragrance chemical found naturally in lavender

TABLE 7.2 (continued)

35	*2-Hydroxy-4-methoxybenzophenone (benzophenone-3)* – Sunscreen and preservative. Found in cosmetics as well as perfumes, dyes, paints, varnishes, pesticides, and plastics to extend shelf life and reduce photodegeneration. May cross-react with ketoprofen, tiaprofenic acid, and fenofibrate. Cause of photoallergy. High cross-reactivity with octocrylene, ketoprofen, and fenofibrate
36	*4-Chloro-3,5-xylenol (PCMX) (chloroxylenol)* – Preservative found in medicated petroleum jelly, EKG paste. Second most common allergy inducer in antibacterial agents
37	*Lauryl glucoside* – Surfactant. Used in toiletries labeled for individuals with sensitive skin. Less likely to co-react with other surfactants
38	*Methylisothiazolinone* – See number 26
39	*Sodium metabisulfite/disulfite* – Preservative. Used as an additive in food (salad dressing, beer, wine) and as a cleaning agent in home brewing equipment and water reverse osmosis systems. Can be a marker of hot tub "shock treatment" allergy (which contains sulfites). Also found in injectable medications, prescription topical products, cosmetics, and personal care products
40	*Methyldibromo glutaronitrile + Phenoxyethanol (MDBGN/PE) (Euxyl K 400)* – Preservative (banned in Europe). MDBGN is the allergen. Found in cosmetics
41	*Diphenylguanidine* – Rubber accelerator. (Part of Carba mix)
42	*Cetearyl glucoside* – Natural, vegetable-based emulsifier derived from plant sugars and fatty acids
43	*Iodopropynyl butylcarbamate* – Preservative. Used in personal care products and industrial products. There are little reactions between this and other sources of carbamates
44	*Ethyl acrylate* – Acrylic monomer; can be polymerized to form plastics and sculptured nails. Rubber gloves do not protect. Acrylates also found in adhesive and dental products

(continued)

Table 7.2 (continued)

45	*Benzophenone-4* – Sunscreen. Photosensitizer
46	*Tosylamide formaldehyde resin* – Preservative. Found in nail polish: added to nail varnish to facilitate adhesion of the varnish to the nail
47	*Methyl methacrylate* – Acrylic monomer. Artificial nails: banned from nail preparations. Orthopedic bone cement. May also be found in dental materials and adhesives
48	*Cobalt chloride* – Metal. Commonly found in metal alloys used to make tools, leather, keys, magnets, jewelry (darker silver), orthopedic and dental implants, and implanted cardiac devices. Dyes (blue green paint, blue tattoos, hair dyes, ceramic dyes). Part of vitamin B12. Added to cement to bind to chromate and decrease its sensitivity. Can be used in plastics manufacturing. Cause poral reaction (irritant). Co-sensitization with nickel. Cobalt spot test with disodium 1-nitroso-2-naphthol-3,6-disulfonate (turns orange-red)
49	*Tixocortol-21-pivalate* – Topical steroid: screen for Class A corticosteroids. Only two topicals in Class A: hydrocortisone and hydrocortisone acetate
50	*Budesonide* – Topical steroid: Screen for Class B corticosteroids: Triamcinolone group. B and D cross-react
51	*Benzisothiazolinone* – Preservative/antimicrobial used in paints, varnishes, adhesives, papermaking, laundry detergents, dish soap, paint, and glues. Cross-reacts with MCI/MI
52	*Disperse dye mix* – Textile dye for synthetic fabrics (e.g., polyester, nylon, acetate). Disperse blue mix (106 > 124) is a mix of two textile dyes. Found most commonly in dark-colored textiles (undergarments and uniforms) and acetate liners of women's clothing
53	*Propolis* – Impurity in beeswax. Also known as "bee glue": a resinous mixture that bees collect from tree buds, sap flows, or other botanical sources that ends up as an impurity in beeswax. It is used by bees in the making of honeycombs. Can be found in Burt's bees products, lip balms, lip sticks, wound care products, and personal care products. Pharmaceutical grade beeswax safe if needed. Often cross-reacts with other fragrances/botanicals/plants

Table 7.2 (continued)

54	*Lidocaine* – Topical anesthetic
55	*Propylene glycol* – Vehicle, humectant, emollient, softening agent, and preservative. Used in personal care products and cosmetics. Can also be found in topical, eye, and ear medications, as well as certain foods (glazing agent, drink mixes, creamers, beverages, packaged foods, processed meats and veggies, lite beer). Found in the base of many medicated ointments. Can be an irritant
56	*Hydroperoxides of limonene* – Major component of oil extracted from citrus rind. In tea tree oil and eucalyptus. Found in up to 97% of essential oils in varying concentrations
57	*Cocamidopropyl betaine* – Surfactant. Foaming agent derived from coconut oil used in bath products like shampoos, hand soaps, and body washes. DMAPA and amidoamine are impurities created in the processing of CAPB (see below in surfactant section)
58	*Formaldehyde* – Preservative and disinfectant in many personal care, household, certain vaccines, industrial products, plywood glue, leather glues, plastics, coatings, fiber board, nail polish, and Brazilian-style keratin hair straighteners. Fixative used in embalming. May be an irritant. Melamine formaldehyde is in many textiles, especially wrinkle-free, permanent-press clothing, or textile with other specific characteristics. Dermabond is hydrolyzed in the body to formaldehyde. Schiff's reagent test: Office screening to detect formaldehyde in clothing. No formaldehyde in nylon. Formaldehyde-containing foods: aspartame (metabolized to formaldehyde/formic acid), coffee (especially instant), smoked ham, cod, caviar, and also in cigarette smoke
59	*Oleamidopropyl dimethylamine* – Emulsifier (a substance that blends together non-mixable liquids like oil and water). Used in personal care products
60	*Ammonium persulfate* – Bleaching and oxidizing agent. Used to lighten hair as well as flour. Used in industrial and consumer disinfectants and bleaches. Common allergens in hairdressers. Marker of pool/hot tub dermatitis to potassium peroxymonosulfate (used to chemically "shock" the water)

(continued)

TABLE 7.2 (continued)

61	*Coconut diethanolamide (cocamide DEA)* – Surfactant. Derived from coconut oils. Used in cosmetics, wipes, shampoos, and detergents to create a creamy texture and provide a foaming action. Less likely to co-react with other surfactants
62	*Compositae mix* – Plant allergen: Mix of five plant extracts from the Compositae (Asteraceae) family, e.g., arnica, German chamomile, lactone parthenolide, tansy, yarrow, daisy, dandelions, ragweed, and sunflower. Includes foods such as lettuce, endive, chicory, and artichoke. Can cause airborne dermatitis and contact dermatitis
63	*Chlorhexidine digluconate* – Antimicrobial cleansing agent. Used in preparation for many surgeries and as a dental rinse
64	*Melaleuca alternifolia (tea tree oil)* – An essential oil obtained from the leaves of the *Melaleuca* plant with antibacterial/mite properties. Toxic when swallowed. D-limonene is the allergen
65	Cananga odorata *oil (ylang-ylang)* – Essential oil obtained from the flower (*Cananga odorata* or ylang-ylang) of the cananga tree
66	*Carvone* – Found naturally in many essential oils used in flavoring and perfumery
67	*Octylisothiazolinone* – Fungicide for use in paints, cutting oils, wallpaper adhesives, etc. Can also be used for leather
68	*Decyl glucoside* – Surfactant. Used in toiletries labeled for individuals with sensitive skin. Less likely to co-react with other surfactants
69	*Sodium benzoate* – Preservative. Widely used in acidic foods such as salad dressings, carbonated drinks, jams and fruit juices, pickles, and condiments. It is also used as a preservative in medicines and cosmetics
70	Mentha piperita *oil (peppermint oil)* – Essential oil from peppermint, used in many flavorings (e.g., toothpaste)
71	*Coco glucoside* – Non-ionic surfactant, used as a foaming, cleansing, conditioning, and viscosity building agent to liquid cleansers and shampoos

Table 7.2 (continued)

72	*Benzalkonium chloride* – Preservative. Used in cold sterilization and in some personal care products
73	*Benzyl alcohol* – Produced naturally by many plants. Commonly used in soap, perfume, and flavor industries as a preservative
74	*Cetrimonium chloride* – Topical antiseptic and surfactant; also commonly used in hair conditioners and shampoos as a conditioning agent
75	*Phenoxyethanol* – Preservative used in many cosmetics and personal care products
76	*Panthenol* – Alcohol form of the B vitamin pantothenic acid. Used in skincare products as a humectant because of its ability to attract and hold moisture
77	*P-toluenediamine sulfate* – Permanent hair dye which is a common source of allergy in hairdressers
78	*Polymyxin B* – Antibiotic used for many gram negative infections (commonly part of triple antibiotic)
79	*Pramoxine* – Used to temporarily relieve pain and itching from insect bites; poison ivy, poison oak, or poison sumac; minor cuts, scrapes, or burns. Found in many anti-itch, hemorrhoid, or other topical creams
80	*Gold sodium thiosulfate* – Common sensitizer with elicitation of symptoms linked to gold in jewelry, occupational exposure to gold, and dental restorations. Common false-positive reaction (no relevance). Classically can cause long-lasting patch test reactions

TABLE 7.3 Other important allergens

α-Methylene-γ-butyrolactone – *Alstroemeria* (Peruvian lily)
Ammonium thioglycolate – Alkaline perm solution. Super rare sensitizer
Carmine – Derived from an insect. Natural red #40, found in cosmetics (blush, lipstick, mascara) and in some artificially dyed foods
Cetylstearyl alcohol – Emulsifier in cosmetics and topical medications
Chloroquinol – Anti-infective topical and systemic agent
Clobetasol-17-propionate – Topical steroid
Ethyl-2-cyanoacrylate – Acrylate in super glues (Krazy glue). Used for press on nails, silk nails, and artificial eyelashes
Cysteamine hydrochloride – neutral perms. Doesn't penetrate latex gloves. Uncommon sensitizer
Desoximetasone – Topical steroid. Lowest likelihood of ACD
Diallyl disulfide – Allergen in garlic/onions
Dimethyl fumarate – Antimicrobial found in sachets (couches, shoe boxes)
Ethylene urea melamine formaldehyde mix – Wash and wear clothing dermatitis
Glutaral (glutaraldehyde) – Preservative used to sterilize medical and dental equipment. Can also be found in waterless hand cleansers
Glyceryl monothioglycolate – perms (acid perms). Can remain in the hair shaft for 3 months. Penetrates rubber and vinyl gloves
Hydrocortisone-17-butyrate – Topical steroids: screen for Class D corticosteroids, clobetasol group
Hydroquinone – Rubber antioxidant and bleaching agent. Used as a topical medication for lightening skin
Lavandula angustifolia *oil* – Essential oil obtained from lavender

TABLE 7.3 (continued)

2-Hydroxypropyl methacrylate – Acrylate monomer in dental composites and sealants
Majantole – Majantole is a flavor and fragrance ingredient that has a lily scent. Found in personal care products and tobacco formulations
Mercapto mix – contains three chemicals used in the manufacture of many rubber products (like athletic shoes). Also found in pesticides/herbicides and sponge makeup applicators
Parthenolide – A type of sesquiterpene lactone and marker of this allergy found in the feverfew herb and used as an anti-inflammatory agent
Phenyl-a-naphthylamine – Rubber antioxidant
Shellac – A resin excreted by an insect. Used mainly in lacquers, varnishes, and wax. May also be used in mascaras, inks, paper, leather finishing, cement, hats, coatings of candy, fruit, medicines
Sorbic acid – preservative for steroid creams. Suspect sorbic acid allergies in patients with dermatitis made work by topical steroids
Thimerosal – Mercury-derived preservative. Used in otic and ophthalmic solutions, in some vaccines. Positive reactions usually a marker of previous vaccines
DL-alpha-tocopherol – Vitamin E. Anti-inflammatory
Triclosan – Preservative. Halogenated phenol classified as a disinfectant, used often in antibacterial soaps
Tulipalin A – Flowers/vegetables, like Peruvian lily, asparagus, hyacinth, and tulips. Common in florists

- Cocamidopropyl betaine (CAPB)
- Amidoamine (AA)
- Dimethylaminopropylamine (DMAPA)
- Oleamidopropyl dimethylamine (OPD)
- Cocamide diethanolamide (CDEA)

N.B.: Cocamidopropyl betaine (CAPB) is formed by reacting fatty acids extracted from coconut oil with DMAPA. This first step yields cocamidopropyl dimethylamine (amidoamine, cocamidoamine), which then reacts with sodium monochloroacetate to give the end products CAPB. There are major known impurities of CAPB including low quantities of the starting material DMAPA and the intermediate amidoamine. Oleamidopropyl dimethylamine results from the reaction of DMAPA and oleic acid. The CAPB and OPD share DMAPA as a starting material.

Rubber

Rubber accelerants
- Thiurams
- Carbamates
- Mercaptobenzothiazoles
- Diphenylguanidine
- Dialkyl thioureas

Rubber antioxidants
- Phenyl-a-naphthylamine
- Hydroquinone
- Paraphenylenediamine (black rubber)

Preservatives
Formaldehyde and formaldehyde releasers

- Quaternium-15
- Imidazolidinyl urea
- Diazolidinyl urea
- DMDM hydantoin
- 2-Bromo-2-nitropropane-1,3-diol (Bronopol)

Other Preservatives
- Methylchloroisothiazolinone/methylisothiazolinone
- Benzisothiazolinone
- Methyldibromoglutaronitrile
- Phenoxyethanol
- Benzalkonium chloride
- Iodopropynyl butylcarbamate

- Parabens
- Tea tree oil

Para-Amino Cross-Reactors

Paraphenylenediamine, benzocaine (ester anesthetics), azo dyes (textile dyes, especially disperse orange), PABA sunscreens, 4,4-diaminodiphenylmethane (in plastic sunglass frames), thiazide diuretics, sulfonamide antibiotics, sulfonylurea antidiabetic agents, PAS, celecoxib, saccharin sweeteners.

Photoallergens

Most common relevant photoallergens are benzophenone-3, octyl dimethyl para-aminobenzoic acid (PABA), and butylmethoxy-dibenzoylmethane.

Fragrance

Fragrances include both perfumes and natural fragrance such as essential oils and other botanical extracts. Products marketed as "unscented" or "fragrance-free" often contain masking fragrances and/or botanicals, respectively, and thus are frequently not truly fragrance free.

Topical Corticosteroids Allergy (Table 7.4)

Corticosteroid Classification Systems

Group 1: (No C16-methyl substitution, no halogen substitution) molecules are more likely to cause delayed hypersensitivity reaction (includes budesonide, hydrocortisone, hydrocortisone 17-butyrate, methylprednisolone, prednisolone, triamcinolone, tixocortol pivalate, prednisone).

Group 2: C16/C17 cis ketal or diol structure, no halogen substitution (except fluocinolone, fluocinonide, halocinonide). It includes desonide, fluocinolone, fluocinonide, halocinonide, triamcinolone acetonide, triamcinolone diacetate, and triamcinolone hexacetonide.

TABLE 7.4 Information and classes of corticosteroid allergy

Topical steroid allergy	Four classes based on frequency of cross-reactions (somewhat unpredictable); metabolites and intermediates can cross-react "Edge effect": Erythema occurs only around the edge of the chamber = true allergy Delayed positive reactions are common; require late readings for proper detection
Class A (hydrocortisone type)	*Screening allergen: Tixocortol pivalate* Hydrocortisone (acetate, succinate, phosphate)[a] (C17 or C21 acetate esters), prednisone, prednisolone, methylprednisolone, cortisone[a], meprednisone
Class B (triamcinolone-type)	*Screening allergen: Budesonide* Triamcinolone[a], fluocinolone acetonide[a], fluocinonide[a], desonide[a] ("-ide" suffix), budesonide
Class C (betamethasone type; *not* valerate)	Betamethasone sodium phosphate (not valerate), dexamethasone, dexamethasone disodium phosphate, fluocortolone, desoximetasone[a]; *least allergenic class*
Class D1	*Screening allergen: Clobetasol-17-propionate* Alclometasone dipropionate[a], betamethasone dipropionate[a], clobetasol propionate[a], clobetasone butyrate[a], diflorasone diacetate[a], fluticasone propionate[a], mometasone furoate, oral/IM betamethasone ("-ate" suffix)
Class D2	*Screening allergen: Hydrocortisone-17-butyrate* Hydrocortisone buteprate[a], hydrocortisone butyrate[a], hydrocortisone valerate, prednicarbate[a]

[a]Topicals

Corticosteroids with lower risk of sensitization

- Class C
- Methylated and halogenated members of Class D
- Newer synthetic steroids like fluticasone propionate (Cutivate) and mometasone furoate (Elocon)

Class A and B cross-reacts with class D2
D1 exhibits quite loss cross-reactivity with other groups
When allergic to one class, test for cross-reactions in all groups

Group 3 (least allergenic): C16-methyl substitution of the D-ring and *halogenation* stabilizes the corticosteroid molecule, protecting them from metabolization and decreasing their sensitization potential. It includes aclometasone, betamethasone, clobetasol, dexamethasone, diflucortolone, diflorasone diacetate, fluticasone, and mometasone. Alclometasone is the most allergenic in the least allergenic group probably because the halogen (chlorine) is far from the C9 position, which is responsible for its molecular stabilization.

Determining Relevance

This is the hardest part – interpreting whether the patch tests are actually relevant to the patient's eruption. The *COADEX* system can help with this.

- *C*urrent relevance – the patient has been exposed to the allergen during the current episode of dermatitis and improves when the exposure ceases.
- *O*ld or past relevance – the patient was sensitized to this in the past, and it caused a rash in the past but has nothing to do with the rash that the patient currently presents for.
- *A*ctively sensitized – the patient presents with a sensitization (late) reaction. The patient may have become sensitized to this through the patch test process.
- *D*o not know – the relevance is not known. Not sure if the exposure is current or old – or perhaps merely an irritant reaction.
- *Ex*posed – (i) cross-reaction, the positive test is due to a cross-reaction with another allergen; (ii) exposed, a history of exposure but not resulting in dermatitis from that exposure or a history of exposure but a definite positive allergic patch test.

If patients are unable to get patch tested or refuse, could do a therapeutic trial of hypoallergenic products to see if their skin clears and could give hint if ACD is playing a role. List of hyporeactive products is shown in Table 7.5.

TABLE 7.5 Hyporeactive product list

Product type	Specific product
Shave cream	Vanicream Shave Cream
Shampoo	Free & Clear Shampoo (with or without zinc), TSal Shampoo
Conditioner	Free & Clear Conditioner
	DHS Color Safe Rinse
	Magick Botanicals Spray on Detangler/ Conditioner
Styling	Free & Clear Styling Gel
	Cleure styling gel
	Pure argan oil
Hair dye	Light Mountain Natural Hair Dye
Cleanser	Aveeno Moisturizing Bar
	Neutrogena Hydrating Cleanser
	Theraplex Gentle Cleanser
	DHS Body Wash
	Cetaphil Gentle Skin Cleanser
Moisturizer	Cleure Body Lotion
	Aveeno Eczema Therapy Moisturizing Cream
	Aveeno Skin Relief Healing Ointment
	Neutrogena Norwegian Formula Hand Cream, Neutrogena Body Oil Fragrance Free
	CeraVe Moisturizing Cream, CeraVe Healing ointment
	Vanicream Moisturizing Cream
	Vaniply Ointment
	Coconut oil, cocoa butter, shea butter

TABLE 7.5 (continued)

Product type	Specific product
Sunblock	Vanicream sunscreen, Cotz sensitivie skin sunscreen
Foundation	Dermablend Smooth Liquid Camo
	Dermablend Cover Crème Foundation
Blush	Cleure Cream-to-Powder blush
Bronzer	Benefit Hoola Bronzer
Powder	Bare Mineral XL Original Veil
	Dermablend setting powder
Mascara	Tarte Lights, Camera, Lashes Mascara
Eyeshadow	Cleure Loose Mineral Eyeshadow
Eyeliner	Sephora Long Lasting Kohl Pencil (black/dark brown shades only)
Makeup remover	Albolene
Antiperspirant	Almay Antiperspirant Deodorant Roll-On
Deodorant	Vanicream Deodorant Stick
Toothpaste	Cleure toothpaste, Tom's Silly Strawberry toothpaste
Topical steroids	Desoximetasone ointment
	Desonide ointment
	Locoid Lipocream or Lotion
	Cloderm Cream

(continued)

Table 7.5 (continued)

Product type	Specific product
Anti-itch	Aveeno Anti-itch Lotion
Bath oil	RoBathol
Laundry detergent	Nellie's Laundry Soda

Adapted from: Scheman A, Rakowski E-M. Hyporeactive products 2015: an adjunct in the treatment of contact dermatitis and other chronic eczemas. Dermatitis. 2015;26(6):293–5
BHT butylated hydroxytoluene, *CSA* cetostearyl alcohol, *PH* phenoxyethanol, *P* parabens, *BAC* benzalkonium chloride, *TEA* triethanolamine, *VE* vitamin E

Chapter 8
Pharmacotherapy

Topical Corticosteroids

Strengths of extend from Class 1 (super-potent) to Class 7 (least potent/weak) (Table 8.1)

S. Hylwa et al., *Pocket Dermatology*,
https://doi.org/10.1007/978-3-030-83602-3_8

Table 8.1 Topical corticosteroids categorized by strength and traditional allergen class (see contact dermatitis section for more information about newer classification systems for ACD to topical steroids)

Structural class	**Class A: hydrocortisone type**	**Class B: triamcinolone acetonide type**	**Class C: betamethasone type**	**Class D1: betamethasone dipropionate type**	**Class D2: methylprednisolone aceponate type**
Class 7: Least potent	Hydrocortisone Hydrocortisone acetate Tixocortol pivalate				
Class 6: Low potent		Desonide 0.05% C,F Fluocinolone acetonide 0.01% C,S Triamcinolone acetonide 0.025% C Triamcinolone diacetate 0.025% C		Alclometasone dipropionate 0.05% C,O Betamethasone valerate 0.1% C	

Class 5: Lower mid-strength		Desonide 0.05% O Fluocinolone acetonide 0.025% C Triamcinolone acetonide 0.1% C, 0.025% O,L Triamcinolone diacetate 0.1% C		Betamethasone dipropionate 0.05% L Betamethasone valerate C,L Fluticasone propionate 0.05% C	Hydrocortisone buteprate 0.1% C,O,S Hydrocortisone butyrate 0.1% C,O,S Hydrocortisone valerate 0.2% C Prednicarbate 0.1% C
Class 4: Mid-strength		Amcinonide 0.1% L Fluocinolone acetonide 0.1%, 0.025% O Halcinonide 0.025% C Triamcinolone acetonide 0.1% O Triamcinolone diacetate 0.1% O	Clocortolone pivalate 0.1% C Desoximetasone 0.05% C	Betamethasone valerate 0.12% F Clobetasone butyrate 0.05% Mometasone furoate 0.1% C,L	Hydrocortisone valerate 0.2% O

(continued)

Table 8.1 continued

Structural class	Class A: hydrocortisone type	Class B: triamcinolone acetonide type	Class C: betamethasone type	Class D1: betamethasone dipropionate type	Class D2: methylprednisolone aceponate type
Class 3: Upper mid-strength		Amcinonide 0.1% L Fluocinonide 0.05% Triamcinolone acetonide 0.1% C, O Triamcinolone diacetate 0.1% C,O		Betamethasone dipropionate 0.05% C Betamethasone valerate 0.1% O Clobetasone butyrate 0.05% Diflorasone diacetate 0.05% C Fluticasone propionate 0.005% O Mometasone furoate 0.1% O	
Class 2: High potent		Amcinonide 0.1% O,L,C Budesonide 0.025% C Fluocinonide 0.05% C,O,G,S Halocinonide 0.1% C,O,S	Desoximetasone 0.25% C, 0.05% G	Betamethasone dipropionate 0.05% O,C Betamethasone valerate 0.1% Diflorasone diacetate 0.05%	

Class 1: Superpotent				Betamethasone dipropionate 0.05% G,OL Clobetasol propionate 0.05% C,O,G,S,F Diflorasone diacetate 0.05% O	
Additional info	Oral: Cloprednol Fludrocortisone acetate Methylprednisolone, prednisolone	Oral: Budesonide Triamcinolone	Oral: Dexamethasone	Oral/IM: Betamethasone	Oral/IV: Hydrocortisone
Cross-reactions	Cross-reacts with B and D2	Cross-reacts with A and D2			Cross-reacts with Class A and B
Patch test screening allergen	Tixocortal-21 pivalate	Budesonide Triamcinolone acetonide		Clobetasol-17-propionate	Hydrocortisone-17-butyrate

Legend: *C* cream, *G* gel, *L* lotion, *O* ointment, *S* solution, *F* foam

Drug Monitoring

Methotrexate

MOA

Antimetabolite and antifolate. Synthetic analogue of folic acid so binds to dihydrofolate reductase with greater affinity than folic acid which thus inhibits and which subsequently prevents the conversion of dihydrofolate to tetrahydrofolate (a necessary cofactor for purine synthesis and thus DNA/RNA synthesis) > inhibition of cell division.

The inhibition of dihydrofolate reductase may be bypassed by leucovorin (folinic acid [naturally occurring version of folic acid (synthetic vitamin B_9)]) or thymidine.

Renal Excretion

Contraindications

- *Pregnancy (category X)* and lactation
- Females or males considering conception
- Recent/active hepatitis, EtOH abuse, cirrhosis, hepatic fibrosis
- History of chronic infection or active infection
- Renal disease (creatinine *clearance* <50 mL/min)

Relative Contraindications

- Unreliable patient
- Renal or hepatic impairment
- Metabolic disease (obesity or diabetes mellitus)
- Severe hematologic abnormalities
- Immunodeficiency syndromes
- Pulmonary fibrosis
- Increased alcohol intake
- Currently taking chronic NSAIDs, dapsone, TMP-SMX (interfere with folic acid) or tetracycline, phenytoin, phenothiazine, barbiturates, NSAIDs, salicylates, and sulfonamides as they displace the drug on albumin (displaces methotrexate on albumin and thus increases methotrexate levels)

Pre-screening Questions

Any history of no history of liver or kidney disease? History of alcohol abuse, cryptogenic cirrhosis, severe illness, blood abnormality such as leukopenia/thrombocytopenia, chronic active infectious disease, immunodeficiency?

Any concern with inability to comply with directions?

Pregnant or planning to have children? *Teratogenic for both egg and sperm* and abortifacient. Females should not attempt to conceive until off the medication for 1 month/one full menstrual cycle; males should wait 3 months.

Pre-screening Labs

CBC, AST/ALT/Bili/albumin/alk phos, creatinine, HIV, hepatitis serologies (B and C), UA, HCG (for females).

Recheck CBC and LFTs 5–6 days after 1/st dose.

Patients with hypoalbuminemia have higher risk of developing pulmonary complications.

Dosing

Weekly dose varies from 5 to 30 mg weekly. Most doses between 15 and 30 mg weekly.

Doses >15–25 mg/week require IM/SubQ injection but can consider for <15 mg in order to minimize GI effects/limited GI absorption at this dose.

- Consider test dose of 2.5–5 mg ×1 with f/u CBC and LFTs in 1 week, then increase by 2.5 mg every 2–3 weeks to 10–15 mg weekly. (Could also go directly to 15 mg/week after test.)
- If not seeing optimal outcome, can consider switching to IM from po as absorption may be a limiting factor in efficacy.
- Pediatric patients may have reduced oral absorption of methotrexate, so consider injectable form of methotrexate.

Folic acid 1 mg/day on the other days of the week recommended

- Decreases methotrexate-induced adverse effects (decreased GI adverse effects, LFT abnormalities, pancytopenia, and increased ability to tolerate methotrexate)

Increased mtx levels with concomitant use of tetracycline, phenytoin, phenothiazine, barbiturates, NSAIDs, salicylates, and sulfonamides as they displace the drug on albumin.

Side Effects

General: Fatigue, dizziness

Gastrointestinal: Nausea/abdominal pain, anorexia > vomiting, diarrhea, stomatitis/mucositis

Cutaneous: Alopecia, photosensitivity, acral erythema, methotrexate-induced nodules of the hands, UV recall

Hematologic: Pancytopenia (leukopenia, thrombocytopenia)

- *Note: leukopenia and thrombocytopenia indicate overdose (leucovorin [folinic acid] rescue required).*
- *Increased risk of pancytopenia with concomitant use of NSAIDs, dapsone, TMP-SMX, or no folate supplementation.*
- Note that cytopenias can occur late, even with stable dose. Can get severe cytopenia if also on TMP-SMX, so advise patients not to take this medication while on methotrexate.
- Methotrexate levels can be increased by displacing it on plasma proteins (albumin) and can occur with tetracyclines, phenytoin, phenothiazines, sulfonamides, NSAIDs, and salicylates.

Hepatic

- Hepatotoxicity (most common significant adverse effect).
- Hepatic fibrosis – causes liver fibrosis without changes in lab abnormalities. Thought to be more common in patients with fatty liver disease.
  - Monitoring per below required after cumulative dose of 3–4gm or 1.5gm if without or with liver disease, respectively.

Reproductive

- *Teratogenic to both egg and sperm: Females must not become pregnant for one whole menstrual cycle (at least*

1 month), and males should wait 3 months before attempting to conceive.

- *Abortifacient*

Pulmonary

- *Acute pneumonitis – idiosyncratic and can be life-threatening if methotrexate is not stopped; can occur any time during therapy even at low doses and is not fully reversible; pulmonary symptoms (especially a dry, non-productive cough) may require interruption of therapy and careful investigation.*
- Pulmonary fibrosis.

Renal: Methotrexate can accumulate in renal tubules and cause renal toxicity when given at high doses (chemotherapy).

Bony: Concomitant use with radiotherapy may increase risk of soft tissue necrosis and osteonecrosis.

Oncologic

- Low-dose methotrexate has been associated with development of lymphoma.
- Radiation recall.

Neurologic: Headaches

Treat acute toxicity with leucovorin (folinic acid)

Monitoring

Calculate cumulative dose at each visit and record in note

CBC at week (1), 2, 4 then q3–6 month thereafter.

LFTs at week 4, then q3–6 months thereafter.

Renal function at month 3, 6, and 12.

Recheck CBC and LFTs as per above after dosage increases.

Monitor cumulative dose at each visit.

Pulmonary symptoms, especially dry non-productive cough; d/c therapy; refer to pulmonology.

Liver Monitoring

- Assess for fibrosis after 3–4 g cumulative dose in patients without history of liver disease or after 1.5–2 g cumulative dose if history of liver disease/non-alcoholic steatohepatitis (NASH).

- Liver biopsy is gold standard but is invasive and can have significant morbid and mortal side effects and, thus, is falling out of favor ((2009 JAAD Liver bx guidelines below for more details).
- Non-invasive monitoring is now preferred. Refer to GI/hepatology. Options include:
  - U/S fibroscan, MR fibroscan (favored)
  - Serum FibroSpect testing (falling out of favor/not typically used as a singular test)

Liver biopsy guidelines (2009 JAAD Liver bx guidelines below)

- See above that non-invasive monitoring is now preferred given risks associated with liver biopsy; however, biopsy can still be considered based on the patient's risk factors.
- If no hepatic risk factors:
  - No pre-treatment liver biopsy.
  - CBC, LFTs qmonth × 6, then q1–3 months thereafter.
    - For LFT elevations <2× upper limit of normal (ULN), repeat test 2–4 weeks.
    - For LFT elevations >2× ULN but <3× ULN, monitor closely, repeat in 2–4 weeks, and decrease dose as needed.
    - For LFT persistent elevations in 5/9 AST levels in a 12-month period or decline in albumin with normal nutrition, do liver biopsy.
  - Consider liver biopsy after 3.4–4 g total cumulative dose or consider switching to another agent or discontinuing therapy after 3.5–4 g or consider following above guidelines without biopsy.
- Patients with risk factors (alcohol use, hepatitis, IV drug use, family history of liver disease, diabetes, obesity, elderly, previous use of hepatotoxic medication)

- Consider another appropriate medications.
- Consider pre-treatment liver biopsy (or after 2–6 months of therapy to establish medication efficacy and tolerability).
- LFT, albumin, CBC every 1–2 months.
- Liver biopsy if AST values elevated over a 12-month period.
- Liver biopsy if albumin falls below the normal setting in well-controlled psoriasis.
- Liver biopsy at 1–1.5 g and every 1 g thereafter.

Mycophenolate Mofetil (CellCept)

MOA

Active metabolite is mycophenolic acid (MPA) (Myfortic).

Inhibits de novo purine synthesis by inhibiting inosine monophosphate dehydrogenase (IMPDH), which is essential for activated lymphocytes.

T and B cells are particularly affected by the inability to use this salvage pathway to make purines and have to make de novo instead.

The drug is a reversible inhibitor; thus administration of guanosine or deoxyguanosine reverses the cytostatic effects.

Pre-screening Questions

No long-term renal or hepatic toxicity (but may require dose adjustment).

Check for drug interactions (below).

Currently pregnant or planning on becoming pregnant? Lactating?

Needs to enroll in REMS if giving to female of child bearing potential (www.MycophenolateREMS.com)

History of chronic or active infection?

History of malignancy?

History of hematologic abnormality?

Drug Interactions

- Salicylic acid and acyclovir/ganciclovir both elevate MMF levels.

- Antacids and PPIs lower MMF levels as gastric acidity is required for cleavage of MMF to its active state.
- Cholestyramine lowers MMF levels as it increases enterohepatic circulation.
- Probenecid inhibits MPA excretion.
- Azathioprine increases bone marrow toxicity.

Contraindications

Pregnancy, lactation, drug allergy, leucopenia, thrombocytopenia, malignancy, active infection, on meds per above

Relative Contraindications

Peptic ulcer disease, hepatic or renal disease (may require dose adjustment)

Fertility: Women of childbearing age must be enrolled in the FDA REMS program.

Do not conceive × 6 weeks after being on the medication.

Pre-screening Labs

LFTs

CBC

BUN/creatinine, electrolytes

Hepatitis B/C serologies

HIV

T-spot/PPD (tuberculosis screen)

HCG for females (serum beta-HCG) - females of childbearing potential must be enrolled in REMS (www.MycophenolateREMS.com)

Dosing

500–1500 mg BID

- Usual dose 1000 mg BID × 12 weeks.
- Increase or decrease dose by 500 mg monthly up to 4 g/day maximum. Don't take with antacids, iron supplements, and vitamins.
- Children's dosing based on body surface area.

Side Effects

Most common: Nausea/vomiting, abdominal cramps, diarrhea (dose related)

Urinary urgency, frequency, dysuria

Tinnitus
Hematologic

- Reversible dose-related bone marrow toxicity (rare).
- Pure red cell aplasia.
- Thrombocytopenia.
- Pseudo-Pelger-Huet anomaly – form of neutrophil dysplasia with nuclear hypolobation and left shift; may predict development of neutropenia.

Progressive multifocal leukoencephalopathy

Increased risk of carcinogenesis (lymphoma and lymphoproliferative malignancies)

Monitoring

CBC with diff and BMP q2 weeks × 2 months, then every 2–3 months once dose stabilized thereafter. Decrease dose if absolute neutrophil count <1300, d/c if WBC <3000.

LFTs at week 2, 4, then every 2–3 months thereafter (can space out further if needed).

Cyclosporine

MOA

Inhibits release of cytokines (IL2) via blockade of calcineurin, which causes decreased *T-cell* activation (Fig. 8.1).

Metabolized by the P450 3A system

Pre-screening Questions

Is this a disease with B-cell activity/antibody deposition? If so, cyclosporine is not a good choice as this affects T cells ⋙ B cells.

History of hypertension, renal disease, gout, electrolyte abnormalities?

On any P450 meds? Do medication interaction check.

On an aminoglycoside, NSAID, amphotericin B, or vancomycin? (increased risk of renal toxicity if on one of these)

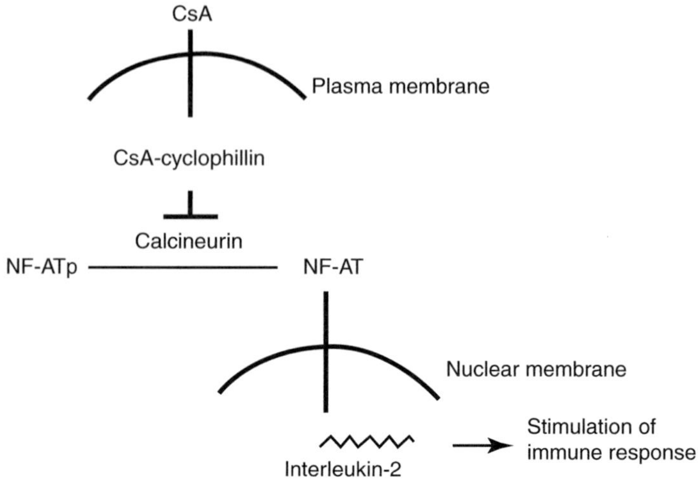

FIGURE 8.1 Mechanism of action of cyclosporine

Drug Interactions

- HMG-CoA may cause rhabdomyolysis.
- ACE-I, beta-blockers, and K-sparing diuretics have increased risk of hyperkalemia.
- NSAIDs increase risk of nephrotoxicity.
- Furosemide can increase uric acid.
- Azoles can increase blood levels.
- H2 blockers and increase CsA levels.

Contraindications

- Malignancy (especially cutaneous lymphoma as there is risk of progression), infection, immunodeficiency, ETOH or drug abuse, abnormal renal function, uncontrolled htn, hepatic dysfunction.

Pre-screening Labs

Blood pressure and renal function (BUN, creatinine, UA) × 2 prior to start of therapy.

CBC, LFTs, lytes, magnesium uric acid, phosphorous, lipids, Hepatitis B & C serologies, HIV × 1 prior to start.

Do med check to make sure no P450 meds as CsA is metabolized by the P450 system.

Advise patients that they should not take aminoglycosides, NSAIDs, amphotericin B, or vancomycin while on cyclosporine as these can potentiate renal toxicity.

Dosing

Comes in 25 mg, 50 mg, and 100 mg capsules; 100 mg/mL solution in 50 mL bottles. Microemulsion formation (Neoral) has greater bioavailability and is the standard.

Dose range: 2–5 mg/kg/day (lipid nanoparticles formulation max dose 4 mg/kg)

- Typical ramp-up: Start at 2.5 mg/kg/day of patient IDEAL body weight divided BID. Keep that dosage ×4 weeks if no adverse effects. If significant improvement hasn't occurred by that time, can increase in 2-week intervals by 0.5 mg/kg/day to a max of 4–5 mg/kg/day. Decrease dose by 25–50% to control adverse effects at any time.
- Dose adjust if creatinine increases 30% from baseline: decrease dose by at least 25% or 1 mg/kg for 4 weeks then.
  - If creatinine drops to <30% of baseline, can continue therapy.
  - If does not drop, then d/c.
- If creatinine increases ≥50% of baseline, d/c therapy.

Treatment durations of up to 6 months have low incidence of renal complications; can be used continuously for up to 1 year according to FDA (2 years by worldwide consensus data).

Cyclosporine should ideally be tapered to prevent flaring.

Side Effects

- *Nephrotoxicity (dose and duration-dependent) – increased risk of nephrotoxicity longer on the medication*
- Reversible hypertension (27%) (dose and duration-dependent) – typically controlled with calcium channel blocker

(e.g., nifedipine or isradipine) as they do not alter cyclosporine levels
- Nausea, vomiting, fatigue
- Arthralgia, myalgia
- Acne, sebaceous hyperplasia
- Gingival hyperplasia
- Hyperlipidemia (triglycerides)
- Electrolyte imbalances: hyperkalemia, hyperuricemia (can precipitate gout), hypomagnesemia
- Hypertrichosis, trichomegaly
- Neurologic (both central and peripheral) changes, including tremors
- Increased risk of non-melanoma skin cancer
- Progressive multifocal leukoencephalopathy
- Reversible posterior leukoencephalopathy (no demyelination unlike PML, but HA, AMS, sz, vision changes)
- Other malignancies

Monitoring
- Blood pressure at each visit.
- BP, CBC, LFTs, BUN/creatinine, lytes, magnesium, uric acid, phosphorous, lipids q 2 weeks × 2 months and then monthly × 2 months. Then, every 4–6 weeks, check creatinine, and every 3–6 months, check all of the above.
- Yearly dental exam.
- If change in dosage, check labs weekly ×1 week and then q2weeks as above. If on long term (>6 months), consult renal and consider creatinine clearance.
- Can get CsA level if necessary.

Azathioprine

MOA

Purine analogue which blocks purine synthesis and thus cell division (particularly in fast-growing cells that do not have a salvage pathway, like lymphocytes) > diminishes T-cell function and antibody production by B cells.

Active metabolite is 6-thioguanine (6-TGN) which is produced by the hypoxanthine guanine transferase pathway. Thiopurine methyltransferase (TPMT) and xanthine oxidase (XO) convert azathioprine into inactive metabolites. TMPT activity is reduced in certain populations; xanthine oxidase function can be decreased by allopurinol or febuxostat; both of these can increase azathioprine levels and increase the risk of life-threatening myelosuppression (Fig. 8.2).

Renal Excretion

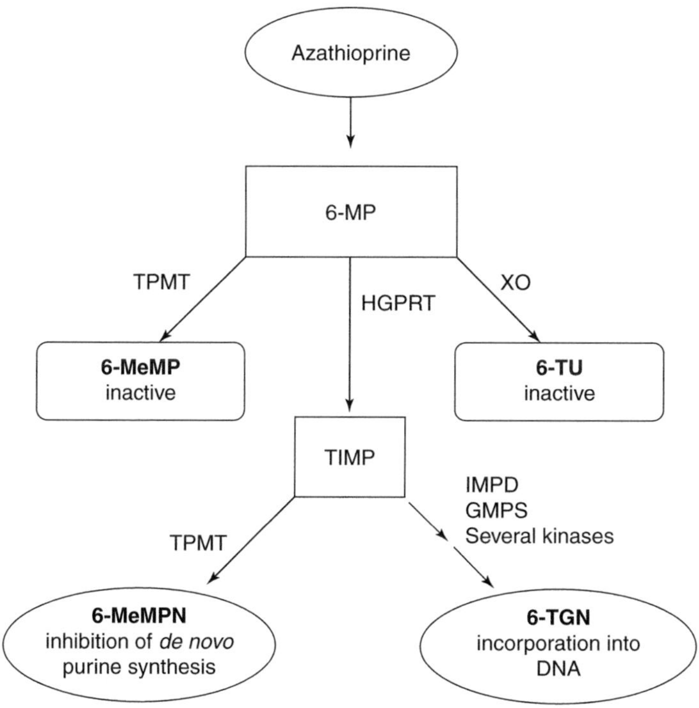

FIGURE 8.2 Mechanism of action of azathioprine. 6-MP 6-mercaptopurine

Drug Interactions

- Allopurinol – significantly reduces the metabolism of azathioprine.
- Febuxostat – significantly reduces the metabolism of azathioprine.
- ACE inhibitors – may induce anemia, severe leukopenia.
- Sulfasalazine – may induce anemia, severe leukopenia.
- Folate antagonists – may induce anemia, severe leukopenia.
- Warfarin – azathioprine decreases the anticoagulant effects.
- Neuromuscular blockers – azathioprine can reverse neuromuscular blockade.
- TNFa inhibitor – can increase risk of hepatosplenic T-cell lymphoma.
- Copper IUD – can render ineffective.

Pre-screening Questions

On allopurinol or febuxostat? If yes, consider alternative med (or must reduce dose by 75%)

On ACE inhibitors or sulfasalazine? If yes, have an increased risk of anemia/severe leukopenia

Have IUD? (Can render copper IUD ineffective)

Of childbearing age or considering becoming pregnant? Consider other medication as it's teratogenic. Can render IUD ineffective

History of lymphoproliferative malignancies or cutaneous SCCs? (Increase risk of these in pts on azathioprine)

On aTNFa inhibitor? Consider an alternative as there is an increased risk of hepatosplenic T-cell lymphoma

Advise patients not to take allopurinol while on this medication as it can lead to severe myelotoxicity.

Lower risk of Hep B reactivation than with other immunosuppressive medications

Pre-screening Labs

TMPT activity level

CBC, LFTs, BMP, UA, TB test (PPD, T-spot, Quant Gold), CXR, Hep B/C serologiies, HIV, HCG for females

Drug Interactions

Allopurinol significantly reduces metabolism of azathioprine.

ACE inhibitor may induce anemia and severe leukopenia.

Warfarin may have decreased anti-coagulation effect. Renders copper IUD ineffective.

Dosing

Comes in 50 mg scored tablets

Dosing based on TMPT level

- If TMPT <5 units, do *not* give AZA.
- If TMPT between 5 and 13.7 units, give up to 0.5 mg/kg/day.
- If TMPT between 13.7 and 19 units, give up to 1.5 mg/kg/day.
- If TMPT is >19 units, give up to 2.5 mg/kg/day.

Based on TMPT level, but generally starts at 1 mg/kg/day. The dose may be increased by 0.5 mg/kg/day, beginning at 6–8 weeks and thereafter at 4-week intervals if needed to a maximum dose of 2.5 mg/kg/day. Therapeutic response after 6–8 weeks of treatment. Once clinical response is obtained, gradual dose reduction should be attempted to reduce the risk of toxicities. If not getting response that you think you should at dose, recheck TMPT level.

Needs acidic milieu for absorption (take with OJ/cola); also take with food to minimize nausea.

Decrease dose by 75% if on allopurinol or do not use at all.

Side Effects

GI upset: Nausea, vomiting – most common side effect. Often present between 1st and 10th day of therapy.

Hypersensitivity syndrome – fever/shock can occur at 14 days. Most common between 1st and 4th week of therapy. More common if also on cyclosporine or methotrexate.

Bone marrow suppression – leukopenia, thrombocytopenia, immunosuppression (correlate with low TMPT level).

Other GI side effects: Gastritis, pancreatitis mucous membrane ulceration, jaundice, biliary stasis

Neutropenia is common, especially in lupus.

Malignancies: SCC and lymphoma (particularly non-Hodgkin's B-cell lymphoma), hepatosplenic T-cell lymphoma if on TNFa inhibitor as well.

Infections: HPV, HSV, scabies.

Transaminase elevation and severe hepatocellular toxicity are rare.

Teratogenic

Monitoring

If not seeing desired effect, or if having side effects, recheck TMPT level to make sure it is still the same and enzymatic activity has not changed.

CBC and LFTs every 2 weeks × 1 months, then q1–2 months thereafter.

Dose increase: check CBC and LFTs every 2 weeks × 1 month after.

LFTs and BUN/Cr should be checked every 6 months.

Physical exam to assess for lymphoma.

Skin check every 6 months to assess for SCC.

D/c if WBC <4000, Hgb <10, Plt <100,0000.

TB testing yearly.

Dapsone

MOA

Antibacterial and anti-inflammatory towards neutrophils by inhibition of myeloperoxidase and their chemotactic abilities

Pre-screening Questions

Allergy to sulfa, especially sulfapyridine?

Anemia at baseline?

History of significant cardiac, pulmonary, liver, renal, or other hematologic disease (anemia or increased methemoglobin may exacerbate pre-existing cardiopulmonary disease)?

Patient with known G6PD deficiency?

Pregnant or breastfeeding? (Excreted in breast milk)

Drug Interactions

Rifampin lowers dose, folic acid antagonists, G6PD depleting agents, didanosine, saquinavir

Pre-screening Labs

CBC with diff, LFTs, BUN/Creatinine, Reticulocyte count, G6PD, HCG/pregnancy test (in females)

Dosing

25–50 mg/days and increase slowly (25 mg/week) to max dose of 300 mg/day. Hgb will fall by 1–2 g/dL and then stabilize.

(For dermatitis herpetiformis: Begin at 50 mg daily and then adjust weekly to control symptoms to a maximum of 300 mg. Reduce to a minimum maintenance level. Typucally, 100 mg is just fine, however).

Patients typically require 100–200 mg daily for adequate control of their skin disease.

Side Effects

Hematologic side effects are the most common (1–2 g drop in hgb, increase retic count, methemoglobinemia)

Three types of blood effects:

1. Hemolytic anemia (especially if G6PD deficient) – dose related
2. Agranulocytosis (usually occurs at 7 weeks (range: 2–12 weeks) – *idiosyncratic and serious*; may manifest as fever, pharyngitis, occasionally sepsis
    (a) Stop dapsone
    (b) Consider giving G-CSF
3. Methemoglobinemia (especially with prilocaine) – dose related
    (a) Symptoms arise as a consequence of hypoxia and are proportional to methemoglobin level.
        i. Peripheral and central cyanosis usually seen at serum methemoglobin level of 15%.
        ii. Levels of 30–45% result in headache, fatigue, tachycardia, weakness, and dizziness.

iii. Levels >60%: cardiac arrhythmia, dyspnea, seizures, coma.
iv. Levels >70% typically fatal.

(b) Serum methemoglobin levels are not always immediately available. An oxygen saturation gap observed between arterial blood gas analysis and pulse oximetry readings is helpful in making the diagnosis. Oxygen saturation levels measured with pulse oximetry are substantially lower than arterial blood gas saturation levels.

i. Pulse oximetry can only measure two hemoglobin species: oxyhemoglobin and reduced hemoglobin. As other hemoglobins arise (e.g., methemoglobin), the oxygen saturation on pulse oximetry falls and plateaus at 85%.

(c) Cimetidine and vitamin E daily reduce methemoglobin formation.
(d) Worsening methemoglobinemia can occur intra- and postoperatively after both local amide and general anesthetic; vitamin C may be helpful.
(e) Treatment.

i. D/C dapsone.
ii. Oral methylene blue 1–2 mg/kg IV used in emergency situations to lower methemoglobin levels. If symptoms persist after 1 h, repeat doses given with caution as accumulation of methylene blue can result in increased production of methemoglobin.
iii. Activated charcoal.
iv. Hemodialysis.

(f) **Reference**: Burke P. *Can Fam Phys*. 2013;59(9):958-61.

Neurologic/Psychiatric Effects (Idiosyncratic)

- *Motor* peripheral neuropathy (usually distal motor) – may present as wasting of hand muscles (reversible if detected early)
- Acute psychosis

Hepatic

- Drug-induced hepatitis

- Cholestatic jaundice

Cutaneous

- Photosensitivity.
- Hypersensitivity reaction (DRESS (may not have eosinophilia))
- SJS/TEN) – patients should be told to stop their dapsone if they have "viral symptoms," such as nausea, vomiting, malaise, and weakness

Metabolic: Note that HgA1c will appear falsely low (older glycosylated cells can't tolerate oxidative stress as well)

Monitoring

CBC with diff and retic count weekly × 1 month, then monthly × 6 months, then q6 months thereafter. Follow more closely if increasing dose. Hgb will fall by 1–2 g/dL and then stabilize.

If patients fail to show some increase in reticulocyte count despite a persistent anemia, the possibility of an associated iron, folate, or B12 deficiency should be considered.

Methemoglobin levels need not be measured unless the patient is experiencing excessive fatigue, headaches, or increasing cardiac or pulmonary symptoms.

LFTs and renal function every 2 weeks × 2 and then every 6 months.

Assess for motor neuropathy at each visit as well.

Colchicine

MOA

Anti-neutrophil: binds to tubulin dimers in neutrophils, preventing microtubule assembly critical for metaphase and neutrophil motility and chemotaxis.

Antimitotic activity.

Pre-screening Questions

GI distress?

On hemodialysis? Contraindicated for those on dialysis

On statin or fibrates? Relative contraindication as colchicine toxicity can be potentiated by concomitant use of cholesterol-lowering drugs

On any CYP3A4 drugs? Do drug interaction check

Pre-screening Labs

None

Dosing

0.6 mg po daily BID

Adjust dosing for renal disease

Side Effects

GI distress with abdominal cramping and watery diarrhea – decreasing from TID to BID dosing may help (26–77%)

Neutropenia, anemia

Fatigue

Dermatologic: alopecia, purpura, rash

Hematologic: thrombocytopenia, leukopenia, granulocytopenia, pancytopenia, aplastic anemia

Elevated LFTs

Musculoskeletal: myotonia, muscle weakness, myopathy, elevated CPK, muscle pain, rhabdomyolysis

Rhabdomyolysis and neuromuscular toxicity have been reported with long-term treatment at therapeutic doses; increased risk with renal dysfunction, elderly patients, concomitant therapy with myotoxic drugs. Symptoms generally resolved within 1 week to a few months upon d/c of drug.

Peripheral neuropathy – numbness or tingling in hands/feet or motor neuropathy; decrease dose or d/c if this occurs

Flare of gout

Reproductive: azoospermia, oligospermia

Monitoring

None

Acitretin

MOA
Vitamin A derivative that acts on retinoid receptors (RAR) which regulate growth and terminal differentiation and anti-proliferation of keratinocytes

Pre-screening Questions
Is this patient a female of childbearing age? If yes, do not prescribe this medication, or else must warn that they must not become pregnant for 3 years.

Pregnancy category X

History of liver disease? Elevated liver enzymes and hepatitis-reported deaths reported.

Alcohol consumption: *Alcohol is contraindicated during treatment and for 2 months after stopping therapy* as alcohol promotes the formation of etretinate which prolongs the half-life and teratogenic risk.

On methotrexate or other liver-toxic medications? Consider other therapy.

Severely impaired renal function? Consider other therapy.

Hyperlipidemia?

Contraindications
Pregnancy: Must have a negative pregnancy test 2 weeks before starting treatment. Also, must *not plan on pregnancy during therapy and for 3 years* (!) after stopping medication.

Use is contraindicated in females with childbearing potential unless patient meets *all* of the following conditions:

1. Two negative urine or serum pregnancy test results (baseline and 1st 5 days of menses immediately before initiation of therapy).
2. Repeat urine or serum pregnancy test monthly during therapy and q3 month during the 3 years following discontinuation of therapy.
3. Committed to use two (at least one should be primary) effective forms of contraception simultaneously unless the

patient is abstinent, is postmenopausal, or has undergone a hysterectomy.
4. Use two effective forms of contraception simultaneously for at least 1 month prior to therapy, during therapy, and for 3 years after discontinuing therapy.
5. Microdosed "minipill" progestin preparations are not recommended because acitretin interferes with contraceptives' effect and it is unknown whether other progestin contraceptives are adequate contraceptive methods during acitretin therapy.

Cannot drink (EtOH) at all while on this medication (especially female) as this will form etretinate, a metabolite that stays fairly indefinitely in the body. No mouthwash, etc. to be safe.

Tetracycline, methotrexate, alcohol, vitamin A supplements

Hepatic impairment

Renal impairment

Elevated blood lipids

Drug Interactions

Alcohol of any kind, isotretinoin, methotrexate, phenytoin, progestin only minipill, St. John's wart, tetracyclines, vitamin A

Pre-screening Labs

Female: negative serum pregnancy test 2 weeks before starting medication, at start, and then every month during treatment and for the 3 years following cessation of therapy

CBC with diff, BMP, phosphorous, magnesium, fasting lipids, and LFTs, CK

Ophtho exam if patient with history of cataracts/retinopathy

Consider in adults lateral spine and calcaneus radiographs + any symptomatic area: repeat only if symptoms

Females with childbearing potential must participate in Do Your P.A.R.T. program and have signed Patient Agreement/Informed Consent for Female Patients.

Inform patients that they should not donate blood during therapy and for 3 years after discontinuation of therapy.

Dosing

Start with 25 mg per day with main meal.

Maintenance dose is 25–50 mg based on clinical response and side effects.

Take with food.

Females with childbearing potential must participate in Do Your P.A.R.T. program and have signed Patient Agreement/Informed Consent for Female Patients.

Side Effects

Dose related: cheilitis, xerosis, peeling skin of palms/soles, hair loss (50–75%)

Muscle and joint pain (especially with exercise)
Hypertriglyceridemia (50–75%)
Dysglycemia (25–50%)
Nail disorders (25–50%)
Pruritus (25–50%)
Rhinitis
Changes in electrolyte levels
Elevated LFTs/hepatotoxicity
Hyperesthesia
Paresthesia
Paronychia
Rigors
Skin atrophy
Spinal hyperostosis
Sticky skin
Xerophthalmia

Retinoid teratogenicity: microtia, hearing loss, microphthalmia, optic nerve atrophy, acral and axial skeletal abnormalities, cardiovascular defects, hydrocephalus, microcephaly, meningomyelocele, thymic aplasia, anal and vaginal atresia

Monitoring

CBC with diff, BMP, magnesium, phosphorous, lipids, and LFTs every 2 weeks to determine response, then monthly for 3–6 months, then every 3 months.

Check glucose with labs if patient is diabetic.

- For triglycerides >800, d/c med or add gemfibrozil. For triglycerides 300–800, reduce dose, decrease diet fats, exercise, d/c alcohol and smoking.

HCG/pregnancy test monthly for females during therapy and for 3 years after cessation of therapy

CK/aldolase if muscle complaints.

Reference: Wolverton. Comprehensive Dermatologic Drug Therapy

Emedicine.com/Medscape https://reference.medscape.com/drug/soriatane-acitretin-topical-343539#5

Isotretinoin (13-cis-Retinoic Acid)

MOA

Vitamin A derivative that acts on retinoid receptors, which regulate growth and terminal differentiation of keratinocytes. Also acts to increase filaggrin production and Odland body secretion of lipids, reduces the size of sebaceous glands, and reduces follicular occlusion; directly inhibits ornithine decarboxylase, so lessens inflammatory hyperplasia.

Pre-screening Questions/Considerations

The physician, the pharmacy, and the patient must be registered with the iPLEDGE program (https://www.ipledgeprogram.com).

All patients – males, females who cannot become pregnant, and females of childbearing potential (FCBPs) – must be aware that this medication can cause birth defects if taken during pregnancy.

Recommended for

- Severe nodular acne
- Moderate acne that is treatment – resistant or for the management of acne that is producing physical scarring or psychosocial distress
- Acne that relapses quickly after discontinuation of oral antibiotic therapy

History of liver disease? Hyperlipidemia?

History of depression? Suicidality?

On a tetracycline-type antibiotic? If yes, must stop this before starting as increased risk of pseudotumor cerebri.

If female, confirm no wish for pregnancy in near future ad two forms of birth control per iPLEDGE (if abstinence, then no second form of birth control).

Will the patient be able to come in for monthly examinations?

Write down iPLEDGE number and last four of the SSN in order to register in iPLEDGE.

Give iPLEDGE packet, get written consent.

Pre-screening Labs

As per iPLEDGE

Weight.

CBC, LFTs, lipids, creatinine, CK (if athletic/work out).

If female, HCG negative × 2 at least 30–37 days apart before starting.

If sexually active, must have two forms of birth control.

Give iPLEDGE handout on information regarding OCPs to females of childbearing potential.

Consider in adults lateral spine and calcaneus radiographs + any symptomatic area: repeat only if symptoms.

Children: height/weight at each visit, bone scan + radiographs of all four limbs + lateral spine baseline and yearly.

Ophtho exam if patient with history of cataracts/retinopathy.

Inform patient that they are not to share their pills with anyone and that they should not give blood while on this medication.

Dosing

The physician, the pharmacy, and the patient must be registered with the iPLEDGE program (https://www.ipledgeprogram.com).

Conventional Dosing

Starting dose: 0.5 mg/kg/day for the first month and then increase to 1 mg/kg/day as tolerated by the patient. Lower doses (0.1 mg/kg/day) may be required in extremely severe cases to prevent worsening.

Note: no difference in efficacy with lower versus higher dosing but significant difference in relapse rates with doses of 1.0 mg/kg/day having less relapse than doses at 0.5 mg/kg/day.

Low dose: 0.25–0.4 mg/kg/day

Relapse rates in patients with moderate acne treated with low dose are equal to those treated with conventional dosing.

Only a 30-day supply of pills can be prescribed; the patient must be seen in back within 30–37 days.

Take with food, especially fatty meals.

One formulation contains isotretinoin + lidose (lipid agent) bypassing the need to take with food.

Goal dose: 120–150 mg/kg; however, doses up to 220 mg/kg may result in lower relapse rates.

- Some practitioners aim to continue treatment for at least 2 months after achieving disease-free activity as this results in a decreased frequency of relapse.

Consider starting OCPs in patients of childbearing potential

Side Effects

Commonly occur:

Cheilitis, xerosis, nose dryness/nose bleeds, dry eyes

- Note that 1 gram/day of omega-3 reduces mucocutaneous side effects of isotretinoin
- Vaseline in the nose, saline nose sprays
- Saline eye drops

Swelling of eyelids or lips

Upset stomach

Thinning of the hair

Unlikely to occur:

Worsening of acne before it gets better (if this happens, start on prednsione)

Muscle and joint pain (especially with exercise) (L-carnitine supplementation may help ameliorate.)

Hyperlipidemia (triglycerides)

Elevated LFTs

Reduced night vision

Photosensitivity

Hair loss

Pyogenic granulomas

Staph colonization

Keloid formation/poor pound healing – conservative recommendation to delay procedures such as dermabrasion or laser resurfacing until for about 6 months after d/c of isotretinoin

Rare:

Pseudotumor cerebri (headache, vision changes, dizziness)

Diffuse interstitial skeletal hyperostosis (DISH)

Premature epiphyseal closure

Depression including suicidality

Cytopenias

Inflammatory bowel disease (controversial)

Retinoid teratogenicity: microtia, hearing loss, microphthalmia, optic nerve atrophy, acral and axial skeletal abnormalities, cardiovascular defects, hydrocephalus, microcephaly, meningomyelocele, thymic aplasia, anal and vaginal atresia

Monitoring

Monitor mood at each visit.

Calculate cumulative dose in mg/kg at each visit.

Lipids, LFTs, CK 1 and 2 months and then with any dosing changes.

Monthly pregnancy tests for females must be performed at a minimum of 28-day cycles.

Children: height/weight at each visit, bone scan + radiographs of all 4 limbs + lateral spine baseline and yearly.

Consider in adults lateral spine and calcaneus radiographs + any symptomatic area: repeat only if symptoms.

Relapse

Acne relapse associated with

- Cumulative dose <220 mg/kg
- Younger age at initial treatment (<16 years old)
- Male sex
- Hormonal acne

References

- American Academy of Dermatology Association. Position statement on isotretinoin. https://www.aad.org/Forms/Policies/Uploads/PS/PS-Isotretinoin.pdf
- Blasiak RC, Stamey CR, Burkhart CN, et al. High-dose isotretinoin treatment and the rate of retrial, relapse, and adverse effects in patients with acne vulgaris. *JAMA Dermatol.* 2013;149:1392–1398.
- Stone SP. *Cutis* 2017;99(6):378–88

Spironolactone

MOA

Synthetic 17-lactone steroid that has antagonistic effects on the androgen and progesterone receptors (decreases testosterone production and by competitively inhibiting binding of testosterone and DHT (dihydrotestosterone) to androgen receptors in the skin). It may also inhibit 5-alpha reductase and increase steroid hormone-binding globulin. Decreases sebum production through inhibition of the androgen receptor on sebocytes.

Pre-screening Questions

Planning on becoming pregnant? If yes, do not give spironolactone. Teratogenic to male fetuses (causes feminization of genitalia).

History of renal disease? If yes, consider using a different med.

On potassium supplementation or an ACE inhibitor? If yes, consider using a different med.

Personal or family history of breast cancer?

Taking trimethoprim-sulfamethoxazole? (See note below)

History of hypertension or heart failure? Do not take without clearance of PCP/cardiologist.

Can be used safely in patients taking drospirenone-containing OCPs.

Male? Typically not used due to risk of feminization.

Drug Interactions

Spironolactone + Bactrim > increased risk of sudden death (mostly in patients >85 years old due to hyperkalemia)

Pre-screening Labs

Creatinine

Potassium

HCG if female

Contraindication

Pregnancy – it has been found to cause feminization in rats with male fetuses at high doses; no human studies of its use in pregnancy.

On other medications which cause hyperkalemia.

Dosing

25–200 mg/day (common dosing 50–100 mg/daily)

Side Effects

Urinary frequency.

Hyperkalemia – at increased risk of this in renal failure, GI distress (nausea, vomiting, diarrhea).

Fatigue, lightheadedness, dizziness, drowsiness, nausea, headache.

Females: Breast tenderness and enlargement, menstrual irregularities (most common but side effect is dose dependent; concomitant OCP use can minimize incidence).

Males: Gynecomastia/tenderness, physical feminization, reversible infertility, sexual dysfunction (loss of libido, erectile dysfunction).

Large-scale studies have shown no association between spironolactone use and the development of breast, uterine, cervical, or ovarian cancers.

Monitoring

If young and healthy, <45 years old, without history of kidney disease, testing for potassium is usually not necessary (unless the patient has another risk of hyperkalemia).

For older patients or those on ACE inhibitors, ARBs, NSAIDs, digoxin, or other medications which cause renal impairment or hyperkalemia, get creatinine and potassium 2 weeks after starting and after changing the dose.

Note: May be a risk for hyperkalemia when spironolactone is combined with trimethoprim-sulfamethoxazole, which can lead to sudden death. The combination should be avoided.

Reference

- Antoniou T *CMAJ*. 2015;187(4):E138–43
- Frideman A. *Cutis*. 2015;96(4):216–7.
- https://www.dermatologytimes.com/dermatology/spironolactone-safe-and-effective-adult-female-acne
- https://www.dermatologytimes.com/dermatology/use-spironolactone-hormonal-acne-women

Finasteride

MOA

Inhibits 5-alpha reductase, which converts testosterone to dihydrotestosterone (DHT)

Pre-screening Questions

History of sexual dysfunction?

Male attempting to conceive? Do not use in men trying to conceive.

Not approved for use in women.

Pregnancy category X – contraindicated in women of child-bearing potential.

Pre-screening Labs

None

Dosing

Androgenic alopecia: 1 mg/day (some prescribe 5 mg pill and have patient divide it into fourths, taking 1/4 pill per day)

Female hirsutism/pattern hair loss (off label): 5 mg/day

Side Effects

- Decreased libido (*may be permanent*) in both men and women.
- Sexual dysfunction in males: Erectile dysfunction, decreased ejaculate volume, orgasm disorders, male infertility and/or poor seminal quality (normalization of quality

has been reported after discontinuation of finasteride); testicular pain.

- Post-finasteride syndrome: Characterized by sexual side effects (i.e., low libido, erectile dysfunction, decreased arousal and difficulty in achieving orgasm), depression, anxiety, and cognitive complaints that are still present despite drug withdrawal.
- Breast tenderness and enlargement: Post-marketing reports of *male breast cancer* associated with finasteride use.
- Depression.
- Lowers PSA and thus interferes with interpretation of PSA. Roughly must double the value to account for being on this medication.
- Probably decreased likelihood of development of prostate cancer, but if develop prostate cancer, more likely to be high grade.
- Female-specific side effects include increased body hair, sweating and hot flashes, and headaches.
- Females should avoid semen of men taking finasteride if trying to get pregnant. Pregnant women should not touch the finasteride pills.

Monitoring

Inquire about sexual dysfunction

IVIg

MOA

Immunoglobulin blood product derived from pooled plasma from 1000+ donors (most is IgG, but there are small and variable amounts of IgA)

Immunomodulatory effects not completely understood: Neutralizes antibodies, Fc receptor modulation, modulation of the production of cytokines and cytokine antagonists, effects on complement (inhibition of complement-mediated damage); inhibits autoreactive T cells; sequesters anti-Fasreceptor Ab; neutralizes bacterial super antigens, acceleration of IgG catabolism

Half-life ~4 weeks

Pre-screening Questions

IgA deficiency or disorder which causes hypogammaglobulinemia?

Renal failure/congestive heart disease? (May not tolerate fluid overload)

Dehydration? Diabetes? May increase risk of renal failure or thrombotic sequelae

Pre-screening Labs

IgA level – get ASAP if even maybe considering to start IVIg.

CBC with diff.

Creatinine/BUN/BMP.

Rheumatoid factor/cryoglobulin – patients with these are at increased risk of acute renal failure.

Hepatitis A, B, C, HIV (mostly medicolegal).

Complete consent for blood products

Dosing

1–2 gm/kg IV divided over a 3–5-consecutive day cycle (0.4/kg/day).

Infusion is usually given slowly over 4–4.5 h.

Monitor vitals during infusion.

Half-life is about 4 weeks (infusions given monthly).

Aggressive disease can be given every 2 weeks.

Maintenance intervals can increase slowly.

(For example, 4-, 6-, 8-, 10-, 12-, 14-, 16-week intervals, then d/c)

Formulations with low sucrose are favored for those with renal disease.

Side Effects

Infusion related

- Immediate adverse reactions following IVIg administration are usually mild and transient flu-like symptoms and include headache (most common), flushing of the face, malaise, chest tightness, fever, chills, myalgia, fatigue, dyspnea, back pain, nausea, vomiting, diarrhea, change in blood pressure, and tachycardia – usually occur within the first 30 min of infusion.

- Can try to prevent by pre-medicate with antihistamines, glucocorticoids, and NSAIDs.
- Slow infusion rate or temporarily discontinue the infusion if develop.
- Hydrate high-risk patients for renal failure, thromboembolic events, and aseptic meningitis.

- Erythema, pain, phlebitis eczematous dermatitis at infusion site.
- Anaphylaxis – rare (most likely to occur in patients with IgA deficiency).
  - Check IgA prior to starting IVIg.
- Fluid overload.
  - May occur in patients with sucrose-containing IVIg.

Late Reactions
Hematologic

- Neutropenia (usually transient; prednisone can help prevent)
- Autoimmune hemolytic anemia
  - Noted in pts with autoAb against blood groups ABO and Rhesus (Rh)

- Neurologic – aseptic meningitis in up to 11% (severe acute headache with neck rigidity, photophobia, fever, lethargy, nausea/vomiting); typically resolves without sequelae
- Thromboembolic events (stroke/MI) – seen with higher doses/higher infusion rates (due to hyperviscosity)
- Infection risk (bc is blood product)
- Acute or worsening renal failure (especially with sucrose containing formulations) – usually oliguric and transient
- Dermatologic
  - Urticaria
  - Morbilliform drug eruption

  - Pruritus of palms
  - Diffuse hair loss
  - Eczema
  - Erythema multiforme
  - Purpuric erythema
  - Petechiae of extremities
  - Mucosa ulcerations
  - Lichenoid eruptions
  - Symmetrical drug-related intertriginous and flexural exanthema (SDRIFE)
  - Small vessel vasculitis (leukocytoclastic vasculitis)

- Arthritis
- Pseudohyponatremia
- IVIg-induced hypersensitivity syndrome

Monitoring

Vitals

Regular neurological exams

CBC with diff

BMP

References

•Orbach H et al. *Clini Rev Allergy Immunol.* 2005;29:173–84.
• Dhar S. *Indian Dermatol* 2009;54(1):77–9

Hydroxychloroquine, Chloroquine, and Quinacrine

MOA

Exact pathomechanism unclear but likely intercalates into DNA, blocking transcription. Proposed mechanisms include:

- Bind to DNA and inhibit superoxide products > inhibiting UV-induced cutaneous reactions.
- Raise intracytoplasmic pH > decrease macrophages to express MHC antigens on cell surface.

- Reduce lysosomal size and impair chemotaxis.
- Inhibit platelet aggregation and cell adhesion.

Has a long half-life and steady-state concentration attained after 3–4 months

Pre-screening Questions

History of porphyria or psoriasis?

History of retinopathy or other eye/vision issues?

History of issues with hydroxychloroquine or chloroquine in the past?

History of hematologic abnormalities?

Currently smoking? (Encourage to quit)

Hepatic or renal dysfunction?

On tamoxifen?

Contraindications

Porphyria

Psoriasis

Hypersensitivity to drug or chloroquine (cross-reaction between chloroquine and hydroxychloroquine)

Retinopathy 2/2 hydroxychloroquine/chloroquine

Relative Contraindications

Severe blood dyscrasias

Hepatic dysfunction

Renal dysfunction (50% reduction in renal function correlates with 2× retinopathy risk)

Women currently taking tamoxifen (increases retinopathy risk 5×)

Neurologic disorders

Retinal or visual field changes

Pregnancy and lactation

Myasthenia gravis (chloroquine)

Pre-screening Labs

Dilated eye examination and visual field testing for baseline documentation

G6PD, CBC

LFT, renal function, pregnancy test, urine porphyrins to r/o PCT if suspected

Dosing

Hydroxychloroquine and chloroquine should not be given together.

Quinacrine may be added to hydroxychloroquine or chloroquine to increase therapeutic effect.

Hydroxychloroquine

- Optimal dosing is ≤5 mg/kg of actual (real) body weight or 400 mg daily, whichever is lower.
- Standard dosing: 200 mg BID then decrease to the lowest necessary dose once control is achieved.
- Conservative dosing: Hydroxychloroquine 100 mg po every MWF for 1 month, then 200 mg po every MWF ×1 month, then if needed, 200 mg po daily × 1 month. Stop increasing dose when disease is under control.
- *Increased risk of retinal toxicity with doses >6.5 mg/kg of ideal body weight*
- If not seeing adequate responses:
  - Check whole blood hydroxychloroquine level with goal for efficacy being >750 ng/mL and for compliance being >500 ng/mL.
  - Can increase to a max of 800 mg/day for a short time period until efficacy seen and then try to back down to standard dosing of 400 mg/day in order to limit retinal side effects.
- *Porphyria cutanea tarda*: WARNING – CONSIDER NOT USING. HIGHER DOSES CAN LEAD TO ACUTE HEPATIC FAILURE. Typical doses in this population are lower 100–200 mg/day

Chloroquine

- Dosing regimens
  - 250 mg po every MWF × 1 month, then 500 mg po every MWF × 1 month, then 500 mg po daily × 1 month
  - Alternatively, chloroquine 250 mg po daily to start
  - Max dose 500 mg po BID

Smoking cessation important

Take with food to minimize GI upset

Side Effects

Gastrointestinal: nausea/vomiting (chloroquine > hydroxychloroquine)

Ocular side effects (not seen with quinacrine):

1. Pre-maculopathy – loss of peripheral vision/changes in visual field without visual loss. *Is reversible if the antimalarial is discontinued.*
2. Corneal deposits (keratopathy) – blurry vision or visual disturbances.
3. *Retinopathy* – "bull's eye" pigment deposition, central scotoma, diminished visual acuity. *Potentially irreversible!!*
4. Neuromuscular eye toxicity (ciliary body dysfunction).

Ocular side effects increase sharply after 5–7 years of use or >1000 gm cumulative dose of hydroxychloroquine and doses > 6.5 mg/kg based on ideal body weight.

Hematologic

- Agranulocytosis (chloroquine)
- Hemolysis especially in G6PD
- Potentially fatal bone marrow toxicity (quinacrine)

Neurologic: Dizziness, headache, irritability, restlessness, excitement, confusion, seizures

Muscular: Myopathy and neuromyopathy (muscle weakness)

Cutaneous: Lightening of hair, alopecia, skin hyperpigmentation (30%: accumulates in melanin-rich tissue = bluish-gray hyperpigmentation over shins, face, palate, and in the nailbeds as transverse bands), lichenoid drug eruptions, morbilliform eruption, erythroderma, SJS, psoriasis exacerbation (especially with chloroquine), yellow pigmentation of the skin (quinacrine)

CNS disease: Infrequency confusion, seizures, restlessness

Cardiac: QT prolongation, ventricular arrhythmias, toxic cardiomyopathy

Monitoring

Assess muscle strength periodically

Inquire any vision changes at each exam

Dilated eye examination and visual field testing within first year and then typically at least yearly after 5 years

Labs

- CBC with diff monthly × 3 months and then CBC with diff every 6 months
- LFTs and BMP (creatinine) periodically
- Methemoglobin level if indicated

Terbinafine

MOA

Allylamine – blocks ergosterol synthesis by inhibiting squalene epoxidase

Works for dermatophytes but not yeast/candida

Pre-screening Questions

History of liver disease? If so, consider other therapy.

Pre-screening Labs

LFTs

Dosing

Pediatrics:

4 years (<25 kg): 125 mg/day PO for 6 weeks.
≥4 years (25–35 kg): 187.5 mg/day PO for 6 weeks
≥4 years (>35 kg): 250 mg/day PO for 6 weeks

Adults: 250 mg/day.

Duration of treatment:

Onychomycosis of fingernails × 6 weeks; 12 weeks for toenails.

Tinea capitis: *Trichophyton* 1–4 weeks; *Microsporum* requires longer duration of therapy.

Side Effects

Headache (13%)

Rash

Pruritus

Nausea/vomiting

Dysgeusia: metallic taste or (possibly irreversible) taste changes

May cause caffeine to have a longer half-life

Worsening of psoriasis/development of psoriasis

Rare:

Liver damage: idiosyncratic and symptomatic hepatic injury and rarely liver failure sometimes leading to death or requiring liver transplantation

Drug-induced lupus or exacerbation of cutaneous/systemic lupus erythematosus

Stevens-Johnson syndrome/toxic epidermal necrolysis (SJS/TEN)

Drug reaction with eosinophilia and systemic symptoms/drug-induced hypersensitivity Syndrome (DRESS/DIHS)

Acute generalized exanthematous pustulosis (AGEP)

Severe neutropenia, thrombocytopenia, agranulocytosis, pancytopenia, anemia

Myalgias/rhabdomyolysis

Vision changes

Serum sickness-like creations

Vasculitis

Photosensitivity

Thrombotic microangiopathy

Hearing impairment/vertigo

Monitoring

LFTs if treating for >6 weeks.

Griseofulvin

MOA

Disrupts microtubule function

Fungistatic

Works for dermatophytes only; *NOT* yeast or bacteria

Possible resistance to griseofulvin by *Trichophyton*

Pre-screening Questions

Do not give to patient with porphyria.

Is the patient on OCPs? (Can render OPCs ineffective.)

On any P450 medications? Induces P450 system – do medication interaction check.

Pregnant? Should not give in pregnancy.

Contraindications

PCN allergy or porphyria

Pregnancy

Hepatocellular failure

Pre-screening Labs

None

Dosing

Dermatophytes only

Microsize

Pediatrics 11 mg/kg/day as single dose or divided q12h

(<2 years old efficacy not established)

Adults:

Tinea corporis, cruris, or capitis: 500 mg/day PO

Tinea pedis or unguium: 1000 mg/day PO as single daily dose or divided q12hr

Ultramicrosize

Pediatrics: 7.3 mg/kg/day (<2 years old efficacy not established)

Can be crushed and given with ice cream

Adults:

Tinea corporis, cruris, or capitis: 375 mg/day PO

Tinea pedis or unguium: 250 mg PO q8hr

Grifulvin V oral suspension – less readily absorbed than above

Treatment Duration

Dependent on infection site

Tinea corporis: 2–4 weeks

Tinea capitis: 4–6 weeks; may be up to 8–12 weeks

Tinea pedis: 4–8 weeks

Tinea unguium: 4–6 months

Microsporum often requires higher doses and longer duration of treatment.

Increased absorption with a fatty meal (whole milk/ice cream).

Resistance seen with *T. rubrum*.

Side Effects

Rash/urticaria (most common)

Nausea/vomiting/GI upset/diarrhea

Headache in up to 50%

Induces cytochrome p450 – look at meds

Will decrease effectiveness of birth control

Paresthesias

Photosensitivity

Drug-induced lupus (rare)

Worsens acute intermittent porphyria

Rare: SJS/TEN, increased AST/ALT

Monitoring

CBC in 4 weeks then every 3 months. LFTs every 3 months.

(Common to not check labs if on med for a short term and the patient is healthy.)

Itraconazole

MOA

Azole – blocks ergosterol synthesis by inhibiting 14-alpha demethylase (blocks conversion of lanosterol to ergosterol)

Good for fungi and yeast and deeper/more serious fungal infections

Blocks the hedgehog pathway

Also has anti-angiogenesis and nail growth actions and modulates inflammatory or immune diseases

Pre-screening Questions

History of congestive heart failure?

History of liver disease?

On any P450 medications?

Pre-screening Labs

LFTs

CBC

Check to see if on any P450 medications – do drug interaction check

Dosing

Onychomycosis

Continual treatment: 200 mg/day for 6 weeks (fingernails) or 12 weeks (toenails)

Intermittent pulse treatment: 200 mg BID for 1 week pulse, then break for 3 weeks, then pulse weekly for 2–3 months

Maintenance therapy: 200 mg po 1 day per month

Tinea Versicolor

200 mg/day × 7 days

For other indications, look up via other sources.

Needs acidic environment for absorption (take with OJ/cola).

Side Effects

Small affinity for the P450 system

Nausea, vomiting (most common), GI upset, diarrhea

Rash/itching

Hypertriglyceridemia

Edema, hypertension

Increased LFTs

Leukopenia

Unusual or unpleasant taste

Impotence/erection problems/hair loss

Changes in menstrual periods

Nephrotoxicity (nephrotic syndrome)

Monitoring

LFTs, CBC, creatinine, UA (to look for proteinuria) at 4–6 weeks of treatment or every 4 weeks if extended therapy

Reference: https://reference.medscape.com/drug/sporanox-omnel-itraconazole-342591#4

Fluconazole

MOA

Azole – blocks ergosterol synthesis by inhibiting 14-alpha demethylase (blocks conversion of lanosterol to ergosterol).

Great for candida, good for dermatophytes, tinea versicolor, cryptococcus.

Candida glabrata is resistant.

Pre-screening Questions

Pregnant or breastfeeding? Avoid

Abnormal liver function?

On an HMG Co-A reductase inhibitor? Avoid

On other 450 activating/reducing medications?

Pre-screening Labs

Check to see if on any P450 medications – do medication interaction check.

Avoid if on HMG Co-A reductase inhibitor?

Dosing

Vaginitis: 150 mg × 1

Tinea versicolor: 50–150 mg weekly for 2–6 weeks

Candidiasis: 200 mg on the first day and then 100 mg daily for 2 weeks

Seborrheic dermatitis: 300 mg weekly × 2–4 weeks

Onychomycosis: 150–300 mg weekly for 6–12 months

For other indications, please see other sources.

Side Effects

Nausea, vomiting, diarrhea, abdominal pain

Dysgeusia

Headache

Rash, urticarial, exfoliative dermatitis

Rarely elevated LFTs (severe hepatitis has been reported rarely)

Endocrine effects: breast enlargement (males), impotence, alopecia if prolonged use at 400 mg

Monitoring

CBC diff, LFT then every 4–8 weeks then every 3 months if prolonged treatment

References

- Cömert A. *Am J Clin Dermatol.* 2007;8(4):235–8
- Gupta AK. *J Dermatolog Treat.* 2013;24(1):75–80
- https://dermnetnz.org/topics/fluconazole/

Doxycycline and Minocycline

MOA
Block the 30s ribosomal subunit

Pre-screening Questions
Is this person 9+ years old? (Cannot use in kids <9 as can cause discoloration of teeth and delayed bone growth)

Pregnant or breastfeeding? Contraindicated in pregnancy and breastfeeding

Pre-screening Labs
None

Dosing
Doxycycline

50–200 mg daily
(Usually 100 mg BID)
20, 75, 100, 150 mg extended release daily

Minocycline

50–200 mg daily
(Often 100 mg BID)
45, 90, 135 mg extended release daily

Doxycycline preferred in patients with renal failure (excreted by GI tract)

Side Effects
Doxycycline
Dental staining in children <9 years old
GI upset/nausea/vomiting/loss of appetite/diarrhea

Pill esophagitis
Photosensitivity and photo-onycholysis
Pseudotumor cerebri, headache, tinnitus (rare)
Vulvovaginal candidiasis
Minocycline
Common

- Vertigo/dizziness (~30%)
- Nausea/vomiting/upset stomach
- Diarrhea
- Headache
- Pigmentary changes
  - Pigmentation of old scars, shins, brown discoloration in sunny areas
  - Gum discoloration
  - Staining of permanent teeth in adults
  - Dental staining <9 years
- Numbness/tingling

Rare

- Pseudotumor cerebri
- Stevens-Johnson syndrome/toxic epidermal necrolysis (SJS/TEN)
- Drug reaction with eosinophilia and systemic symptoms/ drug-induced hypersensitivity syndrome (DRESS/DIHS)
- Hepatic necrosis
- Serum sickness
- Drug-induced lupus
- Photosensitivity
- Tinnitus

Glycopyrrolate

MOA
Anticholinergic

Pre-screening Questions
History of cardiac arrhythmias?

Constipation?
Elderly?
Urinary retention?

Pre-screening Labs
None

Dosing
1–2 mg BID–TID (max 8 mg/day)

Side Effects
Anticholinergic symptoms: dry mouth, dry skin, flushing, blurred vision, constipation, urinary retention; tachycardia, hyperthermia, cardiac arrhythmia/palpitations
Headache
Dizziness

Monitoring
None

Prednisone

Reading: Caplan et al. JAAD; 2017;76(2):201–7.

MOA
Corticosteroid binds to the cytosolic glucocorticoid/mineralocorticoid receptor which activates it. It translocates to the nucleus and then binds to glucocorticoid response elements on multiple genes where the corticosteroids can act as an agonist or antagonist (Fig. 8.3). GCR is ubiquitous throughout the body.

11 beta-hydroxysteroid dehydrogenase in the liver converts steroids to active forms.

Cortisol-binding globulin (CBG) is the main carrier protein. Steroid that is bound to this is inactive; unbound (free fraction) is active.

- Increased CBG: estrogen therapy, pregnancy, hyperthyroidism (decrease free fraction)
- Decreased CBG: hypothyroidism, liver disease, renal disease, obesity (increase free fraction)

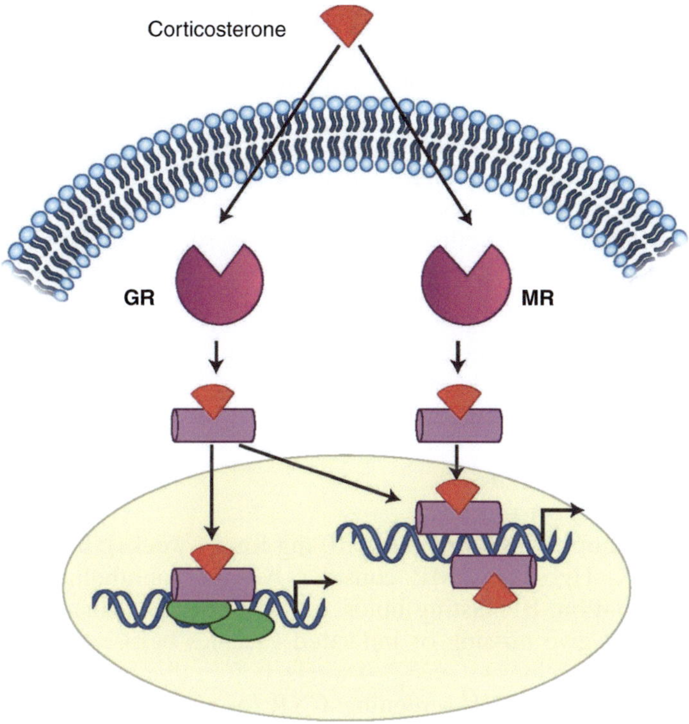

FIGURE 8.3 Mechanism of action of prednisone

Effects: Anti-inflammatory, antimitotic, immunosuppressant, apoptosis induction (autoreactive and neoplastic Tcells), decreased angiogenesis, vasoconstriction, decreased smooth muscle response to histamine/bradykinin. Decreases circulating lymphocytes, eosinophils, monocytes, decreases antibody production, decreases synthesis of pro-inflammatory molecules, decreases fibroblast production of collagen. Increases neutrophils in circulation via less margination.

Basal production of cortisol = ~5–7.5 mg of prednisone per day

Pre-screening Questions

History of congestive heart failure? Diabetes? Use caution/ warn of side effects.

History of peptic ulcers or bowel perforation? On NSAIDs/aspirin – start on PPI.

H/o *H. pylori* infection? Alcohol use? Give concomitant PPI if indicated.

History of osteopenia/osteoporosis?

History of infection/chronic infection?

History of cataracts or glaucoma?

History of neuropsychiatric disorder, depression, suicidality?

Contraindications to Systemic Steroids

- Systemic infections, especially fungal infections
- Herpes simplex keratitis
- Allergy/hypersensitivity reactions

Pre-screening Labs

None for short-term use

If require long-term use (>10 mg for >4 weeks): baseline DEXA, HgbA1c, BMP, consider baseline ophthalmology examination, BP, fasting lipids, get immunization history (if possible, give missing or indicated vaccines before therapy; give live vaccines at least 2–4 weeks before therapy), Hep B, & C serologies, HIV screening; CXR for histoplasmosis if in an endemic area, TB and strongyloides screening as appropriate

There is a higher risk of Hep B reactivation with >10 mg >4 weeks of prednisone.

Based on DEXA, can determine if bisphosphonate is needed (see below for details).

Dosing

Glucocorticoid potencies and duration (based on Caplan et al. JAAD;. 2017;76(2):201–7)

Short duration of action (8–12 h), least anti-inflammatory:

Hydrocortisone: equivalent dose 20 mg
Cortisone: equivalent dose 25 mg

Intermediate duration of action (12–36 h):

Prednisone/prednisolone: equivalent dose 5 mg

Methylprednisolone/triamcinolone: equivalent dose 4 mg

Long acting (36–72 h), most anti-inflammatory:

Betamethasone/dexamethasone: equivalent dose 0.75 mg
Fludrocortisone: equivalent dose

Goals when starting corticosteroids

1. Primary goal is to be off in 2–3 weeks (HPA axis suppression occurs after 3–4 weeks of treatment)
2. If cannot be off of corticosteroids in 2–3 weeks, then goal is to be at physiologic dosing (5–7.5 mg) by 3–4 weeks
3. If cannot meet secondary goal, then plan to change to alternate day dosing or start a steroid sparing agent to transition to

Dosing range: 5–100 mg/day of prednisone

- Advise that should take in the morning and with a meal.
- Divided doses and single dose therapy given at any time other than morning increase risk of HPA suppression.
- Alternate day dosing decreases the risk of nearly all major complications (except cataracts and osteoporosis).

Special Dosing Considerations

Start all on concomitant calcium 800–1200 mg daily and vitamin D 800–2000 units daily supplementation.

If anticipating >1 month of treatment

- Get DEXA scan for baseline and start on bisphosphonate. Note: bisphosphonates are contraindicated in pregnancy, hypocalcemia, renal failure. Read more on prescribing habits before prescribing.
- If >15 mg in patients with immunosuppression or >3 month total treatment
  - PJP ppx according to guidelines below.
  - Get alert bracelet and advise what to do if sick/undergoing surgery as may need to anticipate needing stress dose steroids.

If liver failure, consider prednisolone instead of prednisone as this does not have to be acted upon by the liver.

If prone to ulcers or on NSAIDs/aspirin, start on PPI (see screening questions above).

Monitoring

- Fasting blood glucose/HbA1C
- Blood pressure
- DEXA scans
- Lipids (triglycerides)
- Electrolytes (BMP) including calcium
- Height and weight for children
- TB and CXR if on chronic therapy
- Eye examination every 6–12 months
- AM cortisol or 24-h urine-free cortisol, as required
  - AM cortisol – primary screening tool >10 mcg/dL = good adrenal function
  - 24-h urine-free cortisol – more accurate

When and How to Taper

- Always try to taper if course >4 weeks.
- Begin taper when disease is under control.
- Avoid rapid taper in order to avoid flare of disease.
- Rough guideline is that if corticosteroid has been given for >1 month, taper by 20–30% every 1–2 weeks (if pt. is fragile, extend taper to every 3–4 weeks).
  - Above physiologic CS levels, try to taper more rapidly.
  - Below physiology CS levels (10 mg or less), taper more gradually.
- Prednisone dose increased to last effective dose before flare occurred.
- If after tapering, dose exceeds physiology levels for >1 month, consider alternate day therapy.
- Nearing end of taper, get AM cortisol level to see how you are doing.
  - AM cortisol >10 means adrenals working fine.

Example of Taper (adapted from Caplan et al. JAAD;. 2017;76(2):201–7)

- For patients taking >40 mg/day prednisone.
  - Taper steroids by 10 mg/week to 40 mg prednisone daily.
  - Remain on 40 mg/day for week.
- Starting at 40 mg/day prednisone
  - Taper by 5 mg/week to a dose of 20 mg prednisone daily.
  - Stay on 20 mg prednisone daily for 1 week.
- Starting at 20 mg/day prednisone
  - Taper by 2.5 mg/week to a dose of 5 mg daily.
  - Stay on 5 mg prednisone daily for 1 week.
- Starting at 5m/gday prednisone
  - Taper by 1 mg/week.
  - Continue taper until patient is off of steroids.

Intramuscular Corticosteroids

Posterior placement: be sure to place accurately in order to avoid damaging the sciatic nerve (Fig. 8.4). *Limit to three to four injections per year.*

Intravenous Corticosteroids *(Pulse Therapy)*

Quickly controls serious conditions with minimal toxicity.

MUST ADMIT.

500–1000 mg methylprednisolone IV over 60 min daily × 5 days. *Cardiac monitoring is required.*

Monitor electrolytes, especially potassium.

Alternative day or steroid sparing drug used to maintain improvement after pulse dose steroids.

Risks: sudden death, AFib, anaphylaxis

Side Effects of Corticosteroids

Cutaneous/topical application

- Atrophy
- Telangiectasias
- Striae
- Ecchymoses/purpura
- Skin addiction to topical steroid application
- Poor wound healing

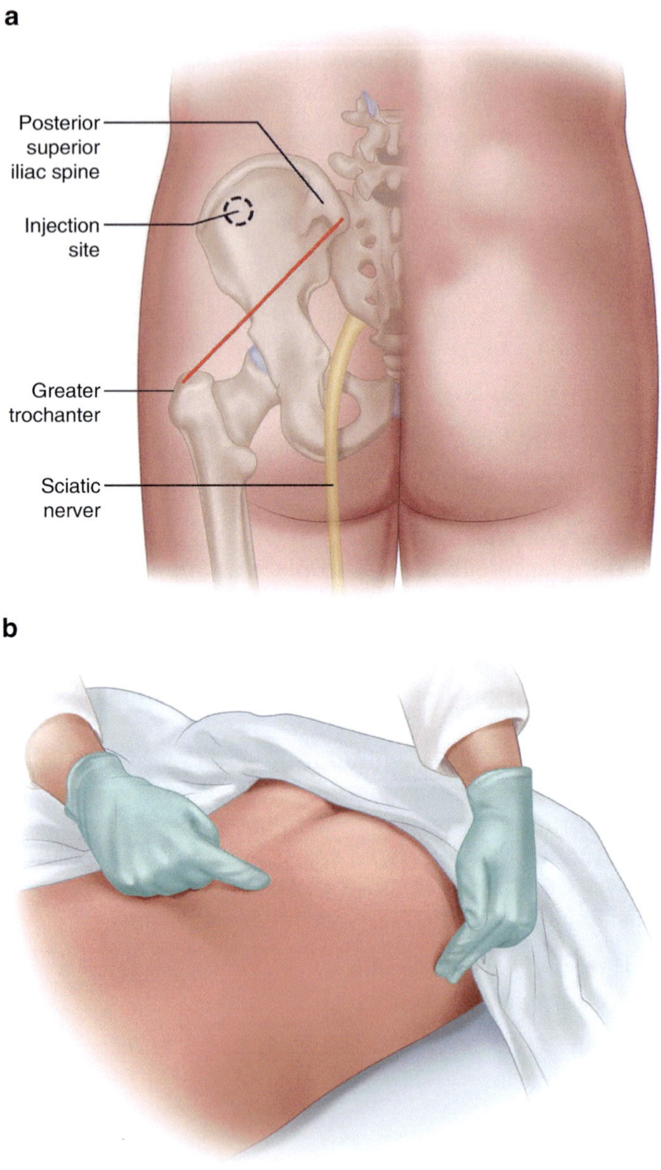

FIGURE 8.4 (**a**) Anatomic landmarks for posterior placement of IM corticosteroid injections. (**b**) Example of finding those locations through palpation

- Hypopigmentation
- Cutaneous infections

Systemic Side Effects
Short term

- Increase appetite/weight gain,
- GI upset/peptic ulcers
- Hyperglycemia/worsening of diabetes
- Hypertriglyceridemia
- Sodium retention/electrolyte disturbances, peripheral edema
- Hypertension
- Worsening of CHF
- Increased energy
- Psychosis

Longer term
General

- HPA axis suppression
- Cushingoid changes/lipodystrophy: moon face, buffalo hump, central obesity
- Failure to thrive

Metabolic effects

- Hyperglycemia/worsening/development of diabetes
- Increase appetite/weight gain
- Hypertriglyceridemia (may result in acute pancreatitis)
- Menstrual irregularities
- Hirsutism

Cardiac effects

- Hypertension
- Increased sodium retention
- Hypokalemia
- Peripheral edema
- Congestive heart failure

Bony effects

- Osteoporosis (although bone loss starts right away, most bone loss in the first 6 months of therapy) – risk does not change with every other day dosing.
- Osteonecrosis (typically 2–3 months into course; proximal femur most common).
- Hypokalemia.

Pediatric effects

- Growth suppression
Ocular effects

- Cataracts (risk does not change with every other day dosing)
- Glaucoma

Gastrointestinal effects

- Nausea/vomiting.
- Peptic ulcer disease (mainly if total dose >1 g); PPI/H2 blockers can help.
- Fatty liver changes.
- Esophageal reflux.
- Bowel perforation.

Muscular effects

- Muscle atrophy
- Myopathy (proximal lower extremity weakness)

Opportunistic infections

- PCP
- TB
- Deep fungal infections
- Prolonged herpetic infections
- Others

Psychiatric effects

- Psychosis
- Hypomania
- Insomnia
- Agitation
- Depression

Neurologic effects

- Pseudotumor cerebri
- Seizures
- Epidermal lipomatosis
- Peripheral neuropathy

Intralesional corticosteroid risks

- Atrophy
- Hypopigmentation
- Striae

Intramuscular administration additional side effects

- Cold abscesses
- Subcutaneous fat atrophy
- Crystal deposition
- Menstrual irregularities
- Purpura
- Damage to underlying tissues/nerves (sciatic)

Pulse IV steroids additional side effects

- Sudden death (thought to be cardiac in origin due to quick electrolyte shifts (monitor potassium))
- Atrial fibrillation
- Seizures
- Anaphylaxis

Steroid Emergencies

- Addisonian crisis – rare and *life-threatening*. Occurs in patients on long-term CS usually with mineralocorticoid activity. Period of stress and the body cannot respond. Patients have *hypotension and very low cortisol levels*.
- Steroid withdrawal syndrome (SWS) – more common. Occurs in patients on long-term CS who undergo short taper. Doses given beyond 2–3 weeks can spur SWS. S/s: arthralgias, myalgias, mood swings, headache, fatigue, lethargy, anorexia, nausea, vomiting. *No change in serum cortisol level* (but rather decreased available intracellular corticosteroid).

Stress Dose Steroids

Major stress (e.g., surgery): Hydrocortisone 100 mg night before surgery and q8h day of

Minor stress (e.g., febrile illness): Take twice basal production (~5–15 mg prednisone) extra

Bisphosphonate therapy

Reference: Caplan et al. *JAAD*. 2017;76(2):201–7.

Osteoporosis with Steroids

Greatest reduction in bone mass occurs in the first 6 months of corticosteroid administration.

Every other day dosing of steroid does not decrease risk of osteoporosis.

Greatest absolute loss of bone mass occurs in young men.

Algorithm to evaluate bone mass:

1. Initiation of glucocorticoids and pt counseling regarding fracture risk, modifiable risk factors, baseline DEXA scan, and begin supplemental calcium and vitamin D
    (a) If low or intermediate risk (DEXA T score -1 to -2.5 and 10 year fracture risk <20%): start bisphosphonates if taking 7.5 mg prednisone or more daily for 3 months or greater.
    (b) If high risk: (T score -1 to -2.5 and 10year fracture risk >20%: start bisphosphonates at any steroid dose.
    (c) If established osteoporosis (T score less than -2.5 or fragility fracture exists): bisphosphonate therapy for osteoporosis.

All patients taking any dose of glucocorticoids with an anticipated duration of 3 months or more should maintain a total daily calcium intake of 800 to 1200 mg daily and vitamin D of 800 to 2000 units daily.

The first-line therapy for treating glucocorticoid-induced osteoporsis is bisphosphonates; alendronate and risedronate are the preferred first-line agents. Intravenous zoledronic acid is reserved for patients who are unable to tolerate oral medications.

Options for bisphosphonate therapy

- Alendronate: 5 mg daily, 70 mg weekly, or 150 mg monthly (generally the 70 mg dose is recommended)
- Risedronate: 5 mg daily or 35 mg weekly
- Zoledronic acid: 5 mg once yearly as an IV infusion for patients who cannot tolerate oral bisphosphonates
  - Monitor for flu-like symptoms 2–3 days after 1st injection; can treat with acetaminophen or NSAIDs; use with caution in patients with history of atrial fibrillation.

Before starting therapy

- Consider referral for dental examination – avoid bisphosphonate therapy when dental work is needed.
- Get calcium and vitamin D levels – correct hypocalcemia and vitamin D deficiencies.
- Get creatinine – avoid bisphosphonate use if creatinine clearance is <30–35 mL/min and refer to endocrinology for management.
- Make sure patient can swallow and stay upright 30 min after taking bisphosphonate.
- Avoid use in patient with active upper GI disease or swallowing difficulties.

Administration

- Take alone on an empty stomach first thing in the morning with 8 ounces of water.
  - Note: enteric coated; delayed release risedronate is taken immediately after breakfast with 4 ounces of water.
- Avoid food and drink and other medications or supplements for 30 min after taking alendronate or risedronate.
- Remain upright for 30 min after taking.
- Discontinue if patients develop esophagitis.

Pneumocystis Pneumonia (PCP) Prophylaxis

PCP is a potentially life-threatening infection caused by *Pneumocystis jiroveci* in immunocompromised individuals.

- Mortality rate from PCP in non-HIV infected patients is 90–100%.

- PCP usually develops within 1 month of glucocorticoid administration (median 12 weeks) with a median dose of prednisone 30 mg/day but can be as little as 16 mg/day.
- Risk factors for PCP
  - Glucocorticoid dose >20 mg of prednisone for >1 month + another cause of immunocompromise
  - Combination of immunosuppressive drugs (TNFa + high dose steroids, mtx + steroids)
  - Treatment of polymyositis/dermatomyositis with interstitial pulmonary fibrosis with glucocorticoids
  - Primary immunodeficiency syndromes (SCID, idiopathic CD4 T-lymphocytopenia, hyper-IgM syndrome)
  - Acquired immunodeficiency syndromes (ALL, solid organ transplant patient on anti-rejection drugs, patients on chemotherapy)
  - Patients with severe malnutrition (especially protein malnutrition)

Prophylaxis

- First line: Trimethoprim-sulfamethoxazole (TMP-SMX) one DS tab daily or three times per week or as one single-strength tablet daily.
  - Patients on methotrexate should not receive TMP-SMX.
- If pt cannot tolerate TMP-SMX, alternatives are atovaquone, dapsone with or without pyrimethamine, pentamidine, clindamycin + primaquine or sulfadoxine + pyrimethamine.
  - Patients who cannot tolerate the use of TMP-SMX can attempt desensitization with allergist.

Caution in SLE

PCP ppx in pts with SLE finds that sulfa-containing antibiotics like TMP-SMX can cause exacerbations of SLE; atovaquone is suggested as an alternative.

Ref: Anevlavis S et al. *Pneumon.* 25(4):348–9.

Reference

- Wolverton, AS et al. *Pneumon.* 25(4):348–9, JAAD CME Jan & Feb 2017 (Caplan et al. *JAAD.* 2017;76(2):201–7)

Oral Contraceptive Pills

MOA

Based on antiandrogen properties: decrease androgen production at the level of the ovary, increase sex hormone-binding globulin, bind-free circulating testosterone thus reducing free testosterone (by 40–50% on average), reduce 4-alpha reductase activity, and block the androgen receptor.

Note: for acne must have a combination pill with estrogen as this is what helps to reduce acne. Progesterone-only pills have been associated with worsening acne.

Combination pills contain both estrogen and progestin components.

Estrogen Component

Ethinyl estradiol: For acne – Reduces the conversion of testosterone to dihydrotestosterone (DHT) in the pilosebaceous unit > decreased sebum production.

For contraception: Reduces LHRH release from hypothalamus, reduces gonadotropin release from pituitary; increases synthesis of DNA, RNA, and various proteins in target tissues; other possible mechanisms include changes in cervical mucus that cause inhibition of sperm penetration and endometrial changes that reduce likelihood of implantation.

Progesterone Component

- First-generation progestins (estranges): norethindrone and ethynodiol diacetate
- Second-generation progestin (gonanes): levonorgestrel and norgestimate
- Third-generation progestin (*less androgenic gonanes*): desogestrel and gestodene
- Fourth generation (antiandrogen): drospirenone

- Drospirenone: spironolactone analogue with anti-mineralocorticoid and anti-androgenic activity

Pre-screening Questions

History of blood clots in the patient or a family member?

Hypertension?

Smoker?

Family history of malignancy, esp breast cancer and/or uterine cancer?

Caution in history of depression, diabetes, hypertension, bone mineral density changes, renal/hepatic impairment, bone metabolic disease, systemic lupus erythematosus or other disorders which are prone to blood clots/hypercoagulability

---

Contraindications to OCPs

Pregnancy
Breast cancer (current)
Breastfeeding: <6 weeks postpartum (caution up to 6 months postpartum)
Age over 35 and heavy smokers (15 cigarettes per day)
Hypertension (>160 systolic; >100 diastolic)
Diabetes mellitus with end organ damage (e.g., renal) or >20 yr duration
Deep vein thrombosis (history of current)
Known thrombogenic mutations
Systemic lupus erythematosus
Migraine with aura at any age
Major surgery with prolonged immobilization
Ischemic heart disease (history or current); valvular heart disease with complications
Stroke
Migraine headaches (with focal neurological symptoms at any age or without focal neurological symptoms but over 35 years of age)
Active viral hepatitis
Cirrhosis (severe) or liver tumor (benign or malignant)
Caution in starting OCPs in patients within first 2 years of starting menses or in patients who are <14 years of age unless clinically warranted due to concerns of decreased bone mass

---

Black Box Warning

Cigarette smoking and risk of cardiovascular disease

- Women >35 years who smoke should not use oral contraceptives.
- Cigarette smoking increases risk of serious cardiovascular adverse effects from combination oral contraceptive use.
- This risk increases with age (>35 yr) and with heavy smoking (15 or more cigarettes/day).
- Advise women taking oral contraceptives not to smoke.

Pre-screening Workup

Blood pressure (contraindicated in hypertension)

HCG if necessary

Dosing

Note: for acne must have a combination pill with estrogen as this is what helps to reduce acne. Progesterone-only pills have been associated with worsening acne.

Four approved OCPs for treatment of acne

- Ethinyl estradiol/norgestimate
- Ethinyl estradiol/norethindrone acetate/ferrous fumarate
- Ethinyl estradiol/drospirenone/levomefolate
- Ethinyl estradiol/drospirenone

Ways to start

- Quick start (preferred): begin on the day prescription is given (as long as pregnancy is reasonably excluded).
- Sunday start: begin on the first Sunday after period.
- First day start - start the pill on the first day of menses.

In general

- Women should be advised to use additional non-hormonal contraception during the first 7 days of therapy.
- Administer tablets in the order directed on the blister pack calendar at the same time each day.

Discontinue therapy 4 weeks before major surgery or prolonged immobilization; may be possible resume 2 weeks afterwards on case-by-case basis.

Side Effects

Breakthrough bleeding (most common) and is associated with missed pills

Nausea, breast tenderness (usually resolve over first two to three cycles of use)

Premenstrual syndrome

Migraine headaches

Menstrual irregularities

Abdominal pain/discomfort

Mood changes

Thromboembolic events (venous thromboembolism)

Other Adverse Associations with Combination Oral Contraceptive Use (references: Cutis Dec 2015; 96(6) and Barbieri et al. JAAD 2019;80:538-49.)

Increased risk of

1. Breast cancer: (RR 1.24 in current users) no longer a risk 10 years after discontinuation
2. Ischemic stroke: increased risk in smoker, HTN, migraines, 50 mcg ethinyl estradiol or greater
3. Hemorrhagic stroke: smoker, htn, 35 yrs or older
4. Diminished bone mass
5. MI: smoker, htn, 35 years or older
6. Venous thromboembolism: smoker, 35 years or older, <21 days postpartum, immobilization, hx PE/DVT, active IBD, hereditary thrombophilia, SLE, antiphospholipid Ab syndrome

Decreased risk of

Decreased risks of colorectal, ovarian, and endometrial cancers

References

- Zaenglein et al. *JAAD*. 2016;74(5):945–73.
- *Cutis.* 2015; 96(6)
- Barberi et al. *JAAD* 2019;80:538–49

Biologics

Vaccines and Biologics

Be sure to give all age appropriate vaccines, especially live vaccines before starting.

If necessary to give vaccine (especially live) while under treatment, for many the general reacmmendation is to stop the biologic 10 days prior to giving the vaccine and then okay to restart 10–14 days after the vaccine.

Should recommend all patients get a flu shot yearly.

Guide to Biologic Names (Table 8.2)

Typically, a monoclonal antibody has four segments and six syllables

- Segment 1 is prefix and is random and distinctive (under control of drug developer).

TABLE 8.2 Biologic nomenclature

Stem	Meaning
-cept	Receptor molecules, native or modified (a receding infix should designate the target)
-mab	Monoclonal antibodies
- xi -	Chimeric (monoclonal antibody)
-xizu -	Chimeric/humanized (monoclonal antibody)
-zu-	Humanized (monoclonal antibody)
-u-	Fully human (monoclonal antibody)
-kin	Interleukin type substances
-kinra	Interleukin receptor antagonists
-ermin	Growth factors
-stim	Colony-stimulating factors
-tide	Peptides and glycopeptides

- Segment 2 denotes the target or disease class.
  - B = bacterial
  - F = antifungal
  - T = tumor
- Segment 3 is the source of the antibody.
  - U = human
  - A = rat
  - Xi = chimeric
  - Zu = humanized
- Segment 3 tag on the "mab" suffice for monoclonal antibody.

TNF-Alpha Inhibitors

MOA

Etanercept: Fully human dimeric fusion protein (TNF type II receptor linked to Fc portion of IgG1) that binds soluble TNFa

Adalimumab: Recombinant, fully human monoclonal IgG1 monoclonal antibody against soluble and transmembrane bound TNF

Infliximab: Chimeric monoclonal IgG; binds both soluble and transmembrane TNFa-receptor

Notable Drug Interactions

- Anakinra
- Azathioprine (increases risk of hepatosplenic T-cell lymphoma)

Pre-screening Information

Contraindications to TNFa-inhibitors: Taking anakinra or azathioprine, active/chronic infection, history of demyelinating disease (e.g., multiple sclerosis and others), CHF (NYHA class III or IV heart failure) (highest risk with infliximab), TB or other granulomatous disease, history of fungal disease (e.g., histoplasmosis, blastomycosis), liver disease (have to get okay from hepatologist before starting if considering).

Chronic disease history: Liver/renal disease?

History of malignancy: Prior or current; may want to consider another agent.

Infection history: Hepatitis? TB? Travel TB? HIV? Grow up in endemic area for infection.

Childbearing status/plans to have children?

Immunization status:

Influenza, hepatitis B, pneumococcal, shingles. Up to date with childhood vaccines?

Vaccines and biologics

Be sure to give all age appropriate vaccines, especially live vaccines, before starting.

If necessary to give vaccine while under treatment, stop the biologic 10 days prior to giving the vaccine and then okay to restart 10–14 days after the vaccine.

Should recommend all patients get a flu shot yearly.

Pre-screening Labs

CBC, BMP, LFTs, hepatitis B/C serologies, HIV, PPD or quant gold/T-spot/PPD

CXR if PPD/T-spot/quant gold positive or if lives or grew up in histo/blasto prone area

Assess vaccination status

Dosing

Etanercept and biosimilar etanercept-ykro

Dosing for psoriasis: 50 mg SubQ two times per week × 3 months, then 50 mg subQ weekly

Adalimumab and biosimilars adalimumab-atto, adalimumab-adbm, adalimumab-adaz, adalimumab-bwwd

Psoriasis: 80 mg SubQ × 1 week, 40 mg subQ 1 week later, then 40 mg subQ every other week

Hidradenitis (no biosimilars)

Induction: 160 mg SC on Day 1 (given in 1 day or split over 2 consecutive days), then 80 mg SC beginning 2 weeks later (Day 15)

Maintenance (beginning Day 29): 40 mg SC qWeek

Infliximab and biosimilars infliximab-dyyb, infliximab-abda, infliximab-qbtx, infliximab-axxq

Dosing for psoriasis: 5 mg/kg IV at 0, 2, and 6 weeks, THEN q8Weeks thereafter

Monitoring

Every 6 months: LFTs, CBC

Yearly: PPD/quant gold/T-spot

Side Effects of TNFa

Injection site reactions (etanercept > adalimumab)

Infusion reactions (infliximab) in ~20%: nausea, headache, flushing, dyspnea, injection site infiltration, taste changes

Infliximab-related infusion reactions

Acute: 10 min–24 h

Delayed: 1–14 days

Decreased infusion rate and premedication may help.

Epinephrine and IV corticosteroids given for serious reactions.

Cutaneous

- May paradoxically induce flares of psoriasis (can be pustular, plamo/plantar) (can often change to another TNFa-inhibitor if this is the case)
- Cutaneous vasculitis

Infections

- Most commonly viral: flu/colds/respiratory infections
- Risk of invasive fungal infections, reactivation of hepatitis, TB reactivations, or other serious infections, especially granulomatous infections
- Opportunistic infections (e.g., legionella, listerial, others)

Rheumatologic

- Development of lupus erythematosus (+ANA, +ds-DNA) (infliximab most commonly)

Neurologic: Worsening of MS, optic neuritis, transverse myelitis, Guillain-Barre

Cardiac: Heart failure worsening (infliximab greatest risk)

Development of antibodies to the TNFa-inhibitor, most common with infliximab (infliximab-associated-antidrug-antibodies): leads to not only decreased efficacy of the drug but can cause increased effusion reactions (infliximab). Breaks in therapy predispose to this. Can add in low-dose methotrexate to minimize Ab formation if this is suspected.

Hepatic: rare liver failure/autoimmune hepatitis (+ anti-smooth muscle autoantibodies)

Hematologic: rare hematologic toxicity

Increased risk of malignancy

- Leukemia/lymphoma.
- Hepatosplenic T-cell lymphoma (fatal) may be seen with TNF-inhibitor + azathioprine.

IL-23 Inhibitors

MOA

Ustekinumab: Fully human monoclonal IgG1 antibody against p40 subunit found in IL12 and IL23

Guselkumab: Human IgG1 monoclonal antibody that binds to the p19 subunit of IL-23 preventing it from binding to cell receptors

Tildrakizumab/tildrakizumab-asmn: Humanized IgG1 monoclonal antibody that selectively binds to the p19 subunit of Il-23 cytokine and inhibits its interaction with the IL-23 receptor

Risankizumab/risankizumab-rzaa: Humanized IgG1 monoclonal antibody that selectively binds to the p19 subunit of Il-23 cytokine and inhibits its interaction with the IL-23 receptor

Pre-screening Information

Immunization status

Influenza, hepatitis B, pneumococcal, shingles. Up to date with childhood vaccines?

Vaccines and biologics

Be sure to give all age appropriate vaccines, especially live vaccines before starting.

If necessary to give a vaccine while under treatment, stop the biologic 10 days prior to giving the vaccine and then okay to restart 10–14 days after the vaccine.

Should recommend all patients get a flu shot yearly.

Infection history (active, chronic, or history of): Hepatitis? TB? Travel? HIV? Grow up in an endemic area for infection? Higher risk of HBV infection and reactivation.

Childbearing status/plans to have children? Consider other agents.

History of malignancy? May want to exclude patients with malignancy within the past 5 years (except for non-melanoma skin cancer).

Obesity? Guselkumab and tildrakizumab seem to have less efficacy in heavier patients.

Pre-screening Labs

CBC, BMP, LFTs, Hepatitis B/C, HIV, PPD or Quant Gold/T-spot/PPD

CXR if PPD/T-spot/quant gold positive or if lives or grew up in histo/blasto prone area

Assess vaccination status

Dosing

Ustekinumab

- <220 lbs (100 kg): 45 mg subcutaneous at week 0, 4, and then every 12 weeks
- >220 lbs (100 kg): 90 mg subcutaneous at week 0, 4, and then every 12 weeks

Guselkumab 100 mg SC at Week 0, Week 4, and q8Weeks thereafter

Tildrakizumab/tildrakizumab-asmn: 100 mg SC at Weeks 0, 4, and q12Weeks thereafter

Risankizumab/risankizumab-rzaa: 150 mg (two 75-mg injections) SC at Week 0, Week 4, and q12Weeks thereafter

Monitoring

At 3 months: CBC
Every 6 months: LFTs, CBC
Yearly: PPD/quant gold

Side Effects

General: Injection site reactions (1%), arthralgias, fatigue

Infections

- Upper respiratory infections and nasopharyngitis (most common for all agents)
- Tinea infections (1.1%)
- Herpes simplex infections (1.1%)

Neurologic

- Headache (common)
- Reversible posterior leukoencephalopathy syndrome (rare, case report)

Pulmonary: Non-infectious pneumonia (ustekinumab: case series, Ekelem et al. *JAMA Derm*. 2019;155(2):229–36)

For tildrakizumab, guselkumab, and risankizumab: "No increase was seen in rates of serious infections, malignancies or major adverse cardiovascular events, with no signals suggestive of an elevated risk of opportunistic infections, active tuberculosis or reactivation of latent tuberculosis infection, mucocutaneous *Candida* infections, triggering or worsening of inflammatory bowel disease, demyelinating disorders or suicidal ideation." Crowley JJ et al. *J Eur Acad Dermatol Venereol*. 2019;33(9):1676–84.

References

- Banaszcyk K. *Reumatologia*. 2019;57(3):158–162.
- Crowley JJ et al. *J Eur Acad Dermatol Venereol*. 2019;33(9):1676–84.

IL-17A: Antagonists

MOA

Secukinumab: Neutralized IL-17A – Human IgG1 monoclonal antibody that selectively binds and neutralizes IL-17A (produced by Th17 cells) and thus prevents it from binding to its receptor.

Ixekizumab: Neutralizes IL-17A – Humanized IgG4 monoclonal antibody that selectively binds and neutralizes IL-17A (produced by Th17 cells) and thus prevents it from binding to its receptor.

Brodalumab: Antagonist to the IL-17 receptor – Interleukin-17 receptor A antagonist inhibits interaction with IL17-A, IL17F, IL17C, IL-17A/F heterodimer, and IL-25, thus inhibiting the release of pro-inflammatory cytokines and chemokines.

Contraindications

Pregnancy – *For brodalumab must enroll in FDA REMS program*

Crohn's disease

Active, chronic, or latent infections

Immunosuppression

Depression/suicidal behavior (brodalumab)

Pre-screening Information

Patient must not be immunosuppressed.

Infection history: Hepatitis? TB? Travel TB? HIV? Grow up in an endemic area for infection?

- Must not have active or untreated latent TB
- Must not have active or chronic infection (HIV, hepatitis, indwelling urinary catheters, chronic leg ulcers)

Childbearing status/plans to have children?

- Not approved for pregnant or nursing women

History of Crohn's disease? Contraindication – although newer studies have shown that perhaps secukinumab does not flare IBD/Crohn's

Immunization status

Influenza, hepatitis B, pneumococcal, shingles. Up to date with childhood vaccines?

Vaccines and biologics

Be sure to give all age appropriate vaccines, especially live vaccines before starting.

If necessary to give a vaccine while under treatment, stop the biologic 10 days prior to giving the vaccine and then okay to restart 10–14 days after the vaccine.

Should recommend all patients get a flu shot yearly.

s Black box warning for suicidal ideation and behavior for brodalumab!

Pre-screening Labs

CXR, PPD/quant gold, LFTs, CBC, Hep B/C, HIV, HCG females.

Be sure to give live vaccines 1 month before starting.

Be sure no h/o Crohn's disease or pregnancy.

If positive PPD, 9 months of INH is recommended before starting treatment.

Dosing

Secukinumab

Administer by subcutaneous injection

- Initial: 300 mg SC at weeks 0, 1, 2, 3, and 4 then
- Monthly maintenance: Beginning at week 8, give 300 mg SC once monthly
  - For some patients, a dose of 150 mg may be acceptable.
  - Note: If you give it more spaced out than that, then your PASI success goes down.
  - Note: Clearance is independent of the kidney and liver so no modification of dose is needed for patients with renal or hepatic impairment.
  - Note: A little less response in people with higher weights. In patients with previous biologic therapy, there is some reduction of efficacy.

Ixekizumab
Administer by subcutaneous injection
Week 0: 160 mg subQ (i.e., as two 80-mg injections), THEN 80 mg subQ q2weeks at 2, 4, 6, 8, and 12, THEN 80 mg subQ q4weeks
Brodalumab
Administer by subcutaneous injection
210 mg subcutaneously at weeks 0, 1, and 2 followed by 210 mg every 2 weeks.

Note: *Requires FDA enrollment in REMS program for monitoring* (requirement for prescribers, pharmacy certification, medication guide for patients with information about risks of suicidal ideation and behavior). Prescribers are required to counsel patients about the risks and patients are required to sign a "patient-prescriber agreement form." www.SILIQREMS.com or call 855-511-6135.

Monitoring
6 weeks after treatment (or based on symptoms) CBC to assess for neutropenia

Every 6 months: CBC.

Due to possibility of neutropenia, check CBC if pt present with signs/symptoms of infection.
Yearly: PPD, quant gold/T-spot
Regularly monitor mood with brodalumab

SE
Infection

- Most common: Increased risk of mild infections – upper respiratory tract infections/nasopharyngitis (27% in tx group vs 23% in placebo group [ixekizumab])
- Increased risk of fungal infections (tinea/mucocutaneous candidiasis)
  - Candidal infections are common in up to 5%.
    - IL-17 is needed in the immunity towards candida.
- Serious infection in 3%

Cutaneous

- Eczema

- Pruritus
- Injection site reactions

  Headache
  Diarrhea
  Rare side effects

- Exacerbation of Crohn's disease
  - Secukinumab: 1/1000 in clinical trials
  - Ixekizumab: 0.1% flare of Crohn's and 0.2% of ulcerative colitis with treatment vs 0% in placebo
- Neutropenia – usually mild, transient, and reversible
- Depression/suicidality – brodalumab
- Severe hypersensitivity reaction
  - Anaphylaxis
  - Urticaria
  - Angioedema
- Anti-drug antibodies
- Arthralgias
- Oropharyngeal pain

Very few infections (not much above placebo), malignant, or unspecified tumors are not much above placebo either.

References

- Culp et al. *Dermatologist.* 2016
  http://www.accessdata.fda.gov/drugsatfda_docs/label/2017/761032lbl.pdf IL
- IL4Ra – Antagonist
  https://pubmed.ncbi.nlm.nih.gov/28985956/

Dupilumab: IL4 Receptor Antagonist

MOA:
Fully human IgG4 monoclonal antibody against the alpha subunit of the IL-4 receptor, which blocks IL-4 and IL-13 –

key inflammatory agents in the triggering of production of IgE and eosinophil activation

Pre-screening Information

Infection history

Childbearing status/plans to have children?

- Unknown if safe in pregnancy/breastfeeding

Immunization status

Influenza, hepatitis B, pneumococcal, shingles. Up to date with childhood vaccines?

Vaccines and biologics

Be sure to give all age appropriate vaccines, especially live vaccines before starting.

If necessary to give a vaccine while under treatment, stop the biologic 10 days prior to giving the vaccine and then okay to restart 10–14 days after the vaccine.

Should recommend all patients get a flu shot yearly.

Pre-screening Labs

None required, perhaps a CBC with diff to check eosinophil count

Dosing

Administered by subcutaneous injection

600 mg (i.e., two 300-mg injections) subQ once, then 300 mg subQ every other week

Monitoring

Not required

Periodic CBC with diff to assess for eosinophilia

SE

- Eye adverse effects – *may need to see ophthalmology for this*
  - Conjunctivitis (9–10%) – most common side effect
  - Blepharitis
  - Keratitis
  - Eye pruritus
  - Dry eyes

- Oral herpes flares (3–4%)
  - Eczema herpeticum
  - Herpes zoster
- Injection site reactions (10–15%)
- Headache (10–17% (but was less than placebo))
- Nausea
- Generalized urticarial/serum sickness-like reactions (rare)
- Hypersensitivity reactions
- Eosinophilia (4–14% vs 1% of placebo) – generally asymptomatic and frequently transient but rare reports of vasculitis and eosinophilic pneumonia
- Cardiovascular events

Treatment with dupilumab results in lower risk of all skin infections.

Reference

- Thibodeaux Q et al. *Hum Vaccin Immunother.* 2019;15(9):2129–39.

Omalizumab

MOA

Recombinant humanized IgE monoclonal antibody that selectively binds to the Ce3 domain of the IgE heavy chain and prevents it from binding to its high-affinity receptor FceRI, preventing surface cross-linking and activation of mast cells and basophils. Administration results in a significant and rapid reduction in serum levels of free IGE with subsequent late downregulation of the FceRI (IgE high-affinity receptor) and FceRII (IgE low-affinity receptor). It possibly may also deactivate allergens and IgE immune complexes and induce apoptosis of eosinophils.

Pre-screening Information

Travel history: Any risk for helminth infection?

Childbearing status/plans to have children?

- Unknown if safe in pregnancy/breastfeeding

Immunization status

Influenza, hepatitis B, pneumococcal, shingles. Up to date with childhood vaccines?

Vaccines and biologics

Be sure to give all age appropriate vaccines and try to give live vaccines before starting.

History of lung disease?

Pre-screening Labs

CBC with diff to check eos.

Stool O&P.

Measure lung function (referral to pulmonology: peak flow, FEV_1).

Sign informed consent on medication given risk of anaphylaxis and prescribe epinephrine auto-injector (see below for Omalizumab Joint Task Force Recommendations).

Dosing

150–300 mg subQ every 4 weeks

- *Give nearby resuscitation equipment.*
- *Must observe the patient for anaphylaxis for a period of 2 h for the first three injections and 30 min for subsequent injections – but symptoms may occur up to 24 h after the dose is given.*
- *Prescribe and train on how to use epinephrine auto-injectors.*

Five steps to consider to ensure safety of patients receiving omalizumab injections (from Omalizumab Joint Task Force) Ref: Cox, Linda, et al. "American Academy of Allergy, Asthma & Immunology/American College of Allergy, Asthma & Immunology Omalizumab-Associated Anaphylaxis Joint Task Force follow-up report." *J Allergy Clin Immun.* 128.1 (2011): 210–212.

1. *Informed consent*: should be obtained from the patient after discussing the risks, benefits, and alternatives to omalizumab (Xolair).

2. *Anaphylaxis education*: educate the patient on the signs, symptoms, and treatment of anaphylaxis.

3. *Epinephrine auto-injector*: prescribe and educate the patient on the proper use of and advise patients to carry an epinephrine auto-injector before and for 24 h after omalizumab (Xolair) injection.

4. *Pre-injection health assessment*: assess health status, including vital signs and some measure of lung function (e.g., peak expiratory flow or FEV_1).

5. *Wait period after injection*: patients should be kept under observation for 30 min after each injection. This time should be extended to 2 h after each of the first three injections; however, it could be modified based on a physician's clinical judgment after discussing the risks with the patient.

Lack of effect may occur in up to 12% of patients.

Monitoring

None mandated.

Periodic CBC with diff.

Monitor closely patients at risk for helminth infection while on this medication.

SE

Warning: Anaphylaxis, including bronchospasm, hypotension, syncope, urticarial, and angioedema of throat/tongue, can occur after administration and can happen with first dose but can occur beyond 1 year of regularly administered treatment. Symptoms may occur up to 24 h after the dose is given.

Most common

- Injection site reactions (45%)
- Viral infections (23%)
- URI (20%)
- Sinusitis (16%)
- Headache (15%)

- Pharyngitis (11%)
- Anaphylaxis (0.09–0.2%)
  - 61% of these reactions occurred in the first 2 h after one of the first three doses.

  Rare

- Pain, arthralgias, fatigue, dermatitis, pruritus, fever, GI upset, epistaxis

References

- Labrador-Horrillo M et al. *Drug Des Devel Ther.* 2015;9:4909–15.
- Godse K et al. *Indian J Dermatol.* 2015;60(4):381–4.
- Cox, Linda, et al. "American academy of allergy, asthma & immunology/American college of allergy, asthma & immunology omalizumab-associated anaphylaxis joint task force follow-up report." *J Allergy Clin Immunol.* 2011;128(1):210–212

Rituximab

MOA

Chimeric monoclonal antibody to CD20 antigen on mature B cells → complement activation and apoptosis of B cells with depletion of B cells occurring within 2–3 weeks of initial treatments with sustained depletion for an average of 6 months. Does NOT affect stem cells/plasma cells.

Contraindication

Active, chronic, latent infections

Relative contraindications

History of cardiac/pulmonary conditions (susceptible to severe infusion reactions), bronchospasm, hypotension, angioedema

Pre-screening Questions

Immunization status

Be sure to give all age appropriate vaccines.

Non-live vaccines to be given at least 4 weeks prior to initiation.

Immune and infection status

History of travel, active/latent/chronic infection? HIV, hepatitis B/C? TB exposure history (travel, occupation, grew up in an endemic area for TB/fungal disease?) Immunosuppressed?

Cardiac history: History of arrhythmias/angina? Perform cardiac monitoring during and after all infusions of Rituxan for patients who develop clinically significant arrhythmias, or who have a history of arrhythmia or angina.

History of anemia, leukopenia, thrombocytopenia?

Pulmonary history: History of asthma, bronchospasm, or other pulmonary disease?

Pregnant? Pregnancy category C

Pre-screening Labs

CXR, PPD/quant gold, LFTs, BUN/creatinine, CBC with diff, hepatitis B/C serologies, HIV, immunoglobulin levels

EKG

Active or latent infections are a definitive contraindication.

Do not administer if low white count or neutropenia.

Dosing

CBC prior to each infusion

All dosing while on cardiac monitoring

Lymphoma protocol: Four weekly infusions of 375 mg/m^2.

RA protocol: Two infusions of 1000 mg 2 weeks apart; repeat courses every 16–24 weeks.

Low-dose protocol: Two infusions of 500 mg 2 weeks apart.

From Drugs.com:

Rituxan should only be administered by a healthcare professional with appropriate medical support to manage severe infusion reactions that can be fatal if they occur.

- *First Infusion*: Initiate infusion at a rate of 50 mg/hr. In the absence of infusion toxicity, can increase infusion rate by 50 mg/hr. increments every 30 min, to a maximum of 400 mg/hr.

- *Subsequent Infusions*: *Standard Infusion:* Initiate infusion at a rate of 100 mg/hr. In the absence of infusion toxicity, increase rate by 100 mg/hr increments at 30-min intervals, to a maximum of 400 mg/hr.
  Initiate at a rate of 20% of the total dose given in the first 30 min and the remaining 80% of the total dose given over the next 60 min. If the 90-min infusion is tolerated in Cycle 2, the same rate can be used when administering the remainder of the treatment regimen.
  Patients who have clinically significant cardiovascular disease should not be administered the 90-min infusion.
- Interrupt the infusion or slow the infusion rate for infusion reactions. Continue the infusion at one-half the previous rate upon improvement of symptoms.

Can premedicate with an antihistamine and acetaminophen ±100 mg IV methylprednisolone or its equivalent 30 min prior to infusion.

Perform cardiac monitoring during and after all infusions of Rituxan for patients who develop clinically significant arrhythmias, or who have a history of arrhythmia or angina.

Monitoring

Time to the depletion of B cells after first rituximab infusion is 1 week to 7 months. Mean duration is 6–12 months. Mean time for the B cells to repopulate the peripheral blood is 6–12 months.

- CBC before each rituximab course.
- CBC and BMP every 1–3 months during treatment period (at least 1 year after last cycle).
- Hep B reactivation has a high risk with rituximab; repeat hepatitis testing during therapy and for several months thereafter as reactivations have occurred several months following completion of therapy (discontinue therapy if reactivation occurs).
- Immunoglobulin levels intermittently.

Can monitor effectiveness by measuring CD 19/20.

Side Effects

https://www.drugs.com/pro/rituxan.html#S6.1

https://reference.medscape.com/drug/rituxan-hycela-rituximab-hyaluronidase-1000306#4

Infusion Reactions (from Drugs.com)

Rituxan can cause severe, *including fatal*, infusion reactions. Rituxan-induced infusion reactions and sequelae include urticaria, hypotension, angioedema, hypoxia, bronchospasm, pulmonary infiltrates, acute respiratory distress syndrome, myocardial infarction, ventricular fibrillation, cardiogenic shock, anaphylactoid events, or death.

Severe reactions typically occurred during the first infusion with time to onset of 30–120 min.

Premedicate patients with an antihistamine and acetaminophen prior to dosing. Institute medical management (e.g., glucocorticoids, epinephrine, bronchodilators, or oxygen) for infusion reactions as needed. Depending on the severity of the infusion reaction and the required interventions, temporarily or permanently discontinue rituximab. Resume infusion at a minimum 50% reduction in rate after symptoms have resolved. Closely monitor the following patients: those with pre-existing cardiac or pulmonary conditions, those who experienced prior cardiopulmonary adverse reactions, and those with high numbers of circulating malignant cells ($\geq$25,000/mm^3).

If reaction is minor, infusion can be restarted at 50% rate reduction and monitored.

Other side effects include the following:

Infections, including serious infections including *sepsis and death* – discontinue therapy for serious infections.

- Hepatitis B reactivation with fulminant hepatitis – discontinue therapy if reactivation occurs
- Large joint infections
- Pneumonia

- Other bacterial/viral infections such as CMV, herpes simplex, parvovirus B19, varicella-zoster virus, hepatitis B and C, and others
- URIs, rhinitis, sinusitis

Cutaneous

- Pruritus
- Alopecia
- Infusion site erythema
- Severe mucocutaneous reactions (SJS/TEN) – discontinue therapy if this occurs.

Neurologic

- Paresthesias
- Peripheral neuropathy
- Progressive multifocal leukoencephalopathy

Cardiovascular

- Hypertension
- Life-threatening cardiac arrhythmias during infusions
- DVT/PE

Renal: Severe, including fatal, renal toxicity can occur after rituximab.

- Gastrointestinal
- Nausea/vomiting
- Constipation
- Diarrhea
- Abdominal pain
- Bowel obstruction and perforation

Cytopenias/myelosuppression

- Neutropenia
- Leukopenia
- Anemia
- Prolonged hypogammaglobulinemia (hypogammaglobulinemia >11 months after rituximab course)

Pulmonary

- Cough
- Dyspnea
- Pneumonia
- Bronchospasm

Other

- Arthralgia
- Pyrexia
- Fatigue
- Asthenia

References

- Zakka LR. *Dermatol Ther*. 2012;2(1):17.
- Drugs.com: http://www.drugs.com/pro/rituxan.html
- Huang et al. *JAAD*. 2016;74:746–53
- Wang HH et al. *Acta Derm Venereol*. 2015;95:928–32.
- Medscape: https://reference.medscape.com/drug/rituxan-hycela-rituximab-hyaluronidase-1000306

Phosphodiesterase Inhibitors

Apremilast
MOA:
Phosphodiesterase 4 inhibitor > intracellular cAMP > protein kinase K > CREB (transcription factor cAMP response element binding protein); inhibition > downstream inhibition of pro-inflammatory markers, including TNF

Pre-screening Questions

- History of diarrhea or GI illnesses?
- Underweight?
- History of mental health issues (depression, suicidality)?
- If yes to any, consider other medication.
- P450 3A4 medication: Thus, many serious drug interactions, so check drug interactions before prescribing.

Pre-screening Labs: baseline weight

Dosing

- Day 1: 10 mg in the AM
- Day 2: 10 mg AM and PM
- Day 3 10 mg AM and 20 mg PM
- Day 4: 20 mg AM and PM
- Day 5: 20 mg AM and 30 mg PM
- Day 6 and thereafter: 30 mg po BID

Renal (severe impairment): reduce dose to 30 mg daily
Monitoring: Check weight at 6 months

SE

- Nausea, vomiting, diarrhea (most common)
  - GI SE are diminished with slow tapering up of the dose.
- Headache
- Nasopharyngitis/URI
- Worsening depression/suicidal thoughts
- Weight loss in up to 10% body weight

Janus Kinase (JAK) Inhibitors: Tofacitinib, Ruxolitinib, and Baricitinib

MOA

Tofacitinib: JAK 1–3 inhibitor (most potent for JAK 3)
Ruxolitinib: JAK 1 and 2 inhibitor
Baricitinib: JAK 1 and 2

JAKs are intracellular cytoplasmic tyrosine kinases that transduce cytokine signaling from membrane receptors via STAT factors to the nucleus. This JAK-STAT pathway is utilized by cytokines (ILs, IFNs, growth factors, hormones). Intracellular JAK proteins are activated by these signals from the cell membrane and become activated and phosphorylate STAT protein, which dimerize and then translocate to the nucleus to regulate gene expression.

In alopecia areata there is increased hair follicle gene expression of IL-15, NKG2D ligands, and MHC-molecules that leads to recruitment of IFN-gamma-producing, NKG2D-expressing CD8 T cells that attack the hair follicle. Because JAK family protein kinases are downstream effectors of the interferon-gamma receptors in keratinocytes, JAK signaling mediates IL-15 activation of T cells and decreases follicular T-cell attack.

There are four known JAKs: JAK1, JAK2, JAK3, and TYK 2.

JAK 1 – mediates signals for a range of inflammatory diseases
JAK 2 – mediates signaling for a range of cytokines, mainly for hematopoiesis
JAK 3 – activity restricted to the lymphoid lineage

There are seven known STATs (STAT1–4, STAT5a, STAT5b, and STAT6).

Pre-screening Questions

On CYP3A4 inhibitors? Do medication interaction checker.
On other immunosuppressants?
History of malignancy?
History of severe or chronic infection?
Are vaccines up to date?

Contraindications

Consider an alternative in a patient with a history of infection or malignancy.

Pre-screening Labs

CBC with diff, BMP, LFT, fasting lipid panel, HIV, hepatitis B and C serologies, PPD/T-spot for TB, CXR

Dosing

Tofacitinib for alopecia areata
Oral: 2 mg, 5 mg, 11 mg tablets

- Standard dose for adults and children weighing >40 kg is 5 mg BID; otherwise 5 mg daily.
- Typical dosing range from 5 mg daily to 5 mg TID (increase risk of anemia at higher dose).
- Typically treat for 1–2 years for alopecia areata; most patients with alopecia areata have a response between 1

and 3 months of treatment although some can take up to 6 months.

- If on strong CYP3A4 inhibitors, not to exceed 5 mg/day.

Topical: Tofacitinib 2% topical

(Tofacitinib 2% cream and ointment; may work better in a liposomal base than something like VersaBase; serologic levels of tofacitinib with topical application were 40-fold lower than with the lowest oral dose of 2 mg BID.)

Ruxolitinib for alopecia areata

Oral: Start 5 mg BID and can go up to 25 mg BID (typical dosing appears to be 20 mg BID).

- Dosing modifications may be required especially for low ANC, thrombocytopenia, renal or hepatic impairment, bleeding, or CYP inhibitor or inducers.
- Please read sources online for more specificities in prescribing.

Topical: Ruxolitinib 0.5, 1%, 1.5%, and 2% cream

Monitoring

CBC with diff, LFTs, lipid panel at least every 6 months

T-spot/TB test and/or CXR yearly

Adverse Effects

Increase in overall infections (20–22%) with serious infections in 2–6%

Low-grade infections (most common): upper respiratory tract infections/urinary tract infections

Headaches

Increases in LFTs

Increase in creatinine

Thrombocytopenia

Decreased neutrophil counts

Anemia

Lipid abnormalities (hypercholesterolemia)

Diarrhea

Diverticulitis

Hypertension

Increased risk of serious infections (fungal, mycobacterial, bacterial, viral) – increased with other immunosuppressants

Lymphoma or lymphoproliferative disorders (0.7 per 100 patient years)

Possible severe infection (TB, invasive fungal infections, opportunistic parasites, bacterial/viral associated with hospitalization/death; 1.7 events/100 patient-years)

Malignancy (0.3 events per 100 patient-years)

Monitoring

CBC with diff, BMP every 2 weeks until stabilized then every 3–4 months thereafter

Modify dose for thrombocytopenia (ruxolitinib)

LFTs and fasting lipid panel at 4 weeks then every 3–4 months thereafter

T-spot/PPD yearly

References

- Wang EHC, Sallee BN, Tejeda CI, Christiano AM. *JID*. 2018;138(9):1911–6.
- Ismail FF and Sinclair R. *Expert Rev Clin Pharmacol.* 2020;13(1):43–51.
- Hosking et al. *JAAD*. 2018;79:535–44.

Vismodegib and Sonidegib

MOA

Hedgehog pathway inhibitor (pathway is important in embryogenesis for cell differentiation and proliferation but in adults is mostly inactive). This pathway is constitutively activated though in BCCs d/t either a mutation in PATCH (PTCH) (85–90%) or smoothened (Smo) (10%)) (Fig. 8.5).

Both vismodegib and sonidegib bind to and inhibit smoothened (interestingly, itraconazole does as well).

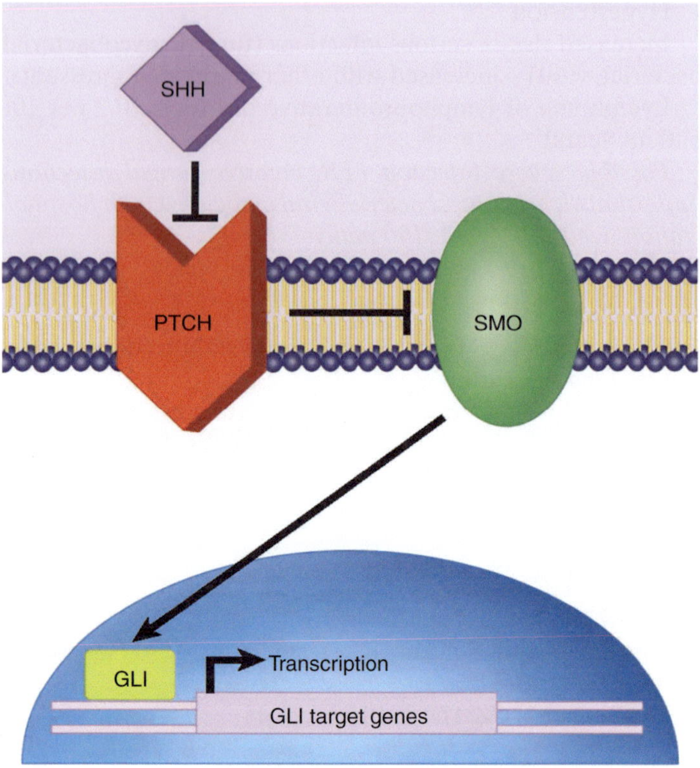

FIGURE 8.5 Hedgehog pathway

Pre-screening Questions

Sexually active/plan on having children? Is the patient a female of child bearing age? Is the patient a male planning on having children? Patient should not conceive or lactate within 24 months after last dose.

Can cause fetal harm when administered to pregnant women or if a pregnant woman is exposed via seminal fluid.

History of electrolyte imbalances.

Contraindications

Pregnancy category X – embryo death and severe birth defects (teratogenic, embryotoxic, fetotoxic).

Pre-screening Labs

CBC, LFTs, baseline CK, and creatinine (especially for sonidegib), baseline weight

If female, pregnancy test

STRICT contraception for BOTH males and females: males should use condoms – even after a vasectomy – to avoid potential drug exposure in pregnant partners and female partners of reproductive potential. *Females must NOT get pregnant for 24 months after the last dose.* Males should wait for at least 7 months.

Patients should not donate blood while taking vismodegib or for at least 24 months after final dose.

Check other CYP3A (P450) medications for sonidegib.

Dosing

Vismodegib: 150 mg po daily

Alternative therapeutic regimens

- 1 week on and 1 week off for 1 month, then 1 week on and 2 weeks off for 2 months, then 1 week on and 3 weeks off for 3 months.
- Monitor for side effects and titrate down or stop if loss of taste leads to weight loss, or other effects which are not tolerable.

Sonidegib: 200 mg po daily

Sonidegib has a longer half-life (~28 days) vs vismodegib (4 days with continuous dosing, 12 days after single dose)

Adverse Effects

Almost all patients will experience >1 adverse effect.

(v = vismodegib, s = sonidegib)

- Muscle spasms (71%v/49%s) – usually occur 2–3 months into taking and resolve 1 month after drug therapy. Exercise, massage, and acupuncture can help. Otherwise, amlodipine 10 mg daily can be tried and usually takes effect as early as 2 weeks. Can decrease the frequency of the muscle cramps but not the severity or duration.
  - Creatinine kinase (CK) elevation – patients should return promptly if they experience muscle weakness,

muscle acnes, and/or dark urine. Get CK and creatinine.
- Sonidegib should be withheld if CK rises above 2.5 the upper limit of normal.
- Recommended fluid intake, magnesium supplementation, simple analgesia, muscle relaxants. When CK returns to normal, pulse therapy for sonidegib should be considered.

- Alopecia (64%v/43%s) – minoxidil topically or orally 1 mg daily.
- Dysgeusia (55%v/38%s) – taste buds have a limited life span of 10–16 days and new taste buds will emerge after treatment cessation. Recommend self-care strategies including smaller and more frequent meals, food at room temperature, stronger seasoning, adjusting salt/sugar level, increasing chewing time for salivary production, avoid metallic plates/cutleries, increasing water intake between foods, maintenance of oral hygiene.
- Weight loss (45%v/27%s) – refer to dietician if needed.
- Fatigue (40%v/29%s) – recommend regular aerobic exercise.
- Elevated creatinine kinase (29% s).
- Nausea/diarrhea/decreased appetite (25–30%v/24%s).
- Constipation (20%v).
- <10%: hyponatremia, azotemia, hypokalemia (v); elevated lipase rhabdomyolysis (1%) (s).

Median length of response is 22.7 months for advanced BCC and 10.0 months for metastatic BCC.

Monitoring

If female of childbearing age: pregnancy tests monthly (and up to 24 months after cessation of treatment).

Consider BMP, LFTs, CK.

Patients should not donate blood while taking vismodegib or for at least 24 months after final dose.

References

- Helpful hints from Practical *Dermatology*. 2017;41(1)
- Migden MR et al. *Cancer Treat Rev*. 2018;64:1–10.

TB Monitoring Guidelines

Risk factors for *M. tuberculosis*

- *Close contacts*
- *Foreign born from high incidence area*
- *Visitors to high incidence area*
- *Residents and employees of congregate settings (long-term care, correctional, shelters)*
- *Healthcare workers who serve patients at high risk*
- *Medically underserved populations*
- *Drug/alcohol abuser*

TB monitoring guidelines (Fig. 8.6)

Pregnancy Categories

Pregnancy risk categories (Tables 8.3)

Sunscreen

Remember: The best sunscreen *is the one that the patient will use.*
Definitions

- SPF = sun protective factor – *only* measures UVB protection
  - SPF = (MED_B with sunscreen)/(MED_B without sunscreen)
    - SPF = Amount of time it takes to produce erythema with sunscreen/time it takes to produce the same erythema without sunscreen.
    - If you normally burn after 10 min, can stay outside 2.5 h before burning (15× longer) with SPF 15.
    - SPF 30 blocks 97% of the sun's UVB radiation.
- Broad spectrum = implies there is some UVA protection in addition to UVB
- Water resistant = for up to 40 or 80 min
  - Can no longer market as "waterproof" or "sweatproof"

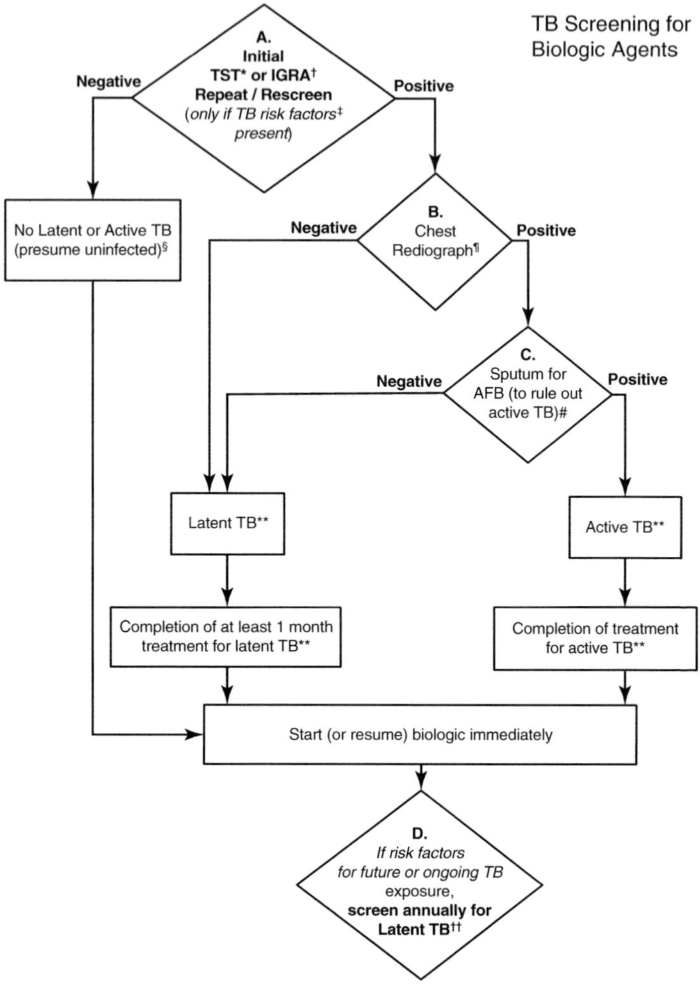

FIGURE 8.6 Stepwise approach to TB monitoring guidelines for patients on biologic therapies (based Duncan. *J Am Acad Dermatol.* 2105;72(4):742)

Table 8.3 Pregnancy risk categories

A	*No fetal risk:* Adequate and well-controlled human studies have failed to demonstrate a risk to the fetus in the first trimester of pregnancy and there is no evidence of risk in later trimesters
B	*Fetal risk not confirmed in human studies but some risk in animal studies:* Animal reproduction studies have failed to demonstrate a risk to the fetus, and there are no adequate and well-controlled studies in pregnant women, or animal studies have shown adverse effect, but adequate and well-controlled studies in pregnant women have failed to demonstrate a risk to the fetus in any trimester
C	*Fetal risk seen in animal studies but not studied in humans; benefits outweigh risks:* Animal reproduction studies have shown adverse effects on the fetus, and there are no adequate and well-controlled trials in humans, but potential benefits may warrant use of the drug in pregnant women despite potential risks
D	*Fetal risk shown in humans, use only if benefits outweigh risks:* There is positive evidence of human fetal risk based on adverse reaction data from investigational or marketing experience or studies in humans, but potential benefits may warrant use of drug in pregnant women despite potential risks
X	*Contraindicated in pregnancy:* Studies in animals or humans have demonstrated fetal abnormalities, and/or there is positive evidence of human fetus adverse reaction data from investigations or marketing experience, and the risks involved in use of the drug in pregnant women clearly outweigh the risks
N	*Unknown:* FDA has not classified this drug

Fetus at greatest risk during the first trimester

- Ultraviolet protective factor = UPF
  - Good: UPF 15–24
  - Very good: UPF 25–39
  - Excellent: UPF 40–50
- Types of sunscreens reviewed in Table 8.4

Table 8.4 Types and properties of sunscreens

Sunscreen type	Mechanism of action	Active ingredients	Advantages	Disadvantages
Physical blockers (inorganic)	Sit on top of the skin and reflect light away from the skin	Zinc oxide Titanium dioxide	Less irritating Hypoallergenic Immediately effective	Leave a white residue on the skin unless micronized or tinted with iron oxide Can feel "thick" May exacerbate acne
Chemical blockers (organic)	Absorbs lights and re-emits energy as small (insignificant) quantities for heat	Benzophenone Avobenzone Oxybenzone Octocrylene PABA[a]	Easier to apply Feel more elegant on the skin Offered in more formulations (gels, sprays, etc.) Water-resistant preparations available	Absorbed into the system Killing coral Physically degraded in the act of protection, so gone after 2 h Don't cover all of UVR

[a]Also can contain stabilizing agents which include Mexoryl, Helioplex (Neutrogena), and AvoTriplex

Avoid sunscreens in children <6 months. Just keep them out of the sun & wear sun protective clothing.

Reapply after exposure to water.

Recommended sunscreens are SPF 30+ and protect against both UVA and UVB.

Recommendations of application

- Average adult should use 1 ounce (a shot glass) per full body application.
- Avoid sunscreens in children <6 months. Just keep them out of the sun.
- Reapply after exposure to water.
- Recommended sunscreens are SPF 30+ and protect against both UVA and UVB (broad spectrum).

Tips

- Mineral makeup, powder sunscreens, or gel sunscreens help minimize breakouts of acne.
- Gel sunscreens are very light and good for athletes.
- Spray sunscreens are advantageous for quick application of children but must make sure that spray is close to the skin to get adequate coverage. Probably not a good idea to breathe the spray.

Sunscreen is just one part of protection oneself from the sun in addition to:

- Sun protective clothing and hats with UPF
- Seeking shade
- Avoiding peak hours of sun: 10 AM–4 PM

Patient education is key. We have found it helpful to use the AAD infographics (available at the AAD website) as well as reminding patients that year round daily protection is important. We will usually highlight that "even on the cloudy days, even just going to the car/driving, or making a quick errand to a store," wearing sunscreen is important.

Gentle Skin Cares

Below is a list of tip and products commonly recommended for gentle skin care:

Bathing
Limiting bathing to a couple of times per week is the best but daily bathing is okay if this is your routine. Shower or bath is fine. Tips for keeping your bathing as gentle as possible:

- Limit the time in the shower to 15 min or less.
- Bathe using warm but not hot water.
- Do not take bubble baths.
- Consider limiting soap to only the "dirty" areas, like the armpits and groin, as much as possible to prevent stripping your skin in other areas of their natural moisture.
- Do not vigorously scrub when cleansing.
- Avoid any soaps with microbeads.
- After showering, pat your skin dry with a towel; do not scrub.
- Make sure you are applying a good moisturizer after bathing every time.
- Use gentle soaps that are free of colors and scents and are not too strong of cleansers.

  Examples of gentle cleansers

- Mild bar soaps: Vanicream bar soap, Neutrogena glycerin bar, Dove sensitive skin (fragrance-free)
- Mild liquid soaps: Cetaphil liquid cleanser, Vanicream liquid cleanser, CeraVe liquid cleanser, Neutragena gentle facial cleaser (creamy)

Moisturizing
It is important to moisturize at least twice per day to the whole body. It is a good idea to moisturize immediately after bathing while the skin is still damp in order to "lock in" the moisture.

Moisturizers come in a variety of types some of which are greasier, heavier, or lighter. The heaviest moisturizers are ointments, which are greasy like Vaseline. The next best are creams, which are usually white and thick but absorb into the skin a little better. The lightest – and thus are not recommended – are lotions which are typically thin and contain more ingredients which can be irritating to your skin.

Examples of moisturizers

- Ointments: Vaseline, CeraVe healing ointment, Vaniply, vegetable oil, coconut oil
- Creams: CeraVe Cream, Cetaphil Cream, Vanicream Moisturizing Cream, Neutrogena Norwegian Formula Hand Cream
- Lotions: not recommended to use

Laundry

Be sure to use laundry products that are free of dyes and fragrances – it is important to note that many laundry products that claim to be fragrance-free actually are not free of these.

Do not use laundry softeners or dryer sheets.

Laundry products include

- 7th generation Natural Laundry Detergent Liquid, 7th generation Free and Clear Natural Laundry Detergent packs, 7th generation Free and Clear Natural 4× Concentrated Laundry Detergent, ECOS Hypoallergenic Laundry Detergent, Free & Clear, ERA Ultra Era Free Liquid Laundry Detergent

Other Gentle Skin Recommendations

- Do not use products such as powders, perfumes, or colognes on your skin.
- Avoid saunas and steam baths – these temperatures are too hot.
- Avoid tight or "scratchy" clothing such as wool.
- Always wash new clothing before wearing them for the first time.
- Sometimes a humidifier or vaporizer, used at night, can help dry skin – but remember to keep it clean to avoid mold growth.
- Avoid applying essential oils to the skin or diffusing in the home.

Laws of Dermatology

Every dermatology residency program has a Dr. Olson, the dermatologist who has seen it all, retains patient minutiae like no one else, is able to generate complete differential diagnoses on the spot, thinks outside the box for treatment and management, and often leaves you wondering "How does she/he do this?" Below the pearls of wisdom from our mentor Cynthia Olson:

Dr. Cynthia Olson's Laws of Dermatology

1. *Morphology is the key to diagnosis.*
2. *Careful, detailed description is the key to morphology.*
   These two are inextricably linked. Try to create a mental picture of the condition with your description – ideally, one should be able to figure out the diagnosis or a limited differential diagnosis before walking into the room. Banish the terms "erythematous" and "lesion" from your vocabulary. There are shades of red and pink (light pink, coral, brick red, violet-red) – try to distinguish between them and also between shades of other colors. Use "macule," "papule," "vesicle," "nodule," etc. as your noun and add as many descriptors as you can. Compare these two descriptions:

   (a) Scattered erythematous lesions on the upper trunk
   (b) Well-marginated, round, 0.5–1 cm salmon pink, flat-topped papules with subtle powdery scale, discrete and confluent on the chest, neck, and upper back
   When one reads b, the diagnosis (tinea versicolor) almost makes itself.

3. *Recognize secondary changes for what they are.*
   If lichenification, prurigo nodularis, or hemorrhagic crusts are all you see, then their geometry and distribution plus history may provide the only clues to the primary process. Do look carefully for primary lesions, though.
4. *Most conditions evolve.*
   Always remember that at any given visit, you are seeing something at one particular point in time. One cannot always make a diagnosis on the first viewing if the process has not fully expressed itself (i.e., in some sense, the con-

verse of Law #2, in that other things are difficult to diagnose if seen too late, after too much secondary change has been superimposed).

5. *A biopsy is just a lab test.*
   Many times, the dermatopathologist is truly "the purveyor of all truth" (as one of my other mentors used to say at Grand Rounds). However, results are dependent on site, lesion stage, and sampling error. Diagnostic features can be obscured by secondary changes on biopsy as well as clinically. If the biopsy results don't fit, go with your clinical instinct (or re-biopsy if necessary).
6. *When in doubt, don't believe the patient.*
   Sometimes history is key, but not everyone is a reliable historian. Again, if the history doesn't make sense, it may not be true. Also, sometimes one has to keep probing to get the important information. As an example, there was a patient who clearly had Stevens-Johnson syndrome who told the resident he was taking no medications. When asked if he has swallowed any pills of any kind in the last week, he said "just the penicillin I always take when I get a sore throat"!
7. *Rare variants of common things are more common than rare things.*
   We all need to be aware of "zebras," of course, to be good dermatologists. However, with experience, you will get to know the different morphologies that common things can appear as. This is especially true in skin of color – e.g., scaly conditions often have a fine papular texture instead, and pink things usually look purplish or grayish. Think about variants of seborrheic dermatitis, eczema, and the link before sarcoid or amyloid.
8. *No pain, no gain.*
   To really get enough benefit to clear a severe or difficult-to-treat condition, many times one must accept some degree of risk. There are a large number of patients with dermatitis of various sorts whose disease is refractory to even the strongest topical therapy. A few months of methotrexate, cyclosporine, or mycophenolate mofetil (usually with about 3 weeks of prednisone to hasten clearing) can

be immensely helpful. With reasonable monitoring, the risks are very manageable for most patients.

9. *Medicines can always be stopped.*
   See Law #8. There are a lot of patients who are very nervous about taking systemic medications. However, it helps a lot to remind them (and yourself) that very few side effects are irreversible once a drug is stopped. One must mention the common and the severe potential side effects, but also assure the patient that you have to take the risks versus benefits into account and you feel this is the best option for him/her.
10. *Treat long enough and strong enough.*
   With dermatitis, especially, it is tempting to back off on topical steroids or prednisone as soon as the worst of the erythema and scaling has resolved. However, the skin barrier will be compromised for some time. I use the campfire analogy frequently. If one throws a bucket of water on the fire, it may appear to be out. However, in many cases, there will be hot embers that will eventually rekindle the fire. Follow the bucket of water with a soaking from the hose. A corollary – give the patient enough of a quantity and enough refills to do the job right (e.g., giving a 30-g tube for a full-body eruption is what is called a "rookie mistake").
11. *Vehicles matter.*
   We all know that ointments are more hydrating and enhance penetration more than less occlusive vehicles. There are other refinements you will learn, too. For example, with retinoids, gels seem to penetrate better and are usually more effective than creams. Lotions and solutions go on better in hairy regions. *Specify* the vehicle and strength in your note and your presentation of the case – it will often make a difference.
12. *Ask the patient what he/she is doing.*
   Even the latest and best regimen will not help if the patient is not following it. Listening to how they describe what they are doing is a good clue to their level of under-

standing and compliance. Write things down, if possible, and explain their importance.

13. *The patient (often) hasn't experienced this before.*
    Although this may be the 800th time you've explained how retinoids help acne and how to cope with the initial irritation, keep in mind that this is the first time this particular patient has heard it. Make sure they hear what they need to know and don't gloss over any anxiety they might have (especially important with non-melanoma skin cancers).
14. *Write diagnoses and instructions down for patients*
    This enables patients to go home with a summary of what you talked about in the office, some reassurance for them, and more spelled out directions on their medications and medication regimens, which can help with compliance. Often, they are not processing everything that you are telling them in the office (per Law #13), and this helps to remind them of the discussion.
15. *The human body is not a machine.*
    This refers to the fact that biological systems are not entirely predictable and patients and their conditions don't all respond in the same way. Once you are reasonably certain of compliance, if something is not working as expected, or is not well tolerated, search for alternatives.
16. *Don't give up on a treatment route too soon.*
    In some ways this is the converse of Law #14. And it doesn't take some experience to know how long to persist. Especially with an anxious patient, it is easy to jump between several treatments in rapid succession. However, skin will only heal so fast, even when the inflammation has resolved, and some medications (especially hydroxychloroquine, azathioprine, and mycophenolate mofetil) take at least 2 months for maximum effect. A corollary – make sure you are at an adequate dose. (Dapsone and cyclosporine are frequently underdosed.)
17. *When in doubt, consult the literature.*
    This has saved many a physician many a time. It may be beneficial to have a file cabinet with paper articles to refer

to as well. Take notes at meetings and at lectures, file them, and don't be afraid to try things.

18. *Tenacity is an all-important virtue.*
    Although nobody can solve every problem, seek ideas from anywhere you can find them, and don't give up easily. 50% of success may be the pure act of being stubborn.
    And two additional points we learned from our work with yet another mentor, Dr. Holmes, that would have Dr. Olson's stamp of approval:
19. *Approach your workday with humility and humor.*
    Dermatology, like all medicine, can get stressful. Patients can bring anxiety and tension as they try to find a treatment or cure. Being a scientist is important to reach empirically based treatments, but in addition the "art of medicine" makes a big difference in your patient's lives. Be there to listen, provide a caring touch, and show them that you see them as a person, not a condition.
20. *Be your patient's best advocate.*
    The patient has to come first in all care considerations. Go the extra mile to ensure a necessary imaging scan is done in a timely manner, a worried patient is able to reach you immediately, call consultants yourself to collaborate, explain everything to your patient in terms that they can relate to, and put in that extra effort beyond acceptable care. Go the extra mile; it will show in your relationships with your patients, increase compliance, and enrich your life tremendously (Table 8.5).

TABLE 8.5 Summary of drug monitoring recommendations

Drug	Drug interactions and other information	Dosage	Side effects	Monitoring baseline	follow-up
Methotrexate	Bactrim, dapsone, and other sulfa meds, NSAIDs, ethanol, minocycline, furosemide, thiazides Take with folate 1 g/day on days not taking MTX	2.5 mg, 5, 7.5, 10, 15 mg tab IV, IM: 2.5 and 25 mg/mL Test dose: 2.5–5 mg Increase by 2.5–5 mg q2–3w until therapeutic dose 10–15 mg weekly	Nausea, fatigue, stomatitis Alopecia Pancytopenia Hepatotoxicity Pulmonary toxicity Pancytopenia Risk of malignancy Acral erythema Teratogen/abortifacient * F (1 cycle), M (3 mos) Recall dermatitis Preg Cat X	1. CBC w/diff 2. LFTs 3. Hep B, C, HIV 4. Cr, BUN 5. hCG 6. TB: (PPD/T-spot), 7. CXR Recheck CBC and LFTs 5–6 days after 1/st dose	1–2 week after test dose or dose escalation: 1. CBC w/diff 2. LFTs Qweekly for 4 wks 1. CBC with diff 2. LFTs Then Qmonthly for 3 mos Then q3–6 mos 1. CBC with diff 2. Cr/BUN - Track total dose at each visit - Liver bx: Low risk: after >4g cumulative dose High risk: after 1–1.5mg cumulative dose

(continued)

Table 8.5 (continued)

Drug	Drug interactions and other information	Dosage	Side effects	Monitoring baseline	follow-up
Azathioprine	Avoid in patients taking allopurinol Absorption may be decreased by antacids Concurrent use with ACI may increase risk of leukopenia May decrease INR in warfarin patients Avoid live vaccines	50, 75, 100 mg tablets IM: 100 mg/vial Empirical dose: 50 mg/day Max: 2.5 mg/kg/day Reduce 25% if GFR 10–50; 50% if GFR <10 Dosing based on TMPT: <5 U, no azathioprine 5–13.7 U, 0.5 mg/kg 13.7–19 U, 1.5 mg/kg >19 U, 2.5 mg/kg Therapeutic response seen in 6–8 weeks Needs gastric acid for better absorption	GI: most common Malignancies: SCC, NHBCL Myelosuppression Neutropenia, esp in Lupus Infection Hypersensitivity syndrome Preg cat D	1. CBC w/diff 2. LFTs 3. Hep B, C, HIV 4. Cr, BUN 5. hCG 6. TB: (PPD/T--spot), CXR 7. TPMP level	Q2 wks for the 1st 2 mos then q1–2 mos thereafter 1. CBC w/diff 2. LFTs - Recheck q2 weeks if increase dose q6 mos 1. LFTs 2. BUN/Cr 3. Skin check - D/c: WBC <4000, Hgb <10, Plt <100,0000

Mycophenolate mofetil	Absorption may be decreased by antacids and cholestyramine Antibiotics that alter gut flora will affect enterohepatic circulation of drug Salicylic acid, acyclovir increase level Contraindicated with pregnancy or must enroll in REMS	250, 500 mg tab Oral soln: 100 mg/mL Effective dose: 1.5–2g daily; possibly higher for immunobullous diseases (3g) Std dose: 500–1500 mg BID Up to 12 weeks for response Do not exceed >2g/day in renal patients Needs gastric acid for better absorption	Malignancies: NMSC, lymphoproliferative GI: most common Agranulocytosis, neutropenia, anemia, TCP Infection (>2g daily) Preg cat D Avoid in breastfeeding, pregnancy, leukopenic, thrombocytopenic, cancer, and infectious patients -Avoid conceiving for 6 weeks	1. CBC w/diff 2. LFTs 3. Hep B, C, HIV 4. Cr, BUN 5. hCG 6. TB: (PPD/T--spot), CXR	Qweekly for 4 weeks, then q2 week for 8 weeks, then monthly 1. CBC w/diff 2. CMP - Q2–4 wks following dose escalation Qmonthly 1. LFTs MPA monitoring if >2g/day D/c or decrease dose if WBC<3500

(continued)

TABLE 8.5 (continued)

Drug	Drug interactions and other information	Dosage	Side effects	Monitoring baseline	follow-up
Cyclosporine	CYP3A4 metabolism NSAIDS, vancomycin, Bactrim, aminoglycosides, amphotericin B increase renal toxicity Hyperkalemia with K supplements or K-sparing diuretics	2.5–3 mg/kg– 5 mg/kg If no improvement by 4 weeks increase by increments of 0.5–1 mg/kg every other week Taper by 1 mg/kg/day every 2 weeks Neoral has better bioavailability Higher dose = rapid onset	Nephrotoxic HTN Malignancy: SCC, NMSC, Lympho d/o Hyperlipidemia Gingival hyperplasia Acneiform eruption ↓ Mag, ↑ K, uric acid Preg Cat C - Avoid in immune deficiency, uncontrolled HTN, renal disease, cancer patients	1. CBC with diff 2. CMP 3. UA 4. Hep B, C, HIV 5. hCG 6. TB: (PPD/T--spot), CXR 7. Magnesium, potassium, uric acid 8. Blood pressure	Q2 weeks for 1–2 mos then monthly 1. CBC with diff 2. CMP 3. Magnesium, potassium, uric acid 4. Blood pressure - Qweekly x1 then q2 week (as above) for dose change Cr >30% baseline, repeat in 2 weeks, if still high > reduce by at least 1 mg/kg for 4 weeks Cr <30%, continue at current dose, if high, stop - Adding amlodipine 2.5–5 mg may ↓ renal risk If >6 mos, check CR clearance

Dapsone	Avoid with Bactrim, MXT Avoid with sulfa allergies Will falsely decrease HbA1C	25 mg, 100 mg tables Usually start w/100 mg daily Most patients require 100–200 mg daily for adequate control	Hemolytic anemia Methemoglobinemia - Treated w/cimetidine, methylene blue Agranulocytosis, idiosyncratic Peripheral neuropathy: distal motor> sensory GI DRESS/DIHS Preg cat C, excreted in breast milk - Avoid in sulfa allergies, G6PD deficient, and severe cardiopulmonary disease patients	1. CBC w/diff 2. LFTs 3. Retic count 4. Neuro exam (walk on tip toes, heels, arm/ leg strength)	Qweekly for 4 weeks, then q2weeks for 8 weeks, then qmonthly for 6 mos then q3–6 mos 1. CBC w/diff 3. Retic count Q2 weeks for 2, then q3–6 mos 1. LFTs Q3-6 mos 1. Neuro exam (walk on tip toes, heels, arm/ leg strength) Methemoglobin level as needed based on sx

(continued)

TABLE 8.5 (continued)

Drug	Drug interactions and other information	Dosage	Side effects	Monitoring baseline follow-up	
Antimalarials: HCQ, CQ, Q	Smoking decreases efficacy Cimetidine may increase level May increase digoxin level	HCQ: 200 mg tabs 4.5 mg/kg/day or 400 mg (lesser one) - Consider ideal BW for petite patients CQ: 250, 500 mg tabs Chloroquine 250 mg po every MWF × 1 month, then 500 mg po every MWF × 1 month, then 500 mg po daily × 1 month. Max dose 500 mg po BID Q: 100 mg tabs 100–200 daily	Eye: corneal deposits, neuromuscular, retinopathy (irreversible); CQ>HCQ Hemolysis, agranulocytosis: Lightening of hair, alopecia Yellowish coloration: quinacrine Blue-gray pigment: shin, face, palate, nailbeds Preg Cat C - Avoid in porphyria or psoriasis	1. Eye: slit lamp, funduscopic 2. CBC w/diff 3. BUN/Cr 4. LFTs 5. G6PD 6. 24-h porphyrin is suspect porphyria	Qmonthly for 3 mos then q3 mos 1. CBC w/diff 2. LFTs Eye exam: 1. yearly, consider stopping medication if >5 year use

Acitretin Isotretinoin	Avoid with excessive ETOH or uncontrolled hypertriglyceridemic patients	Acitretin: 25 mg per day Isotretinoin: 0.5–1 mg/kg/day with goal of 120–220 mg/kg cumulative dose - must enroll in iPledge	Teratogenic Xerosis. Ocular: dry eyes, ↓night vision, blepharoconjunctivitis, infections, corneal deposits ↑cholesterol, TG GI: IBD flare, ↑pancreatitis Liver: transaminitis CNS: pseudotumor, depressoin/suicidality Myopathy Hair loss, nail fragility, xerosis Periungual PGs Preg Cat X	1. hCG - For female 2 tests 1 month apart 2. CBC w/diff 3. LFTs 4. BMP, phos mag, 5. Lipids fasting 6. UA 7. CK if athletic/ work out Don't use acitretin in women of childbearing age Follow iPLEDGE guidelines for isotretinoin	Acitretin: Q2weeks until stable dose, then Q monthly x3-6 mos, then q3 mos 1. CBC with diff 2. LFTs 3. BUN/Cr 4. Lipids Isotretinoin: Q monthly as per iPLEDGE 1. CBC with diff 2. LFTs 3. BUN/Cr 4. Lipids 5. hCG Consider baseline x-ray of wrists, ankles, thoracic spine if plan long-term use Consider eye exam if hx of cataracts or retinopathy

(continued)

TABLE 8.5 (continued)

Drug	Drug interactions and other information	Dosage	Side effects	Monitoring baseline follow-up	
Colchicine	UV light degrade medication	1.5 mg or 0.6 mg 2–3× daily BID dosing if concerned for GI side effects Adjust for renal disease	GI: most common: diarrhea, abd cramping Neutropenia, anemia Fatigue Hair loss fFlare gout Peripheral neuropathy Preg Cat C, excreted in breast milk	No monitoring needed	
	**Can render pts infertile* Allopurinol, cimetidine, chloramphenicol may elevated dose (CYP450 interaction Drink fluids (3 quarts per day) to prevent bladder toxicity Mensa (sodium 2-mercaptoethane sulfonate) to minimize bladder	1–3 mg/kg/day divided to BID dosing Response seen after 4–6 weeks	Nausea, vomiting Bone marrow suppression Darkening of skin/nails Hair loss or changes in color/texture of hair Aphthous ulcers malaise, joint pain Easy bruising/bleeding, poor healing ability, Cystitis with gross or microscopic hematuria Increase bladder cancer Can cause temporary or (rarely) permanent sterility Preg Cat D	1. CBC with diff 2. LFTs 3. BUN/Cr 4. lytes 5. UA	Qweekly x8–12wks then q2 week 1. CBC with diff 2. UA Qmonnthly x6 mos then q3 mos if stable 1. LFTs, lytes Q6 months Stool guaiac, pap smear, CXR Discontinue med if RBCs found in urine. Decrease dose or d/c if platelets <100,000 or WBC <4,000 or 4,500.

Prednisone	Relative contraindications: Active infection: TB, systemic fungal, HSV of eye Active peptic ulcer - Severe depression, psych Hx of psoriasis	2.5, 5, 10, 20 mg tabs Typical: 5–100 mg/d PO Liver failure: use prednisolone instead *IV*: rapid onset Must admit 500–1000 mg methylprednisolone IV over 60 min daily × 5 days. *Cardiac monitoring is required* Monitor electrolytes, especially potassium Risks: sudden death, AFib, anaphylaxis IM: limit to 3–4×/year *Stress dose steroids* Major stress (e.g., surgery): Hydrocortisone 100 mg night before surgery and q8h day of Minor stress (e.g., febrile illness): Take twice basal production (~5–15 mg prednisone) extra Dose in AM qday if possible Single morning dose decrease HPA suppression Alternate day dosing reduces all complications except osteoporosis and cataracts	Cutaneous: atrophy, telangiectasias, striae, poor wound healing Short term: increase appetite/weight gain, GI upset/peptic ulcers, hyperglycemia, hypertriglyceridemia, sodium retention/hypertension, psychosis Longer term: HPA axis suppression, osteoporosis (although bone loss starts right away), osteonecrosis, Cushing syndrome, cataracts, glaucoma, hirsutism, HPA axis suppression, failure to thrive, aseptic necrosis of femoral head, muscle weakness, psychosis, pseudotumor cerebrum, increased risk of opportunistic infections	For long-term use (>4 wks): Blood pressure Weight, height Eye exam Blood glucose/HbA1c Lipid panel TB test DEXA HepB, C, HIV CXR for histoplasmosis if endemic Strongyloides check if endemic If anticipating >1 month of treatment, start on bisphosphonate Start on PCP ppx with Bactrim/inhaled pentamidine If prone to ulcers, consider starting PPI Start on calcium and vitamin D	Blood glucose/HgbA1C Blood pressure DEXA scans Lipids (triglycerides)

(continued)

TABLE 8.6 (continued)

Drug	Drug interactions and other information	Dosage	Side effects	Monitoring baseline	follow-up
Biologics	Contraindications to TNFa inhibitors: Anakinra, active/chronic infection, h/o demyelinating dz, CHF (infliximab), TB, liver disease (have to get hepatology ok). IL17s contraindicated with Crohn's disease Give live vaccines before starting	Etanercept: 50 mg subQ 2 times per week × 3 months, then 50 mg subQ weekly Adalimumab: 80 mg subQ week 1, 40 mg subQ 1 week later, then 40 mg subQ every other week Infliximab: 5 mg/kg IV at week 0, followed by dose at weeks 2, 6, then every 8 weeks Ustekinumab: <220lbs: 45 mg subQ at week 0, 4, and then q12weeks >220 lbs: 90 mg subQ at week 0, 4, and then q12weeks Secukinumab: 150 mg or 300 mg subQ at week 0, 1, 2, 3, 4, and then monthly thereafter	TNFa inhibitors: Paradoxical flares in psoriasis, lupus (+ANA, + dsDNA), infections (colds, flus, or more serious), injection site reaction, serious reactivation of granulomatous disease (i.e., TB), demyelination flares Can develop antibodies to TNFa inhibitors, which can decrease their effectiveness IL12/13: Similar to TNFa + reversible posterior leukoencephalopathy syndrome IL-17: Nasopharyngitis. Increased candida infections.	TNFa, IL12/23, IL17 CBC, LFTs, hepatitis B/C, HIV quant gold/T-spot/PPD, CXR	TNFa, IL12/23, IL17 Q6 months: CBC, LFTs Yearly: PPD/quant gold/T-spot

Apremilast	Relative contraindications: history of GI upset, diarrhea, underweight, serious depression. Many drug interactions	Day1: 10 mg po in AM Day 2: 10 mg in AM and PM Day 3: 10 mg AM and 20 mg PM Day 4: 20 mg in AM and PM Day 5: 20 mg AM and 30 mg PM Day 6 and thereafter: 30 mg BID Renal impairment: reduce dose to 30 mg daily	Headache Nausea, vomiting, diarrhea – GI side effects are diminished with slow tapering up of the dose Worsening depression/ suicidal thoughts Weight loss in up to 10% body weight	*Get a baseline weight* *Monitor for mood changes at each visit*	Check weight in 6 months

Index

S. Hylwa et al., *Pocket Dermatology*,
https://doi.org/10.1007/978-3-030-83602-3

MIX
Papier aus verantwortungsvollen Quellen
Paper from responsible sources
FSC® C105338

FSC
www.fsc.org

If you have any concerns about our products,
you can contact us on
ProductSafety@springernature.com

In case Publisher is established outside the EU,
the EU authorized representative is:
Springer Nature Customer Service Center GmbH
Europaplatz 3, 69115 Heidelberg, Germany

Printed by Libri Plureos GmbH
in Hamburg, Germany